Counseling Skills for Speech-Language Pathologists and Audiologists

Counseling Skills for Speech-Language Pathologists and Audiologists

Lydia V. Flasher, PhD

Clinical Psychologist

Children's Health Council

Palo Alto, California

Paul T. Fogle PhD

Department of Speech-Language Pathology

School of Pharmacy and Health Sciences

University of the Pacific

Stockton, California

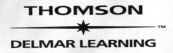

THOMSON

™

DELMAR LEARNING

Australia Canada Mexico Singapore Spain United Kingdom United States

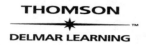

Counseling Skills for Speech-Language Pathologists and Audiologists
by Lydia V. Flasher and Paul T. Fogle

Vice President,
Health Care Business Unit
William Brottmiller

Editorial Director
Cathy L. Esperti

Developmental Editor
Juliet Byington

Marketing Director
Jennifer McAvey

Marketing Channel Manager
Lisa Osgood

Marketing Coordinator
Jill Osterhout

Production Editor
Mary Colleen Liburdi

Editorial Assistant
Chris Manion

Library of Congress Cataloging-in-Publication Data

Flasher, Lydia V.
    Counseling skills for speech-language pathologists and audiologists/ Lydia V. Flasher, Paul T. Fogle
       p.cm.
    Includes bibliographical references and index.
ISBN 1-4018-0910-3
    1. Communicative disorders--Patients --Counseling of. 2. Communicative disorders--Psychological aspects. I. Fogle, Paul T. II. Title
    RC428.8.F56 2004
    616.85'506--dc21

                                2003047388

NOTICE TO THE READER

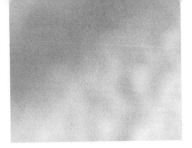

TABLE OF CONTENTS

PART I: FOUNDATIONS OF COUNSELING SKILLS

Chapter 1: THE BASICS

Chapter 2: THEORIES OF COUNSELING AND HOW THEY RELATE TO SPEECH-LANGUAGE PATHOLOGY AND AUDIOLOGY

Chapter 3: THE THERAPEUTIC RELATIONSHIP AND THERAPEUTIC COMMUNICATION

PART II: THE THERAPEUTIC PROCESS WITH CHALLENGING SITUATIONS AND BEHAVIORS

Chapter 10: TAKING CARE OF OURSELVES

Preface

Most undergraduate and graduate training in the communication sciences involves learning about normal development of speech, language, and hearing and the disorders that may arise in a person's life. Typically, relatively little time in academic courses is devoted to people's emotional responses to their disorders and how speech-language pathologists (SLPs) and audiologists can respond in a therapeutic manner. While some counseling skills may be intuitive for some clinicians, all clinicians can benefit from more training in the foundations of counseling skills and effectively using the therapeutic process with challenging situations and behaviors.

Counseling Skills for Speech-Language Pathologists and Audiologists was written to help students and clinicians understand and use counseling theories, skills, and strategies in their clinical training and professional work. Although this book is designed as a textbook and contains many features useful to students and instructors, it is also intended as a practical tool for experienced SLPs and audiologists. Coauthored by a Ph.D. in Clinical Psychology and a Ph.D. in Speech-Language Pathology, the issues and skills covered in this text are invaluable to anyone working with individuals with communication disorders and their families. This teaming of an SLP and licensed psychologist—with over 45 years combined clinical experience in a variety of settings (schools, clinics, home health, private practice), including over 12 years experience in acute, subacute, and convalescent hospitals, county hospitals, Veterans Administration Hospitals, university hospitals, and rehabilitation centers—has allowed for a depth and breadth of information not available in other books on the subject of counseling

One focus of this text is on building counseling skills by placing the theories and practices into "real-life" contexts. SLPs and audiologists working in various schools, medical and rehabilitation centers, home health, and private practices have suggested many of the counseling situations and sensitive issues that are addressed in this book. Similarly, numerous and varied examples of counseling issues and situations are provided that come directly from the clinical work conducted by the author (Dr. Paul Fogle). With the goal of providing applicable, sensible, usable skills to individuals in the communication sciences, the authors present therapy skills, techniques, and strategies in user friendly language without the burden of unnecessary psychological terminology. At the same time, the text shows how clinicians can gain better understanding of client, patient, and family behaviors by employing concepts from a variety of psychological and theoretical perspectives.

Although considerable material is presented in this text, the authors have been selective in what they have chosen to include. Other topics and references that SLPs and audiologists may find useful are provided in References as a resource for more information. Additionally, individuals developing and refining their counseling skills should reflect on their own clinical experiences and how they might manage challenging situations and difficult behaviors in a more therapeutic manner with the techniques outlined in this text.

ORGANIZATION AND FEATURES OF THIS TEXT

Part I of the text is designed to help students and professionals understand the foundational skills of counseling, including the basics: theories of counseling that are particularly applicable to our professions; the counseling relationship and therapeutic communication; and interviewing and therapy microskills. Part II provides information to help students and professionals understand and work with challenging situations and behaviors, including defense mechanisms and various emotional states. Part II also includes topics suggested by clinicians around the United States who have attended seminars on counseling skills for SLPs and audiologists. These include communicating (giving) bad news, resistant and noncompliant attitudes and behaviors, client anger or hostility, managing a crisis, threat of suicide, and reporting child or elder abuse. Additionally, a chapter on taking care of oneself in order to avoid "burnout" is included, and may become increasingly important as one continues in professional work.

Each chapter begins with an outline listing major headings and an introduction that places the material in context, and ends with concluding comments that synthesize the information presented and recap it for reinforcement. A variety of special features bring counseling skills to life. Numerous Personal Experience boxes give readers access to author Dr. Paul Fogle's many years of experience counseling individuals with communication disorders. Written in his personal voice, these Personal Experiences offer glimpses of what it can really be like working with a wide range of clients, disorders, and in challenging situations. The Case Study feature is a more formal presentation of individuals with communication disorders and their treatment, and models how different therapy techniques might be applied in specific situations. Additionally, Counseling Skills in Action boxes demonstrate issues, experiences, and techniques of other SLPs and audiologists, and give a broader foundation of how to apply counseling skills. Each chapter concludes with questions For Discussion. These are thought-provoking questions for use individually or in groups to spark introspection and debate about the topics in each chapter. These questions look for more than right answers by encouraging the sharing of experiences, application of therapy techniques to specific scenarios, and critical thought about how individual clinicians might become more effective therapists and rehabilitation counselors. References listed at the end of the book provide users with a wealth of resources for further reading and research. Finally, a Glossary of counseling terms (in boldface at first use in the text) is included.

A NOTE ON PROFESSIONAL DESIGNATIONS: WHAT DO WE CALL OURSELVES?

A brief discussion about our professional designations is important. Over the history of the profession of speech-language pathology, practitioners have used a variety of terms to describe themselves. Moeller (1975), in her *Speech Pathology & Audiology: Iowa Origins of a Disciple*, discusses the beginnings of our professions in psychiatry and psychology, dating back to the early 1900s. In 1924, Lee Edward Travis, with his training in psychology and medicine, became "the first individual in the world to be trained by clearly conscious design at the doctoral level for a definite and specific professional objective of working experimentally and clinically with speech and hearing disorders" (Moeller, 1975, p. 14).

Travis first used the term *speech pathology* in a catalog course description that he wrote for the academic year 1924–25 for the Department of Psychology at the University of Iowa. Travis had been studying various pathologies in the College of Medicine and apparently began to use the term in reference to speech and voice disorders. However, the training of students was in "speech correction," which also included training in the United States' (if not the world's) first speech clinic. The graduating students became *speech correctionists*, and that professional designation existed widely through the 1940s. Since then (depending on the work setting) we have been referred to as speech therapists (STs), speech clinicians, speech teachers (mostly in the public schools), speech-language therapists, speech and language specialists, speech and hearing specialists, speech, language and hearing specialists, speech and language instructors, the "Speech Teach," Especialistas del Linguaje y Dicion, speech pathologists, and speech-language pathologists (SLPs), and possibly others (Rubalcaba, 2000). The designation speech-*language* pathologist came into existence in the late 1960s with the new emphasis on language disorders of children. At about the same time, the American Medical Association determined that our profession should be under their umbrella (as are physical and occupational therapy) with the intent that a physician's order would be needed for evaluation and treatment of any speech, language, or hearing disorder for children and adults. In order to maintain professional autonomy outside of medical settings, our professional title was changed officially from speech therapist to speech-language pathologist.

Some individuals in our profession are adamant that we be called speech-language pathologists or, at the very least, speech pathologists. Other individuals feel strongly that we are clinicians and not therapists. In most hospitals in which Dr. Fogle has worked, the medical and rehabilitation staff do not use the term speech-language pathologist or speech pathologist; they prefer to use speech therapist or ST, in accord with the other rehabilitation staff (physical therapists, occupational therapists, respiratory therapists, etc.). Likewise, Dr. Fogle tells his students that he does "therapy" not "pathology," believing the word "therapy" has a more positive connotation to lay people than the term "pathology." It is the authors' hope that this text does not offend individuals who feel strongly that only one specific professional designation is appropriate.

Audiologists apparently have not had difficulty with their professional designation. In general, they are commonly referred to as audiologists, although some may prefer the term rehabilitation audiologist because of their area of emphasis. Audiologists do not typically think of themselves as therapists, but may refer to themselves as clinicians. For consistency in this text, SLPs and audiologists collectively are referred to as clinicians, not therapists.

Thank you for your interest in studying counseling skills. The authors hope that this text will serve you well throughout your professional career.

Acknowledgements

FOR DR. LYDIA FLASHER

I would like to acknowledge Dr. Hans H. Strupp and Dr. Ira Turkat for their excellent teaching, support, and inspiration during my graduate school experience. I'd also like to acknowledge my colleagues in the Department of Psychology at the Montreal Children's Hospital, especially Carol Schopflocher and Dr. Phil Zelazo. In addition, I am indebted to my colleagues and the Children's Health Council in Palo Alto, California for their flexibility and support while I finished this manuscript. I am grateful to the students, clients, and families with whom I have worked for many years and who have compelled me to refine my thinking and methods. Special thanks go to my dear and loyal friend Margaret Lovett who has brightened my life for almost 20 years. Finally, I want to thank my husband, Dr. Dawson S. Schultz, for his unconditional love, support, and companionship.

FOR DR. PAUL FOGLE

I would like to acknowledge the people who made this book "real"—the clients, patients, and their families with whom I have worked for over 30 years. They are my best teachers. All of the "Personal Experiences" and "Counseling Skills in Action" actually occurred as described. I would also like to acknowledge Dr. Joseph and Vivian Sheehan for their friendship and training me at the University of California, Los Angeles to work with adults who stutter. Sincerest appreciation goes to Dr. Dean Williams, my mentor and professor at the University of Iowa. Dr. Williams told his students, "I hope all of you find someone who helps you become more than you ever thought you could be." Dr. Williams was that person for me and will be forever missed. Thanks go to Tom Slominski of Northern Speech/National Rehabilitation Services for providing me the opportunity to present seminars throughout the United States to speech-language pathologists, physical therapists, occupational therapists, and nurses on the topic of counseling skills. Finally, I would especially like to thank my wife, Carol Fogle, RN, for her love and support throughout this project.

JOINT ACKNOWLEDGEMENTS

We both wish to express our gratitude to the publisher, Delmar Learning for recognizing the need for a text on this topic and the value of collaboration between a speech-language pathologist and clinical psychologist. Special acknowledgment goes to Juliet Byington, Developmental Editor, who has been supportive and enthusiastic about this book from its inception and has impressed us with her skill and expertise in this project.

About the Authors

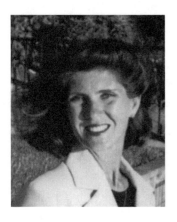

Lydia V. Flasher earned her baccalaureate summa cum laude and Phi Beta Kappa from Duke University, and her masters and doctorate in clinical psychology from Vanderbilt University. Her mentor at Vanderbilt was Hans H. Strupp, a pioneer in psychotherapy research and short-term dynamic psychotherapy. She completed her internship at the Montreal Children's Hospital, a McGill University teaching hospital, and then worked there as a staff psychologist specializing in personality assessment, family therapy, and health psychology in pediatric oncology. Dr. Flasher was a professor at Colorado State University and the University of the Pacific and has eight years of experience teaching graduate students in clinical and counseling psychology. She has been director of a university training clinic for doctoral students in counseling psychology and has over 10 years of experience supervising graduate student clinicians. Currently, she is a staff psychologist at the Children's Health Council in Palo Alto, California where she specializes in multidisciplinary assessments, conducts family therapy, supervises Stanford University child psychology interns, and teaches family therapy seminars. Dr. Flasher lives in the Santa Cruz Mountains above Los Gatos and enjoys hiking and running in the redwood forest.

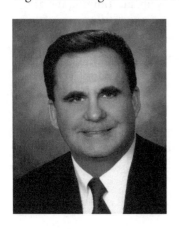

Paul T. Fogle earned his B.A. and M.A. degrees at California State University, Long Beach in Speech-Language Pathology. He minored in psychology during his undergraduate and graduate education. He trained at Rancho Los Amigos Rehabilitation Center with Dr. Chris Hagen. During that time he also worked with the neuropathologist, Dr. Abraham Lu, assisting in brain dissections. He worked for two years after his M.A. in a classroom setting with neurologically impaired (CVA and TBI) adolescents for the Los Angeles County Office of Education. He trained for three years with Dr. Joseph and Vivian Sheehan at the University of California, Los Angeles in the Psychology Adult Stuttering Clinic. He attended the University of Iowa for his doctoral education and training in Speech-Language Pathology and earned his Ph.D. in 1976. He was awarded membership in Sigma Xi, the Scientific Research Society of North America, for his research. Dr. Fogle taught for three years at West Virginia University, and since 1979 has been a professor in the Department of Speech-Language Pathology, School of Pharmacy and Health Sciences at the University of the Pacific in Stockton, California. He currently teaches courses in anatomy and physiology, neurologic disorders in adults and children, motor speech disorders, dysphagia, gerontology, and counseling skills for speech-language pathologists. For almost 20 years he also taught voice disorders and cleft palate. Since the early 1990s, he has been training in counseling psychology and family therapy.

Dr. Fogle has maintained a private practice for over 25 years, working primarily with neurologic disorders in adults and children, voice disorders, and stuttering. He has received the Certificate of Specialty Recognition in Fluency Disorders. During most summers he works in acute, subacute, or convalescent hospitals treating a variety of patients with communication and swallowing disorders. He has worked with the philanthropic "Flying Doctors" organization providing evaluation services for children with cleft palates and cerebral palsy in Mexico. He is coauthor of the *Ross Information Processing Assessment—Geriatric* (Pro-Ed), the *Classic Aphasia Therapy Stimuli* (CATS) (Northern Speech/National Rehabilitation) and the *Safety Awareness Functional Evaluation and Therapy Manual* (SAFE-T Manual) (Lash & Associates, available 2004). He has been involved in forensic speech–language pathology (testifying as an expert witness for depositions, court hearings, and court trials) for nearly 20 years, and has written on the subject. He has given seminars on a variety of topics at various conferences, state, ASHA and international (IALP) conventions and has lectured throughout the United States. Since 1999, he has presented seminars for Northern Speech/National Rehabilitation Services to speech-language pathologists, audiologists, physical therapists, occupational therapists, nurses, social workers, psychologists, and educators on "Communicating with Patients and Families Who Are Angry, Depressed, Resistant or Non-Compliant," and "Evaluation and Treatment of CAPD and ADD/ADHD." His Web site is: *www.PaulFoglePhD.com*

Dedication

*This book is dedicated to
my mentor Dr. Hans H. Strupp
and my husband Dr. Dawson S. Schultz.*

L.V.F.

*This book is dedicated to
the students and professionals who will be using
what they learn to help their clients, patients, and
families, and to David Luterman for his contributions
to counseling in the communication sciences.*

P.T.F.

PART

1

Foundations of Counseling Skills

The first part of this book provides a framework for considering the essential ingredients involved in counseling skills for speech-language pathologists (SLPs) and audiologists. Defining the scope of practice and professional parameters is important for new professionals getting their bearings and for practicing clinicians who want to hone their counseling skills. This section provides an outline of various theoretical frameworks that can help the clinician to better understand and respond to clinical situations. These theories help organize the wealth of information that comes from our interactions with clients. In addition to having good instincts and positive personal characteristics, we need to have a systematic rationale for our behavior with clients.

While the theories may help to orient the clinician and organize certain client phenomena (e.g., existential struggles, family dynamics, and cultural behaviors), the clinician also needs to have a repertoire of basic counseling skills that transcend theoretical boundaries. Chapters 3 and 4 provide detailed information about variables contributing to the therapeutic relationship, therapeutic communication, and microskills, or the specific skill units that provide the foundation of any good therapeutic approach. These variables are practiced unwittingly by many, but we believe that all clinicians can benefit by taking a self-conscious assessment and evaluation of the skills they use. Audiologists and SLPs can learn by taking stock of themselves and the ways that they interact with clients. It is through this never-ending process of self-evaluation that we continue to become better clinicians.

CHAPTER 1

The Basics

CHAPTER OUTLINE

INTRODUCTION

Welcome! You are beginning the study of what is considered by many speech-language pathologists (SLPs) and audiologists one of the most crucial parts of a student's education and training: counseling. Clinicians in the field consistently report that counseling is something they do with every person with whom they work, whether it is a child, adolescent, adult, or elderly person. Often the clinician is involved in counseling family members as well, including parents, grandparents, spouses, siblings, children, and even grandchildren. Any interaction with a client, patient or family member involves using counseling skills, even though you may not be doing "counseling" per se.

Corey (2001) says that counseling is a process of engagement between two people, both of whom are bound to change through the therapeutic venture. Studying counseling and counseling skills will help you develop a deeper understanding of people, their problems, and how they cope. You will also develop a deeper understanding of yourself, your problems, and how you cope. You will learn skills that will help you better manage challenging interactions with family, friends, and co-workers, and you will learn how to help other people cope with life's vicissitudes and challenges.

This text is not a course in psychology or psychopathology; but about helping ordinary people, our clients, and their families deal with problems of communicative disorders. It will help you learn the essentials of counseling as well as the essentials of how to deal with the inevitable challenging situations and behaviors that will arise in therapy. The text is about both you and the people you work with.

DEFINITION OF COUNSELING FOR SLPS AND AUDIOLOGISTS

Counseling began to take form in the early research and writings in psychology by Carl Wundt and Sigmund Freud in the late 1800s (Baron, 1998). Within the broad field of psychology is the specialty of counseling psychology, with its goal of assisting individuals in dealing with personal challenging life situations that do not involve psychological disorders. Even more recent than the development of counseling psychology is the development of Marriage-Family-Child Counseling (now more commonly called Marriage-Family Therapy or Family Therapy). In this text we will draw heavily from counseling psychology literature as well as Marriage-Family Therapy literature.

The American Speech-Language-Hearing Association's (ASHA) 2001 Scope of Practice statement specifically says that counseling is an appropriate function of SLPs and audiologists. Standards for certification and minimal competencies for the provision of audiologic rehabilitation and speech-language pathology services, and best practice patterns all emphasize the importance of counseling in our professional roles. Much of the literature in speech-language pathology and audiology includes references to counseling individuals with communication disorders, particularly stuttering (Van Riper, 1953). However, David Luterman, a clinical audiologist, published his first edition of *Counseling Persons with Communication Disorders and Their Families* in 1984 and his latest in 2001. Most texts on counseling in speech-language pathology have been published since 1990 (Crowe, 1997; Gravell & France, 1992; Lafond et al., 1993; Rollin, 1987, 2000; Scheuerle, 1992; Shames, 2000; Shipley, 1992, 1997).

Maurer and Martin (1997) say that practicing audiologists have expanded their role as counselors in recent years, primarily as the result of the increased emphasis on the fitting of hearing aids and the counseling that takes place in the process. In the last several years there have been an increasing number of texts published in the area of aural rehabilitation with considerable discussion of counseling. Much of the literature in audiologic and aural rehabilitation counseling and the psychology of deafness has been published since 1990 (Alpiner & McCarthy, 1987, 1993, 2000; Clark & Martin, 1995; Holcomb, 1996; Hull, 1992, 1997; Luterman, 1984, 1991, 1996, 2001; Marschark, 1993; McCay & Andrews, 1990; Padden & Humphries, 1990; Paul & Jackson, 1993; Preston, 1995; Schow & Nerbonne, 2002; Tye-Murray, 1998).

The counseling we do in speech-language pathology and audiology is educational and rehabilitation counseling. The terms *counseling* and *interviewing* are often used interchangeably by some professionals. Though the overlap is considerable, interviewing may be considered the most basic process for information gathering. Counseling is a more intensive and personal process concerned with helping people cope with the range of normal to tragic problems (Ivey, 1998). In our professions we do both interviewing and counseling, often without a sharp distinction. The skills used in interviewing and counseling overlap and are used throughout the various stages of the therapy process.

Counseling for the professions of speech-language pathology and audiology may be defined as an applied social science and a helping, interpersonal relationship in which the clinician's intention is to assist a person or family member to understand a hearing, communication, or swallowing disorder, and ways of preventing, managing, adjusting to, or coping with these disorders. As an applied social science, counseling has a considerable body of literature behind it. Counseling is a helping, interpersonal relationship, which means that it involves at least two people and that a relationship, no matter how transient or superficial, always develops. Both the helper and "helpee" have some kind of interaction that leads to opinions and feelings about one another.

The therapist has the intention to assist the person. Our intentions are the moment-to-moment purposes behind our counseling. Every counseling statement, gesture, or silence may be regarded as purposeful (Feltham & Dryden, 2002). However, although sometimes our best intentions may not always be as helpful as we would like, we must always have the client's best interests as our primary goal.

In counseling we attempt to help children, clients, patients, and families understand ways of preventing disorders. For example, we help children and adults understand how they can prevent further loss and preserve the hearing they have. We help parents learn to be better listeners to their young children who are beginning to be unusually dysfluent, to try to prevent the development of stuttering. We also attempt to help individuals manage their communication disorders by understanding what motivates them to improve and what factors, both personal and environmental, may interfere with maximizing their therapy gains.

Counseling involves at times helping individuals and their families adjust to and cope with long-lasting or even permanent communication disorders. A child's severe hearing loss may be life-long; a child's hypernasal speech caused by a cleft palate may affect speech intelligibility throughout life; a young adult with a traumatic brain injury (TBI) may always have difficulty with communicating and problem solving for activities of daily living (ADLs); and an elderly person developing dementia will likely see abilities to communicate and function independently slowly erode over time.

DOING COUNSELING VERSUS BEING A COUNSELOR

Although SLPs and audiologists do counseling and use counseling skills when working with clients, patients and families, it is not appropriate to identify ourselves as "counselors." There are several areas in which we have education and training but which it is not ethical or legal to identify ourselves with those professional titles. For example, we are not anatomists, but we study, understand and use concepts of anatomy and physiology. We are not otolaryngologists, but we study, understand, and use concepts of otolaryngology. We are not neurologists, but we study, understand

and use concepts of neurology. We are not psychologists or counselors, but we study, understand and use concepts of psychology and counseling.

Are You an Anatomist?

I occasionally perform medical-legal work (forensic speech–language pathology), evaluating individuals (often with TBIs or strokes), extensive report writing, depositions and, in some cases, court testifying. One CVA case I was extensively involved with a few years ago required me to be on the witness stand for two and one-half hours, being examined by both the plaintiff and defense attorneys. The plaintiff's attorney brought me into the case. The plaintiff was a woman in her mid-20s. In high school she was an excellent student and a national winner for competitive public speaking. She had been in theater and mountain climbing, and an all-around highly functioning young person.

At the time of her stroke she was a senior in college, within 10 units of graduating with a major in psychology and was going on to graduate school. She was home visiting her mother when she had a stroke and was sent to the local county hospital. The hospital took a wait and see approach and admitted her to the intensive care unit. Over the next four days she deteriorated, died, was resuscitated, and then moved to a large university hospital. Seven hours of neurosurgery were required to repair the damage that had occurred over the previous four days. A medical malpractice lawsuit against the county hospital was filed and a large number of expert witnesses brought in on both sides.

When I first evaluated the young woman she was attending a community college trying to learn how to water and care for plants. Her dreams of completing her B.A. and continuing for an M.A. would never be realized. She had moderate to severe aphasia, moderate dysarthria, and moderate to severe cognitive impairments. No swallowing problems were present.

During the initial portion of the questioning by the plaintiff's attorney my professional credentials were established and I was deemed an expert in the area of speech-language pathology by the court (the judge). Then the attorney proceeded with a series of extensive questions, including questions about the client's neuroanatomy and neurophysiology, neuropathology, speech, language and cognitive impairments, past speech-language rehabilitation, and potential for future rehabilitation. When the plaintiff's attorney completed his questioning the defense attorney began his work.

During the cross-examination by the defense attorney my credentials were challenged (a normal procedure in medical-legal work). The defense attorney asked me, "Are you an anatomist?" with my response being, "No, but I have taught anatomy and physiology, neurology and neuropathology for 18 years." The attorney again asked me, "Are you an anatomist?"

Continues on next page

> *Continued from previous page*
>
> and I responded, "Not by degree, but I have taught anatomy and physiology, neurology and neuropathology for 18 years."
>
> The point of this example is that we cannot claim to be something for which we do not have a degree, whether it is anatomist, neurologist, neuropathologist, or counselor.
>
> P.S.: The plaintiff won the case and was awarded several million dollars.

Rather than say we are counseling a client, patient or family member, we tend to use words such as client/patient/family training or education, conference or consultation, particularly in reports and medical charts. However, in everyday communication with professionals we may use words such as "a conversation" or an "an interesting discussion" when we refer to interactions with a client, patient or family member that we feel involved counseling. We talk about "issues" because that word has no specific professional reference and implies that we do not want to share specifics about the conversation or discussion. We also discuss concerns, situations, or challenges. Most people do not talk about "problems;" they talk about "challenges."

COUNSELING: SCIENCE *AND* ART

Counseling is both a science and an art (Nystul, 1999). The scientific aspect involves the technical understanding of psychological and counseling therapies and skills, and the art is the understanding of when and how to use them. The scientific aspect is unique to professional helpers and differentiates them from nonprofessional helpers. The scientific aspect emphasizes objective observations and inferences, testing hypotheses, and formulating theories about our clients and patients.

We cannot make a clear distinction between the science of counseling and the personality and behavior of the person doing the counseling. Although counselors can learn attitudes and skills and acquire knowledge about personality dynamics and the therapeutic process, much of effective counseling is the product of developing the art. The artistic aspects of counseling suggests that it is a flexible, creative process. Timing of the counselor is often a crucial part of the art; not only saying the right thing but also saying it at the right time. At any given moment when working with an individual, we may need to empathize, teach, model, support, question, restructure, interpret, or remain silent. The therapeutic value of these interventions can depend upon the timing used by the therapist.

The artistic aspect also includes the concept of giving of oneself, such as concern, support, and empathy. This giving of oneself is a delicate, balanced process that is learned over time: when to give, how much to give, in what way to give. This concept is derived from humanistic psychology and emphasizes the importance of being authentic and human in the counseling approach (Nystul,

1999). SLPs and audiologists can give support as they empathize with their clients. Sometimes just listening carefully to clients may be the best gift they can receive at the time, helping them overcome feelings of aloneness and isolation.

Luterman (2001) says that counseling can be demystified so clinicians understand it is something we do, even when we are not aware we are doing it. Counseling skills are used in every encounter, whether intentionally or spontaneously (Crowe, 1997). Strict stimulus-response therapy may not be counseling, but our facial expressions, body language, and tone of voice give strong messages about our acceptance and feelings about the person we are working with. Our feelings about the person always affect the person's interactions with us.

Counseling is not reserved for a particular group of professionals who call themselves counselors or psychologists. The following are brief definitions of various professionals who are commonly seen by individuals seeking what most people typically think of as counseling (Feldman, 2002).

Clinical psychologist.

> Ph.D. or Psy.D. who specializes in assessment and treatment of psychologic disorders.

Counseling psychologist.

> Ph.D. who usually treats day-to-day adjustment problems in counseling setting, such as university or mental-health clinic.

Family therapist (formerly Marriage, Family, Child Counselor).

> Usually M.A. who attempts to change the structure and interaction processes of the client family.

Licensed Case Social Worker.

> Usually M.A. who works with individuals and families, and mobilizes community support systems.

Psychiatrist.

> Physician with postgraduate training in abnormal behavior and psychotherapy who can prescribe medications as part of treatment.

Psychiatric social worker.

> Professional with a master's degree and specialized training in treating people in home and community settings.

Psychoanalyst.

> Either a physician or a psychologist who specializes in psychoanalysis, the treatment approach first developed by Sigmund Freud.

School psychologist/counselor.

> Usually an M.A. in psychology or educational psychology who works in public school settings with children and parents.

Essentially all professionals working with people use some counseling skills as part of their interaction with clients, patients, families. While counseling comes more naturally to some, counseling skills can be learned. Burnard (1999) says counseling is never simply a matter of learning a generic list of skills that you then apply in a range of settings. Instead, counseling involves facing the person in front of you, listening carefully, and using counseling skills to help with the issues at hand. The application of these skills requires the clinician's understanding and selection of which skills to apply, with whom, and at what time.

A client with a delay, disorder, or disability almost always exists within a family context. The communication disorder usually affects more than a single individual. For clinicians to be most effective we must deal with the client and at least some of the important people (family and sometime close friends) in his or her life. The focus, however, must always be on the communication problems and how they are affecting the client and family's coping abilities.

Although Luterman (2001) says that counseling needs to be at the forefront of students' clinical education and our professional research, the professions of speech-language pathology and audiology do not have a history of extensive training in the area of counseling. However, this deficit in education and training is not unique to our professions. In surveys conducted by the author (P.T.F.) of over 3,000 SLPs, audiologists, occupational therapists (OTs) and physical therapists (PTs) throughout the United States who have attended seminars on counseling, fewer than 20% say they had a specific course in their education dealing with counseling. It is interesting to note that most clinicians who attend these seminars have between 5 and 20 years of professional experience, with some having 25 to 30 or more years of experience. Even after decades of working with clients, patients and families, most rehabilitation clinicians still feel uncomfortable with counseling skills that they consider an essential and ongoing part of their evaluations and therapy.

In the counseling seminars an interesting discussion has centered on an SLP who adamantly stated to me in a private conversation, "I don't do any counseling. I just refer everyone to the psychologist (at my hospital)." The discussion centers around how a clinician can effectively do therapy and either ignore or postpone meeting clients' needs at the time they arise. When working with clients, patients, and families we cannot easily interrupt a person who is discussing sensitive issues surrounding a communication disorder and say we cannot discuss the issue, and would like to refer the person to a psychologist. We definitely have our boundaries and scope of practice (to be discussed later), but must work with issues and emotions as they arise. These issues and emotions may become critical in our understanding of the client and our selection of appropriate interventions. Being unresponsive or interrupting the person would be nontherapeutic, and an immediate referral to a psychologist to continue the discussion is seldom practical and can negatively affect your rapport with the client. Cotreatment with a psychologist present is also an unlikely occurrence.

In a study by Culpepper, Mendell, and McCarthy (1994) in which training programs accredited by ASHA were surveyed, it was found that approximately 40% of the programs offered a course on counseling within the department that emphasized relating counseling theories and skills to the profession. Approximately 35% required students to take a counseling course outside of their department, and approximately 25% of programs did not offer or require speech-language pathology or audiology students to have any course work in counseling. Lack of counseling course offerings may reflect a lack of education and training of individuals to qualify them for teaching such a course. Some programs try to infuse counseling into their various course offerings. However, in that model it is difficult for students to get a holistic understanding of counseling as well as specific approaches and counseling strategies that will be helpful with a wide variety of speech, language, cognitive, swallowing, and hearing disorders. The infusion approach follows a top-down model where students try to learn some specific counseling principles or techniques in a course (e.g., aural rehabilitation) and then, along with counseling techniques infused in other courses, attempt to develop a unified approach that fits their world view and ways of working with clients.

When students have a counseling course offered in their major they learn that counseling principles and skills are applicable to all disorders. When clinicians begin to understand counseling approaches and techniques, they begin generalizing them to a variety of disorders and situations. This follows the bottom-up model where a particular approach or technique may apply to a variety of situations. The bottom-up model allows students to build a foundation of knowledge in the area of counseling and see how that knowledge is applicable to all their clinical work.

Beyond education and training in Counseling Psychology or Family Therapy, it is helpful for the individual who teaches a counseling course to be actively involved in the challenges of direct client/patient care. In this way the professor can put into practice and refine what is being taught. Fogle (2001), in an article on "Professors in Private Practice" noted several benefits for professors working with clients and their families on a regular basis. These benefits translate into improved teaching and student training:

- Continual stimulation of working with challenging clients and families
- The direct hands-on experience that cannot be appreciated when observing student clinicians through a two-way mirror
- The satisfaction of working with clients from initial interview to termination of therapy, and knowing that you have been an important part of the person's improvement
- New "therapy stories" for students to help relate theoretical information to clinical practice
- A more realistic empathy with students struggling with therapeutic dilemmas
- The opportunity to collect data for research studies or develop new assessment or therapy materials

OVERLAP IN THE WORK OF SLPS AND PSYCHOLOGISTS: A CONTINUUM

Counseling and psychotherapy have similarities and differences (Rollin, 2000). At no time, however, should the SLP or audiologist say he or she is doing psychotherapy. Some disorders, though, lend themselves to more of a psychotherapeutic or counseling approach. Sheehan (1970) said that stuttering therapy is a modified form of psychotherapy because the clinician is helping the client change attitudes about stuttering as well as the stuttering behaviors themselves. Adults with voice disorders often have interpersonal conflicts and/or anxieties that contribute to vocal fold tension as well as generalized tension. SLPs who address the whole person in a holistic approach are concerned with more than just behaviors; they are concerned with the person's emotions, mind, body, and spirit.

SLPs and audiologists occasionally see individuals with emotional or mental disorders who have diagnoses specified in the *Diagnostic and Statistical Manual of Mental Disorders Fourth Edition, Text Revision* (DSM-IV TR) (American Psychiatric Association, 2000). We work with individuals who have substance abuse problems, adjustment disorders, mood disorders such as depression, conduct disorders, alcohol abuse problems, and anxiety disorders. However, we do not focus on or address those emotional or mental disorders per se; we work with the speech, language, and cognitive problems that may be a part of those disorders.

There are, however, several DSM-IV TR (2000) classifications that we as a profession frequently encounter. SLPs are qualified to make some of these diagnoses, but we are not qualified to make the vast majority of them. In some cases we may be the main professional treating a client who has been diagnosed by a psychologist. For example, the DSM-IV TR (2000) discusses in considerable detail "amnestic (amnesia) disorders" (294.0) that are characterized by memory impairment which affects the person's ability to learn new information or to recall previously learned information or past events. These memory disturbances must cause marked impairment in social or occupational functioning, and must represent a decline from a previous level of functioning. This DSM-IV TR diagnosis reflects the memory impairments SLPs work with when patients have had strokes, TBIs, tumors, or other neurologic damage. The DSM-IV TR also has a considerable discussion of various types of dementia, such as Vascular (Multi-infarct) Dementia (290.4x) and Alzheimer's Disease (290.0). SLPs working in convalescent hospitals see many residents with dementia.

Attention Deficit Disorders (ADD/ADHD) (314.00 and 314.01) are a DSM-IV TR (2000) diagnosis. We see many children in our public school case loads who have ADD or ADHD who also have language disorders, including problems with pragmatics. The DSM-IV TR manual has specific sections on Expressive Language Disorders (315.31), Mixed Receptive-Expressive Language Disorders (315.32), Phonological Disorders (315.39), and Stuttering (307.0). There are DSM-IV TR classifications for Learning Disorders, including Reading Disorders (315.00), Disorders of Written Expression (315.2), and Mental Retardation with severity levels ranging from Mild (317) to Profound (318.2). Autistic Disorder (299.00) and Pervasive Developmental Disorder (299.80) are DSM-IV TR classifications. It is clear that there are a variety of disorders that psychologists, psychotherapists, and psychiatrists are able to diagnose, but the SLP may be the professional who is most involved in the habilitation or rehabilitation of these disorders.

PERSONAL QUALITIES OF EFFECTIVE HELPERS

Before we begin discussing personal qualities of effective helpers (counselors), we should first explain what is meant by "helper." The term "helper" tends to show up in the counseling and psychotherapy literature and refers to to several professionals who are trained in and use counseling as their way of helping people. As clinicians we know that we are helpers, but it is a term we do not typically apply to ourselves. Ultimately, our goal for helping a client is for that person to not need our help any longer, to become independent of us, to become a self-helper (Brammer, 1996, in Nystul, 1999). Like most helpers, our job is to work ourselves out of a job.

The term helper is useful to us in our understanding of counseling. Rogers (1957) identified three core conditions as "necessary and sufficient conditions" to help individuals with personal growth (these will be discussed further in Chapter 2 in the section on Humanistic Therapy). These conditions must first be characteristics of a counselor before they can be conditions the counselor brings into the client-clinician relationship.

- Congruence: Means the clinician is genuine in terms of what he or she is experiencing and communicates. Congruence implies that the clinician is in touch with thoughts and feelings, voices them when it is perceived to be helpful, and that body language and tone of voice mirror words and statements.

- Empathic understanding: The clinician attempts to understand the client from the client's point of view (i.e., trying to understand what the person is thinking, feeling, and experiencing, and communicating this understanding back to the client).

- Unconditional positive regard: The clinician needs to communicate a sense of acceptance and respect to the client. The clinician is consistently nonjudgmental, which allows the client to relax, trust and be open with the clinician. It means being accepting of the client, but not necessarily all the client's behaviors; to "Separate the deed from the doer" (Martin, in Nystul, 1999).

The challenge with these characteristics is that they are difficult to teach. SLPs and audiologists typically have a good helping of these characteristics before their training begins, which may be one of the reasons they have gravitated to these professions. Their training helps to further develop their natural tendencies.

Clinicians, like other people, often have difficulty with congruence. It is sometimes difficult to know just what we are thinking or feeling, or to put this into words. It is even difficult sometimes to know the difference between a thought and a feeling. Feltham and Dryden (1993) define thought as cognition or mental activity, using words such as thinking, remembering, reasoning, concentrating, questioning, figuring, calculating, projecting, and pondering. Feeling is defined as affect or emotion, using words such as happy, joyful, delighted, sad, depressed, lonely, eager, apathetic, surprised, curious, indecisive, fatigued, courageous, protective, powerful, satisfied, overwhelmed, loved, hopeful, angry, and fearful. Like primary colors, there are primary emotions of joy, anger, and sadness. Many of our emotions are variations or degrees of these primary emotions.

Clinicians sometimes struggle with understanding their own thoughts and feelings and how they interact and influence each other. Baron (1998) and Burgoon, Buller, and Woodall (1996) discuss how affect influences cognition and how cognition influences affect. For example, our affects (feelings) and affective states (moods) influence our perceptions of ambiguous stimuli or experiences. In general, we perceive and evaluate these stimuli and experiences more favorably when we are in a good mood than when we are in a negative mood. Positive and negative feelings exert a strong influence on memory. In general, when we are feeling positive we tend to retrieve positive memories, and vice-versa. Clinicians need to be aware of how their feelings and affective states may be influencing their thoughts and interactions with a client.

At the same time, clinicians are trying to have their body language, facial expressions and tone of voice be congruent (match or in agreement) so that listeners do not get a mixed message. Clients and patients (particularly those with neurological disorders) are often confused enough without us confusing them more by saying one thing with our words and something else with our body language, facial expressions, and tone of voice.

Empathic understanding, that is the attitude and skill of following, grasping, and understanding as fully as possible the client's subjective experience (Feltham & Dryden, 1993) can be very challenging. We need to try to see the client's world from his or her perspective and appreciate that we can never totally see the world as he or she does, any more than someone can see our world as we see it. No one has lived our lives, and we have never lived our clients' lives. Sometimes, at best, we may identify people's thoughts and feelings but not be able to identify *with* them.

We can better identify with some of the thoughts and feelings our clients and patients have if we have had similar experiences. May, Remen, Young, & Berland (1985) use the phrase "wounded healer" to suggest the ability of a clinician to work from a perspective of resolved emotional experience that has sensitized a person to self and others. It is paradoxical to some people but logical to others that individuals who have suffered and have been able to go beyond or transcend that suffering and gain insight into themselves and the world can be more helpful to others who are dealing with similar emotional and/or physical trauma or loss. While the clinician's personal experiences increase her depth and insight into another person's experiences, it is important not to assume too much similarity between the client's and one's own experiences and responses to them.

We emphasize to students that there are many experiences we do not want to identify with our clients and patients. We do not want a stroke or TBI. We do not want to begin to stutter, develop vocal nodules, or have Parkinson's disease. However, even though we have not experienced these conditions, we can still do our best to imagine the situation to better empathize with the people we try to help.

Unconditional positive regard is an ideal we can strive for: accepting, respectful, and nonjudgmental. However, our own values, ethics, and morals can affect our best intentions to remain accepting, respectful, and nonjudgmental. Clinicians working in some settings, particularly county hospitals, may see patients who have had TBIs or strokes who are murderers, rapists, child abusers, or child molesters. It can be difficult to have or maintain the unconditional positive regard for these individuals that we more easily have for other people. The clinician's ability to have and maintain unconditional positive regard may also be challenged with more ordinary people who have behaviors or attitudes that are quite dissimilar to our own.

The Moonshiner's Son

While working in a skilled nursing facility one summer an SLP worked with an 81-year-old man who was born and raised in Tennessee. During a conversation about his youth the patient said, "I shot two of 'em." The SLP asked him what he meant and he told the SLP that when he was 14 years old he shot two "revenuers" who had found his father's moonshine still out in the woods. As it had been 67 years since the incident, and the SLP knew the patient might not live much longer, he decided not to inform the proper authorities. He also did not change his positive view of the man and his unconditional positive regard for the patient. However, had the patient been a young man and the SLP was working with him, and had the patient just committed two murders, the SLP likely would have had much more difficulty maintaining his unconditional positive regard.

We know that some clinicians tend to be very genuine, warm, accepting, and sensitive to their clients, while others are more business-like, cool, matter-of-fact, objective and distant. Much depends on the clinician's personality style. In some cases students need to be tempered in one direction or the other; to be more objective and business-like (professional), or to be more warm and sensitive to their clients. We must also change our style depending on the type of client or patient we are working with, for example, a child who stutters versus a child with spastic, quadriplegic cerebral palsy, or an adult with a TBI versus an adult with severe developmental delays.

According to Riley (2002) and Gladding (2000) a clinician's personality is at times a crucial ingredient in determining the effectiveness of counseling. Corey (2001) explains that if counselors possess wide knowledge, both theoretical and practical, yet lack human qualities of compassion, caring, good faith, honesty, realness, and sensitivity, they are merely technicians. Kottler (1993), Nystul (1999) and George and Cristiani (1995) summarize the counseling and psychotherapy literature on the topic of personal qualities of effective helpers, including:

The Dean and the Client with Cerebral Palsy

In my private practice I work with a range of types of cases. For several months I worked with a woman who had been referred to me by a home health agency. The woman had a TBI from a motor vehicle accident and was now back on her job but needed additional high level cognitive therapy. The client had a Ph.D. in political science and was a Dean at a university. She was functioning at a higher level than most clients, so I used some of her "Dean work" in her university office as the therapy, and maintained a very professional demeanor when working with her. However, one-half hour later I was working with a two-year old boy with severe spastic quadriplegic cerebral palsy. I was down on the floor playing and laughing with him in a child-like manner, maintaining a very different professional demeanor. The therapy time with these two vastly different clients reminded me how flexible we need to be in order to adapt to working with a wide range of clients.

Encouraging

The ability to be encouraging may be one of the most important qualities of clinicians. We need to be the client/patient's cheerleader. Encouragement helps people learn to believe in their potential for improvement. Being encouraging also implies that we have some confidence that our clients can improve and that we can be helpful in this process. If we cannot be encouraging, then we need to question whether we are working with a client who has a poor prognosis, or whether we are the best clinician to work with that client.

Emotionally Stable

Most SLPs and audiologists appear to be at least fairly well-adjusted people who are coping with life's challenges adequately to maintain their mental health. However, we, like every other person, have stresses in our lives and have days where we feel less focused and energetic. We may even feel sometimes that our problems are worse than those of the people we are trying to help, although we never want to suggest or imply that to them.

Sometimes the problems we are working on with clients may be similar to those that we are working on in our own lives. For example, an SLP may have a child with ADD, a spouse with a stroke or head injury, or an elderly parent with dementia. We may identify with the struggles the client, patient or family members are trying to manage, and sometimes have to work hard not to allow our personal emotions to come forward. We may have to try to distance ourselves just enough to maintain our professional stance in order to be helpful to the people who have come to us for therapy. However, when we feel we cannot be sufficiently objective and professional because of issues in our own lives, we need to consult with a supervisor, coworker, or mental health professional to try to help us better manage ourselves so we can meet the needs of our clients. If we find we cannot be effective clinicians because of temporary personal or professional interferences, we need (if at all possible) to make appropriate referrals to other clinicians. We may later be able to effectively help such clients, but for a time we may be too fragile or self-absorbed to be of use.

As professionals, we need to actively practice those things we find helpful to maintain our own good mental health. Many clinicians think in terms of staying centered, meaning knowing: "I'm OK. I usually do things right. I'm an honest person. I'm a good person. I complete tasks. I'm a good clinician. People usually like me. I'm basically a happy person. My family loves me. People are basically good. My faith will sustain me. Tomorrow is a new day." Clinicians in seminars have suggested a variety of ways they find helpful to center themselves, for example, going outside for a few minutes to look at the grass and trees; going for a brief walk; exercising; deep breathing, praying, meditating, or talking to a friend. We need to always be in the process of learning how to take better care of ourselves so we can take better care of others.

Self-Aware

Self-awareness appears to be related to other concepts of self, such as self-acceptance, self-esteem, and self-realization. Having a sense of self and being comfortable in our own skin is important for us to maintain our emotional stability. Self-awareness also helps us appreciate our strengths and limitations as clinicians. We have awareness that we can do good therapy with certain kinds of clients and a realization that we may do merely adequate therapy with others. We are aware of what areas we need to seek further training and continuing education. We also are aware of areas where we can be helpful to other clinicians in their attempts to continue their training and education. There is a general sequence in our professional lives that is passed on from generation to generation. The sequence is: "I need help" (education, training, experience); "I can do it alone" (I'm able to be independent now); and "I can help you" (I'm ready to help educate, train, and provide experience for you).

Positive Self-Esteem

A positive self-esteem, tempered with humility, can help clinicians cope with the trials of therapy. Also, when clinicians feel positive about themselves they tend to see the positive attributes of their clients. When clinicians feel negatively about themselves they are more likely to demonstrate defenses when suggestions are being made by supervisors about how to improve their work.

Patience

One of the hallmark characteristics of SLPs and audiologists is patience. It is the ability and willingness to persevere during the often long, slow road of speech and language development or rehabilitation of our clients and patients. We need to practice "patience."

The challenge for many people we work with is their impatience to improve, to be able to communicate without difficulty. Our ability and willingness to be patient gives them a model and someone to help temper their anxiety and frustration about their pace of improvement.

Tolerance for Ambiguity

There are few absolutes in our professions, although there are three that should be emphasized to students: you are going to make mistakes; you are going to get tired; and you are never going to know enough. Ambiguity is a part of our incomplete knowledge and understanding of every area of our professions. The data are never all in. At the end of most every research article is the standard statement, "Further research is needed." Speech-language pathology and audiology, like medicine, are inexact sciences. Ability to tolerate ambiguity reflects our flexibility and ability to work at the fringes of our knowledge and competencies. As David Luterman said in a seminar on counseling at the 1999 ASHA Convention, "In our professional lives we need to always be working on the fringes of our competencies. If we wait to be 'certified' in everything we do we have probably missed helping a lot of people." The only way we become competent is by doing what we are not yet competent to do.

Spirituality

Although this may seem like an inappropriate personal quality to discuss, spirituality is an emerging concern in the counseling and psychotherapy literature. The value of addressing and utilizing spiritual-religious dimensions in the helping process is being recognized. Characteristics of spirituality include being sensitive to religious-spiritual issues of our clients, patients, and their families, as well as ourselves.

Amazing Grace

One day after finishing work at a convalescent hospital I was about to leave the facility when the Director of Nursing (DON) came running up to me and grabbed my hand. She had me in tow when she grabbed another SLP's hand. As we were rushing down the hall she said, "We are going to sing 'Amazing Grace' to a resident." I thought to myself, my singing is *not* going to be therapeutic. One of the resident's last requests was to hear his favorite hymn (even if it was poorly sung). The DON, the other SLP and I stood at the end of the resident's bed, his wife and son behind us. We gave our best rendition of the hymn and it seemed important to everyone present. We honored his request and spirituality. Not long after that he rested in peace.

The majority of people in this country profess some belief in God, as they know it. For many of our clients and patients, their spiritual beliefs provide comfort and support beyond what any person can provide. In many cases, our own beliefs may be similar to theirs, and it can be comforting to the people we are working with if they have the sense that we are on the "same wavelength." No matter what the spiritual or religious beliefs are of the people that we are working with, we need to honor and respect them, not just tolerate them.

Riley (2002) and Gladding (2000) define several other personal qualities of an effective counselor, including:

- Curiosity and inquisitiveness—a natural interest in people
- Ability to listen—finding listening stimulating
- Emotional insightfulness—comfort dealing with a wide range of feelings, from anger to joy
- Introspection (self-awareness)—the ability to see or feel from within
- Capacity for self-denial—the ability to set aside personal needs to listen and take care of others' needs first
- Ability to laugh—the capability of seeing the bittersweet quality of life events and the humor in them

SLPs and audiologists may choose their professions partly because they naturally have many of the personal qualities that are important in being good counselors. However, much of their clinical training with children and adults either directly or indirectly helps enhance or strengthen those qualities, and the training continues throughout their professional careers.

PURPOSES OF COUNSELING FOR THE SLP AND AUDIOLOGIST

Riley (2002) says that the goal of counseling is to facilitate individuals to find their own answers, experience an internal sense of control, and leave with new perspectives and the confidence that they can continue to care for themselves. She lists several outcomes expected from counseling with a SLP:

1. The client will be more self-aware and able to observe him- or herself with some objectivity.
2. The client will exhibit reduced limitations that inhibit choices.
3. The client will experience increased internal (vs. external) control.
4. The client will be able to recognize and accept responsibility for his or her feelings.
5. The client will demonstrate an increased use of "I" statements rather than "you" statements.
6. The client will be able to deal with uncertainty with less anxiety.

7. The client will have a more positive view of self and others.

8. The client will have made a commitment to continue to grow.

Crowe (1997) identifies seven purpose of counseling for our professions:

1. Gather and convey information (e.g., interviewing and presenting diagnostic information).

2. Prevent disorders from developing or from becoming more severe and involved (e.g., teaching parents how to listen to their child who is at risk for stuttering).

3. Help clients adjust emotionally to their disorders and to resist developing counterproductive behaviors in reaction to them (e.g., helping a child with a repaired bilateral complete cleft lip accept her appearance and recognize other kinds of beauty in herself).

4. Help be supportive of families and significant others in coping with a client's disorder or disability (e.g., helping the parents of a child with traumatic brain injury deal with the new and difficult behaviors of their once loving child).

5. Help clients improve their overall function and independence by learning decision-making and problem-solving skills, and maintain high motivation levels for therapy (e.g., helping patients with strokes recognize their abilities and appreciate the small gains they are making).

6. Provide an environment for clients that is optimal for change and improvement (e.g., helping a family realize the negative impact of their chiding and criticism of the client as an ineffective way of encouraging him or her to work harder.)

7. Help clients develop the self-reinforcement behaviors and coping strategies that are critical to successful carryover and generalization of therapy results (e.g., helping clients see their progression of improvement and ways they can continue to help themselves once they are discharged from therapy).

Overall, every aspect of our work as diagnosticians and clinicians includes counseling as an integral part of interaction with clients, patients, and their families. The people we try to help may not remember our therapy techniques that helped them improve their abilities to communicate as much as they remember how we listened to them and talked with them about the sensitive issues surrounding their hearing, speech, language, cognitive, or swallowing problems.

BOUNDARIES AND SCOPE OF PRACTICE WITH COUNSELING

In order for SLPs and audiologists to do our work professionally and ethically, we need to understand our scope of practice. As mentioned earlier, ASHA (2001) includes counseling our clients, patients, and their family members as within our scope of practice *as the counseling relates to the com-*

munication problem. Stone and Olswang (1989), Stone, Shapiro, and Pasino (1990) and English (2002a) say that in order to better understand our scope of practice we can divide boundaries into "within our boundaries," "out of our boundaries," and "challenges to our boundaries." The ideal stance is to have a firm understanding of the within-boundaries and out-of-boundaries areas for our professions, and to recognize the situations that present challenges to our boundaries and require our thoughtful discernment about how to best manage those challenges.

Within Boundaries

Within-boundaries areas are the legitimate areas within the scope of practice of SLPs and audiologists, including but not limited to:

- interviewing the client/patient or family
- presenting the diagnosis of delays or disorders
- providing information about the delays or disorders
- discussing interventions for the delays or disorders
- dealing with the client/patient and family's reactions to the diagnosis
- planning for obtaining educational or health care needs beyond our therapy
- supporting the strengths of the person and his or her efforts to regain function and to be independent
- supporting the strengths of the family to help them interact optimally with the client/patient
- creating supportive empowerment for the client/patient and family to develop the ability to manage their own problems and be independent of the clinician

The within-boundaries areas are broad and most young clinicians learn to develop some level of comfort with these during their clinical training. However, new clinicians sometimes do not realize that all their clinical work in some way involves counseling skills, and that their counseling must relate to the communication problems of their clients.

Beyond Boundaries

Beyond-boundaries areas for SLPs and audiologists are areas or issues that are clearly out of our scope of practice to work on directly, although we know they may have contributed to the cause or continuation of the communication problems with which we are working. Several of these issues need immediate referral to other professionals. Examples of issues beyond our scope of practice include (in alphabetical order):

Chemical dependence

Child or elder abuse

Chronic depression

Legal conflicts

Marital problems

Personality or character disorders

Sexual abuse and sexual problems

Suicidal ideation

Challenges to Boundaries

Challenges to our boundaries can occur in our first interactions with any client. We cannot avoid possible encounters with situations that challenge our boundaries, so we need to recognize them and have the tools to respond to them appropriately. We sometimes start therapy working within our boundaries but find that there are issues affecting our therapy that are beyond our boundaries. In these cases, we may find ourselves on a slippery slope. For example, a mother may appear angry or displeased with the clinician about the way he or she is working with her child. After the clinician discusses with the mother her concerns, the mother begins to disclose marital difficulties that are increasing her irritability. The clinician needs to be alert not to slide into a discussion of her marital issues, even though they may be affecting the mother's perception of the clinician's work.

Another type of challenge to our professional boundaries occurs when we must make a decision about whether we are equipped to accept a particular client or venture into a particular discussion with a client or family member. In these cases, we may not have preset boundaries, but must assess our resources in the moment and decide whether or not to work with that client or venture into a discussion of a very challenging issue. We must ask ourselves what resources (knowledge, experience, understanding of the problem, or support from other professionals) we have to address these problems.

Education Versus Recent Experience

I had been out of acute and subacute hospital work for several years and knew that I had much to learn about working with tracheostomized and ventilator-dependent patients. During my summer hospital work I was fortunate to have a very experienced supervisor who was both knowledgeable and willing to teach me. Even though I had a degree beyond hers and 10 years more clinical experience, I knew that she had information and experience I did not. I recognized that this was an excellent learning opportunity and was willing to be a student and welcomed being closely supervised while developing new skills. It would have been unethical of me to pretend that I had expertise in an area I did not.

Other challenges to our boundaries are when parents want us to help them with behavior problems of siblings of the child we are working with, or individuals who want a diagnosis of a problem over the telephone. Many of these challenges to our boundaries involve ethical issues, which are dis-

CASE STUDY

He–She

The Department of Otolaryngology at Stanford University Medical School in Palo Alto, California provided a patient with my name and telephone number and instructions to contact me for voice therapy. The patient called me to briefly discuss the need for voice therapy and to schedule an appointment. The client was a man going through a gender change. I admitted to the individual that I really had no experience in that area, but was willing to meet "her" to discuss her voice.

The person came to my home, where I see occasional clients, and when I opened the door I was confronted with a rather tall woman dressed in a dark skirt and white blouse, flats, hair of moderate length, and pilot sunglasses. Her handshake was strong and very masculine.

I invited her in and when she was comfortable she began to tell her story. She had served in the Army, had been a police officer, and was now a computer programmer. When she was a man, she was married and was the father of two children, a boy and girl. In her mid-40s she realized that she had been born the wrong gender and eventually decided to make the change from a man to a woman. She was currently receiving hormone therapy and living as a woman (she had not had the surgical alterations). She wanted to change her voice to sound more feminine.

I discussed the fact that just raising the pitch would not necessarily make her sound feminine, and that there were differences in voice inflection and intonation, choice of words, and overall ways of talking that significantly influenced a feminine presentation of a person. At one point I asked if she had ever watched the movie "Tootsie" with Dustin Hoffman making a remarkable temporary transition from male to female. She admitted that she had not, so I suggested she rent the movie and study some of the things Dustin Hoffman did to appear so convincingly as a woman.

I met with the client two more times while I searched for a SLP who had both an interest and experience in this unusual area of voice therapy. I recognized that I could not meet her needs and I was not particularly interested in developing skills in this area. I also felt it was important for her to have a female SLP to help her learn nuances of feminine speaking and body language.

cussed in more detail in Lubinski and Frattali (2001), and Shipley (1997). Stone et al. (1990) gives the following rule of thumb: if a clinician is feeling tense or anxious, developing headaches, and so forth, from working with a particular client, patient or family, it may be a red flag that the clinician is in a beyond-boundaries area for our profession, level of training, or expertise.

Stone et al. (1990) use the metaphor of a concentric circle model to represent the boundaries for counseling within our professions (see Figure 1-1). They say to think of the circles as an ocean and that as professionals we are willing to go into the water. The boundaries are the depth of water. The outer circle is within our boundaries; the middle circle challenges our boundaries; and the inner circle is out of our boundaries.

A modification of the model may help better visualize the concept. Rather than smooth concentric circles, the model may be seen as the challenges to our boundaries having a jagged, serrated, concentric circle. The jaggedness represents areas we may venture into to varying degrees, and that it is difficult to know all the challenges in advance (see Figure 1-2).

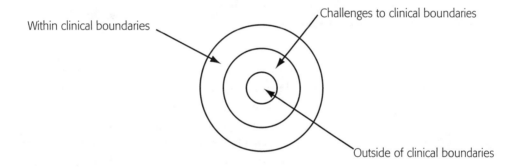

Figure 1–1 Concentric circles representing clinical boundaries for counseling (adapted from Stone et al., 1990)

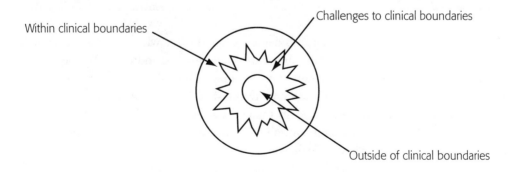

Figure 1-2 Concentric circles with jagged edges representing clinical boundaries for counseling (adapted from Stone et al., 1990).

Stone et al. (1990) present the following metaphor. When we are students or newly graduated we tend to stay very close to the shore. As we gain more experience we venture out farther but we must first know how to swim. The water can get choppy and even have big waves. It can get deep very rapidly and we can quickly be in over our heads. It is more comfortable for us if we always know where the shoreline is (within boundaries). If we get too deep in the water (e.g., discussing marital relations) we start to thrash around and may even drown, but if we keep our heads clear and start to swim back to shore we will be safe. If we are working with complex family dynamics, we are in very strong weather and need to stay close to shore. There also may be sharks (challenging issues) in the water or a strong undertow, which means we should not be swimming alone (we need another professional we can talk to about challenging issues). We may need a lifeguard (a supervisor who can help us better manage a situation). The better and more experienced swimmer we are, the farther out we can go. If we are going to swim we are going to get wet, and jumping in the water can be very uncomfortable. However, to become a stronger swimmer we need to get wet often, practice our various strokes, and build our strength.

Heart Burn

A woman referred to me by an otolaryngologist for voice therapy was very responsive to therapy. However, she began to increasingly discuss some issues she was having with her husband that caused mental and physical tension, including tension in the laryngeal region. I was willing to listen to but not discuss some of her marital difficulties. After one of our sessions in which she had tried to triangulate me into taking her side on an issue (I refused to take sides), I had a symbolic somatic response—I had heart burn. I learned from that experience to be more mindful of when I was going beyond boundaries and to be willing to redirect the client to areas I could more appropriately listen to and address.

If both the clinician and client bring considerable strengths (knowledge, experience, understanding, insight, patience, etc.) to the relationship, more issues may be addressed. We need to ask ourselves, What baggage (things that are bothering us) may potentially affect our best therapy with clients? (See discussion of transference and countertransference in Chapter 3.) Some days we can work with certain emotional issues more easily than others, but we still must do our professional job no matter how we are feeling and maintain stable, predictable boundaries and therapeutic environments. Sometimes the client or family's pain will be similar to pain we have felt or are currently experiencing. However, we need to stay focused on our client's experience and not our own so the person we are trying to help does not think we have a bigger problem than he or she has. Baggage can be present in other areas of our professional lives as well.

Personal Baggage

In 1969 I served in Vietnam as a Combat Medic, with all that that implies. In my graduate level Neuropathologies in Adults course I discuss TBI. In that section I sometimes relate a couple of personal experiences fighting in a war. I recall one day I was going to tell the students a story but stopped because it was bringing back some well-suppressed emotions, so I started to tell a different story and it had the same effect. I tried to tell a third story and realized, for whatever reason, I could not handle sharing any such experiences that day. I told the students I would try to tell them some experiences another day. It is part of the baggage that I have had to work on and accept.

Setting Boundaries in the Therapeutic Relationship

Pipes and Davenport (1998), say that "boundary" does not mean "wall" (with all the pejorative connotations accompanying such a term). Rather, from a counseling perspective, it refers to the characteristics of the relationship along the dimensions of (a) role behavior and (b) identification with the person with whom we are working. The concerns often are whether we are "getting too close" to the client and not maintaining our professional role, or whether we are identifying too closely with the issues the client is working on and losing our objectivity.

Counselors and psychotherapists use the term **therapeutic alliance** (Greenson, 1967) to mean the helping relationship and the factors involved which maximize therapeutic effectiveness. It is frequently thought of as the bond or rapport between the client or family and the therapist (Feltham & Dryden, 1993), but also includes mutual respect, honesty, trust, and the agreed upon goals of therapy. The therapeutic alliance can be threatened or damaged, rather than enhanced, if the therapist tries too hard to establish rapport (e.g., too vigorous of a handshake, too warm of a greeting), or the therapist goes beyond professional boundaries in his or her discussions and interactions with a client.

The therapeutic alliance involves the establishment of the appropriate **therapeutic distance**. Therapeutic distance refers to distinguishing between what the client's problems are and our own. If we are emotionally too involved with our clients we are probably too close to be able to assess their situation with reasonable objectivity. For example, if a mother is discussing the family conflicts that have been occurring because of her child's ADD, and you start recalling and focusing on the emotional difficulties in your own family with your younger brother who had similar problems, you may not be able to continue listening to the mother with sufficient therapeutic distance. However, if we are too distant and detached from our clients we are unable to appreciate their problems with the necessary sensitivity. For example, if you cannot be empathic toward a client because of his or her lifestyle, you may feel that the client brought the problem (e.g., TBI) on himself and treat the client in a detached, distant manner.

Optimal therapeutic distance places a priority on the client's needs rather than our own and always respects the professional nature of the relationship. Optimal therapeutic distance means looking at the person holistically. Gladding (2000), and Carlson and Ardell (1988) say that if a person is to be evaluated completely we need to understand some of the person's physical (e.g., general health, pain or discomfort), intellectual (educational level), social (friendships and support systems), emotional (anxieties, fears), and environmental (home life and work) processes. The ideal is to understand the person as a whole, including beliefs, perceptions and goals, and to realize that the mind and body are interacting systems, not separate entities (Nystul, 1999).

Mr. M. and His Mittens

After beginning summer work in a skilled nursing facility, I was asked to evaluate an elderly gentleman for potential oral feeding. The patient had had a nasogastric tube (NG tube) for several months and was wearing "mittens" on both hands as a restraint to prevent him from removing the NG tube (pulling it out), which he had been able to do on many occasions before the placement of the mittens. My evaluation revealed that he was not a safe oral feeder and that nothing by mouth (NPO) was the safest method of hydration and nutrition. He also had severe dysarthria and receptive aphasia.

The patient's wife was present during my evaluation and shared her frustration and sadness about not being able to hold her husband's hands to comfort him because of the interference of the mittens. I suggested that a stomach feeding tube (percutaneous endoscopic gastrostomy [PEG] tube) might be a consideration as her husband had had the NG tube for so long.

I wrote my evaluation results in the patient's medical chart with a recommendation to the physician for consideration of the placement of a PEG tube. Later I received word from nursing that my recommendation had been denied. I followed up and spoke with the physician who told me that the patient was going to die soon and there was no need to change from NG tube feeding to PEG tube feeding. I discussed with him the wife's frustration and sadness, but this did not sway the physician. I later discussed with the wife the physician's decision and encouraged her to speak with him for further understanding of the decision.

As an SLP I was looking at the patient holistically rather than just physically. Had the patient received a PEG tube months before he could have had the comfort of his wife's hand on his, meeting both of their emotional needs. Sometimes we can only watch in sadness as medical decisions are made that we may not feel take into consideration the patient as a whole person.

Another way of talking about excessive therapeutic distance is to identify the person's actions and behaviors that create this condition. Therapeutic distance is not just an attitude or frame of mind. Some professionals use distancing techniques (being aloof, cold, detached, monotone, having little facial expression, or showing lack of interest or concern about the person's thoughts and feelings) to prevent or decrease emotional involvement. Adams (1993, p. 35) says, " 'Distance' may be another term for repression" (i.e., some professionals repress their feelings about another person's pain so they do not need to confront their own feelings). Although this use of the word repress is not a psychologically exact definition, Adams does convey that excessive therapeutic distance involves the person's refusal of vulnerability, and the deleterious effect this has on the client-therapist relationship.

Adams (1993, p. 35) also says that "Bedside manner has nothing to do with information about the patient. Bedside manner is the unabashed projection of love (of all people), humor, empathy, tenderness, and compassion for the patient. Scientific brilliance is an important tool, but it is not the magic inherent in healing." Many clients and patients are motivated to work in therapy and to practice their exercises not just to see their own improvement, but to please the clinician who has established a healthy and mutually rewarding therapeutic relationship.

In the following sections Stone et al. (1990) discuss levels of a working, therapeutic relationship as they apply to SLPs and audiologists.

LEVEL I: "I CAN WORK WITH YOU"

When considering boundary issues we need to not only consider our expertise in an area but also safety issues of the clinician. The clinician must create conditions in order to feel physically safe. A realistic assessment of safety means knowing whether you are in a safe part of town (but not being complacent about alertness even in a safe area), whether there is sufficient lighting, what distance needs to be walked, the possibility of severe weather. Inside a building (e.g., a hospital) the therapist needs to be alert to patients who have a history of acting out or violence. (The code 5150 is often used to denote a patient who has potential for harming staff. In some hospitals Code Green is used to alert personnel that a patient is being unusually uncooperative and that people in nearby areas should come to assist the health care provider with a silent show of force rather than physical intervention or combativeness.) In home health care the wise clinician is very alert to any signs that reflect potential danger. School settings are considered generally safe but they are not without violence. For example, in the late 1990s there was a series of random shootings in junior and senior high schools around the United States.

Beyond our casual to systematic assessment of the environment, we may use our gut-level feeling to alert us to potential dangers (De Becker, 1995, discusses the importance of listening to our fear). Clinician physical safety is always the first consideration. However, SLPs and audiologists need to go about their business and provide their services with an awareness of safety issues but not be paralyzed with fear.

A Client in a Bad Area of Town

An insurance company asked me to evaluate a young man in his home (apartment) who had sustained a TBI from being accosted with a baseball bat. When I scheduled the appointment I learned that the 19-year-old young man was from Southeast Asia and spoke little English since the trauma. His girlfriend agreed to translate during the evaluation.

I knew the area where he lived was not the safest part of town, but I was willing to do the evaluation. The young man lived with his family in a small second floor apartment. When I was invited into the living room I noticed that all the furniture was against the walls (this may have been a cultural arrangement, but it was somewhat disconcerting to me). The father brought me a folding chair and set it in the middle of the room and invited me to sit down to wait for the client. The girlfriend and young man later came out of a back room and she showed me to what had been a laundry room where a small table had been set up for us to work. A second visit was needed to complete the evaluation.

The young man definitely needed therapy and I referred him to the University of the Pacific Speech, Hearing, and Language Center. However, because of transportation difficulties he was not able to attend. In my report to the insurance company I made note of potential safety issues for a SLP doing home health care with this client, such as the high crime rate in his area, including assaults and rapes. I was not willing to continue going to the young man's home and I would not recommend that another SLP take risks.

We structure our environment to create a formal or casual atmosphere. An informal or casual structure invites more testing of the boundaries while increased structure increases the clearness of the boundaries. The clinician must be the one to structure the session and environment. We can do this by staying focused on the communication disorder (behaviors) but still deal with the emotions and other issues that arise. Our general demeanor, the way we dress (professionally or inappropri-

Seeing Clients in Their Homes or Offices

I find that working in private practice is ideal for working with clients in their homes. I typically work with a child in his or her room with toys on the floor. I get to know the child's brothers and sisters, pets, and sometimes friends. I also get to work with the parents (e.g., the parents of a child who stutters) at their kitchen or dining room table where they are com-

Continues on next page

Continued from previous page

fortable and perhaps more their real selves. (I have had fathers offer me a drink or beer while we are talking. I *always* decline the offer.)

With adult voice cases and adults who stutter I get to see and better understand some of the family dynamics that I would not be able to observe in a more sterile clinic environment. With clients who had a CVA or TBI I often work at the kitchen table and have their own household items available to incorporate into therapy.

By seeing a client with vocal nodules in her home I was able to observe the floor plan and acoustics of the home. I observed that the floors were hardwood with no carpeting or rugs, and that the walls were sparsely decorated, causing excessive reverberation of sound. I noted that I automatically raised my voice volume, as did the client, when in her home as a natural effort to talk over the reverberation and ambient noise. I suggested that constant loud voice use in her home, along with other factors, may have contributed to her vocal nodules. She discussed this with her family and they decided to make some changes by adding some throw rugs and sound-absorbing wall hangings.

Another voice case was a high-powered attorney with an otolaryngology diagnosis of muscular tension dysphonia. I saw her for several sessions in her home and then she asked me to have a therapy session at her law office. The client had a very large, imposing (distancing) desk. With the client on one side of the desk and me on the other, I noted how automatically we both raised our voice levels to be more easily heard. I then noticed that there was a heater/air conditioner vent almost directly over her desk that was very noisy. I suggested that it would be easier to talk with her, as well as easier on her voice if she sat closer to me on the client's side of the desk. I also noticed a small conference room adjacent to her office and asked if we could try working there. With both of us at the small round conference table we were away from the noisy heater/air conditioner vent and we automatically lowered our voice loudness levels. She stated that she was willing to begin working with her clients in the smaller room to help conserve her voice.

ately casual), and body language (posture, gestures, facial expressions) are important in structuring the therapy environment and maintaining a professional stance.

Private practice and home health care may be settings that most challenge our structuring of therapy because of their typically inherent casual atmospheres compared to clinics, offices, hospitals, and so forth. It is wise for clinicians working in private practice and home health care to be particularly cautious of their own and the client's behavior, and to maintain appropriate structure and boundaries.

LEVEL II: "I CAN CONTINUE WORKING WITH YOU, BUT . . . "

Once again, we may not choose to say these words aloud, but we may need to consciously consider what we need to do to restructure the therapy environment. Whenever we restructure the environment our tone of voice and body language are essential components of our messages. The clinician needs to restructure or refocus the therapy session to work on the problems and issues that he or she can comfortably work with. The clinician might say, "Let me stop you there and ask you about . . . " or "I would like to stay focused on . . . " The client usually will follow the clinician's lead, but if not the clinician may need to redirect or refocus the client again. In some instances a more direct approach may be needed, such as stating that the conversation is going into areas that are outside a clinician's scope of practice or that the area of conversation is not really appropriate in the therapy setting. (See Chapter 4, Interviewing and Therapy Microskills, for more detailed discussions of skills and strategies that may be helpful in this situation.)

Mr. C. and His Suggestive Stories

Occasionally while supervising students in a university clinic, an adult male client with a cerebral vascular accident (CVA) or TBI, has begun to make comments or tell stories and jokes to the female clinician that are not appropriate. After the session I have discussed with the clinician that if the client continues to be inappropriate that she needs to set boundaries. The clinician was told to say to the client after the next time such an incident occurred that it was not appreciated when he made any suggestive remark or told a joke that had a sexual reference or innuendo. If the client continued such behavior then the clinician was to terminate the session with the client understanding the reason. I also discussed with the clinician that in acute care hospitals when patients with TBIs are at various levels of the Rancho Scales they often have inappropriate behaviors. However, in a university clinic adult male clients sometimes attempt to flirt with a female clinician or intentionally lead a conversation in a direction that could potentially embarrass her or cause awkward interaction.

In medical settings clinicians need to always be alert to patients who may potentially be harmful to caregivers. For example, patients with TBI at Level 4 (Confused, Agitated) on the revised Rancho Levels of Cognitive Functioning (Hagen, 1998) may be verbally abusive or strike out at a person as a result of their neurological impairment (see Chapter 8 for management techniques). Although the striking out is understandable behavior as a condition of the neurologic damage, therapists can be injured. We should consider that the patient is, even with his or her worst behaviors, doing the best he can to manage himself. When the patient cannot manage his behaviors appropriately we need to structure the environment and our responses and to minimize inappropriate or potentially injurious behaviors.

Kriege (1993) emphasizes that we can best help patients by accepting them exactly where they are (cognitively, emotionally, and physically), and to treat them with respect, and give sufficient personal space. If we are seeing a patient at bedside we need to approach the patient confidently, but cautiously, and in a nonthreatening manner. We need to try to understand what triggers the patient's behaviors and what the risks are for harm to himself or us. We need to know our own reactions when our emotional buttons are pushed. The threat may be more psychological than physical, with our professional qualifications or self-worth being attacked. We need to know our limits, be in complete control of ourselves, and remain outwardly calm.

It is very helpful to speak to the patient in a soothing, calm, and reassuring tone of voice. Speaking slowly and using short, simple sentences (Rule of fives: five-letter words, five-word sentences) help decrease the amount of information the patient has to process and, therefore, the amount of frustration. We need to try to decrease noise and confusion in the patient's room. Dimming the lights can be soothing to the patient. Gently touching the patient can help him or her adjust to our presence. We need to share with the other rehabilitation team members and health care providers what we find helpful when working with a particular patient. We need to encourage other staff to interact with the patient who has difficult or challenging behaviors. A patient who feels avoided or isolated can trigger defenses, with one of the defenses being aggression. As always, it is a team approach.

Confabulation of a 17-Year-Old

I was asked to evaluate and then provide private therapy for a 17-year-old high school student who had sustained a severe TBI when hit by a car as she was crossing the street after leaving her school bus. I learned during the interview with the parents that the girl had made accusations about sexual abuse by a family member, but that the accusations were unfounded and the likely result of confabulation secondary to the head injury. I told the parents that I would be willing to evaluate and provide therapy for their daughter as long as there was another adult in the room able to observe every moment while I was present. This structuring allowed me some level of comfort and feeling of professional safety.

LEVEL III: "I CAN'T CONTINUE WORKING WITH YOU"

When a client continues to try to take us beyond our boundaries and we have repeatedly tried to stay focused on the communication problems the person presents, we need to make explicit statements and give clear messages that we cannot help the person in general or specific ways. In most cases a gentle voice is sufficient, but in others a firmer voice is needed. For example,

> Gentle voice: "I have really enjoyed working with you and I care about you, but what we are dealing with is beyond what I can work with (my scope of practice)."

> Firmer voice: "I know that this is important to you, but I cannot be a resource for you in this area. It is beyond my scope of practice. We need to find someone else who can help you with these issues."

In such cases where we feel that the client's needs are beyond our scope of practice, we have a few options. The first, of course, is to refer the client to another professional such as a family therapist, counselor, or psychologist. The client may need to work with that professional before we can continue our therapy or we may continue working with the client concurrently while the client is seeing the other professional. Another option is for the client not to bring up with the clinician issues that are clearly outside of our scope of practice or realm of expertise.

In summary, the within-boundaries areas are legitimate professional areas for SLPs and audiologists to communicate with clients and families. The beyond-boundaries areas are issues that are clearly out of our scope of practice. Challenges to our boundaries are not always clearly delineated and may arise at any time in our work. We need to be very careful not to go beyond our education, training, and skill levels.

CLIENTS AND FAMILIES SOMETIMES QUESTION THE CLINICIAN'S LIFE EXPERIENCES

Occasionally our credibility will be questioned on the basis of inadequate life experiences. This concern may be voiced in the form of questioning the clinician's apparent youth, status as an unmarried person, lack of experience in raising children, and so forth. Whatever the concern, the clinician needs to keep in mind the value of not reacting defensively. What clients are usually most concerned about when asking these kinds of questions is, "Are you competent to work with me with my kinds of problems?" The inquiry is likely one for information about the clinician and not necessarily an expression of resistance. (Note: Young psychologists, counselors, and psychiatrists have similar experiences.) A possible response to this challenging situation may sound like this: "That is a reasonable question (observation), and I believe you and I will get along fine. You are right in saying I'm younger than you (have not raised children, etc.), but I believe I can help you. My education and training have provided me knowledge and skills designed to help you, and I have been helpful to other people with similar problems. However, if you feel I am not able to do that, I will help you find someone you feel will be more helpful to you." Such a response is usually sufficient for the client to decide to continue working with the clinician. However, if the client persists with feelings of uncertainty about the clinician's qualifications then the clinician should make reasonable effort to find another clinician to work with the client.

ETHICAL AND LEGAL ASPECTS OF COUNSELING FOR OUR PROFESSIONS

Nystul (1999) says that ethical-legal issues reflect on both the art and science of counseling. In general, ethical codes and legal statutes are not absolutes but serve as principles to guide clinicians' interactions with the people they are trying to help. Corey (2001) says that professionals cannot rely on ready-made answers given by their professional organizations because such organizations typically provide only broad guidelines for responsible practice. Ethical and legal aspects cannot always be clearly separated. What is unethical is not always illegal, but what is illegal is likely unethical. However, there are specific legal statutes that apply to our work, for example, the reporting of suspected child abuse or elder abuse.

"*Ethics* is generally defined as a philosophical discipline that is concerned with human conduct and moral decisions" (Van Hoose & Kottler, 1985, p. 3 in Gladding, 2000). Garner (2001) in *Black's Law Dictionary*, says ethics relate to moral obligations that one person owes to another. Law is the precise codification of governing standards that are established to ensure legal and moral justice (Hummell, Talbutt, & Alexander, 1985 in Gladding, 2000). Garner defines law as "The regime that orders human activities through systematic application of the force of politically organized society, or through political pressure" (p. 363). *Illegal* refers to an act that is not authorized by law, while *alegal* means outside the sphere of law and not classified as being legal or illegal, such as a contractual agreement between a client and therapist that the therapist will provide the best therapy of which he or she is capable (Garner, 2001). The scope of this text does not include an extensive discussion of ethics, law, illegality, or alegality. We will focus on the most common ethical and legal issues dealing with clients in regards to counseling that SLPs and audiologists may encounter. For a more detailed discussion of ethical and legal standards of conduct the reader is referred to Shipley (1997) and Lubinski and Frattali (2001).

The American Speech-Language-Hearing Association (ASHA, 1994) Code of Ethics is what we follow in our professional work. If a clinician is uncertain about ethical or legal issues related to work, he or she should review ASHA's Code of Ethics and Scope of Practice statements, and, if necessary, contact the ASHA Headquarters to discuss the matter with an appropriate person.

In 1994 ASHA published "Professional Liability and Risk Management for the Audiology and Speech-Language Pathology Professions" (*ASHA*, 36 (Supplement 12), 31–32). The following outlines specific areas that are particularly applicable to our counseling efforts.

Confidentiality and Patient Records

Two provisions that apply to patient records and confidentiality are:

1. Individuals shall maintain adequate records of professional services rendered and products dispensed and shall allow access to these records when appropriately authorized. (Principle I-H).

2.   Individuals shall not reveal, without authorization, any professional or personal information about the person served professionally, unless required by law to do so, or unless doing so is necessary to protect the welfare of the person or the community (Principle I-I).

Recently, federal guidelines also have been described in the Health Insurance Portability and Accountability Act of 1996 (HIPAA). The accountability portion of this act provides funding for, and strengthening of, enforcement of compliance with health care regulations, including those pertaining to privacy rights of clients. Professionals can access information about this federal code on the Web site: *http://www.access.gpo.gov./nara/cfr/index.html*

Flarey (2001) states that medical records are under common law (the body of law derived from judicial decisions rather than from statutes or constitutions), state law, and federal law. Any written words, from reports and computers disks or hard drives to Post-It Notes, are a legal document. Legally, the client owns any written information about him or her and the professional owns the paper or computer disk on which the information is written. The professional is the legal guardian of all documents, which requires us to safeguard those documents. Whoever is physically holding the record is the legal guardian, whether it is the professional, secretary, or family member.

Because SLPs and audiologists frequently interact with family members, educators, nurses, physicians, other rehabilitation specialists (PTs, OT, respiratory therapists, etc.), as well as other SLPs and audiologists to best serve the needs of our clients and patients, we frequently share our information and reports with other professionals. However, such sharing should only be done with the client or patient's approval. Consent authorization forms are needed to have a written statement on file that the client has approved sharing specific confidential information.

Morrison and Anders (1999) and Nystul (1999) discuss counseling issues relating to children and adolescents, and that there are special ethical and legal issues in terms of confidentiality. Confidentiality with minors is a gray area for professional counselors as well as SLPs and audiologists. Conflicts can result from the clinician's legal responsibility to respect a parent's right to be informed about what occurs in the therapy session with a child, and the ethical responsibility to maintain the confidentiality of the minor. Occasionally, a child might ask a clinician specifically not to tell his or her parents about something talked about in therapy. For example, a child who stutters may admit that he or she has more difficulty talking with his father than his mother. The question then becomes, how do we disclose that information to the parent without violating the child's confidentiality? If we choose not to disclose that information, how can we use it in a therapeutic way to help the child's speech? There are no specific guidelines for answering such questions, and each situation needs to be considered individually. One method of using information therapeutically that the child has shared in confidence (but without attributing the information to the child directly) is to use a third person approach. For example, you may say to the parents, "Many children who stutter have more difficulty talking to one parent or the other, and quite commonly these children have more trouble talking to the parent whom they see as the rule enforcer in the family, which may be either the father or the mother. In your family, whom do you think your child sees as the rule enforcer?" From the parents' responses you could say that that might also be what their child feels and that he or she might see that parent as more difficult to talk to than the other parent.

Gladding (2000) suggests that counselors establish guidelines with parents and the minor about the nature of information that can be released to parents. The American Counseling Association (ACA) (1997) provides an ethical code that can help structure guidelines for SLPs and audiologists: "When counseling minors or persons unable to give voluntary informed consent, counselors act in these clients' best interest" (Section A:3). The counselor can therefore release confidential information to parents when the counselor believes it is in the child's best interest.

Concurrent Therapy with a Mental Health Professional

Some private clients I have worked with have voluntarily informed me that they are also concurrently working with a counselor, psychologist or psychiatrist. I have, quite appropriately, not received reports from the other professionals working with these clients. However, brief 10–15 minute telephone calls to the psychologists can sometimes add or clarify relevant information about the clients that can help me with my therapy. The clients' work with the other professionals is confidential and clients choose what, if anything, to share with me. The reports I write on my evaluations of clients and their progress in therapy are provided to the clients who have the option then of sharing them with other professionals in any way that they choose.

For the protection of both the client and clinician, it is wise to state the terms of confidentiality within the work setting, including who will see any information and why (Shipley, 1997). If a court (judge) requests your documentation you *must* submit all documents (Fogle, 2000). If, however, an attorney subpoenas your records you do not have to submit them until there is a court order. The clinician must be the interpreter of his or her own reports, that is, the attorney or court will likely call upon the clinician to interpret the findings and specific statements in any subpoenaed reports.

Team Approach

SLPs and audiologists always work as team members with clients, families and other professionals. The most important person on the team is the child, client, or patient, and without that person no other team members are necessary. Therefore, at a minimum the team includes the child, client, or patient and the clinician. Additional team members may be parents, grandparents, spouses or partners, teachers, other school personnel, psychologists, administrators, nurses, physicians, PTs, OTs, respiratory therapists, social service and discharge planners, counselors, or psychiatrists.

Professionally, we do not work in a vacuum. What we communicate and how we communicate to the other team members about our clients and patients can have significant impact on the other team members' interactions with the people we are trying to help. Much of what we communicate is data and observation based information, for example, what is included in an evaluation of a child's speech, language, and hearing report or a medical note. However, as objective as we may try to sound or appear, our feelings about the child, client, or patient may emerge. If we have very positive feelings about the person we are trying to help, our choice of words, tone of voice, facial expressions, and body language will likely reflect our feelings. The same is true if we have negative feelings.

As team members, we need to be aware of the primary and secondary messages we are communicating. For example, we may be discussing our evaluation results about a client (primary message) and at the same time unknowingly revealing our negative feelings about the person (secondary message). Listeners (observers) note our words as well as our affect. If we are trying to sound positive about a client but our tone of voice, facial expressions or body language belie our words, the other team members will receive mixed messages and may "believe" our nonverbal communications more than our verbal. The unintended messages that have "leaked out" may influence or alter their perceptions of the client or patient, and therefore possibly their interactions with the person. It is appropriate for us to alert other team members about concerns we have about a client or patient's behaviors, affects and cognitions; however, we need to be particularly careful to not unduly bias the other team members against the person.

Making Referrals

Shipley (1997) says that the referrals SLPs or audiologists make to other professionals mean the clinician is attempting to serve the client's best interests. We may make referrals to educational specialists such as reading specialists, or medical specialists such as otolaryngologists. We may refer a client to a psychologist or counselor when we feel the client's problems are beyond our scope of practice. We also may refer clients to other SLPs or audiologists who have greater expertise in a particular area than we might have.

Another Therapist Was a Better Match

Over the years I have referred a few private clients to other SLPs whom I felt would be better suited (a better match) for a particular client. For example, I began working with a young adolescent girl with a voice problem and by the second session had the feeling that she could be better helped by a female SLP. I discussed this with the client and her mother, and then found a SLP to whom I felt confident referring the client.

Continues on next page

> *Continued from previous page*
>
> In another case, I began working with a five-year-old boy with language problems, particularly word finding. I saw the young boy in his home. He was cooperative and willing to work with me, and I liked him. However, after several sessions I felt that I was not the best SLP for him and could not pinpoint just what was lacking in our working relationship. I discussed the issue with the parents and the child and, although they wanted me to continue, agreed that if I did not feel I was the best SLP to serve his needs, they would be willing to have another SLP take over. The SLP I chose to replace me developed an excellent working relationship with the child and family, was his SLP for quite a long time, and accomplished the goals that were needed.

When we make referrals to other professionals we need to give clear, straightforward, but tactful reasons for our recommendations. Lavorato and McFarlane (in Shipley, 1997), note that some clients may be reluctant to see another specialist, particularly a psychologist, psychiatrist, or other mental health professional. Clients may be concerned about the cost of other therapy, whether insurance will cover it, and/or the imagined stigma of seeing such a professional. Lavorato and McFarlane suggest the client consult with or talk with another specialist, avoiding words such as be evaluated by or consider psychotherapy. "Talk with" is less threatening and likely to be more easily accepted by the client. The word counselor is less threatening than psychologist, psychotherapist, or psychiatrist. Another method is to use descriptive phrases such as "see a specialist who can help with problems like you are experiencing."

Referring a client or patient to another professional means that you have provided the best service you can to that individual. It does not mean that you are inadequate or that your professional scope of practice is too narrow. It means that you recognize your professional limitations (we all have them) and that you are working within our profession's scope of practice. When you receive referrals from another professional such as an otolaryngologist, psychologist, or education specialist it means that he or she also recognizes professional limitations and scope of practice, and that your education and training in speech-language pathology or audiology is the expertise wanted for the client or patient.

CONCLUDING COMMENTS

This chapter provides a definition of counseling for SLPs and audiologists and explains the major points in the definition. Counseling is both a science and art, and we begin our study of it by learning the science so that we can better develop the art. There are several DSM-IV TR diagnoses that psychologists or psychiatrist may make, but then refer to SLPs for the actual treatment. By being enrolled in a course on counseling skills for our professions, you are likely to already have many, if not most, of the personal qualities of effective helpers fairly well developed. However, knowledge of relevant psychological concepts and counseling skills can facilitate the process of striving to become better clinicians. We must always keep in mind our personal and professional boundaries so that we can effectively and ethically serve those who put their trust in us.

Discussion Questions

1. How can you apply concepts from counseling to your personal life?

2. How would you define counseling for our professions of speech-language pathology and audiology?

3. Discuss the differences between doing counseling and being a counselor. When you are doing counseling are you also at that time being a counselor?

4. What do you feel is more important to effective and successful counseling, the science or the art?

5. Why do you think counseling courses have not been an integral part of speech pathology and audiology curriculums throughout the history of our professions?

6. Do you think it is helpful for professors to also be practicing clinicians? Why?

7. Why do you think SLPs and audiologists are often the professionals who are most involved in the habilitation or rehabilitation of several DSM-IV diagnoses that may be made by psychologists?

8. Of the numerous personal qualities of effective helpers discussed in this chapter, which ones do you feel are some of your strongest? Some of your weakest? How might you strengthen your weakest personal qualities?

9. Discuss how counseling skills could be used with each of the within-boundaries areas for our professions.

10. Think of additional beyond-boundaries areas for our professions.

11. What are some challenges to boundaries you have been confronted with in your clinical work thus far?

12. What is some baggage you have that might affect your counseling with clients and families?

13. How do you distance yourself from clients, patients, and family? From other people?

14. How do you structure your therapy environment to maintain the boundaries you are comfortable with?

15. What life experiences do you lack that you feel may affect your credibility with the parents of a child? An adolescent who stutters? A married woman with a voice disorder? An elderly man with aphasia?

16. What would you say to:

    a. a parent who asks you how you could know anything about raising a child with problems when you are not even a parent?

    b. an adolescent who stutters who asks you how you know anything about what it feels like to stutter when you have never had the problem?

    c. a married woman whose voice disorder appears to be partly the result of family stress when she asks you how you could know anything about what it is like to be married or have children when you are not married or do not have children?

    d. an elderly man with aphasia who communicates that you do not understand what it is like to be old and not be able to understand or talk to other people.

17. Discuss a counseling issue you had relating to a child or adolescent when you were uncertain about breaking confidentiality by sharing information with a parent.

Theories of Counseling and How They Relate to Speech-Language Pathology and Audiology

CHAPER OUTLINE

INTRODUCTION

Gladding (2000) says that exceptional practitioners on the basis of their experiences and observations formulated counseling theories and therapies. However, no one theory or therapy approach fits all situations and a clinician may actually apply multiple therapy approaches with any one client, patient, or family. What theoretical and therapy approaches an individual clinician uses often depends on the clinician's personal orientation (e.g., humanistic, behavioral, etc.), what the clinician has learned in his or her training, and what has worked for the clinician in the past. There is no one right theoretical or therapeutic framework. As it is impossible to learn and use the over 400 counseling and psychotherapy approaches that are currently in the literature (Prochaska & Norcross, 2003), speech-language pathologists (SLPs) and audiologists can be most effective by learning a few of the most applicable approaches to our professions. The theories presented in this chapter are among those that are considered to form the conceptual and clinical bedrock of the fields of psychology and counseling (Gurman & Messer, 1995).

There is much value in a clinician having multiple theoretical and therapeutic frameworks from which to work. If a clinician only has one or two to draw from, he or she is limited in ability to understand and help clients, patients, and families. ("If a person only has a hammer, then everything looks like a nail.") Theoretical purity (following only a particular approach) is seldom helpful with the vast variety of people and problems we work with. Lazarus and Beutler (1993) found that 60% to 70% of professional counselors identify themselves as eclectic in the use of theory and techniques. However, beyond just an eclectic approach we can use an integrative approach in which we tie together approaches that have commonalties. For further reading in the area of psychotherapy and counseling theories, the student or clinician may wish to refer to one of many excellent textbooks in the area, for example, Capuzzi and Gross (1995); Corey (2001); Corsini and Wedding (2000); George and Cristiani (1995); Gurman and Messer (1995); Prochaska and Norcross (2003). A personal favorite of the author (L.V.F.) is Prochaska and Norcross, which inspired the format for this chapter and the presentation of a case example seen through the lenses of various theoretical perspectives.

This chapter begins with two therapy approaches that emphasize the clinician-client relationship: understanding it and working with it. It then moves into therapies that emphasize helping people change their ways of thinking about particular issues and their problematic behaviors as they relate to our professions. Additional therapy approaches are discussed that help enlarge our way of seeing the client/patient's world as well as our own.

HUMANISTIC THERAPY

Carl Rogers (1951, 1957, 1961, 1980) developed in the 1940s and 1950s what is known today as humanistic therapy and client-centered (person-centered) therapy. Rogers emphasizes that people are rational and inclined toward positive growth or **self-actualization** (realizing one's potential). This viewpoint is considered the central assumption of humanistic therapy. Healthy personality development occurs if the person receives sufficient **unconditional positive regard**, that is, love and acceptance from parents or significant others for his or her unique, individual self. Often times the best example of unconditional positive regard is the love and acceptance a parent has for his or her child. For example, the parents of a hearing impaired child who show consistent love and acceptance helps the child to grow and develop feelings of self-worth. The child learns **congruence**, that is, to be in touch with his or her own thoughts and feelings, and communicates them with facial expressions and body language that mirrors verbal or sign language.

Unhealthy personality development occurs when an individual experiences conditions of worth, repeatedly receiving messages from parents that he or she will be loved and accepted only if certain conditions are met; for example, the individual must never cry or show anger and, instead, must be compliant, studious, and easy to get along with. As a result of these experiences, the child learns to conceal his or her real self, present a façade that is incongruent (discrepant between what the child thinks, feels, and expresses verbally or nonverbally) with genuine feelings. In presenting a façade, the child sacrifices natural tendencies toward positive growth in order to receive conditional love and approval. For example, a child with a hearing loss may not feel accepted by parents when the child observes that they give more attention and love ("regard") to siblings. The hearing impaired child may try to conceal from parents that he or she could not hear or understand them in order to appear more like siblings.

The SLP or audiologist using humanistic or person-centered techniques attempts to promote the person's natural positive striving and growth. The clinician's role is **nondirective** (not trying to influence, being primarily reflective) and supportive. The therapist avoids engaging in confrontation or direct attempts to change the person's behavior.

Conditions Necessary and Sufficient for Therapeutic Change

Rogers (1957) discussed therapeutic conditions that he regards as necessary and sufficient for therapeutic change, which are outlined in the following sections.

GENUINENESS

The genuine clinician presents herself in an open manner and is not showing a façade. The clinician behaves in a way that is congruent (consistent and genuine) with real feelings. For example, if a client comments to the clinician, "You look tired today," the clinician may say, "Yes, you're right, I am a little tired today." In this response, the clinician validates the client's (correct) perceptions.

Presenting a congruent response is challenging when how we feel toward a client is not congruent with how we think we should feel toward the client. For example, we may feel irritated with a client who has not followed through with exercises or comes late to sessions. Yet we are striving to respond respectfully and therapeutically. If we are not careful, what the client may experience is a mixed message from our real feelings leaking out. Our behavior may be polite on the surface but contain undertones of anger or resentment. Another example of incongruency is when the clinician may not be aware of how angry or annoyed he or she actually is.

In either case above, the clinician focuses on presenting a positive and warm response to the client. However, the client may perceive both levels of the clinician's response: the polite surface behaviors and the angry, irritated undertones. The incongruence between the two levels of communication will likely cause discomfort in the client, and the client may respond negatively. The clinician, unaware of the client's perceptions, may view the client as uncooperative, unappreciative, or difficult. In order to work with this challenging situation, the clinician first needs to become aware of any tendency toward an incongruent response, and work through the negative feelings toward the client rather than just trying to conceal them. The clinician may also choose to express feelings to the client in a nonthreatening manner using "I-messages" (e.g., "When you do . . ., I feel . . . " As we have seen in the above example, trying to conceal negative feelings often does not work.

Working through negative feelings towards a client involves trying to better understand the client's viewpoint (empathy). The clinician may want to ask him or herself some questions, such as,

What stops the client from coming on time? What is the client afraid of? Usually if the clinician can better understand the client's fears, she will feel more empathic and less annoyed with the client. The point is that the clinician needs to reflect on her own behavior toward the client and not simply blame the client. By taking these steps the clinician will be better able to develop or return to a stance of unconditional positive regard toward the client. It is important to note that Rogers' (1957) concept of clinicians' genuineness has sometimes been misunderstood as a license for clinicians to talk about themselves or engage in excessive self-disclosure. This was not Rogers' intention; he was primarily concerned with the idea that clinicians should not feign interest or caring as this façade is likely to be detected by clients and family and damage the therapeutic relationship.

EMPATHY

Empathy involves "being with" the person and his or her experiences on a moment-to-moment basis. It is a personal encounter, not simply an objective appraisal of the person's problems. In order for the clinician to experience and show empathy, the clinician must understand not only the clinical condition, for example, stuttering, but how the stuttering is affecting the person's self-image and life. Although we can never truly feel what the client feels, we can try to get a sense of what the person must cope with most every time he or she tries to talk.

In striving to be empathic, clinicians should take care not to go overboard. Sometimes excessive efforts to appear friendly, caring, and empathic, especially in the early stages of the working relationship, can appear phony and ungenuine to the client. This is a different kind of incongruence than discussed above. In this case the clinician is trying to appear warmer and more empathic than how she is truly feeling. She may have a saccharine presentation that usually is viewed negatively by clients.

UNCONDITIONAL POSITIVE REGARD

When the SLP or audiologist communicates genuine respect and caring to the person he or she is demonstrating unconditional positive regard. This allows the person to experience a nonjudgmental environment for considering what is being asked in therapy, even if the person cannot (or will not) perform the task with maximum involvement or effort.

In humanistic therapy there is an emphasis on providing a positive relationship rather than on therapeutic techniques. As the person expresses him or herself, however, the clinician is alert for statements pertaining to the self (for example, "I haven't felt like doing my exercises lately." or "I don't understand how these exercises will help."). The clinician also attends to the person's nonverbal communications that are incongruent with verbal communications, (e.g., smiling while discussing a significant personal loss).

In order to help both the client and clinician understand the client's feelings, the clinician may provide reflections that paraphrase the statements or, when needed, point out discrepancies in the communications (these skills, rooted in Rogers' theory, are expanded in Chapter 4, Interviewing and

CASE STUDY

Reflecting Empathy to a Child Who Stutters

A 13-year-old boy was brought to therapy by his parents because of the child's stuttering problem.

Clinician: "Tell me what it's like to talk in different situations."

Child: "I don't talk much at school. It makes me nervous."

Clinician: "You don't talk much because it makes you nervous."

Child: "Yeah, and I get *really* nervous about speaking out in front of the class."

Clinician: "Speaking out in front of the class. Is that one of the hardest things for you to do?"

Child: "Uh huh, especially if the teacher wants me to read from the science book."

Clinician: "You don't like to read out loud from the science book." (The clinician is staying very close to what the child says, but not sounding like a mechanical parrot.)

Child: "Yeah, the words are tough and I get stuck on them and I make a fool of myself."

Clinician: "So you are afraid of stuttering or making a mistake and looking like a fool in front of your classmates."

Child: "The guys will laugh at me."

(The reflections gently encourage the child to continue to provide helpful information, and to do so without feeling judged or criticized by the clinician.)

Therapy Microskills). To provide a simple reflection the clinician should let the person know he or she has been heard, and that the clinician is interested in hearing more. The clinician's reflection's should, however, not simply mimic or parrot the client's last words. For example, a patient may mention symptoms that reflect penetration of food or liquid into the larynx (e.g., episodes of coughing or choking), and then deny that they are a problem. The clinician may reflect on both of these statements and then ask about the person's feelings. The patient may be feeling embarrassment or fear about meal times. For example, the clinician might say, "You say you are doing some coughing and choking while eating, but that it's not really a problem for you. Are you sometimes a little embarrassed about coughing and choking, or are you a little afraid that you won't be able to continue eating regular food?" Providing an environment where all the person's feelings and experiences are respected and validated is central to humanistic therapy.

CASE STUDY

Michael and a Humanistic Therapy Counseling Approach

Throughout this chapter Michael and his family will be used to illustrate how various therapy approaches and strategies can be used with a fairly complex case.

Michael is a 12-year-old seventh grade boy who sustained a closed head injury from a motor vehicle versus bicycle accident. He was not wearing a helmet at the time of the accident. He is in an acute care hospital in his small hometown. The child, according to the parents and teacher, was well-adjusted, well-liked by his peers, and a good student with no learning disabilities. He was athletic and enjoyed soccer and baseball.

Michael's father, John, is a computer programmer and his mother, Margaret, is a third-grade elementary schoolteacher at the school the child attends. Michael has a 14-year-old brother, Steven, and eight-year-old sister, Lisa. Steven has reportedly always had difficulty in school and has been a challenge at home. Lisa is doing well in school and has no significant behavioral or family problems. Michael's maternal grandparents (Joe and Martha) live near the family and are very involved in the lives of all three grandchildren.

Michael's neurological injuries include frontal lobe damage, contracoup damage, and damage to both left and right temporal lobes. He has been diagnosed with moderate receptive and expressive aphasia, moderate cognitive impairments affecting his attention, immediate and recent memories, and sequencing and organizational abilities. His judgment, reasoning, and problem solving are also moderately impaired. His speech is characterized by mild to moderate dysarthria with respiration and phonation within normal limits, but mild hypernasality and moderate weakness of the mandible, lips, and tongue. He is approximately 90% intelligible at the single word level, 80% at the phrase and short sentence level, and 70% at the conversational level. He does not have dysphagia.

Michael is currently at a Rancho Level 6, Confused-Appropriate with some emerging Level 7, Automatic-Appropriate, behavior as evaluated from the Revised Rancho Levels of Cognitive Functioning (Hagen, 1998). Michael shows the following signs and symptoms from the Rancho Scales: inconsistent orientation to person and place; able to attend to highly familiar tasks in nondistracting environments for 30 minutes with moderate redirection; remote memory has more depth and detail than recent memory; vague recognition of some staff; emerging awareness of appropriate responses to himself, family, and basic needs; emerging goal-directed behavior related to meeting basic personal needs; lack of awareness of impairments,

Continues on next page

Continued from previous page

disabilities, and safety risks with unrealistic planning for the future; follows simple commands; and verbal expressions are appropriate in highly familiar and structured situations.

The parents are experiencing guilt related to not requiring Michael to wear a helmet when riding his bicycle. His older brother is concerned that Michael may now be retarded and an embarrassment to the family. His sister is confused about why Michael does not understand what she says, why he sounds so different and acts so funny. Michael's grandmother, Martha, has been concerned for some time about the freedom his mother has given him, which has been a source of tension between the parents and grandparents. The grandfather just wants his favorite grandson to get better.

Patients with traumatic brain injury (TBI) commonly have behaviors that are disagreeable to both the family and the rehabilitation staff. Michael's father, who is known for his impatience and somewhat intolerant attitudes, is having difficulty accepting the "new" Michael. John is demonstrating cold and distancing behaviors (aloofness, detachment, monotone voice, little warmth in facial expressions, and stiff, noncomforting touch) toward Michael. The SLP notices the father's behaviors and knows that it is important for Michael to receive as much warmth and acceptance as possible from everyone in contact with him. The SLP also knows that the father is an important communication partner for Michael, and the father's withdrawal may interfere with Michael's improvement in rehabilitation. The SLP shows genuine empathy for the father and his difficulty accepting his son as he is now. The SLP does not distance herself from the father, but rather presents unconditional positive regard so the father does not feel judged. The therapist realizes that her relationship with the father is very important for the total team approach, where not only the rehabilitation staff are there to help Michael, but all the family and other caring people in his life.

Some clinicians may feel distressed by the father's withdrawal and lack of involvement with his son. They may even feel irritated with the father for not providing more unconditional love and support. In experiencing these responses to Michael's father, the SLP may find it challenging to maintain a congruent relationship. The SLP may feel a need to suppress the urge to criticize the father for his failure to provide more support in Michael's time of need. The SLP will need to empathize with the father's fears and anxieties in order to feel less judgmental toward him. Once the SLP can do that, she has a better chance to approach the father with a genuine and caring manner, even if she does not approve of all his responses toward his son.

Continues on next page

Continued from previous page

The father's behaviors may also contain incongruencies. He may indicate that he is having difficulty spending time with Michael and seeing him as the same son who he was before. John tries to smile while saying this to the SLP. The SLP may offer a reflection by saying, "It's hard to spend time with Michael now because he just isn't the son you have always known." This response helps the father feel validated and may also encourage him to explore a little further why he is distancing himself from his son. The father needs to feel accepted for his thoughts, feelings, and behaviors, just as we are hoping the father can learn to accept Michael's thoughts, feelings, and behaviors.

INTERPERSONAL THERAPY

Interpersonal therapy was founded by Harry Stack Sullivan (1953, 1972) whose ideas emerged in the 1950s (Gladding, 2000; Corey, 2001; Prochaska & Norcross, 2003). The emphasis in this therapy approach is upon observable interpersonal interactions, styles of communication, and self-defeating communication patterns (Anchin & Kiesler, 1982; Klerman & Weissman, 1993; Weissman & Klerman, 1991). According to interpersonal therapy, learned and rigid styles of communication are what cause emotional disorders or disruptions. People do not develop emotional disorders from a single trauma, but from ongoing problems in communication and problematic relationship patterns with important people in their lives (Benjamin, 1993; Strupp & Binder, 1984). In interpersonal therapy it is believed that these roles were learned in childhood; however, the SLP does not need to try to investigate the person's early childhood history. The clinician may assume that the person's interpersonal patterns were learned early in life and that they represent the person's best attempts to interact and gain approval of others, and to protect himself from overwhelming anxiety (Wachtel, 1993). For example, a child who is developing stuttering behaviors may become anxious and exhibit more dysfluency when his achievement-oriented parents ask him to perform in front of guests. His anxiety may be a result of fearing disapproval from his parents if he does not perform to their expectations. As an adult, this person may continue to be more dysfluent when performing or speaking in front of a group. In addition, the adult who stutters may perceive his employer as having expectations similar to his parents.

Another brief example of this concept is an adult who is having difficulty making decisions about beginning therapy, continuing therapy, or doing what is asked by the clinician. This adult may have had early childhood experiences with parents who were unusually critical of his ideas and decisions, and so learned to please parents by being indecisive and allowing parents to make choices for him. Another example is a man who shows passive-aggressive behavior toward the clinician. This man may smile and nod every time the clinician gives a recommendation or instruction, but the clinician later learns that he has not followed through with any of the recommendations. This person may also have had critical and controlling parents, but his style of coping was to try to develop some autonomy while still appearing compliant. Thus, he developed a pattern of relating by saying one thing to please the listener but without the intention of doing what he says. From the clinician's perspective, the client's current **interpersonal style** is understandable in view of his earlier experiences and learned ways of coping. This perspective makes us less likely to simply apply derogatory labels to the person (e.g., he's a passive-aggressive person, or she's manipulative); and makes it more likely that we will view the person more positively and interact in an empathic way. When we label the person (rather than the behaviors) in a derogatory way, we are less likely to try to understand the situations that elicit the behaviors. Interpersonal behavior is always understood in the context of learned styles of communication and interaction.

Particular interpersonal styles tend to elicit (pull for) predictable responses from others (Kiesler, 1982). For example, friendly listening tends to elicit friendly and open disclosure from others, while authoritative commands and critical monitoring of a person tend to elicit deferring and overconforming behavior, and rejecting behavior is likely to elicit withdrawal. This principle has important implications for the clinician who may consider the type of responses he is pulling from clients and patients. A clinician who behaves in an authoritative and directive way may pull for unquestioning compliance. In some situations this kind of unquestioning compliance may be initially desirable, for example, with a TBI patient who has swallowing problems and the therapist wants the patient to do swallow safety maneuvers before fully understanding why and how they can help. However, as the patient improves cognitive abilities for reasoning and judgment and is getting ready to be discharged home, it is increasingly important for the patient to understand what is being asked and to demonstrate higher level cognitive abilities. The change of condition of the patient means the clinician needs to be able to modify an interpersonal approach from being authoritative to being more collaborative with the patient. Clinicians need to be aware of their own behaviors and how they may influence the responses of their clients and patients. In others words, what the clinician observes in a person's behavior reflects a combination of the person's learned style and what is elicited in the current interaction (Kiesler, 1982).

Another important principle in interpersonal therapy is that how we take care of ourselves is based on how we were once treated by significant others (e.g., parents) (Strupp & Binder, 1984; Benjamin, 1993; Henry, 1997). If we were treated well and nurtured by our parents in times of distress, illness, or crisis, we tend to nurture ourselves later in life. The clinician who has a history of working reasonable hours and taking vacations may be less prone to professional stress and burnout than the therapist who tends to neglect him or herself. The same is true for clients; those who take good care of themselves may have been well cared for as children. Another example is the client who is open and responsive to suggestions from the clinician; the client may have had important people early in life who were open and responsive to him or her.

Using interpersonal therapy techniques the clinician may share with a person the clinician's impressions of what transpires between them. This intervention is referred to as **metacommunication** (Kiesler, 1988). Thus, the clinician might say to a client, "You know, I feel a 'pull' to write out an exercise schedule for you, but I think it is best if you come up with a schedule yourself." In this way, the dialogue focuses on the process (what is happening between the two of them) rather than only the content (e.g., the client's next exercise schedule). This way of speaking to clients often feels awkward to novice clinicians because it seems to ignore our social rules and taboos regarding direct communication with others about our feelings toward them. However, it can be very useful to clarify what is happening in the interaction between the client and clinician.

Another example of metacommunication may go as follows: an elderly woman residing in a skilled nursing facility objects and resists the exercises designed by her clinician who appears extremely young to her. The resident demands to know how many people like her the clinican has seen. The clinician has an option of giving a "content" response and telling the resident how many similar residents she has seen. Or she may chose to give a "process" response to this patient, "Mrs. Williams, I'm wondering if you are unsure about my qualifications and expertise, and not quite ready to trust my recommendations. Is that what you are asking me?" With such a response the clinician tries to deal with the **complex interpersonal message**. This response is often a surprise to the person, but can give the person permission to talk about the "real" concerns and thus disrupt maladaptive interpersonal patterns that the person unwittingly may create with the clincian. Otherwise, these maladaptive communications may interfere with treatment. It is important to recognize that there can be a variety of reasons underlying this type of patient challenge. First, the patient may have earnest and legitimate questions about the clincians's experience. Alternatively, the patient's questions may serve the function of resistance and, in effect, stall her treatment process. In either case, helping the patient talk about his true feelings may help to move the therapy process in a productive direction.

CASE STUDY

Michael and an Interpersonal Therapy Counseling Approach

Michael, the 12-year-old boy with a TBI, was known for being a good boy and was caring toward his family. The dramatic changes in his behavior after the accident are reflective of his TBI more than of a long-standing way of interacting with family and friends. The SLP may want to explain to the family some of the behavioral changes that are reflected in the Rancho Scales, and that Michael has progressed as much as would be expected. His current Level 6, Confused-Appropriate with some emerging Level 7, Automatic-Appropriate behaviors, indi-

Continues on next page

Continued from previous page

cates that even though he is not functioning and behaving as he did before the accident, he still has several levels to progress through, that is, Levels 8, 9 and 10. Although Michael may not return completely to his premorbid personality and behavior, because he had such a good foundation before the accident, the family may be hopeful that Michael will become more like his previous self.

Michael's mother, Margaret, is having some difficulty supporting him in ways the SLP feels would be helpful. Margaret has important history that may shed some light on her current ways of responding to Michael and his multiple problems. Margaret is the oldest of three children and her two-year-old sister drowned in the family pool when Margaret was eight years old. Margaret's mother had asked her to watch her little sister closely while she was out shopping, and somehow the toddler fell into the pool. After this tragic incident Margaret's mother became angry and withdrew from her. Margaret started giving extraordinary attention and developing overinvolvement with her four year-old younger brother to help ameliorate some of her guilt.

In the current crisis Margaret is feeling John is withdrawing from her and interprets the withdrawal as his anger and disappointment with her. Out of her guilt and trying to regain her husband's attention and affection, she is "smothering" Michael by trying to do things for him that he is developing the ability to do for himself. It is difficult for her to see Michael's progress and need for increased independence.

Michael's father is not involved enough and his mother is involved too much. Neither parent is able to respond to Michael's true needs. The problematic interpersonal patterns in this family are affecting the parents' ability to support the speech-language therapist's goals by following her instructions as well as the goals and instructions of the other rehabilitation team members (PTs and OTs). If there is agreement among the rehabilitation therapists, it suggests the difficulty with the parents is more of an interpersonal problem with the parents rather than an individual clinican not communicating well with the parents.

When parental education strategies are not working, it may reflect long-standing interpersonal patterns of the parents. Clinicians should not assume it is resistance from the parents and possibly respond to them in ways that do not promote better interaction.

In this case the rehabilitation team would benefit from requesting nursing or Michael's physician to have a psychologist consultation. Having a psychologist involved increases the scope of the team to address the needs of the parents that go beyond the other rehabilitation team members' training. The psychologist can also help the child, nurses, and the rehabilitation team learn how to better cope with the parents as they are working through their "issues."

BEHAVIORAL THERAPY

Behaviorism emerged as a school of American psychology and became popular in the 1950s and 1960s (Skinner, 1953; 1974). Behaviorists ally themselves with objective, empirical science and the prediction of behaviors (Corey, 2001; Craighead, Craighead, Kazdin, & Mahoney, 1994; George & Cristiani, 1995; Gladding, 2000; Prochaska & Norcross, 2003). They are concerned with universal, elementary laws of behavior (e.g., people do what they are reinforced for doing) and place ultimate importance on the role of the environment in creating, modifying, and maintaining particular behaviors. The primary clinical emphasis is on translating symptoms (e.g., anxiety about stuttering or loss of speech after a CVA) so that they can be understood in terms of concrete behaviors that are observed by the clinician (Bellack, Hersen & Kazdin, 1982; Ciminero, Calhoun, & Adams, 1977; Goldfried & Davison, 1976), such as fear of speaking in front of a class or avoiding interaction with friends. These behaviors can then be addressed by modifying environmental consequences such as asking the other students to praise the child's attempts at speaking rather than teasing or ridiculing him.

B.F. Skinner (1953, 1974) described how an individual's behavior develops through the process of **operant conditionin**g. Simply stated, individuals learn to behave in ways that are reinforced. Skinner believed that all behaviors are controlled by patterns of reinforcement. For example, behavior that is followed by rewards or **positive reinforcement** will increase in frequency. Therefore, to understand a certain behavior, the clincian must identify the reinforcers in the environment. A classic example is the parent who buys his child an ice cream cone as a reward for going to therapy. This positive reinforcement may increase the child's cooperation with the therapy. However, reinforcement can also serve maladaptive goals, for example, a parent who speaks for his dysfluent child reinforces the child's avoidance of speaking.

Skinner (1953, 1974) also identified different types of **reinforcement schedules**, for example, an **intermittent reinforcement schedule** to show how certain behavior is maintained even though it is only reinforced on some occasions. For example, the clinician may reinforce the child's correct productions of a sound after every five productions (a primary reinforcer). On the negative side, intermittent reinforcement can perpetuate a problem behavior, for example, a parent may occasionally speak for his dysfluent child, which reinforces the child's avoidance, and the child comes to expect that reinforcement. As the therapy progresses, the child's target behavior may be reinforced, not through obvious means such as ice cream cones, tokens, or explicit praise such as "Good job!" but through **secondary reinforcers** such as a smile, head nod, or an approving gesture made by the clinician.

Social learning theory (Bandura, 1968, 1969; Dollard & Miller, 1950), which is a perspective adopted by many behaviorists, emphasizes that much of human behavior is caused by **observational learning** (modeling). Many behaviors are acquired through a process of social imitation of a person (a parent, older sibling, or teacher) who has prestige or upon whom the individual is dependent, for example, a new laryngectomee meeting a successful esophageal speaker.

Joseph Wolpe (1958, 1987) applied principles of **classical conditioning** to understanding human emotional problems and anxiety (Baron, 1998). He is best known for developing a behavioral treatment approach called **systematic desensitization** to treat people with phobias that he considered learned anxiety responses. In this treatment approach, people learn to face feared objects (e.g., dogs, bridges, or injections) gradually and to employ relaxation techniques that lessen the physiologic arousal associated with anxiety. The SLP can help people learn to face fears as well, for example, a child who stutters and avoids certain sounds, words, topics, people, or situations.

Clinicians often intuitively know to start with the least feared speaking situation (e.g., talking with a parent) and advance to the most feared speaking situation (speaking in front of a class). By progressively moving from easiest to hardest, the child, in effect, has become systematically desensitized to feared speaking situations and more relaxed about approaching the next more difficult situation.

As all behaviors are learned and dependent upon how other people respond, behaviorists do not use personality descriptors such as lazy, disrespectful, honest, or generous, which suggest that people possess these inherent traits. Abnormal, inappropriate, or problematic behavior is considered learned behavior. Therapy is often a process of extinguishing old behaviors (e.g., a frontal lisp) and learning new behaviors (correct production of /s/).

Behavioral therapy tends to be very structured, focusing on techniques rather than simply "being with the person" (Goldfried & Davison, 1976; Bellack, Hersen & Kazdin, 1982). Behavior therapists take an active role in structuring treatment programs to address particular behaviors. This is very consistent with the training received and therapy conducted by SLPs. Although behavior therapists are increasingly recognizing the importance of the therapeutic relationship, their main concerns in this area are to increase compliance with treatment plans and to model appropriate behavior for the client (Sweet, 1984). For example, a clinician teaching a child with language and pragmatic problems appropriate turn-taking behaviors during a conversation. Another example would be a clinician who models appropriate verbal responses to frustration in front of a patient who swears frequently since her CVA.

Assessment focuses on discovering the current conditions under which certain behaviors occur, that is, the **stimulus-response chains** (Cautela, 1977). If excessive or inappropriate behaviors are occurring (e.g., a child gets out of his seat frequently during therapy), then the clinician may focus on altering **reinforcement contingencies**, that is, changing the consequences associated with the person's response. The clinician may, for instance, reward the child with a sticker for sitting in his or her seat for five minutes. In this way, the child learns that appropriate behavior results in positive attention (reinforcement).

The SLP must also be alert to the possibility that a person's behavior is being maintained by a pattern of **negative reinforcement.** This concept is different from the notion of punishment and means that a behavior is more likely to occur if it results in the removal of an unpleasant or aversive stimulus. For example, an elderly patient who is restricted to pureed food and protests with cursing or abusive behavior (throwing food) learns that these behaviors result in the clinician terminating the therapeutic feeding attempts, and the patient is left to manage by himself.

Clinicians may attempt to shape desirable behaviors (e.g., increasing fluency in a child who stutters, or increasing speech intelligibility to decrease the perception of nasal resonance in a child with velopharyngeal incompetence) by reinforcing the person's gradual improvement and **successive approximations** to the desired behavior. The clinician using behavioral approaches will help the client **generalize** his newly learned skills (behaviors) in the therapy session to the home environment by giving homework assignments.

In conducting behavioral assessments, clinicians place behaviors in three categories: excesses, deficits, and inappropriate. For example, repetitions of sounds for a child who stutters could be considered excesses, a loss of expressive language in a CVA patient could be considered a deficit, and certain undesirable behaviors after neurological damage could be considered inappropriate. The clinician will identify the specific behaviors that need to be modified and write specific behavioral goals. In the case of excesses the goals will involve decreasing certain behaviors, in the case of deficits the goals will involve increasing certain behaviors, and in the case of inappropriate behaviors the goal will be to modify the behaviors.

CASE STUDY

Michael and a Behavioral Therapy Counseling Approach

Michael has a variety of excesses, deficits, and inappropriate behaviors. Michael tends to have perseverative behaviors, responding to different verbal stimuli with the same answers. He has deficits in his immediate and recent memory, making it difficult for new learning. He has inappropriate behaviors such as swearing and occasional striking out at caregivers.

In patient care conferences and rehabilitation team meetings the SLP will want to describe specific behaviors Michael is demonstrating that can then be care planned where all the team members respond to Michael's behaviors in consistent, nonpunitive ways. The family and other visitors should be informed of how the rehabilitation team members are managing various behaviors of Michael and how the family can respond to Michael in ways that are consistent and reinforce the work of the therapists.

COGNITIVE THERAPY

Behavioral therapists now include the role of cognitions (thoughts) in determining behavior (Beck, 1995; Mahoney, 1974; Meichenbaum, 1977; Wilson & Franks, 1982). However, cognitive therapists have always recognized that thoughts influence behaviors. People do not just respond to events but to their interpretations and beliefs about events. For example, when a student clinician arrives late to a therapy session one supervisor may feel the student has a legitimate reason for being late and, therefore, treats the student in an accepting manner. Another supervisor, however, may interpret the student's lateness as a sign of the student's irresponsibility and lack of professionalism, and therefore respond to the student in an aloof, cold manner.

Cognitive therapists recognize that there are countless perspectives or interpretations of any given event. Furthermore, the way in which people think about events (their perceptions) determines how they feel about themselves, others, and the future (Beck, 1995; Corey, 2001; George & Cristiani; 1995; Gladding, 2000; Prochaska & Norcross, 2003). For example, a patient who is discharged from therapy before feeling he has reached maximum potential may interpret the discharge to mean that he is not worth the clinician's time, the clinician is uncaring, and the patient will never get better now. It is clear that this sequence of thoughts can affect a patient's mood and behavior.

Cognitive theorists believe that certain core beliefs affect our behavior with others (Beck, 1995). These core beliefs are often learned early in life and become part of the assumptions we make about people. For example, "People are basically good." and "I can trust medical professionals to take good care of me." These thoughts and beliefs are "automatic" and we are not likely to evaluate them, so they persist in an unscrutinized form. In many situations a person's core beliefs work to the clinician's advantage. The person may have had an earlier positive experience with a SLP (e.g., the person's child benefited from speech therapy), and now the person has sustained a traumatic brain injury and maintains the automatic belief that a SLP too will help him. Any previous experience with a clinician, whether positive or negative, may influence the person's thoughts and behaviors toward a clinician.

Cognitive therapy has been applied to understanding and treating depression (Beck, 1967, 1995). Depressed individuals are regarded as having made pessimistic assumptions about themselves, other people, and the future in general. For example, a depressed individual might think, "I can't win," "People don't like me," and "I can't control what happens to me." Further, they might be inclined to selectively attend to negative experiences that confirm their beliefs and to ignore experiences that are inconsistent with their beliefs. For example, a child with a central auditory processing disorder (CAPD) and attention deficit disorder (ADD) who has had numerous failures in school and poor peer relationships may have negative expectations for the new school year that has just started. He may tend not to notice positive expressions such as a teacher's praise or classmate's attempts to get him involved in play activities. What the child tends to notice (or misinterpret) are the behaviors that confirm his negative beliefs about himself.

The essential idea of cognitive therapy is to help the individual recognize and examine tightly held but problematic beliefs and replace them with more adaptive and flexible ways of thinking. The goal in therapy is to examine the evidence that these beliefs are true, to refute them if erroneous, and then to construct rational, behavioral steps for coping with the erroneous thinking (Beck, 1970, 1976; Craighead et al., 1994; Ellis & Grieger, 1986; Prochaska & Norcross, 2003).

Many times SLPs and audiologists work with a person's faulty beliefs surrounding the communication problem. This is frequently seen in children and adults who stutter (Conture, 2001; Guitar, 1998; Zebrowski, 2002). For example, children and adults may have negative beliefs that affect their expectations of their ability to improve. The child or adult who has been stuttering for years will likely have low expectations of his potential to ever be much more fluent. The person may have had no interactions with someone else who stutters and, therefore, thinks that his stuttering problems are unique. The clinician may want to help the person recognize that he is not alone, and that there are many people who stutter, even though the person has not encountered them. In this way the clinician is helping the person to recognize and modify his faulty beliefs.

Cognitive Distortions

Common types of erroneous thinking or **cognitive distortions** include (Beck, Rush, Shaw, & Emery, 1979; Craighead et al., 1994; Prochaska & Norcross, 2003):

1. **Catastrophizing.** The person frequently believes the worst will happen, or, if something bad can happen, it will happen to him. For example, "If I don't get my voice back by next week, I may lose my job." A cognitive therapy intervention may include helping the person see the actual probabilities of the worst happening and focusing on evidence that the worst will not likely happen.

2. **"I Should" Statements.** These typically reflect perfectionistic tendencies and an intolerance of personal flaws. For example, a patient with dysphagia may say, "I should be able to eat my meals without any help." Or a patient with speech apraxia declares, "I should be able to say it, but I can't." A cognitive therapy intervention may include helping the person understand that what he has been able to do easily before his swallowing or communication problem cannot be done safely or easily now because certain parts of the brain are not working the way they used to.

3. **Dichotomous Thinking.** The person views events and experiences as one extreme or the other (all good or all bad). For example, the client talks very negatively about another clinician or a physician. A cognitive therapy intervention may include helping the person view people and experiences on a continuum, where even the worst experience or person has some good attributes.

4. **Overgeneralizations.** The person believes that if something is true in one case, it applies to any case which is similar. Dysfluent children, for example, overgeneralize fears of speaking situations, such as speaking up in class to speaking in front of small groups of children. Many discouraged patients make incorrect inferences based on one or two isolated events. After a new patient with a laryngectomy fails to easily learn esophageal speech, the patient may think, "I'll never be able to do this." After one hospital staff member treats a patient rudely or sternly, he concludes, "Everyone here is a jerk. No one here cares about me." A cognitive therapy intervention may include helping the person understand that his logic (thinking) may not be accurate and to help the person recognize exceptions to his rule.

SLPs using cognitive therapy techniques vary in how confrontational they choose to be with individuals who are demonstrating various forms of faulty thinking. However, the common theme is that they do not take a person's beliefs at face value; they question them and help the person develop more positive and realistic interpretations of experiences. While recognizing that people may have developed their negative beliefs early in their lives, the clinician using cognitive therapy techniques focuses on challenging and changing the current beliefs that interfere with a logical and rational approach to the communication problem.

CASE STUDY

Using Cognitive Therapy Techniques with a 13-Year-Old Girl

Lisa, a 13-year-old girl with a repaired cleft lip and palate who continues to have some hypernasality is anticipating a future surgical revision of her lip. She says, "If I don't get my lip repaired perfectly I'll never be pretty and no one will like me. I won't get invited to a prom, no one will ever marry me, I'll never have children, and I'll die alone." The SLP may begin to gently challenge the girl's beliefs in the following way.

SLP: "It sounds like you are really feeling discouraged now. I'm wondering, though, how much of what you are saying is actually true. For instance, when you say no one will like you, I'm wondering if you have some friends now, despite the scar on your lip and your speech problem."

Lisa: "Yes, I do have a couple of friends."

SLP: "And have they seen the scar on your lip and heard you talk?"

Lisa: "Well, of course. Who could miss it or not hear me sound like I talk through my nose?"

SLP: "So they haven't refused to be your friend because of your lip and speech."

Lisa: "Well, I guess not."

SLP: "Even though your lip and speech bother you, they don't prevent your friends from liking you. What do you think they like about you?"

Lisa: "Well I like to do a lot of things, so we play volleyball and go shopping together."

SLP: "So if these girls like you, what are the chances that you will find other friends in the future, even boyfriends?

Lisa: "Well, maybe you have a point. Maybe I was getting a little carried away."

CASE STUDY

Michael and a Cognitive Therapy Counseling Approach

As you recall, Michael is a 12-year-old seventh grade boy who sustained a closed head injury from a motor vehicle versus bicycle accident. He has been in rehabilitation receiving speech therapy, physical therapy, and occupational therapy for the past four weeks, making steady but slow progress. However, for the past two weeks Michael has refused to actively participate in his speech therapy as well as physical and occupational therapy. Michael is showing depressed affect and expressing a sense of hopelessness about his future, getting back to school, and playing soccer and baseball again.

Michael is making statements such as, "If my speech doesn't get better I'll fail school and lose all of my friends" (a catastrophizing statement). "I should be able to talk right by now" (an "I should" statement). "You're not helping me" (an overgeneralization). The SLP may begin by gently challenging Michael's perceptions that he is not making progress in therapy. The clinician may ask Michael if his speech and memory are better now than they were a few weeks ago. The clinician may also show Michael a graph with his improvement in various areas of his speech therapy. The clinician may ask how often he now has to repeat what he says in order to be understood by others. Michael may then realize that he has to repeat himself much less frequently than he did a few weeks ago. Through these various methods of providing evidence of Michael's progress, the clinician challenges the patient's pessimistic beliefs and helps him to develop more positive and realistic beliefs about his therapy.

FAMILY SYSTEMS THEORY

A variety of schools of family therapy emerged in the 1950s to 1960s, which presented a radical alternative to mainstream approaches to clinical psychology and the study of mental illness in individuals (Bateson, Jackson, Haley, & Weakland, 1956; Bowen, 1978; Haley & Hoffman, 1968; Minuchin, 1978; Satir, 1964, 1976, 1983). Pioneers of these theories emphasized that a person's emotional problems must be viewed in the context of the family's roles, communications and interactions. Individuals do not have emotional or behavioral symptoms in a vacuum, but rather develop and maintain their symptoms in a dysfunctional family context where there are faulty communication and interaction patterns, and/or faulty family structure. Because these theories focus on family relationships and systems rather than individuals, they are often referred to as systems theories.

A basic premise of the family therapy model is that each person (family member) in the system (family) affects all other members and that the system is *inter*dependent. Within the family system are subsystems, for example, mother-father, mother-son, father-son, grandparent-grandchild, and so forth. Another basic premise is that separate elements (e.g., an individual's behavior) cannot be understood apart from the whole system (the family). Thus, a person's behavior that appears problematic or puzzling may be better understood by examining it in the family context.

While there are at least a half dozen separate schools of family therapy, some concepts are universally accepted (Gladding, 2000; Goldenberg & Goldenberg, 2000; Prochaska & Norcross, 2003). Many of these were developed by two institutes in Palo Alto, California which shared the assumption that communication is the key to understanding human behavior. Some of the well-known pioneers of this communications approach to family therapy include Bateson et al. (1956), Satir (1964, 1976, 1983), Watzlawick (1978) and Weakland (1976). These individuals studied the complex patterns of communication occurring in families, looking at verbal and nonverbal dimensions, and overt versus covert messages. They believed that emotional and behavioral symptoms might develop in children and adults because of repeatedly receiving "mixed messages" from family members. Typically, these mixed messages are ones in which the verbal and the nonverbal (covert) messages are contradictory. The covert message may be conveyed through voice inflection, body language, and facial expression.

Jack and His Parents

A six-year-old boy with moderate to severe dysfluency was referred to me by the Stuttering Foundation of America. When I work with a child who stutters much of my focus is on the parents, helping them identify attitudes and behaviors they may have that may be contributing to dysfluencies of their child, and how they can change those attitudes and behaviors (Fogle, 1978; Zebrowski, 2000). Parents are often unaware of many of the overt and covert attitudes and behaviors they present to their children. Therefore, when working with the parents I use the *Modified Children's Report of Parental Behavior Inventory* (MCRPBI) (Fogle, 1978; Schaefer, 1965; Yairi, 1970; Yairi & Williams, 1971) to identify many of these attitudes and behaviors. The MCRPBI is a 192-item questionnaire which is divided into 19 scales that assesses various areas of attitudes and behaviors parents may have toward their child, for example, acceptance, rejection, positive involvement, hostile control, withdrawal of relations, positive attitudes toward speech, and negative attitudes toward speech. Assessing parental attitudes and behaviors can help to identify areas for needed change.

Jack's parents told me that their son's stuttering sometimes annoyed, upset, or embarrassed them, but that they did not think he noticed their feelings. When Jack tried to talk to his parents they would tell him how much they enjoyed hearing his stories about school, but their tense body language and facial expressions and loss of eye contact telegraphed a dif-

Continues on next page

Continued from previous page

ferent message to the child. The overt message was an invitation for the child to tell the parents about his school day, while the covert message was the parents' communication of disapproval, anxiety, and embarrassment about his stuttering.

The child's natural response to the perceived covert messages was to withdraw. Such mixed messages placed the child in a quandary where he might be punished (reprimanded for not talking about his school day) for correct interpretation of covert messages. After several weeks of therapy with the parents they became aware of and were able to modify many of their attitudes and behaviors that were contributing to Jack's dysfluency, and the child's stuttering diminished significantly. This left fewer changes for the child to make in his stuttering and allowed for a more permanent improvement of his speech problem. Had the therapy focused mainly on the child the family dynamics would likely have changed little, resulting in more difficulty in the child maintaining the improvements he made in his fluency.

Hospitalized patients may also receive mixed messages that make it difficult to know what to do. Elderly people and stroke survivors, in particular, may receive contradictory messages that cause them to wonder just what their family truly wants. For example, many people stoically accept that when adult children say that the parent can come to live with them but do nothing to help the parent make the transition, the real message is unstated but clear. When stroke survivors or elderly people are able to return home, they are often excluded from normal family activities, some because they cannot physically or communicatively become involved, and others because no one makes sufficient effort to include the person. When a person is unnecessarily excluded from family activities, the communication disorder becomes a true handicap (Tanner, 1999).

Individuals like the patient in the following case study may become especially sensitive to covert messages that are expressed repeatedly and, as a result, develop behavioral symptoms such as food refusal or incontinence. The key ideas here are that mixed messages (e.g., "I really want you to come home, but . . . ") put the recipient in a bind where no course of action seems acceptable. Meanwhile, the person who gives the complex communication is typically unaware of the double-sided nature of the message. However, the complex message may reflect internal conflicts and feelings that are viewed as unacceptable such as, "I really don't want to take care of my mother after she leaves the hospital," or "My child's stuttering embarrasses me." Rather than directly expressing feelings that may go against a person's principles, they "leak out" in the form of mixed messages. A clinician who understands this communication process can help the family to identify the incongruent messages being conveyed and to work towards therapeutic decision-making without negatively labeling any of the family members.

CASE STUDY

Mom and Her Son

An elderly person who is convalescing after a stroke may hear her grown son's invitation, "Mom, we want you to come live with us now so that you have someone to help take care of you." At the same time, however, the elderly patient hears her son's heavy sighing and worries about space in the home and financial matters. The patient may experience this as a lose-lose situation. Neither response (i.e., to accept her son's offer or to decline it) solves the dilemma. If she accepts her son's offer, she may feel (correctly) that he will be burdened by her presence and needs. If she declines his offer and tries to live alone, she may contribute to his further worry and rumination about her safety. The patient in this situation may act strangely, refuse medication, or behave in other ways that postpone medical recommendation for hospital discharge. In effect, her behavior serves to stall decision-making in a no-win situation. The SLP who is aware of the patient's situation is likely to be empathic and better understand her occasional difficult behaviors. The clinician can reflect his or her understanding of the predicament to the patient, and this reflection may result in increased compliance and cooperation in therapy.

SLPs and audiologists have used Family Systems therapy concepts with language-impaired children (Andrews, 1986; Andrews & Andrews, 1990, 1993). Mary Andrews, a trained family therapist, and James Andrews, an SLP, described techniques for helping children with language disorders within a family-based approach. The blueprint for family-centered early intervention is the Individualized Family Service Plan (IFSP), which includes 1) making a contract with the family, 2) planning for and conducting an assessment of the child, 3) identifying family strengths and needs, 4) developing outcome statements, 5) implementing the plan of treatment, and 6) evaluating the plan. This process is discussed in detail by McGonigal, Kaufman, and Johnson (1991). Andrews and Andrews emphasize the value of encouraging all family members to participate in the evaluation and treatment of a child with a hearing or communication impairment. Family members are likely to accept an invitation to participate when it is made clear that they can be helpful to their child by being involved from the initial evaluation and throughout therapy.

Family Systems concepts can also be used by paying attention to the labels that family members give to one another (e.g., my bright child, my problem child, my handicapped child) and the way those labels affect the therapist's perceptions of the client. Negative comments or innuendoes from family members may bias the clinician in subtle ways about the client. Novice clinicians may have a tendency to be compliant to family members who present themselves as the authority in the family, affecting the therapist's perceptions of the client and their treatment efforts.

Family Therapy emphasizes concern about the negative labels family members use to describe the client or patient that may bias the clinician (Minuchin, 1978). Often clinicians interview family members to obtain information about the client, their concerns, and goals for treatment. Potential problems arise when the family members' comments and labels regarding the client bias the clinician's perceptions. In addition, the family member's statements may diminish the client's credibility in describing his or her own strengths and weaknesses, and therefore, reduce the clinician's perceived need to have an extended dialogue with the client. For example, the parent who describes his child as motivated and loving versus the parent who describes his child as unmotivated and difficult. The parent who describes the child in positive terms is likely to be having better experiences with the child and will be supportive of the child's best interests in therapy. However, the parent who uses negative terms and descriptions may present more challenging attitudes and behaviors for the clinician.

We also need to be aware how labels may be used to control a family member's behavior (e.g., my hard-working child, my lazy child, my demented father). Typically, assigning a label gives one family member power over another. If a family member informs a clinician that the client is lazy, unmotivated, uncooperative, or demented, it gives that family member the appearance of a legitimate basis for claiming power over the labeled person and taking authority and control over the person's treatment. The actions, opinions, or preferences of the client or patient then may be disqualified or disregarded. Clinicians who accept at face value the family labels of a person (e.g., lazy, demented) may not be as open and willing to take into consideration the client/patient's perceptions and requests.

Another broadly accepted concept in family therapy concerns recurrent behavioral patterns that keep the family system functioning within tolerable limits. Each family has a predictable pattern of behavior that serves to maintain its balance or **homeostasis** (Bateson et al, 1956). Serious illness or injury inevitably disrupts the family's current homeostatic equilibrium. Even in crisis, healthy families are able to maintain homeostasis, but still be flexible enough to adapt to change. For example, a family of four may function well until the father sustains a TBI. In response to this event, the wife and two teen-aged children may shift roles and responsibilities in order to take care of mortgage payments and daily household chores. In contrast to this family, other families may exhibit less flexible and more rigid patterns of behavior, for example, a father with a TBI where the family members deny the severity of his impairment and maintain unreasonable expectations for his recovery, and refuse to take on new household responsibilities.

Family therapists such as Ackerman (1984) and Bowen (1978) examined family patterns that were repeated in one generation after another. The concept of multigenerational transmission of symptoms states that symptoms are caused by the family's failure to separate themselves from the immediate family and the problems of prior generations. The family's ability to cope with a current illness or crisis may be strongly and negatively affected by their previous experiences with illness and crises that may have occurred in previous generations (usually grandparents). The SLP and audiologist need to be aware of this possible family dynamic which limits the family's current coping and make a referral to a family therapist.

Concepts originally defined by Minuchin (1974) in his description of **structural family therapy** are also widely accepted by family therapists. Minuchin was primarily interested in the structure of family systems and the belief that unhealthy family structures support emotional symptoms. He believed that a healthy family has a **hierarchy** wherein the parents are in charge and in control of the children. The parents also form a subsystem where they are close to each other and communicate clearly with each other about the family's functions. Siblings generally get along harmoniously, have a special bond with one another, and thus form another subsystem within the family.

A family with healthy organization also has clearly marked **boundaries** (Goldenberg & Goldenberg, 2000; Minuchin, 1974). Boundaries help to demarcate and maintain family member roles. A father who needs comforting after learning of a serious medical diagnosis goes to his wife, rather than his daughter, for solace. A mother who is upset by her husband's hospitalization goes to her siblings or adult friends for support. Boundaries in a family may be assessed by finding out who spends time with whom, especially in times of emotional distress.

Frequently seen in educational and medical settings are cases where well-meaning but overly protective parents "speak for" and exert excessive control over the behavior of their children. **Enmeshed** families occur when boundaries between members are blurred and members are overly concerned or overly involved in each other's lives (Goldenberg & Goldenberg, 2000; Minuchin, 1974). When parents are overly involved in their child's life the child may not be allowed to make independent decisions. An enmeshed parent-child relationship may serve to lower the parents' anxiety regarding their child. This may, for example, inhibit the child from using the problem-solving skills that the SLP has been working on in therapy that are also designed to help the child develop self-confidence in his or her own abilities.

At the other end of the family dynamics spectrum, excessive **disengagement** where family members have overly rigid boundaries in which members feel isolated or disconnected from each other (Goldenberg & Goldenberg, 2000; Minuchin, 1974). Each member may function separately and autonomously, and with minimal involvement in the day-to-day activities of the family. There is little sense of family loyalty and interpersonal distance is significant, with little ability to ask for or receive much needed emotional support. Communication among family members is often strained and guarded. In some cases this can lead to a child's behavioral difficulties and inappropriate age roles in a family. This may occur when there is a severely medically ill or chronically depressed and withdrawn parent who is relatively unavailable to the child, either physically or emotionally. The child may become parentified; that is, he or she takes on adult-like responsibilities. The SLP may want to encourage the parents to resume some of the activities the parentified child enjoyed before the child began taking on the more adult-like roles. In a disengaged family, parents may be encouraged to become more involved in their child's school and play activities.

Triangulation refers to the process where two family members recruit a third family member into an unhealthy alliance, often in order to avoid conflict with one another (Bowen, 1978; Goldenberg & Goldenberg, 2000; Minuchin, 1978;). There are at least two common versions of triangulation. In the first, the parents avoid conflict with one another by banding together and focusing upon the misbehavior of the child. Here, the child is a **scapegoat** and treated as though he or she is responsible for all the family's unhappiness. Scapegoating helps the family avoid conflict that is perceived as more threatening to them (e.g., the father's disability) than the conflict with the child. In the second common version of triangulation, a parent may develop a close alliance with a child in order to keep the spouse at a distance. The parent may choose to spend an inordinate amount of time with the child to avoid spending time with the spouse. In this case, the parent-child alliance often does not serve the child's best interests but keeps the child entangled in the parents' conflict. In both versions of triangulation, the child is used to avoid conflict between the parents. SLPs and audiologists need to be alert to a parent's attempts to triangulate the clinician or to take sides against the other parent or the child. A signal that such a triangulation attempt is eminent is when a parent asks to meet with the therapist in private or wants to share some confidential information about a spouse.

In general, clinicians working from the family therapy perspective realize that they cannot remain the neutral outsider when working with families. Family members tend to compete for an alliance with the clinician, and certain family members may try to monopolize the therapy time. Thus, the clinician inevitably becomes part of the family system, and must use this position carefully. It is important for the clinician to decide when to "join" with a particular family member in order to gain compliance with an educational or medical recommendation, or to encourage a child, client, or patient to assume increased responsibility for self-care during therapy.

In some situations it may be most important for the SLP or audiologist to join with the mother or father who is supportive of therapy and can help structure the child's treatment exercises (Goldenberg & Goldenberg, 2000; Minuchin, 1974). In other situations it may be most important for the clinician to join with the child who appears motivated to increase his or her independence by developing problems-solving skills. In this way the clinician makes conscious decisions about with whom to join and when in order to achieve the best therapeutic results.

The legacy left by the pioneering family therapists is profound; they have helped us to "de-pathologize" the family members and to see an individual's behavior as both affecting and being affected by the family. SLPs and audiologists, like family therapists, can look at the communication, roles, and meanings of life experiences that families develop to try to achieve balance and coherence. Our interventions often focus on trying to get families to interact and communicate in healthier ways with one another.

EXISTENTIAL THERAPY

Existential therapists are interested in the ultimate conditions of life and how people deal with the tragedies of existence (Corey, 2001; Gladding, 2000; Prochaska & Norcross, 2003). Yalom, (1980) describes existential psychotherapy as a dynamic approach to therapy which focuses on concerns that are rooted in the individual's existence. People face conditions of existence that are awesome and profound. We grow up, we grow old, we become ill, we die. Yet knowing these conditions, we still strive to be good children, good adults, good workers, and good to our neighbors. Somehow we strive to find meaning to pursue our goals and to be responsible despite the inevitability of our

CASE STUDY

Michael and a Family Therapy Counseling Approach

Michael, as you recall, is a 12-year-old seventh grade boy with a TBI from a motor vehicle versus bicycle accident. His hospitalization and impairments are having a profound effect on the homeostasis of the family. Both parents have lost significant time from their jobs and, although they have not lost income because of the nature of their jobs (father is a computer programmer and mother is an elementary teacher), there are numerous expenses that are created when a family member is hospitalized. Although insurance will cover a significant portion of Michael's hospital stay and rehabilitation, it will not cover all of it, and the parents have to make up the difference. Financial concerns, although not spoken about directly, are always in the back of the parents' minds, thus creating additional tension in the family. The parents are talking about possibly needing to discontinue eight-year-old Lisa's ballet lessons. To keep things balanced, they are considering not sending Steven, the 14-year-old brother, to science camp this year. The parents have already decided not to take a much-needed family vacation. Both siblings sense an eminent loss of some of their favorite activities and are developing some resentment toward Michael for doing something dumb on his bicycle, like not wearing his helmet. The grandparents know the parents' financial struggles and wish they could help, but they are on a fixed income with little or nothing to share. They are happy to take care of Steven and Lisa while the parents are at the hospital.

The SLP recognizes that when a child or adult has a significant impairment, the entire family is affected—the family system. The therapist observes the parents' warm and loving interactions with Michael, but also recognizes the stress on the parents' faces that Michael can likely see also. The parents reassure Michael that everything will be all right but, even though he is in an egocentric state because of his TBI with a Rancho Level 6 (Confused-Appropriate), he senses some mixed messages from his parents. He asks if he can take his bicycle on the vacation the family was planning and hears his mother say, "Of course," but sees his father turn his head and look away. The therapist checks Michael's medical chart to make certain that social services are involved with the family, as this is an area outside her scope of practice.

Reduction in the family leisure and quality time together also disrupts the family's homeostasis. Margaret has always attempted to make dinnertime the opportunity for the family to be together and to tell their stories about their days' events. She used it as a time to gauge how each child was feeling about school, friends, and family. Her dinnertime is now usually spent

Continues on next page

Continued from previous page

at the hospital with Michael and the mother knows that she is not as available to her other children as she would like to be. She is hoping that they can manage for awhile on their own. "Child watch" is taking the time of both parents; one parent is always at the hospital while the other one is trying to carry on at home. The SLP recognizes that both parents are sleep-deprived, anxious, and exhausted. Some of the negative comments made by the parents likely reflect their exhaustion more than any true negative feelings they may have about their child's medical care and rehabilitation. The father complains about the physician's lack of interest in Michael and the physical therapist's impatience with his son. The SLP knows to be alert to potential triangulation in this conflict and to avoid siding with the father against either the physician or the physical therapist.

The parental subsystem is disrupted because of lack of time together; when the parents are together their conversations are always about Michael. There appears to be some bickering between the parents that they are trying to hide from their children, but not successfully. The SLP confers with social service staff and the hospital psychologist to ask if there is a way the parents can be encouraged to take a day off and just take care of one another rather than taking care of Michael.

The SLP hears Michael's parents tell him that he is "still our bright boy," wondering how often that is said to Steven with his difficulties in school and being a challenge at home. Does Steven feel equally validated and appreciated by his parents? The SLP may take care to present praise to the child who appears to get less parental attention. This simple SLP intervention may remind the parents to pay attention to the healthy children as well. The SLP can discuss with the parents the need to praise their other children and model desired behaviors, such as acknowledging the accomplishments of the healthy children as well as the gains Michael is making in therapy.

Some degree of enmeshment appears to be present. The parents, particularly the mother, are overly involved with Michael and are doing things for him that he is capable of doing himself, such as speaking for him and helping him dress when he can generally manage these tasks but with considerable difficulty. The SLP recognizes, however, that in times of crisis families often pull together so tightly that they appear enmeshed. This enmeshment is usually temporary and will decrease as the child improves. However, the SLP knows that she needs to encourage both parents to allow Michael do to all that he can for himself even though he struggles.

The SLP recognizes that while she is involved with Michael's rehabilitation she is not a neutral outsider. The mother is competing for the SLP's attention, trying to get the SLP to address

Continues on next page

Continued from previous page

comments about Michael to her rather than the father. The SLP takes care to join with all family members. For example, the SLP tries to look at both parents when conferencing with them, and not just the parent who asks most of the questions. She makes certain that she asks each parent individually what questions the parent might have. She also speaks to Michael's brother and sister and his grandparents, sharing information with them so that they do not feel left out of Michael's rehabilitation. The SLP tells and shows each family member how to best communicate with Michael; how to use the "Rule of 5s" (5 letter words, 5 word sentences), and how to be alert to possible agitation when he is feeling overwhelmed. She explains her goals to the family and provides hope that Michael will make maximum improvement because of the excellent medical care and strong rehabilitation team working with him.

own demise. Understanding and finding meaning in our existence, despite its sometimes bleak conditions, was the focus of early existential writers (Bugenthal, 1965; Frankl, 1959; May, 1953, 1961).

SLPs and audiologists inevitably encounter existential issues in their work: when a clinician counsels parents of a child whose seizure disorder is contributing to his impaired speech and language, and the impairments are altering the parents' expectations of their child's future; when the clinician is working with an adult patient who is struggling with his cognitive losses and the meaning of life after a stroke; and when the clinician grows fatigued because she has encountered so many cases where human loss and suffering takes an increasing toll on her abilities to cope with and manage anxiety about dealing with more loss. However, for many SLPs and audiologists existentialist principles may become more relevant as they encounter increasing losses in their own professional or personal lives.

Existential therapy is concerned with each person's unique experience of being-in-the-world (Boss, 1963), how people perceive themselves and their surroundings, and how they manage to create meaning in their lives. In this context, people are understood to be in a constant state of flux and this is reflected in how they deal with their lives. This includes how we treat and take care of ourselves and others, as well as our relationship to the existential conditions of life such as the uncertainty of our own health, the meaninglessness of tragedies, and the isolation of losing loved ones (George & Cristini, 1995; Prochaska & Norcross, 2003; Yalom, 1980). The following describes some of the specific concepts considered by existential therapists that are relevant to clinicians.

Existential Uncertainty

Existential uncertainty involves the fact that as much as we attempt to control events in our lives, we discover that many events are outside our control. We may lead a healthy lifestyle, practice good nutrition, exercise regularly and wear seat belts when driving. Yet we may develop a brain tumor or a chronic illness or be struck by a drunk driver. In an attempt to protect disabled loved ones we may provide protective devices in the home. However, we still cannot eliminate all uncertainty regarding when or how they may fall. We cannot eliminate uncertainty even though we can try to decrease the risk of harm or danger to our loved ones and ourselves. Our beliefs that we should be able to eliminate uncertainty can leave us with feelings of guilt when we are unable to control tragic events, especially for those whom we love. For example, a grandparent has a serious fall in the shower resulting in a TBI, even though the adult children had just installed safety bars. Or a mother briefly loses sight of her two-year-old who falls into the swimming pool and has a near-drowning that results in severe anoxia.

Existential Meaninglessness

Once a tragic event occurs, questions and doubts around meaninglessness emerge. **Existential meaninglessness** refers to our anxieties about the meanings we have created for ourselves that may be obliterated by a single event. If a child is born with severe neurological impairments, or a person has a TBI from a motor vehicle accident, or an adult has a severe stroke, previous meanings may be challenged or destroyed and we may be left with a sense of meaninglessness. Such tragedies may lead to the terrifying thought that there is no meaning, no significance in existence. The challenge we all face is to find meaning in our lives despite the adversities in order to endure life on a daily basis. Frankl (1959) emphasized that the primary force in life is one's search for meaning. Each person must create a unique and specific meaning that gives life coherence and significance. While some people look to religious ideas to give their lives meaning, others develop secular meanings which provide them with direction and dignity in an indifferent world. Many health care professionals may find meaning in their efforts to help others.

Many existential issues came to the forefront in the tragedy described on the next page and in the responses of the individuals involved. Tragedies of this kind challenge our usual, day-to-day beliefs and leave us face-to-face with these universal concepts of meaning, uncertainty, isolation, and death. Some individuals are able to modify their beliefs in healthy ways, so that they accept what they cannot control but still feel a sense of effectiveness and meaning in their lives.

Existential Isolation

A third existential concern is isolation or our ultimate aloneness in the world (Fromm, 1956; Yalom, 1980). Yalom says that **existential isolation** refers to an unbridgeable gulf between any other person and ourselves. We can have close family or friends who share important events in our lives with us, but ultimately, no one knows what it is like to be us, to undergo the pain and loss caused by our illness or our process of dying. For many people, it is not death itself that is so frightening, but the sense that it highlights our ultimate aloneness. No matter how close we become to another person, each of us must depart our existence alone. No one can go with us on that journey (Yalom, 1980).

COUNSELING SKILLS IN ACTION:

Air Force Major Janet Deltuva

On September 11, 2001 Air Force Major Janet Deltuva, an SLP assigned to the Pentagon in Washington D.C., was in her office directly across the courtyard from the point of impact of the jetliner that flew into the Pentagon that morning. Major Deltuva had been trained in medical readiness and her role was to assist senior medical officers, who immediately set up a triage area in the center courtyard.

Major Deltuva performed a variety of extraordinary tasks that day that went beyond her normal speech-language pathology training and duties. She comforted injured victims, handed out surgical gloves, distributed glucose saline and other supplies, and did whatever was asked. Major Deltuva sought out victims who were alone and assisted them in any way she could, helping them make cell-phone calls to family and giving reassurance to the injured. Later that day she was asked to find volunteers to separate the living from the dead, and then was sent to count body bags.

In spite of tragedies, including terrorist attacks, Major Deltuva stated, "We have to establish a new 'norm' in our lives. If you choose to live in fear, the enemy has achieved their objective. And unlike many things in our lives, we do have control over how we deal with fear" (Moore, 2001, pg 6).

Elderly people in convalescent hospitals may represent a readily apparent example of feelings of isolation and aloneness. They often have lost most of their family and close friends, and may have few if any visitors. The only interactions they may have with people are the brief nursing care and meals that come throughout the day. Beyond this physical isolation and aloneness, elderly people are likely to feel existential isolation of going through their own demise—alone. However, SLPs and audiologists need to be aware that nonhospitalized people may be experiencing a profound sense of isolation in the midst of their illness and suffering, even when surrounded by loving family and friends.

Another example of isolation is the hearing impaired or deaf child whose parents choose not to learn sign language. The child's only extensive conversations may be with other hearing impaired children who sign or perhaps his or her classroom teacher. However, the hearing-impaired child who is fortunate to have parents and siblings who have learned sign language may still be isolated during some family time, such as visiting family or friends who do not sign, or watching television when there is no closed captioning. The child may be left out of important conversations, the humor of programs, or important news messages.

Both of these children inevitably experience isolation, even though the second family has tried to minimize the child's physical isolation. The sense of isolation felt by these children stems from feeling different from other children and that their families, no matter how loving, can never fully understand what it is like to be hearing impaired. No matter how well meaning an SLP or audiologist is she can never completely close the gap of existential isolation. Even if the clinician has a similar experience, for example, a hearing loss, the clinician can still never know what that experience is like for the person she is working with.

Maurer and Martin (1997) say that no communication environment is a positive one for people with hearing impairments. Environments where older people reside or spend much of their time such as private homes, high-rise apartments, nursing homes, extended-care facilities, and senior centers, often are located in high-traffic areas where average outside noise levels exceed that of normal conversation. Interior noises of buildings negatively affect a person's hearing as well. In turn, older adults often feel isolated because of their hearing loss which is compounded by the unmanageable environmental noise levels. Hearing-impaired adults often find themselves isolated from family and friends because people communicate less with them, and what is communicated may not be heard accurately or completely.

False reassurance that the SLP or audiologist understands or knows what it is like to have a particular impairment is not helpful; the person with the impairment really knows better. Such false reassurance makes the person feel even more isolated. We can never fully understand all of a person's emotional pain and suffering. Also, clumsy attempts at empathy where the clinician says, "I understand." may sound arrogant to the person who knows that the clinician does not truly understand. Therapeutically, it is better for the clinician to say, "I'm trying to better understand how you are feeling and what you have to deal with." In the face of these existential conditions of life, as well as others, emotionally healthy people try to find meanings that make their lives worthwhile. They also try to find a balance between facing the dread brought on by these conditions versus a less healthy denial of these existential facts of life.

It is not necessarily the professional responsibility of the SLP or audiologist to have extended conversations with clients or patients and their families about their struggles with uncertainty, a sense of meaninglessness, or isolation. However, the clinician, particularly in acute-care settings or other crisis environments may be confronted with patients and families who are dealing with such issues. Statements that signal such struggles may be: "Why is my family suffering so many tragedies all of the time?" "How can I ever forgive myself for letting this happen to my child?" "What did I miss that could have made me aware that my husband was having little strokes?"

In response to the client's struggles to find meaning, the SLP or audiologist may want to make empathic responses acknowledging the person's anxiety and distress by saying, "It's understandable that it is difficult to make sense of this experience." This statement helps the person feel understood. If the person continues to ruminate along these lines, the clinician may wish to go a step further by helping the person regain a sense of meaning by asking, "What has helped you in the past make sense of difficult situations?" The clinician should not feel compelled to impose his or her own meanings on events, such as "I'm sure your family will become stronger and closer by dealing with this together." or, "I'm sure God has a plan for you."

Existential Nonbeing (Death)

Yalom (1980) discusses **existential nonbeing** and death anxiety in his classic text, *Existential Psychotherapy*, and Luterman (2001) cites Yalom extensively. Although death arguably is the single most important issue of life, it is a topic that most people avoid. In fact, most people spend considerable energy avoiding the terror of death, losing oneself, and becoming nothing. The experience of the inevitability of our end, of our death, is referred to as the realm of nonbeing. This experience or death anxiety motivates many people to turn to diversions in life, a lust for lasting fame, and reckless activity which seem to defy the possibility of death (e.g., race-car driving and extreme sports).

Although the physicality of death destroys a person, the idea of death and the closeness of death saves him. The awareness of death encourages a mindfulness of being, that is, attempting to live authentically and living life to the fullest. Near-death experiences (resulting from automobile accidents, heart attacks, etc.) often lead to a strong sense of the shortness of life and how precious it is; a greater sense of zest for life, a heightening of perceptions and emotional responsiveness; an ability to live in the moment and to savor each moment as it passes; and a greater awareness of life and living things and the urge to enjoy life now before it is too late (May, 1975; Yalom, 1980).

Anxiety and fear of death may occur on many levels, for example, the act of dying, fear of pain during dying, causing grief for family and friends, loss of caring for other people, regretting unfinished business (personal and professional), mourning the end of personal experiences, and being forgotten. Death anxiety and difficulty discussing death may contribute to the limited discussion of death of clients and patients in the speech-language pathology literature on counseling. Luterman (1984, 1991, 1996, 2001) and Scheuerle (1992) have brief discussions of the topic. Other writers on counseling in speech-language pathology and audiology do not include discussions of death.

The reality is that clients, patients, and their families likely think about death much more than might be imagined. Patients, given the slightest encouragement, will often discuss their concerns about death. They may discuss the death of family members or friends, or themselves. Because clinicians may have had limited experience with death or are uncomfortable with the subject, they may avoid any conversations or reference to death. Denial-based strategies (e.g., suppression, repression, displacement, and belief in personal omnipotence) are ubiquitous and powerful defenses that play a

Facing Death with a Client

I have been willing to openly discuss death with many of my patients in hospitals, particularly those in convalescent hospitals where death becomes a way of life. Also, the topic of death has seemed relevant and/or imminent for some private clients. Other professionals and family members have appeared too busy or unwilling to talk with patients about their thoughts and feelings on this important area of life.

Continues on next page

Continued from previous page

I worked with a private client, a woman in her mid-60s with Parkinson's disease, for several months in her home at her kitchen table. Over the months her physical strength and ability to ambulate and communicate deteriorated. While she was still able to verbally communicate she occasionally, with no other family members present, would begin to talk about her imminent death and that she did not fear it. She said that she welcomed it. My willingness to listen and openly talk about death helped create richness in the therapy relationship. A few months after I had ended my therapy with her she died and I was asked by her family to do the eulogy at her funeral. It was a tremendous honor and responsibility to prepare the lengthy eulogy for this prominent figure in the community.

central role in selective inattention to potential conversations about death. This denial is present in many of the helping professions (Yalom, 1980).

Children often have a pervasive concern of death that exerts far-reaching influence on their experiential worlds. Death is a great enigma to them, and one of their major developmental tasks is to deal with fears of helplessness and obliteration. "All gone" is one of the first phrases in many children's language, and "all gone" is a common theme in childhood fears. Young children often fear being devoured, flushed away, or sucked through the bathtub drain. Perhaps the true facts of life for children involve the realization of death. However, adults confuse children about death with their idioms, for example: "My car died on the way to work." "I was just dead at the office today." "I'm feeling dead. I'm going to take a little nap." Many children are confused about the permanence of death.

Children with chronic (e.g., asthma) or life-threatening (e.g., cancer, leukemia, severe burns) medical conditions are often more knowledgeable and even precocious in their understanding of death than the adults around them believe. SLPs working in school settings may have children on their caseloads who may have severe asthma attacks or seizures during therapy. Children may bring up discussions about death at unexpected times and it is important for the clinician to be willing to engage in these discussions. Children often feel isolated about their concerns of death, and it is important for clinicians to inform the parents about discussions they have had with children about this matter. If a child brings up the topic of death more than occasionally, or if the child appears troubled by thoughts of death, it may be important for the SLP to contact the school psychologist. In medical settings, particularly acute-care hospitals and children's hospitals, ongoing death concerns and fears may be prominent in children's thoughts and conversations. It is important to listen to the children and speak openly with them but mainly rely on each child's knowledge about death. Adding to their knowledge of death may be counter-therapeutic as it may create new fears or exacerbate existing fears.

Death of a Child

I worked with a girl with severe, spastic, quadriplegic cerebral palsy for 18 months. I received the referral when she was about two years old. She had been born without neurodevelopmental impairments but had a heart defect that required open-heart surgery when she was six months old. All went well with the surgery; however, she had severe complications afterwards, died, but was resuscitated after many minutes without oxygen, which resulted in the cerebral palsy.

Neurodevelopmental Therapy (NDT) was appropriate for this child with primitive reflexes and no functional form of communication. I worked with the child twice a week in her home on the living room floor with her mother present. One week the child developed a bladder infection and died suddenly. On a Thursday afternoon at one o'clock when I would normally be doing therapy with her I attended her funeral.

Yalom (1980) expresses a fundamental principle in this beautiful and profound passage:

Count your blessings! How rarely do we benefit from that simple homily? Ordinarily what we *do* have and what we *can* do slip out of awareness, diverted by thoughts of what we lack or what we cannot do, or dwarfed by petty concerns and threats to our prestige or our pride systems. By keeping death in mind, one passes into a state of gratitude, of appreciation for the countless givens of existence. This is what the Stoics meant when they said, "Contemplate death if you would learn to live." The imperative is not, then, a call to a morbid death preoccupation but instead an urging to keep both figure and ground in focus so that being becomes conscious and life richer (p. 163).

CASE STUDY

Michael and an Existential Counseling Approach

Michael and his family are experiencing classic existential conditions: uncertainty, meaninglessness, isolation, and death anxiety. Michael is likely feeling some existential isolation: feeling alone, not understanding what other people are saying to him, not being able to communicate his wants, needs, thoughts and feelings easily or clearly. He is likely experiencing a

Continues on next page

Continued from previous page

sense of meaninglessness about the accident that has left him with so many impairments; he may be asking himself why this has happened to him or what he has done to deserve this. He is probably feeling uncertainty about his future, whether he will be able to do well in school again, be as athletic as he was before the accident, and whether he still will be liked by his friends—or whether they will abandon him because he is not the same old Michael. He may be thinking about how close he came to dying. The SLP needs to be willing to listen to Michael's confused and sometimes disorganized conversations about himself that are occasionally punctuated with existential concerns. It is important to listen empathically, although the SLP may not be able to help him fully process his concerns. The SLP may want to discuss openly with the parents Michael's concerns as well as make a referral to the hospital psychologist for ongoing sessions to give Michael the opportunity to process his concerns.

Each of Michael's family members will likely be going through their own existential crises, including uncertainty as to how Michael's impairments will not only affect him, but the entire family; whether Michael will be accepted by his peers or will he be socially isolated; and how meaninglessness this tragedy is—how could it serve any good purpose. They are thankful that he survived the accident, but are very aware of how close they were to losing their son. The parents will likely have a heightened sense of gratitude for Michael's life and their relationship with him.

The SLP needs to be willing to listen to each of the family member's existential concerns and make appropriate referrals to the hospital psychologist. It is very important for the SLP to not trivialize any of the family's concerns by making what could be construed as condescending, naive statements. See Figure 2-1 for examples of therapeutic and nontherapeutic statements.

It is important for clinicians to acknowledge the family's existential concerns rather than deny them. Overly optimistic response to the family may quell the clinician's anxiety, but may feel invalidating to the family.

MULTICULTURAL THEORY

The development of multicultural theory since the 1960s has coincided with the increase of cultural diversity in the United States, particularly in the increase of African-American, Hispanic, Asian, and Middle Eastern populations (Prochaska & Norcross, 2003). These groups have challenged the traditional male European perspective that has dominated North American thinking in areas as diverse as science, social policy, ethics, and family values. These groups have not always expe-

Nontherapeutic Statements	Therapeutic Statements
"I understand what you must be going through."	"I understand that you are going through a lot of difficult adjustments right now." (This response makes fewer assumptions that the clinician knows exactly what the child's family is feeling.)
"I'm certain that some good will come out of all this."	"It sounds like you are considering how all this is going to affect Michael and the whole family." (In this statement the therapist is encouraging the family to find their own meaning for this experience rather than the clinician imposing his or her own meaning.)
"I'm sure that Michael's friends will welcome him back and he will be just as popular as he ever was."	"You're concerned about Michael's relationships with peers and hoping he won't be isolated, teased, or rejected." (The clinician acknowledges the possibility of isolation rather than denying it.)
"Michael is a survivor. He is going to come out of this better than any of us might expect."	"Michael has made it through the acute phase. The medical and rehabilitation teams will do all we can to help him realize his potential." (The clinician acknowledges the uncertainty rather than denying it.)

Figure 2-1 Nontherapeutic and therapeutic statements

rienced the European/North American perspective as fair or applicable to them, and therefore have called for a re-evaluation of traditional attitudes and beliefs, a striving for equality for all people, and an appreciation of diverse beliefs and lifestyles (Saba, Karrer, & Hardy, 1995).

The role played by culture has increasingly come to be recognized in all aspects of counseling, from assessment to intervention. The cultures of both the clients and their families as well as the cultures of the clinicians influence the counseling process both pervasively and profoundly. Salas-Provance, Erickson, and Reed (2002), for example, confirmed the general concept that culture plays an important role in folk- and medical-belief systems regarding health and illness within a multi-generational Hispanic family. Their study also pointed out that the experiences and beliefs professionals hold may be in stark contrast to those held by clients. Overall, it is recognized that all counseling occurs in a multicultural context and the cultures are crucial components of the counseling experience. Multicultural theory and principles are applicable to all counseling approaches used by clinicians, whether behavioral, humanistic, interpersonal, family, existential, or others (Gladding, 2000; Kuo & Hu, 2002; Pedersen, Draguns, Lonner, & Trimble, 1996).

Much of the recent speech-language pathology literature on multicultural populations focuses on children and the demands for services in the public schools (e.g., Battle, 2002; Langdon, 2002; Roseberry-McKibbin, 2002); however, we need to keep in mind that many adult clients, patients and their families have diverse cultural backgrounds as well.

The 2000 U.S. Bureau of the Census (cited in Battle, 2002; Kuo and Hu, 2002; and Roseberry-McKibbin, 2002), reported that racial and ethnic minorities accounted for up to 80% of the growth in population in the 1990s for the United States. Analysis of the resident population of the United States by race showed that 75.1% were white; 12.3% were black or African-American; 3.6% were Asian or Pacific Islanders; 0.1% were American Indian, Eskimo, or Aleut; 0.2% were native Hawaiian; 2.4% were two or more races; and 5.5% were identified as other. The ethnic composition of the country showed that 87.5% were non-Hispanic, and 12.5% of the residents of the country were identified as Hispanic.

The terms race and ethnicity are often used interchangeably, although they have different meanings. Race is defined as a classification that distinguishes groups of people from one another based on physical characteristics such as skin color, facial features, and hair texture. Two people can be the same race but differ widely in cultural identity. Ethnicity (ethnography) is a term that is sometimes confused with race, but is the social definition of groups of people based on various cultural similarities, and includes race as well as factors such as customs, nationality, language, and heritage. Understanding of ethnicity implies a developed sense of the complexity of perceptions, symbols, meanings, and behaviors of a culture (Battle, 2002; Roseberry-McKibbin, 2002).

Culture may be defined in several ways, including ethnographic variables such as ethnicity, nationality, religion, and language; demographic variables of age, gender, place of residence, and so forth; status variables such as social, economic, and educational background, and a wide range of formal or informal memberships and affiliations (clubs, organizations, etc.). A broad definition of **culture** is any group of people who identify or associate with one another on the basis of some common purpose, need, or similarity of background (Gladding, 2000). Culture means there are shared beliefs, traditions, and values of a group of people. Culture is a term that implies explicit behaviors such as clothing and ways of dressing, food preferences, customs, lifestyle, and language. Implicit cultural variables include such areas as age and gender roles within families, child rearing practices, religious and spiritual beliefs, educational values, and attitudes. Speech, language, and communication are embedded in culture. The social rules of discourse and narratives are culturally determined (e.g., who speaks to whom, when, where, the physical distance between communicators, eye contact, who initiates the conversation, who selects the topic, who ends the conversation). Communication and language are reciprocal: culture and communication influence each other (consider the "deaf culture"). Culture is the lens through which people perceive and interpret their worlds (Canino & Spurlock, 2000).

Multicultural societies contain a diversity of cultures with varieties of religions, languages, customs, traditions and values, and where there are numerous racial and ethnic backgrounds living and working together (Battle, 2002; Roseberry-McKibbin, 2002). Multicultural counseling involves two or more people with different ways of being socialized and perceiving their social environment being brought together in a helping relationship (Nystul, 1999).

Acculturation refers to the learning, incorporating, and adopting of some of the values, customs and beliefs of the dominant culture in order to fit in and get along with the society in which a person is living. It does not mean people must give up their cultural or religious heritage. People who retain their original cultural identity but simultaneously become acculturated to the American way of life have achieved **bicultural adjustment**.

Distress often occurs in the family context when certain family members (usually the younger ones) are more acculturated to the dominant culture than its elder members. This may lead to conflicts in decision-making when, for example, a parent's wishes reflect their culture's traditional beliefs but their child's preferences reflect their more acculturated status. Here, the clinician should listen to, respect, and strive to understand the different worldviews that are expressed so that a culturally sensitive decision can be made.

Multicultural theory emphasizes the importance of taking into account culturally diverse world views. **World view** pertains to an individual's assumptions and perceptions about the world (i.e., existence, history, society) from a moral, social, ethical, and philosophical perspective. It is the source of a person's values, beliefs, and assumptions. These are derived from cultural, social, religious, ethnic, and/or racial perspectives (Pedersen et al., 2002). Multicultural theory rests on the assumption of cultural relativism, that there are few universal standards for evaluating right or wrong, healthy or unhealthy human behavior. What people believe and how they behave is significantly influenced by the culture in which they are raised.

A Japanese-American Boy Who Stuttered

I received a rather desperate telephone call from an American man who was born and raised in Stockton, California, but was now living in Japan teaching English in the schools. He had been in Japan for ten years, married a Japanese woman, and they had a five-year-old son who had begun to stutter. The father contacted the Stuttering Foundation of America to receive the name of an SLP in the Stockton area who had experience working with individuals who stutter. My name was provided to him. The family planned to return to Stockton for the summer and was hoping their son could receive therapy while here. I explained to the father that much of the therapy would include working with the parents and not just the child. Appointments were scheduled, and in their second week in Stockton I began working with the child and parents on a regular basis.

In this case I was working with three cultures in the same family: the father, Caucasian American; the mother, Japanese; and child, Japanese-American. I had a fair understanding of

Continues on next page

Continued from previous page

Japanese culture from spending some time in Japan many years ago, and having five Japanese foreign exchange students live with my family over part of various summers. I understood how a child with a handicap or disability might be perceived by some Japanese parents as a reflection on their parenting or a reflection on their family. Extra sensitivity was needed when talking with both parents, but particularly the mother, about their child's speech problems and things they could do when interacting with the child that could help improve his self-esteem and speech fluency.

Lack of knowledge or inability to communicate fluently in the host society's language may contribute to members of other ethnic groups experiencing a disadvantaged status. In a medical setting, a language barrier may inhibit a patient's attempts to communicate and therefore his silence mistakenly may convey consent, or the patient's medical questions may go unanswered. If at all possible, it is helpful to have a translator present in these cases to facilitate medical communication and understanding.

Multicultural Work Environments

In many of the hospitals I have worked there have been numerous cultures involved with a single patient. I recall a female Vietnamese patient who had a male Indian physician, several female and male Filipino nurses, female and male African-American and Hispanic CNAs, and me, a Caucasian male SLP from California. This example illustrates that clients and patients may receive medical care and treatment from a variety of cultures with varying languages, dialects, accents, and world views. It also points out that as SLPs and audiologists we not only work with clients and patients from different cultures, but that we also work with other professionals from diverse cultures.

A primary issue of concern for multicultural counseling is the dominance of theories and perspectives based on European/North American cultural values. Some of the predominant beliefs of European/North Americans are the value of individuals, an action-oriented approach to solving problems, the work ethic, the scientific method, and an emphasis on strict time schedules (Gladding, 2000).

Flying to Mexcico

I have been involved with the Flying Doctors, a philanthropic organization that provides medical treatment to people in small cities and towns in Mexico. The volunteers pay all their own expenses and fly into Mexico in private planes. Professionals who make these trips usually include plastic surgeons, ophthalmologists, orthopedic surgeons, anesthesiologists, and nurses. I was invited to be on the team as their first SLP. During the flight from San Francisco into a small city a few hours south of the Mexican border, when I was not flying the six-passenger, twin engine Piper Cub, I worked with a young woman who spoke fluent Spanish. She had lived in Mexico, but did not know the necessary medical terminology for the work we would be doing with children and adults with cleft palates and cerebral palsy. While I was getting to know the translator I developed confidence in her ability to accurately translate the information to the families, and to do it with the understanding and sensitivity of a person who knew and understood the Mexican culture.

Stereotyping and overgeneralization are inherent dangers when considering culture, race, and ethnicity. Stereotyping may be defined as rigid preconceptions individuals hold about other people who are members of a particular group. Stereotyping fails to take into consideration logic or experience, and distorts all new information to fit preconceived ideas (Nystul, 1999). To avoid stereotyping and overgeneralizing it is important for clinicians to treat clients as unique individuals first and as people from a particular culture second. Part of being a culturally competent professional is the ability to recognize that there is tremendous diversity that exists within each culture and that each person in any cultural group must be viewed first and foremost as an individual (Battle, 2002; Kuo & Hu, 2002; Pedersen et al., 2002; Roseberry-McKibbin, 2002).

As clinicians we need to be aware of our own cultural, racial, and ethnic backgrounds, and how they influence us. Even individuals who deny any form of racial or ethnic prejudice often implicitly value certain types of people and devalue others. We are also a part of a variety of subcultures that may influence our beliefs, values, and assumptions. Some subcultures may include the part of the country and the state we live in; whether we were raised in or work in an urban or rural area; our family's educational and economic backgrounds; the type of university or employment setting we are in; and many others. We need to be very aware of the influences of our larger cultural and ethnic backgrounds and the subcultures we have been, and are, a part of, and how they affect our interaction with clients, patients, and their families, as well as other professionals.

Roseberry-McKibbin (in Shipley, 1997, pp. 158–164) discusses numerous assumptions and values of Americans with mainstream backgrounds that may differ significantly from other cultures. For example:

1. "Punctuality is important and is an intrinsic part of a professional relationship based on mutual respect."

2. "In professional situations such as meetings, it is important to 'get down to business' as quickly and efficiently as possible."

3. "Informality and social equality are the ultimate goals in all interactions between professionals and clients."

4. "Frankness, openness, and honest discussion of situations and feelings is important."

5. "The gender of the clinician and the client is not important; the clinician's competence is the most important variable."

6. "The age of a clinician, relative to the client, is unimportant as long as the clinician is competent."

7. "Written documentation is a necessary and intrinsic part of professionals' interactions with clients and families."

8. "Speech and language therapy are usually necessary even if the client does not have an overt physical handicap."

9. "Rehabilitation is usually necessary because the goal for all individuals, including those with speech and language impairments, is to be as independent as possible."

10. "When clients display speech-language disabilities, Western forms of intervention are the most effective and appropriate."

11. "When a particular client is receiving rehabilitative services or therapy, the family must be as active as possible in collaboration with the clinician."

12. "Individuals have control over their own destinies."

13. "Families who speak other languages at home need to speak English to their children so that the children will learn English."

14. "Counseling individuals in isolation can be quite effective."

These assumptions are often such a basic part of the way we think about the world and interacting with people that it may not occur to us that other people may make different assumptions. We also tend to elevate these values and consider them ideals, and may judge negatively people who have different or opposing values. For example, a person who does not value punctuality and is late for appointments may be judged negatively.

There is no one multicultural theoretical perspective or approach that is appropriate for working with all cultures. Realistically, it is impossible for any SLP or audiologist to be well-educated and understand the numerous cultures and subcultures within his or her community, much less the countless variations and nuances within any recognized cultural group. However, Battle (2002) presents several helpful "dos" and "don'ts" when considering a person's cultural background:

1. Consider your own personal cultural beliefs, attitudes, and values and how they may be contributing to the clinical encounter.

2. Learn the name of the person's cultural or geographic group that is commonly used by that group. For example, use Japanese for someone from Japan, not Asian. Use Guatemalan for someone from Guatemala, not Hispanic or Latino. (It may be helpful to inquire about the client's preferences, for example, how the client would like to be addressed.)

3. Avoid using questionable or negative connotations such as culturally deprived, culturally disadvantaged, or minority.

4. Do not overgeneralize or stereotype individuals or groups of individuals.

5. Be aware of the nonverbal sources of miscommunication between people from different cultural groups, such as styles of greeting behavior, the role of touch during conversation, and appropriate topics of conversation.

Culturally sensitive clinicians clearly have multiple responsibilities. One is to learn about cultural diversity (Kuo & Hu, 2002). Clinicians cannot possibly learn all the values and customs of all societies of the world. They can, however, learn about common beliefs and values held by people belonging to the major ethnic groups in their communities. This provides a foundation for learning about other cultural groups and respecting diverse systems of thought.

Roseberry-McKibbin (in Shipley, 1997) makes several suggestions for effectively communicating when interviewing and counseling clients who are experiencing difficulties communicating in English.

1. Loudness. Do not increase the volume of your loudness. Unnecessary loudness may make clients feel they are being treated like children.

2. Rate of speech. Decrease your rate of speech and pause often. The slower rate makes it easier for individuals to understand, and the pauses between sentences allow them time to process the information.

3. Articulation in connected speech. Articulate each word clearly, but do not exaggerate mouth movements. Avoid using contractions such as "don't," "wouldn't," and so forth.

4. Sentence length and complexity. Avoid multisyllabic words. (Using the "Rule of 5s," i.e., 5-letter words, 5-word sentences, may be helpful.) Avoid slang and idioms, technical jargon, and abstract terms.

5. Repeat key information. Clients typically need to hear key words and concepts several times, especially clients for whom English is not their primary language.

6. Nonverbal cues and body language. Proxemics (the use of physical distance) and kinesics (the use of gestures and facial expressions, including eye contact) differ among cultures.

7. Size of interaction groups. During interviews clients may be more comfortable and bolstered by having other family members or close friends present.

8. Allow extra time for meetings and be patient. Avoid appearing hurried.

9. Use translators when needed. Be cautious to choose translators who have good communication skills and act in a professional manner, including maintaining confidentiality.

Fortunately, many departments of communicative disorders in universities and colleges around the country are providing education and training in the area of multicultural populations to assist SLPs and audiologists to begin to develop multicultural competencies. There is a need for clinicians in all work settings to have extensive and ongoing education in this important area to better help our clients, patients, and their families. Awareness and understanding of multicultural issues also can help us with our interaction and sensitivity with colleagues and coworkers.

CASE STUDY

Michael and a Multicultural Counseling Approach

In order not to stereotype Michael and his family's racial, ethnic and cultural backgrounds, and to avoid stereotyping the SLP's racial, ethnic and cultural backgrounds, the authors have chosen not to continue this case study in relationship to multicultural theory. The reader is encouraged to consider his or her race, ethnic and cultural backgrounds and to imagine how they may influence interaction with Michael and his family by varying their backgrounds, for example as an African-American family, an Hispanic family, an Asian family, and so forth.

INTEGRATION OF THEORIES

A number of prominent theorists have attempted to integrate or combine elements from various theories (Safran & Segal, 1990; Wachtel, 1977), or have traced this movement (Goldfried, 1982). There is also a journal entitled *Journal of Psychotherapy Integration*.

During interactions with a client or family, an SLP or audiologist may apply various theoretical concepts discussed in this chapter (Humanistic, Interpersonal, Behavioral, Cognitive, Family Systems, Existential, and Multicultural). The clinician may integrate theoretical principles and use what is believed to be the most therapeutic intervention at the moment. Integrative counseling is the process of selecting concepts and methods from a variety of therapeutic approaches (Corey, 2001). Surveys of clinical and counseling psychologists report that 30% to 50% of the respondents consider themselves to be integrative or eclectic in their therapeutic practice (Norcross & Newman, 1992; Norcross & Prochaska, 1988; Prochaska & Norcross, 2003). As SLPs and audiologists working with a wide variety of hearing, speech, language, cognitive, and swallowing disorders of individuals of all ages, we need to be able to draw upon concepts, strategies, and techniques from a variety of counseling frameworks to communicate effectively with our clients, patients, and their families. The integrative approach is characterized by openness to various ways of integrating diverse theories and techniques. An integrative approach to counseling attempts to look beyond and across the confines of single-theory approaches to see what can be learned from—and how clients can benefit from—other perspectives (Corey, 2001).

There are three primary methods for achieving integration: **technical eclecticism, theoretical integration,** and common factors (Arkowitz, 1997; Corey, 2001). Technical eclecticism is a collection of techniques chosen from a variety of different approaches. The clinician chooses at any moment during an interaction with a person the technique that will be most helpful without necessarily subscribing to the theoretical position from which the technique is drawn. Theoretical integration refers to development of a conceptual or theoretical framework that synthesizes the best of two or more theoretical approaches with the assumption that the synthesis will be richer than the individual theories alone. The common factors approach attempts to distill from different theoretical systems, nonspecific elements (Frank, 1973, 1979, 1982) that are common among the theories. Nonspecific elements include such factors as positive expectations, a warm, trusting relationship, and faith in the clinician. This perspective on integration is based on the premise that these common factors are at least as important in accounting for therapy outcomes as the unique factors that differentiate one theory from another (Corey, 2001). Patterson (1986) cites seven commonalities among counseling approaches:

1. The counseling approaches agree that humans can change or be changed.

2. The approaches agree that some behaviors are undesirable, inadequate, or harmful, or result in dissatisfaction, unhappiness, or limitations that warrant change.

3. Counselors expect people to change as a result of their particular techniques and interventions.

4. Individuals who seek counseling experience a need for help.

5. Clients generally believe change can and will occur.

6. Counselors expect clients to be active participants.

7. Intervention characteristically includes encouragement, support, and instruction.

Overall, because no one theory, strategy or technique is always effective when working with a wide range of ages, delays and disorders, and personality types, it is wise to not limit ourselves to a single theory (Corey, 2001; Kelly, 1991; Lazarus, 1996). Corey states,

> Practitioners who are open to an integrative perspective will find that several theories play a crucial role in their personal counseling approach. Each theory has its unique contributions and its own domain of expertise. By accepting that each theory has strengths and weakness-

es and is, by definition, "different" from the others, practitioners have some basis to begin developing a theory that fits for them. Developing an integrative perspective is a lifelong endeavor that is refined with experience (p. 459).

CONCLUDING COMMENTS

Several theories and therapy approaches of counseling have been presented to help clinicians develop a framework from which they can work with clients, patients and their families. Clinicians need to remember that no one counseling theory or therapy approach fits all situations and that clinicians will likely draw upon several therapy approaches with a particular client or family member.

The foundation of counseling is the clinician-client relationship; therefore emphasis is first placed on "connecting" with the client and family (including appreciating cultural differences), and second on cognitive and behavioral changes. Existential concepts may seem unusual for SLPs and audiologists to consider when working with clients and their families, but many of the life problems we are trying to address often involve uncertainty, meaninglessness, isolation, and sometimes even death. Most of the other theories and therapy approaches discussed involve analysis of culturally influenced behavior, family functioning, and values development, while these existential concepts tend to address more universal life experiences. Finally, it is important to remember the theories and therapy approaches presented here are just a few of the hundreds in the counseling and psychotherapy literature, and that there are other theories and approaches that contain relevant concepts as well.

 Discussion Questions

1. Discuss why no one theory or therapy approach fits all situations.

2. Discuss a few of the therapy approaches that you would likely use with any counseling interaction.

3. What does unconditional positive regard mean to you? How do you show it to people?

4. How do you think some of the roles you learned in childhood may influence how you interact with clients of different ages, for example children, adolescents, young adults, older adults, the elderly?

5. How have your interactions with people been shaped in your training to be an SLP or audiologist?

6. What types of erroneous thinking or cognitive distortions do you occasionally use?

7. Discuss a client with whom you had to work closely with other family members. What were the subsystems that were involved? Was there any triangulation involved?

8. How do you respond to existential uncertainties in your life?

9. Discuss the death of someone with whom you were close. How did that affect the way you see life and relationships?

10. Discuss the primary cultures and subcultures you are a part of. How do those cultures affect the way you interact with people from other cultures? Discuss whether you think that being an SLP or audiologist places you in another subculture.

The Therapeutic Relationship and Therapeutic Communication

CHAPTER OUTLINE

INTRODUCTION

Technical expertise is necessary but not sufficient to be a competent speech-language pathologist (SLP) or audiologist. It is not only the clinician's knowledge of our profession and therapeutic techniques that define what we do, but the ability to enter into the person's world and to develop a therapeutic relationship. The child or adults' subjective experiences of communication problems are inevitably affected by the quality of the relationship with the clinician (Brammer & MacDonald, 1999; Luterman, 2001; Rollin, 2000; Shames, 2000; Shipley, 1997). The quality of the relationship, once it begins, has its own dynamic quality that inevitably is affected by what the clinician and client bring to it. The client and the clinician continue to influence each other as their relationship evolves.

How clients behave toward us is inevitably linked to how we think, feel, and behave toward them. This chapter describes some of the essential relationship factors and communication strategies that can be used to enhance the cooperative, working alliance between client and clinician.

VARIABLES CONTRIBUTING TO THE THERAPEUTIC RELATIONSHIP

The variables contributing to the therapeutic relationship are illustrated in Figure 3.1. The client-clinician relationship is dynamic, meaning that it is constantly changing. The relationship emphasizes the *affective* mode because, like any relationship, there is an emotional quality of the interaction. Ideally, a positive working relationship begins upon the initial contact of a client and clinician. However, for new and inexperienced clinicians, there is often a feeling of anxiety when meeting a new client, or working with a disorder for the first time, or working with an adult for the first time. This is normal. Clinician anxiety, however, can interfere with how we are perceived by clients and their willingness to trust and work with us.

Inexperienced and experienced clinicians enter into evaluations and therapy with clients with self-perceptions of their education and knowledge, training and competence. Clinicians have needs to feel good about their clinical work and that their clients respect them. Clinicians have values about what is important to them (and may impose those values onto the client). Clinicians have feelings of uncertainty, anxiety, and even fear about how the evaluation and therapy sessions will go, including considerable anxiety about what their supervisors will see and like. Clinicians have experiences with other children and adults that they draw upon to help them feel comfortable with clients. Clinicians have expectations of themselves, sometimes hoping to do a "perfect" evaluation or therapy session, and soon find that perfection is elusive even to the most well-educated and experienced clinicians. Clinicians often have expertise in areas other than speech-language pathology or audiology that help give them confidence that with enough education, training, experience, and time, they also can develop expertise in their profession.

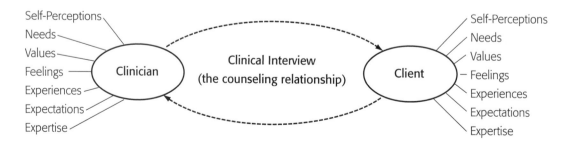

Figure 3-1 The counseling relationship in the clinical interview (adapted from Brammer & McDonald, 1999).

It is important to keep in mind that the client, child or adult, also is likely to have some level of anxiety upon meeting a clinician. It may be the client's first experience with an SLP or audiologist, and there may be considerable uncertainty about how much benefit he or she will receive. Clients who come to us for help may have self-perceptions that are not positive. Children sometimes have had years of frustration because they cannot be understood easily, or have difficulty communicating with peers, teachers, and even their family. Adults who have functioned well all their lives but now have a significant loss of hearing, speaking, understanding, communicating, or swallowing may have negative self-perceptions because they compare themselves to how they used to be and may not appreciate their potential for rehabilitation, and for some clients whose potential for rehabilitation is poor even with the best of care, their negative self-perceptions of their communication or swallowing problems may be accurate.

Many clients, however, have overly optimistic and unrealistic expectations for improvement, the rate of improvement, and the clinician's ability to facilitate those improvements. While clients' positive expectations can initially contribute to a positive client-clinician relationship, the client may experience disillusionment with the clinician and the therapy if the clinician does not during the interview, evaluation, or therapy discuss the amount, rate, and durability of improvement that is likely.

Clients have needs to feel they are getting the best of care and that they have potential for improvement. Clients have values about what is important to them in therapy and, ideally, will be in agreement with what the clinician also feels is important. This agreement is an important element of the therapeutic alliance. Clients have feelings of uncertainty, anxiety, and even fear about how they will do in the evaluation and work with the clinician. They frequently have considerable anxiety about the qualifications and skills of the clinician. Will the clinician be able to help? Clients, like most people, hope that the other person will like them. Clients have experiences with other adults and professionals that they draw upon to help them feel comfortable with the clinician. Clients have expectations of themselves, sometimes expecting that they will be "cured" quickly of their hearing, speech, language, cognitive, or swallowing problems. Adult clients often have expertise in a variety of areas in their personal and professional lives, often having raised a family, been a valued employee for many years, and a contributor to society. Clients can often draw upon successes in other areas of their lives to experience self-confidence and motivation to address the challenges in therapy.

Both clinicians and clients enter the therapeutic relationship with these variables, but approach the therapy from different perspectives. They are, both literally and figuratively, on opposite sides of the table. It is important for clinicians to get their own concerns and anxieties out of the way so that they can better attend to their clients. When clinicians understand their clients' self-perceptions, needs, values, feelings, experiences, expectations, and areas of expertise, they can begin to tailor their behaviors, communication, and treatment strategies so that the potential for success is optimal.

In addition to the variables discussed above, clinicians have general styles and ways of approaching clients that can affect their relationship. How clinicians talk about and think about their clients in general can set the stage for how a particular clinician-client relationship develops. Some ways of talking about clients "objectify" them (i.e., as though they are objects rather that people). ASHA has a "person first" policy, for example, referring to the person with a hearing impairment rather than the hearing-impaired person, or the person who stutters rather than the stutterer, or the patient who had a TBI rather than the TBI patient. In medical settings patients are particularly vulnerable to feeling decreased worthiness. While we know that most SLPs and audiologists are empathic, they may inadvertently objectify patients by using objectifying language. Sometimes patients hear this language when clinicians and medical personnel are discussing them, and may perceive it as dehumanizing. Patients' emotional suffering is increased when therapists treat them as objectified anatomic parts and, conversely, suffering can be alleviated when clinicians acknowledge and respect their personhood (Frank, 1991).

One remedy to the overemphasis on medical technology and the increasing neglect of the human side of illness and treatment is a renewed appreciation and attention to the therapeutic relationship. This focus is consistent with the writings of medical ethicists (Schultz & Carnevale, 1996; Zaner, 1993), psychologists (Burnard, 1999), nurses (Bishop & Scudder, 1990; Keltner, Schwecke, & Bostrom, 1999), and physicians (Cassell, 1996) who have urged health care professionals to put the "care" back into medical care. Caring for patients may not cure illness but it can contribute to the lessening of patient suffering and provide the foundation for a trusting and cooperative patient-clinician relationship. For these reasons, clinicians should be guided by an ethic of health care.

For SLPs and audiologists, the question is not whether they have time to develop a relationship with a client. The client-clinician relationship is an inevitability and, therefore, the question is how therapeutic that relationship will become. Clinician-client relationships can either enhance or diminish treatment gains.

Personal qualities of effective helpers have been discussed. There are also guidelines to follow to develop better therapeutic relationships with our clients and patients. It is helpful to analyze some of the skills that can contribute to a positive working relationship. Increased awareness of these skills can help clinicians be more mindful and intentional in their interactions with people, especially with those individuals who are challenging. Although the elements of a therapeutic relationship are intertwined in our daily work, they are discussed in sequence here to understand them better.

TRANSFERENCE AND COUNTERTRANSFERENCE

We have all developed a pattern of feelings, expectations, perceptions, and attitudes that shape our new experiences with others. Some people refer to this phenomenon loosely as the emotional "baggage" they are carrying. These person templates or schemas typically operate automatically and can have a powerful impact on the process and outcome of a new relationship. The client's feelings, expectations, perceptions and attitudes are referred to as transferrence, while the clinician's feelings, expectations, perceptions and attitudes are referred to as countertransferrence. Both are inevitable experiences (Butler, Strupp, and Flasher, 1993; Kahn, 1999), and it is wise for clinicians to understand these forces that can exert a powerful influence over the therapeutic climate. Depending upon the type of transferrence or countertransferrence responses, these can either facilitate or interfere with the therapeutic process.

Transference

In addition to the conscious needs, values, and expectations that each person brings to the therapeutic relationship, the client also brings a set of unconscious wishes, perceptions, and fears. These unconscious forces that shape the client's perceptions of the therapist are referred to as **transference** (Freud, 1912; Gill, 1982). While this concept was originally used by psychoanalytic theorists, it has in more recent years been understood in broader terms by psychologists from many theoretical camps (Kahn, 1999; Safran & Segal, 1990). While this concept has many ramifications for the therapy process that are beyond the scope of this text, a basic understanding of transference phenomena can provide SLPs and audiologists with important tools for understanding and nondefensively addressing certain aspects of the therapeutic relationship.

The basic idea is that people view others through the lenses of their past experiences. The transference, then, simply refers to the lenses through which we perceive new situations and people. We all are influenced by our past relationships and, for example, have grown to trust easily or remain skeptical of others based upon our past experiences. Every time we meet a new person, we encounter a multitude of incomplete or ambiguous stimuli that we must organize in some way. Our transferences can be thought of as organizing principles (Stolorow, Brandcraft, & Atwood, 1987; Kahn, 1999) which help us to filter, organize, and attend to certain characteristics or behaviors in other people. Becoming sensitive to transference phenomena can help clinicians make sense of situations and avoid defensive counter moves when clients behave in puzzling or irritating ways.

In some therapeutic situations, the transference may be "invisible" or unnoticed by the clinician, and not require any special skills or interventions. These are often situations where a relatively well-adjusted client approaches the therapist with a trusting and positive therapeutic relationship. In a specific case, a child may have a positive impression of the SLP or audiologist who reminds her or him of a gentle and loving mother or aunt, or an elderly patient may respond to the younger clinician "as if" he were a loyal son. In these cases, the client takes in a certain amount of information about the new clinician, and then fills in the blanks with the old experiences. The fact that transference is occurring does not mean that the client is blind to the actual characteristics of the clinician. To some degree, there is a hook or peg on which the transference is hung (Wachtel, 1993, p. 58).

With some clients, however, the transference interferes with the development of the therapeutic relationship and accomplishing therapeutic tasks and goals. These cases are often ones in which a negative transference develops. Here, the client's perceptions of the clinician are colored or clouded by past negative experiences. For example, a child may respond in a guarded and tense fashion to a new speech teacher as if the SLP were her critical mother or teacher, or an adolescent may respond argumentatively to the clinician as if she was an authoritarian parent. Bearing in mind Wachtel's (1993) point about needing a peg on which to hang the transference, the clinician should always reflect on his or her behavior to examine what he or she may have done that was interpreted as authoritarian or critical.

Clinicians may learn to use special caution with some clients so that their behavior is not misinterpreted. What is important to remember is that we all establish transference relationships in our everyday lives. Therefore, clients should not be criticized or told that they are wrong for how they perceive us. It is not appropriate, for example, to declare "I am not your critical (or authoritarian, punitive, etc.) parent!" If you sense that your client perceives you in a negative way, you might ask (in a nondefensive tone) what you have done or what makes it seem that way to them. For example, "I'm wondering what I may have done or said that sounded critical to you." In this way, you gather information about your client's perceptual style, sensitivities, and your impact on the client. In some cases, talking about their perceptions resolves the tension. In other cases, you may need to calibrate your future behavior, for example, making certain to discuss recommendations in a collaborative tone so that you are not perceived as authoritarian.

COUNSELING SKILLS IN ACTION:

Client Romantic Transference

A female client asked her male SLP in private practive to schedule an appointment at her home. The SLP did not know her husband would be at work. Once they were seated at her dining room table, the client began to compliment the SLP's gentle manner and sensitivity to her feelings and to lament her husband's shortcomings in these areas. The client had apparently begun to develop a romantic transference onto the SLP. It was likely the SLP's kind and sensitive manner that stimulated her fantasy. In cases like these, it is extremely important to maintain professional boundaries and to recognize and avoid responding to the client's projections, for example, that the clinician will be the knight in shining armor who rescues the client from a less than satisfactory relationship.

Countertransference

The counterpart to the transference concept is **countertransference**. Since its introduction (Freud, 1910), this concept has undergone many changes in meaning and has become increasingly important to an understanding of the therapeutic relationship (Butler, Flasher, & Strupp, 1993). The countertransference concept originally referred to the clinician's personal psychological "baggage" which interfered with the therapy. For example, a clinician who avoids giving a clear and detailed explanation of a child's communication disorder to the parent, may have his own issues with loss and giving bad news. She may have experienced personal losses that make it difficult to face losses in her professional work. In such cases, countertransference is viewed as an impediment to therapy because it prevents the clinician from adequately performing aspects of clinical work. Historically, the clinician's personal psychotherapy was viewed as the appropriate forum in which to work through and eliminate these interfering emotions and behaviors.

More recently, the countertransference concept has been expanded to include all the clinician's emotional responses to the client (Anchin & Kiesler, 1982; Kernberg, 1965). Many of these responses do not reflect the clinician's psychological problems and short-comings, but are understandable responses to certain kinds of client behavior. For example, friendly and agreeable clients typically elicit a friendly response from the clinician. An SLP or audiologist may do extra favors for a well-behaved child who reminds her of a younger sibling, or a clinician may consider providing extra help to a client, thinking of her as if she were a kind, elderly grandparent. These examples demonstrate that some countertransference responses involve positive emotional reactions to clients.

Other countertransference responses involve negative emotional reactions to clients. A clinician who dislikes a particular sullen and suspicious client may "forget" to reschedule the client's missed appointment. A client who speaks in a harsh, critical manner to the audiologist may elicit a more terse and less friendly greeting than the audiologist offers other clients. In these cases, the clinician's countertransference responses represent deviations from the clinician's usual, friendly and professional style.

An important concept articulated by the interpersonal theorists (e.g., Anchin & Kiesler, 1982) is that countertransference responses should not simply be concealed or eliminated. They can be used as a tool to understand clients better. The clinician's countertransference response may provide important clues about what the client is feeling or thinking about the clinician. For example, a clinician who is bored with a particular client may realize that the client appears apathetic and unmotivated to put forth effort in therapy. The clinician who gets angry with a particular client may reflect (privately) on what that client has done and what she or he may be trying to communicate. Is the client resisting the clinician's recommendations because she or he feels efforts will be futile? Is the client feeling rejected by the clinician who appears hurried or preoccupied? What can we learn about the client based upon our countertransference responses? Clients are often responding to how we have treated them or what they perceive we have communicated to them.

The goal here is to become comfortable and nondefensive about our own emotional responses so that we can reflect on what factors have triggered them. As human beings, our reactions to clients are seldom neutral even though we are trained to maintain a professional stance. This does not mean that we should feel free to express all our emotions to clients, but rather that we should admit them to ourselves. Once we do this, we may develop insight into the factors that are impeding a particular therapy or therapeutic relationship. For example, if a clinician finds herself feeling angry with a client, she may reflect on this emotional response and realize that it is a reaction to the client's chronic lateness for therapy appointments. The outcome may be that the clinician discusses this (lateness) issue with the client or asks the client how he is feeling about the therapy. In countless situations, the clinician's countertransference can be used as a tool to analyze what is happening in the therapeutic relationship.

ATTENDING AND LISTENING

A foundational and prerequisite element of a therapeutic relationship is attending to the client through both auditory and visual channels. The purpose of clinical observation is to take in as much information as possible about the client. Riley (2002) provides several suggestions about what the clinician should observe when the client enters the room. For example, does the client smile or is she serious? Does she start talking or wait for the clinician to ask a question? Is the client open in her comments or cautious? Does her body language appear tense or relaxed? Is there appropriate eye contact or avoidance? Are the arms crossed or in a relaxed position? Is the voice tense or natural? If the voice becomes tense, what is being discussed? When asked what the client observed about herself since the last session, how does she respond? Does the client appear interested in observing herself in an objective manner? First impressions during an interview or the beginning of a therapy session provide clues as to how the initial portion of the meeting may be focused. Riley says that through observations the clinician looks for signs of fear, anger, sadness, interest, excitement, reticence, eagerness, and so on. When a clinician reflects back to the client something that he or she perceives but that the client is not aware of, there is the experience of being heard. For example, if the clinician observes tension in the client's voice and body when the discussion is about work being difficult, the client is often pleased and surprised, wondering how the clinician knew. Schow and Nerbonne (2002) say that rehabilitative audiologists need to begin their work by listening to their clients' attitudes toward hearing loss and their goals in seeking help. By listening to the hearing-impaired person, the audiologist begins to build a bridge between the client's life experiences with a hearing loss and the audiologist's understanding of the results of the formal audiologic assessment.

Barkley (1998) says that attending (attention) includes arousal (being alert), selective attention (choosing what to attend to), sustained attention (staying focused), and how much information can be attended to or processed at one time. Clinicians must first attend to their clients before they can listen to them. Most clinicians have had the experience of clients speaking to them while the clinician is attending to something else. There are a variety of obstacles to attending and listening to clients, a few of which are:

- the clinician's stress and anxiety
- negative value judgments of the client
- the clinician is so eager to respond that he or she listens only partially to what the client is saying
- rehearsals of what the clinician is planning to say
- problems the client is presenting are very similar to problems the clinician is personally trying to manage, resulting in splitting the clinician's attention between the client's problems and his or her own problems
- the client's experiences are very different from the clinician's and the clinician is having difficulty relating to the client

▪ the clinician not feeling well or being preoccupied by his or her own physiological needs, such as hunger

Listening to a person may sound deceptively simple, but it may be partially or completely omitted when clinicians feel pressured by a busy schedule and demanding environment. Under these circumstances, clinicians may be too fatigued or distracted, or simply forget to genuinely listen to their clients, patients and their families. Instead, they may operate on automatic pilot, explaining to clients about their communication problems and the intended therapy procedures rather than listening to the clients for information about how they are currently feeling and thinking about their impairments. To listen to a client or patient, the clinician should take note of the person's responses to stimulation (e.g., the therapeutic exercises). Is the person physically and psychologically ready to engage in therapeutic tasks? Is the person motivated to take part in therapy? Does the client understand the purpose of the therapy or exercises?

Joseph Wepman's conceptual model for therapy for the processes involved in recovery from aphasia considers the previous questions (Brookshire, 1997; Chapey, 2001; Wepman, 1951). Wepman discusses *stimulation* as the auditory, visual, or tactile stimuli the clinician presents to the patient. *Facilitation* refers to the patient's physical and psychological readiness to benefit from the stimuli (therapy) presented. *Motivation* is the patient's interest and even enthusiasm to attend and work for improvement both in the therapy session and outside it. Wepman's overall conclusion is that when stimulation, facilitation, and motivation are operating optimally, therapy has its best opportunity for success.

Listening to our clients and patients will probably take more time in the short-run than simply going about our preplanned therapy; however, time may be saved in the long run. Listening to people also requires emotional stamina and investment on our part. When we listen to people, we open ourselves to the experiences of human tragedy, loss, and suffering. Hearing our clients' and patients' stories "touches" us and reminds us that we are vulnerable to life's vicissitudes as well. To listen to people involves being attuned to their messages and needs, no matter how bluntly or subtly expressed. It means listening to a person's clear statements about physical discomfort as well as listening for nonverbal messages, for example, a cough that signals reluctance to comply with the clinician's request, or a raised finger that signals that the person wants to say something. Our attunement to people involves paying attention to the main channels of communication (both verbal and nonverbal) they use and learning to recognize their needs, so that we are less likely to miss important signals.

On a pragmatic level, careful listening can lead to a modification of our therapy plans to better meet the client's needs and preferences. For example, a client may hint at a desire to focus on an area in therapy that is important to him or her, such as remembering grandchildren's names, that helps the clinician better understand what is motivating to the client. On an interpersonal level, our listening helps people feel understood, appreciated, respected, and cared for. Simple listening can go a long way toward building the person's trust in the clinician and therapy. At the same time, it is sometimes necessary to put limits on listening to a person's concerns. Because of time constraints, as well as professional scope of practice, a client or patient's concerns (complaints) may need to be directed to another health care or mental health specialist, for example, a nurse, psychologist or pastoral staff. Careful and therapeutic listening involves making decisions about what is relevant to our area of practice and what information warrants another professional's evaluation.

TONE OF VOICE

In professional as well as personal relationships, tone of voice communicates an immense amount of information and can be even more powerful than the content of the message. Throughout the life span, the sound of a person's voice often mirrors the person's emotional state (Boone & McFarlane, 2000). How we feel may be heard in the sound of our voices as well as in changes in our prosodic rhythm patterns. Our emotional status plays a primary role in the control of respiration; for example, nervousness can be heard in our shortness of breath.

From the client's perspective, the clinician's tone of voice may be recalled long after instructions or therapy is forgotten. A warm and friendly, yet confident and authoritative, voice helps clients both like and respect clinicians without fully knowing how competent they may be. A tone of voice that sounds blaming, belittling, or critical may discourage clients from following recommendations, no matter how good they are. A gentle and accepting voice tone may make it easier for clients to accept the clinician's words, even when difficult news or information has to be shared. However, the clinician should avoid sounding saccharine or excessively sweet. This may be perceived by clients and professionals as being artificial and in some settings (particularly medical) can quickly diminish professional credibility. On the other hand, a tone of voice that reflects false confidence or bravado can sound equally artificial and diminish respect for a clinician.

EMPATHY

Empathy is central to the development of a therapeutic relationship. It is the principal route to understanding clients and their families and helping them to feel understood. Adler (1956) characterized empathy as the ability to "see with the eyes of another, hear with the ears of another, and feel with the heart of another" (p. 135). Empathy involves careful listening, understanding, *and communicating* that understanding to the client. Important skills for empathic understanding include attending, listening, paraphrasing, reflection of feeling, and summarizing (these skills will be discussed further in Chapter 4, Interviewing and Therapy Microskills). The clinician strives to accurately paraphrase the client's main thoughts or feelings, often using the important words of the client, and distilling and condensing the principal thoughts and feelings (Nystul, 1999). The clinician tries to communicate to the client that she not only has technical expertise and understands the communication problems, but is trying to understand what it is like to walk in that person's shoes. The clinician, while maintaining a professional posture, is allowing herself to feel something of the person's distress or emotional suffering and what it might be like to go through that experience (Brammer & MacDonald, 1999; Ivey, 1998).

A distinction needs to be made between empathy and sympathy. Sympathy does not require as much interpersonal connection with someone as does empathy. We may genuinely feel sorry for someone's loss (sympathy), but we may not engage in the dialogue that is required to achieve true empathy. To have sympathy, a person feels sorry for another's situation or loss, yet remains relatively detached (e.g., we send sympathy cards, not empathy cards). With sympathy, friends or families may cry with one another, but there is not necessarily a personal responsibility to become involved and an ongoing responsibility to help. Sympathy often includes sharing mutual or similar experiences in commiseration. Sympathy is not a professional stance with clients, patients, and families, and in counseling it may be nontherapeutic. For example, if, while listening to a particularly tragic case history, a clinician begins to cry in front of a client, the client may view the clinician's response as somewhat unprofessional. The client may change the topic or edit the information he or she is presenting to avoid further upsetting the clinician.

Therapeutically, empathy is the better response to clients' and families' difficulties and tragedies. Although you may genuinely feel sympathy toward a person (you can cry after the person leaves), empathy allows you to feel, as best you can, what the person is experiencing, but function at an interpersonal level that is sufficient to maintain your professional composure. Your composure assures people who are suffering that you can maintain the professional perspective necessary to help them.

An important skill in determining an appropriate empathic response is reading the client's nonverbal behavior (Brammer & MacDonald, 1999). Body communication of feelings and needs often is more revealing than words. By carefully attending to clients' and family members' verbal messages, tone of voice, facial expressions, and body language we can answer important questions that will help guide our responses to the person. For example, What is the person feeling right now? How does the person view this problem? How does the person view his or her world right now? Other important questions include, Why is the person so upset? What is causing this strong emotional reaction from the person? With all these questions the clinician needs to be nonjudgmental of the person and, therefore, more therapeutically responsive.

Ivey (1994, pp. 145–147) discusses different levels of clinician empathy, from subtractive levels to basic empathy to additive levels. Subtractive responses are less-than-desirable responses and subtract something from the client's experience. They do not adequately capture the client's story and usually indicate poor listening skills on the part of the clinician. Basic empathy indicates that the clinician's responses are compatible with the client's experience; the clinician is using good attending skills with paraphrasing, reflection of feeling, and summarization. In additive empathy the clinician adds congruent ideas and feelings and furthers the depth of understanding in order to facilitate client exploration of additional or alternative thoughts. By deepening the client's understanding, the additive level of empathy also opens up some degree of hope. The following are examples of five levels of empathy to a client (modified from Ivey, 1994, pp. 145–146):

> Client: "I don't know what to do with my son since he was in the car accident. He doesn't seem to want to be part of the family anymore and he just stays in his room all of the time. I've tried everything I can think of and everything anybody else can think of!"

Clinician (Level-1, *subtractive response*): "You seem to have a rather negative view of your son. I think you ought to consider the fact that he has had some neurological damage."

Clinician (Level-2, *slightly subtractive response*): "It sounds like you are very frustrated and maybe feeling like giving up on your son."

Clinician (Level-3, *basic empathy*): "You're discouraged and confused about how to help your son become more involved with the family. The things you have tried so far haven't worked, and you're not sure what to try next."

Clinician (Level-4, *slightly additive*): "You have tried every way you can think of to get your son back involved with the family, but nothing is working. You've tried hard and are getting tired and a little frustrated with the situation. What does all this effort that you've made for your son tell you about your feelings for him?"

Clinician (Level-5, *additive*): "I sense your confusion and frustration right now, and your feeling that maybe you should give up. Based on what you have told me, your thoughts and feelings make a lot of sense. It is also understandable that you keep trying to bring your son back into family activities together (hope for the future, and suggestion that the parent's efforts are not futile). You have told me how loving and happy he was before the accident and how different he is now. It sounds like the adjustment to these changes has been very difficult for you. I imagine it takes a while to adjust your expectations, especially because you care so much for him.

This last response, at the level 5 additive level, takes a risk of adding the clinician's perceptions. It is always important to observe how the client responds to empathic statements so that you can return to safer, level 3 responses if needed.

Overall, empathic responses involve the use of nonblaming language so that the client or family member can feel that whatever they have done, or whatever they are thinking or feeling is normal. SLPs and audiologists' training helps them learn to avoid subtractive responses (levels 1 and 2); use effectively basic empathic responses (level 3); and occasionally employ slightly additive empathic responses (level-4). Psychologists and counselors may more appropriately use additive (level-5) responses.

Providing empathic responses follows a 1-2-3 pattern (Ivey, 1998) and requires that we listen to the client's responses to determine whether our statements should be recalibrated.

1.   The clinician attends to, listens to, and observes the client's verbal and nonverbal behaviors. The clinician selects a thought or feeling the client has communicated, and paraphrases, reflects, or summarizes the thought or feeling to the client.

2.   The client responds to the clinician's statement (observation) with verbal and nonverbal behaviors. The client's response may indicate general agreement or disagreement with the clinician's empathic remark.

3.   The clinician again attends to, listens to, and observes the client's verbal and nonverbal behaviors and responds to the client's behaviors. For example, "That observation seemed

to have resonated with you in some way," or, if the clinician's response was not sufficiently empathic she might say, "The observation I just made got a reaction from you. Can you tell me what you are thinking?" This question provides an opportunity to continue the dialogue with the client and to repair the empathic error if necessary.

Empathic responses are often important to communicate as the clinician is sharing a diagnosis with a parent or client. Many times children with hidden problems such as central auditory processing disorders are brought to the clinic for an evaluation. The parents may have no idea what is wrong with their child, why he is not listening, learning, or obeying them. Parents have typically given much thought to their child's difficulties and tried to figure out the problems. They may have taken the child to various specialists, a pediatrician, reading specialist, or maybe even a psychologist. However, often it is not until the child is seen by a SLP or audiologist that a consideration or determination is made that the child may have an impairment of central auditory processing (Bellis, 1996; Chermak & Musiek, 1997; Iskowitz, 1999; Kelly, 2001; Roeser & Downs, 1995).

After the child has been evaluated and the clinician and parent(s) are in the exit interview, the clinician may want to reinforce the parents for all they have done to try to determine the nature of the child's problems. It may be helpful for parents who are experiencing guilt for not getting an earlier evaluation or therapy to say, "Don't be hard on yourself. You have been searching for a long time to discover what your child's problems are. It has been perplexing, but I think we are beginning to understand some of the foundational problems that are creating a lot of the other symptoms he has. There are strategies that can improve your child's communication."

It is not necessary that clinicians have gone through situations and experiences identical to their clients and patients in order to empathize with them; clinicians who have openly faced loss and suffering in their own lives are capable of feeling and expressing empathy for others. Along these lines, a clinician may respond to a client with, "I know that this slow process of recovery is really hard on you." This example highlights the point that empathy needs to be communicated, not just privately felt by the clinician. Empathy is not a static quality or a personality trait of the clinician; it occurs in an interpersonal context. Clients are not likely to know that their clinicians are feeling empathy unless it is communicated (Ridley & Lingle, 1996).

Two types of cautions regarding clinicians' expressions of empathy need to be described. The first caution involves failures in empathy that occur when a well-meaning SLP or audiologist unwittingly projects her or his own reactions to a situation onto a client. An SLP may think it would be terrible not to be able to read newspapers, magazines, or books. Yet this client, who did little reading anyway, is not particularly concerned about decreased reading ability. In this case, it would not sound empathic for the clinician to tell the client, "Not being able to read must be very hard on you." This may not accurately reflect the client's appraisal of the situation.

The second caution involves expressions of empathy which side with the client's pessimism instead of fostering hopefulness. While it is important to communicate to people an understanding of their experiences, a clinician's communications should avoid excessive indulgence in their pessimism or self-pity. The clinician should try to balance empathy for how the person feels at the moment with expressions of hopefulness that are realistic and appropriate to that person's situation.

COUNSELING SKILLS IN ACTION:

Expressing Empathy

A 14-year-old boy sustained a severe traumatic brain injury when hit by a drunk driver as he and his family were walking along a country road while on vacation. He was taken to a large children's hospital in Northern California where he remained in a coma for several months. When he was capable of receiving rehabilitation, physical therapy, occupational therapy and speech therapy professionals began working with him. After a few months of rehabilitation he was discharged home and the hospital referred him to an SLP, Peter, for continued speech, language and cognitive therapy.

Upon Peter's initial interview with the parents he learned that Jason (not his real name) was a very bright high school freshman (academic records supported this), was very well liked, and athletic. Although both parents appeared to have gone through the grieving process, bringing the child home with his numerous severe physical, speech, language and cognitive limitations made the reality of his impairments and disabilities even more grievous. Both parents were understandably lamenting the loss of the child they knew (just as the child was lamenting the loss of the self he knew). The parents appeared to have considerable pessimism and fear about their son's future improvements, his eventual independence, and quality of life. The father was particularly concerned that his son could not continue being the athlete he was before the TBI and to play football as the father had done in high school and college. The child, understandably, also had considerable pessimism and self-pity about his future in school, athletics, and socially.

Peter felt it was important when talking with both the child and parents to be both empathic ("It's understandable how frightening it must be not knowing how much recovery can be made."), realistic, and hopeful. Over the many months that he worked with the child, he frequently conveyed to Jason and his parents that he was likely going to continue having problems with his speech, language, and cognition, but with supportive parents, hard work, and continued therapy he would maximize his potential.

With a lot of support from his family, and from Peter, his SLP, Jason eventually graduated from high school and community college, and is now living semi-independently.

RESPECT FOR THE PERSON

Another crucial building block for the therapeutic relationship is the clinician's respect for the person. Clinicians' questions, suggestions, and interventions should always convey respect for individuals and should affirm that they are doing the best they can under difficult circumstances. The delicate balance is always between acceptance of individuals for who they are (and how they feel at the moment) and encouragement to change (Linehan & Kehrer, 1993). For example, a SLP can convey empathy and respect to a client who is dysfluent, but simultaneously present therapy that instills hope and encourages the person to develop healthier attitudes toward dysfluency and ways of improving speech. One can hope that, over time, the client will internalize the SLP's messages and become both more self-accepting and more encouraging of self-change.

Respect for the person is most often communicated through daily interaction rather than through direct statements. In other words, the clinician's behaviors convey an implicit respect for the person's dignity, privacy, autonomy, and vulnerability. In medical settings, in particular, patients may feel that their dignity and privacy are invaded because of needing assistance with dressing and toileting. They may feel that they have lost autonomy because doctors, nurses, and rehabilitation staff make decisions for them. SLPs, for example, may decide what food textures and liquid consistencies are safe for the patient, thereby taking charge of areas the patient has controlled most of his life. The patient may feel vulnerable to the "whims" of the medical staff caring for him, and even the rehabilitation staff who are attempting to help the patient return to his home and community. The patient may feel that the SLP is being arbitrary in his or her decision about the patient's limits in problem solving and reasoning through safety issues in the home. Clinicians need to act in ways that protect and support people's basic human rights by giving them adequate information, respecting their physical modesty, and providing them with an environment where they are encouraged to develop their potential.

One way that SLPs and audiologists protect their clients' and patients' rights is by maintaining professional boundaries. The clinicians' actions should serve the clients' needs rather than their own. Although clinicians should relate to clients as people who are sensitive to life's trials, relationships with clients are generally nonreciprocal. Therefore, clinicians should not slip into a social posture of reciprocal sharing of feelings and problems. Occasional clinician self-disclosures may enhance the therapeutic relationship and the clinician's credibility. Self-disclosure can best be used sparingly and on occasions when the client expresses doubt in his or her direction of treatment. On these occasions, the clinician might let the client know that he or she is not alone and that the current obstacles can be surmounted. Empathic self-disclosures may be meaningful to the client if they accurately reflect the client's current feelings and simultaneously instill hope. Clinician self-disclosures are not likely to promote the therapeutic relationship when they are used to help the clinician increase her or his self-confidence, credibility, or need for a social connection with the client.

Occasionally a clinician may work with a client who has a similar disorder or problem as a clinician's family member, such as a parent or grandparent. For example, the clinician may be working with a young girl who has an attention deficit disorder and significant language problems, and the clinician may have a daughter with similar problems. It would not be therapeutic to commiserate with the parents of the client about the mutual challenges they experience with their daughters. However, it may be helpful to mention briefly that the clinician has a child with similar problems and how important it has been to get a thorough diagnosis and ongoing therapy. Similarly, if the clinician has a parent or grandparent who suffered a CVA it may be therapeutic to mention to the patient or family member the experience and how important it has been to have the help of an SLP, but not to present details of how the clinician has coped with the challenges.

THERAPEUTIC COMMUNICATION

Communicating in a therapeutic manner with clients can help support, develop, and maintain a therapeutic relationship. Therapeutic communication refers to the actions, utterances, and behaviors that contribute to the therapeutic relationship. While the therapeutic relationship describes the context in which therapy occurs, dimensions of therapeutic communication provide therapists with the "how to" skills or the methods for conveying respect, empathy, understanding, and warmth to our clients.

Therapeutic communication encompasses our verbal and nonverbal communication; it includes our physical presentation, body language, tone of voice, and wording of responses or interventions. The moment we meet a client we begin to communicate both nonverbally and verbally. Even when a person has no voice or ability to speak, he or she is "shouting" nonverbally to anyone and everyone (Tanner, 1999). The old adage is true: we cannot not communicate. In other words, even our silence is not neutral (Anchin & Kiesler, 1982); it can convey respect and patience or indifference and disrespect. The following discussion addresses different aspects of therapeutic communication.

Nonverbal Communication

Our nonverbal communication can convey our professional role and authority in a friendly, nonintimidating manner (Burgoon, Buller, & Woodall, 1996). Our nonverbal communication can also convey respect and acceptance for people. Nonverbal channels of communication include our physical appearance and dress, our postures and movements, and how we position ourselves in relation to our clients. Clients are not the only ones who may develop a guarded posture in the therapeutic setting. Sometimes, clinicians present themselves in a guarded fashion, either because they lack confidence with certain types of clients or because they are uncomfortable with a client's interpersonal style (e.g., angry, hostile, or sullen). Optimally, our nonverbal communication should convey our professional confidence and poise, and it should be consistent with our verbal messages.

PHYSICAL APPEARANCE

Obviously, there are aspects of our physical appearance that we cannot change, for example, our height and general body type. However, we can choose to dress professionally to enhance our credibility, particularly when working on sensitive issues with clients, patients, and family members. Some hairstyles and colors, excessive piercings or tattoos may look unprofessional or even threatening to some people. The task here is to balance personal preferences with the demands of our professional roles. In our professions of speech-language pathology and audiology being well groomed is an asset; however, we do not want to appear to be prima donnas to our clients or coworkers.

Deciding upon our physical presentation (e.g., hair and dress) may also depend upon the particular setting, client population, ethnicity, and regional standards. Wearing a white coat, for example, may enhance professional credibility in some settings (i.e., medical) but unnecessarily intimidate or distance clients (e.g., children) in other settings. Dressing very casually may convey comfort and poise with clients in some settings, but disrespect in others.

Children often wear clothing and styles to project particular images, and adults often do the same. However, hospitalized patients usually have that form of expression curtailed when they are required to wear unattractive and often uncomfortable and poor-fitting gowns. Patients can reestablish some of their self-image when they are allowed and encouraged to wear clothing that reflects their personal style.

Helping Clients Feel Good

In convalescent hospitals some residents choose to wear clothes that may appear unnecessary for the environment. Some women like to dress in their finest attire before going into public areas, and some men wear a tie throughout the day, much like they may have worn through much of their professional careers. When I see a resident well-groomed and dressed I like to compliment him or her and make a little fuss over how nice the person looks. Residents seem to always appreciate people who notice when they are dressed up. They may have precious few opportunities to express their pride and dignity and to garner positive comments from others.

BODY LANGUAGE

There are other aspects of our physical presentation that affect clients and these generally are referred to as body language. We convey to people how we feel about them through an assortment of macrogestures (e.g., body postures, arm and hand positions, and gestures), and microgestures (e.g., eye contact, eye blinks, and intentional and unintentional facial expressions). Clients are keen observers of clinicians' movements and gestures that convey comfort versus tension in their presence. Clinicians who feel comfortable with their clients typically have an open body language, for example, their arms and legs are uncrossed. Clinicians who are tense or unsure of themselves may communicate these feelings with more of a closed body language, for example, crossing their arms over their chest or holding their note pad as if it is a shield between them and their clients. Clinicians can monitor the degree of confidence, comfort, and engagement that is conveyed by their body language with clients. Clients can be very sensitive to the emotional barriers clinicians create with their arms, note pads, or other objects. In general, clients feel you are interested in them if you face them squarely and lean forward slightly, have an expressive face, and use encouraging gestures (Burgoon et al., 1996; Ivey, 1998).

Clinicians can also monitor how they pace themselves (e.g., walking or arm gestures) with different kinds of clients; for example, adjusting your pace to be consistent with an elderly client's slower pace can communicate empathy. On the other hand, maintaining a pace that is much faster than a client's may communicate impatience or intolerance. Slowing your pace or adjusting it to be more similar to a client's may pose a challenge to clinicians who are extremely energetic and achievement or activity (versus relationship) focused.

PROXEMICS

One of the first signals we give people about how we feel about them is where we stand or position ourselves in relation to them. Burgoon et al. (1996) discuss personal space and interpersonal or conversational distance (proxemics). Personal space refers to the minimum amount of spatial distance a person needs to feel comfortable, which can vary considerably depending on the relationship, interaction, or activity with another person, as well as cultural backgrounds.

A Stranger at the Door

I received a request from a home health agency to evaluate and treat an elderly woman who had sustained a CVA. The woman lived in an older part of town and it wasn't generally safe when strangers came to the door. I had scheduled the appointment with a lady friend of the client who was planning to be present during my visits. I followed my typical procedures which include immediately after ringing the door bell, stepping back two paces so that when the door is opened I do not present a physical threat by having invaded the person's comfort zone. I am also out of arms' reach. (This procedure was learned during my ambulance driving and attending years; the driver and attendant never knew what to expect when a door opened.) I handed the client's friend my business card and she looked it over carefully. She then asked to see my driver's license (a very wise request) and I took it out of my wallet and handed it to her. She told me to wait a moment while she showed them to my new client. The door was closed, but after a couple of minutes the woman returned and invited me into the home. I was very aware that both elderly women were initially uncomfortable with a strange man in the home, and that the utmost decorum was needed in their presence.

Appropriate distance can convey respect, but standing too far from a person can convey (accurately or inaccurately) discomfort or dislike of the person. According to Hall (1959, 1966, as cited in Burgoon et al., 1996), public distance is about 10 feet or more apart; however, this is not considered a distance for effective therapeutic interaction or communication. Social-consultive distance (4 to 10 feet) is used for both social conversations and business transactions. However, social conversations frequently occur in the close range (4 to 6 feet) and business transactions in the far range (6 to 10 feet). Both people are out of touching range. Counseling clients and family members is often done within the social close range. SLPs and audiologists frequently use the personal-casual distance (1 1/2 to 4 feet) when working with clients and patients, for example, when doing table work. The far range (2 1/2 to 4 feet) is often a range used when doing counseling with clients and families.

The intimate distance (0 to 18 inches) is often needed during evaluations and therapy, with a direct hands-on approach necessary to assess oral-motor or swallowing functioning and to assist the client or patient to achieve particular oral-motor movements or swallowing procedures. Giving a warning that you are about to touch the client shows respect for personal space. Patients in medical settings often feel that physicians and clinicians disregard their need for personal space and privacy. Giving a patient advance warning, such as, "Mrs. Cohen, I would like to place my fingertips on your throat while you are chewing and swallowing to see how you are doing with your swallowing today. Is that okay?" communicates respect and a desire to avoid being overly intrusive to the patient. When entering the client's intimate zone observe his or her nonverbal messages. Note the client's facial expressions and body language for signs of how the person is tolerating your close presence and physical contact. It helps to verbally express appreciation of the client's willingness to let you come near and touch the person's face or neck. Although counseling is not done in the close range, counseling skills are being used, including eye contact, appropriate facial expressions, choice of words, and tone of voice. We need to keep in mind that the various proxemic distances and the comfort levels of both the client and clinician are culturally based and often gender based, and what may be comfortable to the clinician may be very uncomfortable to the client.

Evaluating Mr. T.

An attorney contacted me and requested that I evaluate a man's language and cognitive functioning because he had a history of various closed head injuries. The man I was to evaluate was in jail. I had to pass through various levels of security and entered into a small visitor's room. My client was brought into a small holding room. Cameras recorded everything being done. We both sat on hard, round stools separated by a low wall and a heavy wire mesh. I had to lay all the testing material on the metal counter on my side of the wire mesh. No physical contact with the materials was possible for the examinee other than during a writing task where I slipped a piece of paper and pen through a narrow slot. Although we were within the personal-casual distance, there was nothing personal or casual about the interaction. The environment was highly structured and not particularly well-suited for developing rapport.

Hospitalized individuals, particularly those in skilled nursing facilities, often stake out their territory in the hallway, near the nursing station, or the activities room. Many residents have their place to eat in the dining room area and they become upset if someone inadvertently sits in that place and, because of inability to communicate well, may give strong nonverbal messages to indicate their displeasure. A sense of personal territory helps patients feel that they have some control over their environment and that they possess something. Asking patients if you may join them shows respect and consideration for their territorial needs (Tanner, 1999).

The Holocaust Survivor

I received an order to evaluate a patient's swallowing in a skilled nursing facility. I was advised by nursing that the patient was an elderly woman who had survived the Holocaust and that she was still very fearful of men, particularly men wearing any kind of uniform. I chose to take off my white lab coat before entering the room. At the doorway I knocked and softly said her name to get her attention. Her bed was next to the door and I made certain she was watching me as I approached so that I would not startle her. I bent down slightly as I walked toward her so my eyes would be nearer her eye level, and to try to make myself appear less threatening. I pulled up a chair and sat beside her bed so that I was not standing over her, and I did not touch her. This approach apparently worked well, along with noninvasive gestures, a soft tone of voice, and quiet conversation. I did not attempt to evaluate her swallow during this time, but only gain her trust. I came back later and was able to successfully do a bedside swallow evaluation.

SEATING ARRANGEMENTS

Seating arrangements and postures can have an influence on our clients' level of trust and comfort. Frequently, clinicians and clients sit across from one another in therapy with a table between them. Various assessment or therapy materials may be scattered over the table. However, when counseling with an individual it is often better not to have a table (a physical barrier) between you and the person. Sitting at right angles facing one another with just the corner of the table to one side and an open area on the other can facilitate a sense of openness in the communication. Sitting on the same side of the table facing one another is also helpful for a feeling of openness. If a table must be between you and the person to whom you are talking, try to have the evaluation or therapy materials moved to the side so they are not distracting or adding to the physical barrier.

When discussing sensitive issues or presenting bad news, it is helpful to have cups or glasses of water on the table for each person present, including yourself. Sometimes when we are uncomfortable about what we are sharing with someone our mouths may become dry and a sip of water can give us some moisture as well as help soothe our nerves. During extended counseling, clients and families may also need a little water to drink to relieve a dry mouth or to sip during anxious moments. Having water available to clients and families is a small gesture that reflects thoughtfulness and sensitivity.

EYE CONTACT

Positioning ourselves so that we can make direct eye contact can show respect, interest, and sensitivity to clients. Standing up while the client is sitting down interferes with comfortable eye contact and may appear intimidating, especially to children. (Children often are more comfortable if a clinician drops down on one knee to be more eye-to-eye.) Clients may interpret how well clinicians like them based upon the clinicians' amount of eye contact. Clinicians can also stay alert for signs that certain clients are uncomfortable with eye contact and this may reflect different cultural or ethnic backgrounds and social customs.

By maintaining good eye contact with the people to whom you are talking, you can more easily note their responses to your comments. Good eye contact allows you to observe their facial expressions and helps you interpret what they may be understanding, or how they may be feeling in response to your statements. Clients often look away when discussing topics that particularly distress them, and we, ourselves, may find that we tend to avoid eye contact when we are uncomfortable with a topic or uncertain of our information (Ivey, 1998).

When talking to clients or family members, as well as professionals such as teachers and administrators, nurses and physicians, it is often helpful to establish eye contact for one to two seconds before speaking. This can help listeners recognize that you are serious about what you are going to communicate and also can help you appear more confident than you may actually be feeling. A clinician who has poor eye contact when communicating may be perceived as less confident or trustworthy than one who establishes and maintains good eye contact (Burgoon et al., 1996; Sheehan, 1970).

TOUCH

As SLPs and audiologists we typically must touch clients and patients in our work with them, for example, during oral-peripheral and swallowing examinations, oral-motor exercises, and audiological testing and tympanography. It is respectful to clients of all ages to ask them if you may touch them, particularly around the head or face, areas that are often the most sensitive for many individuals. A surprise touch from a clinician can be startling and offensive to many clients. Some clinicians typically have warm hands, which may feel comforting to clients and patients. Other clinicians may tend to have cold hands that are at first uncomfortable to the person they are touching. Individuals who tend to have cold hands can tell the client that they are going to warm them up by rubbing them together for a moment. This sometimes amuses clients, but they also appreciate the clinician's thoughtfulness.

The amount of touch that is comfortable to give or receive in social environments (which also may carry over to professional environments) may depend on the region of the country the client or clinician is from. A 1985 study by Riseberg (cited in Burgoon et al., 1996, p. 99) of Northwestern University Medical School included surveying approximately 20,000 people in 25 states. Riseberg's finding (percentages apparently were rounded) include:

- In the Northeast: 90% of people are from low-to-medium-touch backgrounds, and 5% each are from high-touch and no-touch backgrounds.

- In the South: 80% of people come from medium-to-high-touch backgrounds, 15% from low-touch, and 5% from no-touch backgrounds.

- In the Midwest: 80% are from low-to-medium-touch backgrounds, 10% each from high-touch and no-touch backgrounds.

- In the West: 85% are from medium-to-high-touch backgrounds, 10% from low-touch, and 5% from no-touch backgrounds.

Although it is difficult to generalize about touch when working with clients and patients, we need to appreciate that even though we are accustomed to touching both children and adults on and around their faces and even inside their mouths, such touching may be very uncomfortable to the client or patient because of their cultural, regional, or family backgrounds. A client's personal (and possibly traumatic) experiences may also sensitize them to touch. In addition, some patients with CVAs or TBIs may have either hypersensitivity or hyposensitivity to touch, and therapists need to be aware of this possibility. Those with hypersensitivity may not appreciate or easily tolerate touch around the face and neck. Those with hyposensitivity may not perceive the tactile cues that are presented.

COUNSELING SKILLS IN ACTION:

Hypersensitivity to Touch

After a particularly emotional session with her clinician, the mother of three children stood up and began walking towards the door. The clinician followed behind her and gently reached out to momentarily put his hand on her shoulder in a gesture of support. The sobbing woman whirled around and glared at the clinician and ordered him to "never do that again!" A review of the client's records revealed that she had been raped years earlier and had therefore developed a hypersensitivity to touch, especially unexpected touch.

CONSISTENCY OF COMMUNICATION

Consistency of communication is extremely important in creating a therapeutic climate. There are two types of consistency: 1) communication consistency in-the-moment and 2) communication consistency over a period of time (Ivey, 1998). The first, communication consistency in-the-moment refers to the clinician's ability to send a consistent message through both verbal and non-verbal channels of communication. If a client perceives inconsistent messages from the clinician, the efforts at therapeutic communication may be negated. For example, if the audiologist is careful to use friendly, nonblaming language but has her arms folded and a tense jaw, she may betray a negative attitude toward the client. Any positive efforts may go unnoticed by the client and the client may feel mistrustful of the audiologist.

Initially, this may sound like too much for a clinician to keep track of; however, consistently positive communication skills will probably come automatically to the reflective and well-trained clinician in most circumstances. When a clinician notices inconsistencies in her or his own communication with a client, it may signal ambivalence or suppressed feelings (e.g., frustration) toward a client. It is time, then, to reflect on one's own feelings and reactions toward the client so that consistent communication can be resumed.

Consistent communication over time is also very important to the maintenance of the therapeutic relationship. This involves clinician stability of attitude and behavior toward clients. We should treat clients the same way next week as we did this week. Clients should be able to predict how we will treat them rather than wonder what mood we will be in, how kind or understanding we will be. Clients are inevitably experiencing uncertainty in their lives because of their hearing, communication, or swallowing problems, and our relationship with them should contrast with that uncertainty. The professional relationship should offer a safe haven from all the other unpredictable events in their lives.

NONBLAMING LANGUAGE

When clients do not follow through or complete assigned therapeutic tasks (or when the nature of their symptoms/complaints is unclear), the clinician's manner of inquiry can either encourage the client to examine his or her behavior or increase the client's resistance or defensiveness (Wachtel, 1993). Clinician's language can encourage the client to open up or it can create an adversarial climate. Even if the clinician feels frustrated by the client's low motivation or lack of commitment to the therapy, clinicians should resist the urge to sound disapproving or blaming toward clients. Such messages are not likely to encourage clients to work harder in therapy. On the contrary, clients who feel blamed are more likely to feel ashamed or embarrassed, and more likely to hide their true feelings from the clinician.

It is important to maintain focus on the tasks of therapy without blaming the client for noncompliance or behaviors that interfere with therapy. Blaming clients (even when done unintentionally) can cause them to feel even worse about themselves and therefore less likely to follow through with future tasks. Instead, the clinician can try to reflect the client's reluctance, mixed feelings, or reasons for not following through with the recommended exercises and therapy. For example, the clinician may respond to noncompliance with therapeutic tasks by wondering aloud: "I'm wondering if you are concerned about whether you will succeed on these exercises" or "I'm wondering if you are upset about not seeing faster improvement." This technique allows the clinician to side with the client's struggles while allowing him or her to maintain his or her dignity. Another approach is to assume that the client had good reasons for not doing something asked, for example, "You usually do most (some) of the exercises during the week that I give you. This week must have been extra hard for you not to do any them. Are there any thoughts about the therapy you would like to talk about?" Once the client feels understood (rather than blamed), he or she will be much more likely to follow through on the tasks of therapy.

MAKING CLEAR STATEMENTS

An important principle when communicating with clients and their families is to use clear, unambiguous language so that there is no questions about your intent and message. Your effectiveness will be increased by eliminating vague words or statements. Such words and phrases as *I think*, *maybe*, and *sort of* convey uncertainty (Zaro, Barach, Nedelman, and Dreiblatt, 1995). There is considerable difference in impact between saying, "I think this might possibly help you," and saying, "I believe this will be helpful." Statements such as "I'm not really sure; I don't have much experience with this, but it may possibly be helpful. I don't know about this, but let's try it out and see what happens." burdens the client with the therapist's own insecurity and uncertainty. The clinician could be more effective by saying, "Research and experience show that this type of approach can be helpful and will likely be of assistance to you."

COUNSELING WITH CHILDREN AND ADOLESCENTS

It is important to gauge your choice of words for the age of the individual with whom you are talking. As presented later in Chapter 4, we need to modify our interviewing and counseling techniques with children and adolescents (Novak, 2002; Zebrowski, 2002). Young children generally respond better to a directive, structured style of interviewing with simple questions, rather than a nondirective, unstructured style with open-ended questions (Morrison & Anders, 1999). Our questions and messages to them need to be particularly clear, using words and language structures that match their language abilities. Observing successful preschool and elementary school teachers' interactions with children can provide good models of how to talk with children at their levels.

Reflecting children's positive feelings seldom presents problems; reflecting their negative feelings often requires more skill. With children it is helpful to use language that is simple, clear, concrete, and direct. Clinicians should use words that cannot be misunderstood and that are not vague or evasive. When you are trying to identify the particular mood a child might be struggling with, try to be as specific and accurate as possible. Select the word that seems to describe what is going on with the child, the word that reflects the child's feelings at that moment. If a young child appears anxious you might say, "You look scared (or afraid)," because that is the childhood word. The words fearful, frightened, tense, anxious, nervous, edgy, jittery, alarmed, worried, uneasy, or apprehensive may not fit because those are more adult words. Also, try to gauge the intensity of the affect as accurately as possible. If the child is very angry, "You seem annoyed," may underestimate the child's current feelings; whereas, "You seem hopping mad" or "really angry" may better capture the child's current emotional state. Adult words such as incensed, infuriated, irate, outraged, or enraged are not meaningful to many children. It is also important to remember that children do not need their feelings agreed with; they need them acknowledged. By giving words to children's feelings, they begin to trust that you understand them and are not judging them, only identifying what they are feeling and how deeply (Faber & Mazlish, 1980; Novak, 2002).

Zebrowski (2002) presents many important points about building clinical relationships with teenagers who stutter, and these points are applicable to teenagers with other communication problems as well. Communicating with adolescents can be very challenging, and it is often even more challenging when the adolescent has a communication disorder. Teenagers frequently cannot or will not respond with a direct answer to a direct question. Zebrowski says that this may be because the adolescent may not know the answer, may be processing the question and the response slowly, and/or may be reticent to divulge information. Zebrowski recommends an "advance-retreat-advance" approach when trying to obtain information from adolescents. For example, when asking a direct question such as, "What are some of the things you would like to change about the way you talk? (advance), the adolescent's response may be, "I don't know" or "I'm not sure." This may indicate the clinician needs to retreat by making a statement of acceptance such as, "That's okay" or "That's fine. It's something to think about." A general comment about either real or hypothetical clients may then be made, for example, "Sometimes teenagers want to learn how to talk more easily on the phone." This can be followed with an advance such as, "Is that true for you?" If the adolescent continues to be noncommittal, the clinician should move on to another topic (retreat), but return to the question later when it appears the adolescent will be more interested and responsive (advance). Using the adolescent's own comments as a bridge back to a previously asked but unanswered question helps the clinician obtain information when the adolescent is willing to share or divulge it. Conversely, pushing adolescents for responses or information that they are not willing to share can create power struggles that parallel relationships with their parents. These power struggles can usurp therapeutic efforts and lead to a stalemate in the therapeutic progress. In general, adolescents cannot be pushed, but they can be led.

Humor can be helpful in communicating with clients of all ages, but clinicians must be cautious about how it is employed (Manning, 2001; Zebrowski, 2002). When clients are struggling with their symptoms and prone to shame or embarrassment about them, they may not yet have the critical emotional distance that will allow them to laugh at their own foibles. When clients are not ready to laugh at their own mistakes, it would be a therapeutic error for the clinician to do so. Even if done in a light-spirited manner, clients who are still very insecure about their symptoms may regard them as no laughing matter and may (mis)interpret the clinician's laughter as cruel teasing. On the other hand, once the client begins to gain some self-confidence as well as trust in the clinician, the client may begin to laugh at some of his or her own communication errors or dysfluencies. The clinician, at this point, may smile or laugh with the client as long as the client is laughing at the problem. This moment of humor and laughter may deepen the clinician-client relationship. Humor, though, is best occasionally interspersed through a therapy session and not necessarily a significant part of it.

Humor can reflect insight and perspective about a communication problem, and indicate the realization that even with significant problems there can be a lighter side that may be appreciated (Manning, 2001; Zebrowski, 2002). Humor also reflects a person's ability to distance him or herself from the problem or current situation and indicates positive coping with a problem rather than avoiding or hiding from it. Stuttering therapy often involves helping the person desensitize him or herself to various aspects of stuttering and decrease emotional reactivity to dysfluencies. The child or adolescent's ability to use and accept humor that relates to the communication problem reflects development of insight and positive emotional distance. Some general cautions about using humor with clients are:

1. Be certain you are not laughing *at* your client, or that you are not interpreted as doing so.

2. Do not use humor to avoid important topics related to the client's therapy.

3. Do not go overboard with laughter—use it sparingly.

4. Your manner of laughter needs to sound adult, not giggly or raucous.

5. Do not laugh at behavior or topics that you do not wish to reinforce, for example, an adolescent's sexual innuendoes.

When talking with adolescents it is generally best to avoid using the latest slang or jargon because teenagers often feel such language sounds artificial or phony when coming from an adult, particularly a professional. Also, avoid using profanity because you feel it might help you sound in-tune with the young adult. In place of saying, "You look p———- off!" you might say, "You look *really* angry!" If you sense the adolescent is depressed, he would likely relate to the word "sad," "unhappy," or "miserable" more than depressed, disconsolate, glum, gloomy, lugubrious, sorrowful, or melancholy.

When communicating with adults, consider their age, education, and professional background when known. Clear, concise, and precise wording, no matter what the person's background is always appreciated. It is best to use ordinary and vivid words to express the mood you think the person is experiencing. When trying to identify an adult's mood, use adult words so that the person feels you are not talking down to her or him. For example, rather than saying, "You seem scared." you might say, "You look apprehensive." Most adults do not like their negative feelings to be exaggerated or amplified by someone else, for example, "You look *really* apprehensive!" It is usually best to understate an adult's feelings rather than overstate them.

COUNSELING WITH OLDER ADULTS

There are a number of counseling challenges that are commonly encountered when working with older patients (Boles, 2002; Toner and Shadden, 2002). Older patients are often seen in medical settings where there are time pressures and the clinician has insufficient time to conduct a thorough evaluation. Strict time limits can pose problems when working with the elderly because of their often-slowed response times, tendency to engage in tangential or unrelated conversation, attempts to extend conversation with the therapist in order to maintain social contact, and difficulty hearing which results in the need for frequent repetitions and rephrasing of statements and questions.

Many older people are most comfortable relating information in stories, which can be time-consuming and difficult to follow (Boles, 2002; Ryan, 1995; Toner & Shadden, 2002). Older people's narratives often have ambiguous references (e.g., using him, her, or it in place of a name or noun), which may be the result of word-finding difficulties. However, in order to obtain important information, clinicians need to be willing to listen to the form of communication the client prefers to use, which may also require the clinician teasing out the important information from an ongoing, ambiguous narrative. Older people often begin an interview with informal conversation about casual or familiar topics. This encourages a more balanced, humanistic interaction with the professional rather than a question-answer format which may seem abrupt or even rude to the older person. Older clients sometimes address professionals as "Dearie," "Honey," and so forth, especially if the clinician is much younger than themselves. Although the clinician may prefer to be addressed in a more professional manner, it may be prudent to accept such labels in order to maintain rapport. However, older people often appreciate being addressed as Mr., Mrs., or Dr. as a sign of respect.

Dr. M...

A resident I worked with in a skilled nursing facility had been a prominent physician in the community. After a CVA he had a variety of speech, language, cognitive, and swallowing problems. Most of the nursing and rehabilitation staff spoke to him using his first name; however, I always called him Dr. M... He appeared to appreciate hearing his professional designation and responded quite favorably to what I asked of him.

Many people adjust their style of speaking (accommodation) when talking to different age groups, for example young children, older children, adults, and older adults. However, overaccommodation occurs when individuals modify their speech style to a stereotypical pattern as a result of their perception of the person to whom they are talking, such as an elderly person (Shadden &

Toner, 1997; Toner & Shadden, 2002). Inappropriate speech registers or styles may be used, including oversimplification of language form and vocabulary, exaggerated suprasegmentals or intonational patterns, increased loudness, slower speaking rate, higher pitch, and frequent repetitions or redundancy. Such overaccomodations are variously referred to as elderspeak (Cohen & Faulkner, 1986; Shadden & Toner, 1997; Toner & Shadden, 2002), patronizing speech (Ryan et al., 1991; Shadden & Toner, 1997; Toner & Shadden, 2002), and/or secondary baby talk (Caporael, 1981; Shadden & Toner, 1997; Toner & Shadden, 2002).

Ryan, Hummert, and Boisch (1995) and Toner and Shadden (2002) describe how many individuals use patronizing communication styles of either caring or controlling when "talking down" to older people. The following are examples of these communication styles.

Baby Talk

Baby talk may be considered both caring and controlling. In this communication style, elderspeak is used with generic terms of endearment (e.g., Sweetie, Honey, and even Mama or Pops). The younger person speaks in a tone (often with a high pitched, saccharine voice) as though talking to an infant or very young child. A clinician may attempt to reinforce (control) desired behavior in an older individual by saying "You are working *so* hard today. I am *so* proud of you."

Overly Personal Talk

Overly personal talk is often accompanied by an endearing touch such as a pat on the shoulder, hand-holding, or light hug. It is high in caring and low in controlling. The younger person may compliment the older person's appearance, such as, "You look so cute in that outfit" or "That color looks so good on you." It is important for SLPs and audiologists to gauge their level of communication based on their familiarity and relationship with the client.

Directive Talk

Directive talk has the intent of having an elderly person carry out a specific task, such as taking a medication, doing a specific exercise, or stopping a particular behavior such as moaning, crying, or using the nursing call button frequently. This form of communication is primarily controlling with little or no caring. The speaker's goal is to obtain compliance from the elderly person by being controlling while having minimum interaction (caring). For example, "You have already used the call button five times today. What do you want?"

Superficial Talk

Superficial talk is neither caring nor controlling; however, it can be considered rude. This may occur when an individual discusses an older patient as though the person is not present, or when a professional discounts the elderly person's expressions of feelings or needs by abruptly changing topics. Rather than seeing superficial talk as neutral (neither caring nor controlling), it may be perceived as uncaring and disrespectful.

Additional Guidelines for Working with Older Clients

Beyond the general guidelines of basic counseling skills, it is helpful when talking to elderly individuals to provide an environment that is communication-friendly and age-sensitive. Consider the arrangement of furniture to ensure safety, easy access, and comfort. Ensure adequate lighting, eliminate glare and use backlighting when possible to help the older person better attend to your facial expressions and possibly help them with lip reading. Older people often have more difficulty hearing and understanding in noisy, distracting environments; therefore, working in a quiet room may facilitate interaction. Avoid a question-answer format (particularly closed questions) for obtaining information and allow adequate time for the person to respond to open-ended questions. Provide opportunities for the person to initiate topics and ask questions.

Older clients and caregivers appreciate being included in decision-making about their care, which helps create a sense of partnership when planning goals, strategies, and therapy activities (Toner & Shadden, 2002). When clinicians make recommendations that older clients may not be ready to accept (e.g., an augmentative communication system or a hearing aid), they may appear to have not heard the recommendations or suggestions. Even when the clinician is confident that the recommendations have been heard, the client may choose to ignore them by directing the conversation away from the clinician's focus. Seeking input from older clients rather than being directive helps them feel that they are still in control of their lives and that some young professional is not determining what the client must do.

Counseling with older clients and caregivers often requires negotiating (Toner & Shadden, 2002). In some cases the SLP and social service staff will need to work together to help the client and caregiver reach agreement about in-home care. What clients want may not be what caregivers in the home can provide. Sometimes a compromise must be negotiated where neither person is completely satisfied, but where an agreement can be reached that is mutually acceptable (or tolerable). For example, an older client may want to live with his or her children, but because of the client's difficulty with communication and self-care, family members may not be able to provide the time and attention the client needs. Other living arrangements such as a board and care facility may be the best option for both the older client and family caregivers.

Overall, communicating effectively with older individuals often requires greater than usual amounts of sensitivity and patience. By keeping in mind the changes in hearing, speech, language, and cognition that are part of the normal aging process, coupled with the impairments seen by the audiologists and SLPs, communication and counseling strategies can be optimized.

AVOIDING "PATHOLOGIZING" THE PERSON OR FAMILY (SYMPTOMS VERSUS DISORDERS)

Although our scope of practice covers numerous diagnoses, it does not include emotional disorders. As discussed in Chapter 1, there is some overlap in disorders that psychologists and SLPs diagnose (e.g., receptive and expressive language disorders, phonological disorders, stuttering, etc.). We need to be cautious, though, about "pathologizing" a client by saying the person is depressed, anxious, paranoid, schizophrenic, narcissistic, histrionic, has a dependent personality disorder, and so forth. Such labels and diagnoses are beyond our scope of practice. We also do not want to elevate symptoms to disorders. However, we do see individuals who have such characteristics and symptoms, and some aspects of our observations may need to be included in our description of these individuals. In such cases it is prudent to use descriptions of behaviors that reflect our observations rather than global pathologizing terms.

SLPs and audiologists can use **action language** (Schafer, 1983) to describe the behaviors of clients rather than drawing conclusions that objectify and pathologize clients. We can describe situation specific behaviors (i.e., a state) but not label the complex of behaviors that may constitute a certain personality style (i.e., a trait) or a disorder. Even though a client has a certain set of behaviors that we see in a particular situation, this does not mean that these are typical of the person. For example, rather than saying the child looked depressed, it is better to describe his behaviors, such as he walked slowly with his head down, slumped in his chair, gave minimal verbal responses, frowned during many tasks, did not show pleasure or enjoyment during play activities, or did not give evidence of a sense of humor. The SLP or audiologist may conclude based on observing these behaviors while with the child, plus collateral information from the parents, teachers, or other professionals (e.g., reading specialists, resource specialists, school nurse), that the child appears to be exhibiting depressive symptoms that may warrant further evaluation by another professional such as a counselor or psychologist. In the case of an adult, rather than saying a client or patient is anxious, the clinician might describe the person as having rapid speech, tense facial expressions, repetitive behaviors such as wringing hands or tearing paper into small pieces, or excessive perspiring. The clinician may conclude that the client exhibited symptoms of anxiety.

SLPs and audiologists may note whether behaviors, characteristics, or symptoms are understandable reactions to a particular situation (e.g., during an evaluation), or whether they appear excessive and may be causing impairment in the client's functioning. By being careful to describe a person's behaviors rather than inferring the client's overall emotional state or disorder, SLPs and audiologists can work within their scope of practice and avoid negative legal repercussions. Finally, it is important to keep in mind that many psychological symptoms mask medical disorders (Morrison, 1997) and it is beyond the scope of the SLP and audiologist to make this determination.

NEGOTIATING

Negotiating is a skill that is used by all SLPs with clients, patients, family members, and even with other professionals (for example, clinicians with classroom teachers, clinicians with nursing staff, clinicians with administrators, clinicians with other clinicians) (Cohen, 2002). In all our professional work it is helpful to present a negotiating posture. Negotiating connotes being empathic and understanding the other person's perspective. Clinicians who collaborate well with others may intuitively use negotiating skills, but even so, it is useful to have a framework to think about how to structure negotiation dialogues. The need for these skills becomes even more apparent when the client or family member demonstrates noncompliance or resistance. These challenging situations may be the result of the therapist dogmatically pursuing a therapy plan without considering the client's feelings, wishes, or desires. Noncompliance or resistance may occur when the SLP or audiologist has not been sufficiently flexible and willing to negotiate with the client or family, or has failed to check with them to find out what they are interested and willing to do in therapy.

Pruitt (1981) and Fein (1993) state that it is only when negotiators (people attempting to resolve an impasse) are concerned about the interests of both parties that they have an opportunity to solve problems with some mutual satisfaction. The most productive posture is firm flexibility, that is, asserting one's own goals while being pragmatic about the means through which they are achieved. It may then be possible to construct an agreement in which both parties make adjustments that allow them to receive more than they would have had they not cooperated. For example, when an SLP attempts to help a parent understand the importance of speech therapy for a child, the SLP needs to maintain a firm stance about the importance of therapy, but flexible enough to help the parent feel that she or he has important input into the decision about whether the child should receive therapy. Another example is an audiologist who attempts to have a child begin wearing his first hearing aids. The child may recognize that they help him hear better, but is reluctant or unwilling to wear them because of embarrassment around his friends.

Concepts and techniques from the Harvard Negotiation Project (Fisher & Ury, 1991) can be helpful to clinicians in their attempts to work with clients and their families. The Harvard Negotiation Project is a research project at Harvard University Law School that works on negotiation problems and develops and disseminates improved methods of negotiation and mediation. The principles and practices developed by the Project are used at all levels of professional interaction as well as in state, national, and international negotiations. The following information is derived primarily from that source.

One of the basic principles of negotiating is that any method of negotiating may be fairly judged by three criteria: (1) it should produce a prudent agreement if agreement is possible; (2) it should be efficient; and (3) it should improve or at least not damage the relationship between parties. A prudent agreement can be defined as one that meets the legitimate interests of each side to the extent possible, resolves conflicting interests fairly, is durable, and takes into account all the people involved (Fisher & Ury, 1991).

When people (including clinicians and clients or family members) negotiate over positions, they tend to lock themselves into and defend those positions. Egos become identified with the position and "saving face" makes it less likely that any agreement will reconcile the parties' interests. Any agreement reached may reflect a mechanical splitting of the difference, which may be less than satisfactory to either side. Position bargaining may become a contest of wills with an "I'm not going to give in" approach. As clinicians, we need to avoid viewing the other side as adversaries and use a more congenial style of negotiating. In the case of the mother who is reluctant to have her child in therapy or the child who does not want to wear his hearing aids, taking strong positions may include having feelings of winning ("I got my way!") or losing ("I gave in and the clinician got her way). In either case, the parent, child, SLP, or audiologist may feel that losing the argument means a loss of ego or self-esteem.

Fisher and Ury (1991) stress "principled negotiation" or "negotiation on the merits" with the emphasis that the participants are problem-solvers, and the goal is a prudent outcome reached efficiently and amicably. Negotiating on the merits is based on four principles: (1) People—separate the people from the problem, that is, be soft on the people, firm on the problem; (2) Interests—focus on interests, not positions, that is, explore interests and avoid having a bottom line; (3) Options—consider as many as possible, that is, generate a variety of possibilities before deciding what to do; and (4) Criteria—evaluate the results based on some objective criteria, that is, try to reach an agreement based on criteria independent of will and personal feelings, and be open to reason but do not yield to pressure.

For example, some parents may doubt the value of speech therapy or may be reluctant to make the time commitment. Trying to understand parents from their perspectives can help the clinician be more empathic, but at the same time maintain a firm position on the value of therapy. Both the parent and the clinician are interested in what is good for the child's speech and language development. The parent and SLP have options that can be explored to resolve the impasse, and objective criteria may be considered to determine the benefits of therapy for the child. The child who is reluctant or unwilling to wear his or her new hearing aids is understandably embarrassed about wearing them, but still needs to wear them to hear the teacher better and to improve communication with friends. Both the child and the audiologist are interested in the child having more positive experiences in the classroom and with friends. The child and audiologist have options that can be explored to achieve their mutual goals.

In all negotiating there are two kinds of interests: the substance (the problem) and the relationship with the people negotiating (i.e., the clinician and client or family). When negotiating with a client or family member, present the facts as each of you view them as well as the feelings behind the facts. In the long run, the facts may not be as important to the ongoing working relationship as the feelings. (*Note*: After I complete the evaluation of a client and finish explaining my findings and answering the client's and family's questions, I always ask, "How do you feel about the information I have just given you?" People usually remember the feelings they leave with more than the facts that were presented.) The mother who is reluctant for her child to receive therapy (the substance of the problem) may still be reluctant to alienate the therapist who may eventually provide therapy to her child. The child who does not want to wear his hearing aids may still want to stay on good terms with the audiologist who may test his hearing in the future.

No matter what the problem is that is being negotiated, we are always working with three basic categories: perceptions, emotions, and communication (Cohen, 2002). Understanding the client or family members' perceptions means understanding the problems as they view them. Trying to understand the problems from the other person's perspective can help us have a more empathic view of what the client is thinking and feeling. However, as objective and professional as we try to be when in a dispute or negotiating with a client or family, our own emotions may come into play. Anxiety, fear, and even anger are not uncommon emotions to feel in such circumstances. The client or family may be feeling similar emotions. It is helpful to ask ourselves what is causing these emotions. Why are we angry? Why are they angry? Are we feeling insecure? Is the client or family responding to past grievances (e.g., goals that were unmet, an insensitive comment)? Are emotions spilling over from one issue to another (e.g., difficulty with a teacher or physical therapist)? Are personal problems (on either side) interfering with "taking care of business"? Applying the principles and techniques presented in Chapter 8 on Angry or Hostile Attitudes and Behaviors may be helpful with several of the strong emotions people express when negotiating.

Underlying all fair and reasonable negotiations is participation and disclosure by both parties. Involving the client or family in the ultimate decision-making is essential to their acceptance and treatment compliance. When a decision is made unilaterally by the clinician, it may be rejected by the client or family members who feel excluded from the decision-making process. Prior to entering a negotiation meeting, it is very helpful to carefully think through, "What do I want to come out of this meeting?" When communicating during your negotiations, try to sit on the same side of the table as the other person. A table between two people becomes both a physical and psychological barrier. Open body posture is very important, even if we are feeling somewhat anxious about the situation. Be aware that the other person may hear something quite different from what we are saying, and *we* may hear something quite different from what the other person is saying, particularly if our emotions are strong.

The basic problem in a negotiation process usually is not in conflicting positions; that is, the client, family, and clinician all want what is best for the client (e.g., the child to receive the help she needs to develop her speech and language, or the child to hear as well as possible in the classroom and with friends, or the adult to receive the maximum amount of therapy for which she will benefit). The conflict is likely between each person's needs, desires, concerns, and fears; ultimately, their interests (Fisher & Ury, 1991). For example, the mother may have concerns that her child already has too much time out of the classroom with the reading specialist and resource specialist, and that speech therapy will just be "too much." The child who does not want to wear his hearing aids has a desire to "look normal," even at the expense of hearing well, and is fearful that he will be teased by the other children.

Reconciling interests rather than positions is productive because both parties typically have many similar interests, although they may be taking opposite positions. Recognize what the common interests are, for example, wanting the child to have the best speech and language the child can develop, or having adequate hearing to have the best classroom and social experience. We can ask the child, client, or family members what their interests are and discuss ours openly with them as well. Be as specific as possible. Validate the other person's interests and follow up with a statement about our interest. For example, "Like you, I want Maria to do well in school and develop the best speech and language she can." Another example occurs when a patient or family member insists on the patient being discharged from the convalescent hospital (their interest). We can validate their interest by saying, "Like you, I am interested in Mr. Berger being discharged to his home when he is cognitively safe to be able to manage himself independently." These statements validate our client's interests while connecting them to our therapy goals. In this way, our respective positions can be viewed as compatible rather than as mutually exclusive.

If we want someone to listen and understand our reasoning, it helps to give our interests and reasoning first, and our conclusions and recommendations later. If we present our conclusions and recommendations initially, the other person may be thinking about arguments to counter them rather than listening to our reasoning. Many of our clients may not be well-educated (at least in the areas of speech-language pathology or audiology) and may not fully understand or appreciate our reasoning about their problems. If the client or family feels threatened by our education and knowledge, they may become defensive and may cease listening to us. Our warmth and openness can help balance the strength of our statements. Successful negotiating requires being firm *and* open. When negotiating with clients, families, or other professionals, using the skills presented in the following chapter on Interviewing and Therapy Microskills can help foster a mutually successful outcome.

CONCLUDING COMMENTS

The therapeutic relationship and communication are intertwined and can enhance or diminish the potential effects of the SLP or audiologist's treatment. The therapeutic relationship provides a basis for trust, motivation, and compliance in our professional work. Prerequisites for developing a therapeutic relationship are recognizing our clients' perceptions, needs, values, feelings, experiences, expectations, and expertise. Understanding and being attentive to transference and countertransference experiences can give clinicians tools with which to better manage therapeutic relationships. Attending and listening are foundational to the therapeutic relationship. Our tone of voice often conveys as much of the meaning as our choice of words. Empathy is central to the development of a therapeutic relationship and involves careful listening, understanding, and communicating that understanding to the client. Respect for the person should affirm that the person is doing the best he or she can under the circumstances. The challenge is to convey acceptance of the person and still encourage change.

Therapeutic communication involves both verbal and nonverbal communication. Nonverbal communication includes our physical appearance, body language, proxemics, seating arrangements, eye contact, and touch. Consistency of communication helps create and maintain a therapeutic climate so that clients and patients can anticipate the way the clinician will present her or himself in dress and manner, and attitude and behavior. Nonblaming language is an important element in therapeutic communication. Clinicians need to resist sounding disapproving or frustrated when clients do not do as much as we expect. Being clear in our communications will help clients and their families better understand our intentions and messages. Using descriptions of behaviors rather than "pathologizing" a person communicates respect and keeps us within our scope of practice. Negotiating is a skill that is used by all professionals with clients and patients, and sometimes even among themselves. Principles from the Harvard Negotiation Project can be helpful in our professional work with such challenging situations.

 Discussion Questions

1. What does the following statement mean to you: "Technical expertise is necessary but not sufficient in order to be a competent SLP or audiologist."

2. What are some of your self-perceptions about your knowledge, training, and competence that might affect your interaction with a client?

3. When have your values clashed with the values of a client? Explain.

4. What are some of the feelings you have when you begin therapy with a new client? A type of client you have never worked with before? An adult client?

5. What expectations do you have of yourself when doing an evaluation? A therapy session?

6. What expertise do you have in other areas of your life that helps give you some confidence that you can eventually develop expertise in speech-language pathology or audiology?

7. How do you show clients that you are attending to them?

8. When talking with people, what behaviors do they exhibit that help you feel they are listening to you?

9. Practice with your voice tone with another person how you convey empathy. Friendliness. Warmth. Confidence. Blame. Belittling. Criticism. Saccharine Quality. Bravado.

10. How can communicating empathy help clients?

11. Provide examples of subtractive, basic, and additive empathy levels.

12. How do you like people to show respect for you? How do you show respect for others?

13. What do you think your physical appearance conveys to a client?

14. Show how you stand and sit when you are feeling comfortable with someone. Show how you stand and sit when you are feeling uncomfortable, guarded, or anxious with someone.

15. What distance is comfortable to you when working with clients? When counseling with them?

16. With various people in the room, practice establishing eye contact for about two seconds before you begin to speak and maintain good eye contact even when you are uncertain of what you are saying (e.g., while discussing the anatomy and physiology of respiration).

17. Based on where and how you were raised, how comfortable are you with professionals touching your head, neck, and face? Inside your mouth?

18. How consistent are you in your communication and interaction with clients? How well do you think they can predict what mood you will be in and how you will respond to them?

19. Describe an occasion where you talked "over" a child's level of understanding. What was his or her reaction? What did you do to repair your error?

20. What are some of the psychological terms you tend to use loosely to describe people? For example, do you use terms such as depressed, paranoid, and so forth?

21. Do you sometimes feel that negotiating means simply splitting the difference? How might you look at negotiating differently now?

22. Discuss a time when you had difficulty negotiating with someone? What would you do differently now?

Interviewing and Therapy Microskills

CHAPTER OUTLINE

- Introduction
- Counseling Microskills
- Questions
- Accurate Observations and Listening
- Selective Feedback
- Concluding Comments
- For Discussion

INTRODUCTION

Microskills is a term used in counseling psychology that refers to specific communication skills that help clinicians interact more intentionally with clients; that is, to thoughtfully but quickly choose responses to clients from a wide range of possibilities (Ivey, 1998). The assumption is that there is no one right therapeutic response to a person. The range of possible responses emerges from the clinician's assessment of the whole person and the situation.

Microskills form the foundation of interviewing and obtaining information throughout our interactions with clients and family members. Microskills are transtheoretical; that is, they are useful and necessary with any theoretical or therapeutic approach a therapist follows. Microskills have been considered technical skills used to understand how a client experiences and makes sense of his or her world. The intention is to gently enter the world of the client—seeking to understand the client through his or her perspective rather than our own. How is the client constructing his experiences and what sense is the client making of those experiences? From this understanding, the clinician and client can jointly search out new ways of helping the client think, feel, and behave with regard to the problems being experienced (Brock & Barnard, 1992; Corey, 2001; Ivey, 1998).

Within the broad heading of microskills are several general and specific skills, including verbal and nonverbal encouragers, asking questions, paraphrasing and reflections, clarifications, reframing or relabeling, interpretations, suggestions, and the use of silence. The clinician's process of learning and developing these skills follows much the same sequence that occurs in therapy with many of our clients. For example, a dysfluent client who is trying to become aware of, monitor, and then eliminate stuttering behaviors may follow this sequence:

1. Is made aware of a particular behavior by the therapist.
2. Becomes aware of the behavior after doing it.
3. Becomes aware of the behavior while doing it.
4. Becomes aware of the behavior before doing it but does it anyway.
5. Becomes aware of the behavior before doing it and intentionally does not do it.
6. Speaks naturally without the behavior.

As clinicians learn and develop microskills they often become self-conscious and aware of what they say, how they say it, and what they are doing with their bodies while talking with clients. Being aware of what you are doing can interfere with being natural. However, the rehearsal and practice of these skills helps them become integrated into the way you communicate with clients (and everyone else) and they become natural strategies for communicating.

COUNSELING MICROSKILLS

The following interviewing and therapy microskills are integrated from a variety of sources, including Brammer and MacDonald (1999), Burnard (1999), Corey (2001), DeJong and Berg (1998), Evens, Hearn, Uhleman, and Ivey (1993), George and Cristiani (1995), Gladding (2000), Hackney and Cormier (1999), Ivey (1998), Morrison (1995), Morrison and Anders (1999), Mosak and Maniacci (1998), Nystul (1999), Pipes and Davenport (1998), Shipley and McAfee (1998), Sommers-Flanagan and Sommers-Flanagan (1993), Wachtel (1993), and Zaro, Barach, Nedelman, and Dreiblatt (1995).

Verbal Encouragers

Verbal encouragers are prompts the therapist uses to try to elicit more information from the client, such as "Uh-huh," "Yes," "Ummm," and simple repetition of a word the client has said. When women are speaking with one another they tend to use many verbal encouragers, such as "OK" and "All right," which help them feel they are being listened to and understood. Men, however, may feel that when a female clinician says "OK" or "All right" she has heard all she wants or needs to hear about that topic and he should move on to something else. Therefore, an encourager for a woman may be a discourager for a man. During interviews and therapy we need to consider adjusting our verbal encouragers to the gender we are talking to.

Nonverbal encourages such as smiling, eye contact, leaning forward, open body posture, and nodding the head may be used alone or in conjunction with verbal encourages. It is important to appreciate how much our verbal and nonverbal encouragers influence the direction of the conversation. What we encourage we will likely hear more about, and what we do not encourage we will likely hear less about. However, excessive verbal or nonverbal encourages (e.g., excessive "Uh-huhs" or head nodding) can actually inhibit the client from talking. The use of too many encouragers can appear wooden and unnatural and the client may not see the clinician as genuine (Morrison, 1995).

"Therapist Noises"

"Therapist noises" is a term Wachtel (1993) discusses, and we as speech-language pathologists (SLPs) and audiologists need to be aware of these as well. One of the classic "noises" that clinicians might use when we do not know quite what to say (or do not want to say what we are really thinking) is, "That's interesting." "Interesting" is one of those words that seems to convey the neutrality that is believed to be the proper stance for clinicians to maintain. By commenting that the client's behavior or thought is interesting may seem that we are simply calling attention to it and, in a way, hoping that the client will also look at the behavior or thought in more depth and be curious about why it is "interesting." However, for most clients it is not too difficult to detect that the real message conveyed by our expression of "interest" is a form of subtle disapproval. Often there is a subliminal message in the phrase, such as "That's really weird," or "That's really stupid." We all have images of psychoanalysts in old movies saying to a person in a heavy Viennese accent, "Verrry interressting," which we know is not a compliment. As we do not want to sound rude, we merely comment that the idea or behavior is "interesting."

"Huhm" is a noise that can mean anything we want it to mean, and therefore really means nothing. There is usually some slight evaluative tone, either negative or positive, that goes with it. It is the tone that reflects the meaning.

Counselors, psychologists, and psychotherapists like to use the word *sense* in place of feel, feeling, thought, opinion, or idea. For example, "I have the sense that you are . . .," "It is my sense that . . .," "I sense that you are angry with . . .," and so forth. *Perhaps* is another word that therapists tend to use, for example, "Perhaps you're feeling a little such and such." *Perhaps* gives the client permission to disagree with the therapist's statement, although it tends to have a stilted quality to it compared to the more common and informal word, *maybe*.

When we are working with clients we tend to use words and phrases such as "That's interesting." "How did that make you feel?" and "Perhaps." We need to be careful about not overusing such words and phrases because they can begin to sound like cliches. They may boost the therapist's fragile sense of expertise but may not sound genuine to the client. If in doubt about what to say next, a moment of silence might sound more respectful than one of these overused phrases.

QUESTIONS

There are a variety of types of questions used in counseling which allow clinicians to understand clients and their families better. Clients, patients, and family members generally expect to be asked questions by a professional who is involved in helping them. Questions are essential tools in interviewing and counseling because they help focus the client or family on issues that need clarification and understanding. Understanding the person assists the SLP or audiologist to enter into the world of the client, that is, to understand the world through the client's perspective—how the client sees, hears, and feels the world. Understanding how the client makes sense of his or her experiences is one of the most important considerations for effective helping (Morrison, 1995; Ivey, 1998).

Asking questions of clients and families also can be therapeutic because it allows them to think about their situations and experiences in new or different ways, and helps them look deeper into their own thoughts and feelings, and, we hope, solve their own problems rather than expecting the clinician to solve them. Clinicians who have a more cognitive-behavioral orientation toward counseling are likely to use more questions than those with a person-centered orientation (Feltham & Dryden, 1993). Clinicians with a person-centered orientation also want to encourage clients to solve their difficulties but do not view the clinician's systematic questions as critical to this process. If the clinician feels that a client is becoming tangential with a response or moving in a direction that is not productive to the session, the clinician can use a question to redirect the focus and gain more control of the session.

Cautions When Asking Questions

The following section highlights some of the cautions emphasized by Ivey (1998) that need to be considered when asking questions.

BOMBARDMENT OR GRILLING

Too many questions may overwhelm clients and put them on the defensive. The person who asks the questions is usually in control of the interview or conversation. The questioner determines who talks, when, and about what. Too many questions may make clients feel controlled, manipulated, or criticized.

MULTIPLE QUESTIONS

If we ask several questions at once clients may become confused and not know which one to answer or how. It is better to ask a single question and then wait patiently for the person to respond, and, when the person appears to have finished responding, to wait a moment longer. This extra moment allows clients not to feel rushed and they may begin to add useful information that would not have been offered had the clinician rushed in too quickly with another question.

LEADING QUESTIONS (QUESTIONS AS STATEMENTS)

Clinicians sometimes try to make points or lead clients to the correct behaviors by being indirect, using a question rather than a declarative statement. Leading questions tend to encourage specific responses, which may differ from what the client truly feels. For example, "Based on what we have discussed, don't you think therapy would be helpful?" "Don't you think practicing your oral-motor exercises would help your speech be more intelligible?" "Wouldn't working on listening skills help your son feel less rushed when he is talking and maybe help his fluency?" "Would wearing your hearing aid help you enjoy social situations more fully?" Such leading questions or indirect statements tend to sound condescending, and there are more direct and respectful ways to communicate with clients. A general rule of thumb is that if you are going to make a statement, it is best not to frame it as a question.

Questions and Cultural Differences

WESTERN CULTURES

Western cultures tend to use rapid-fire questions more than some other cultures, which may be perceived by some cultures as aggressive or offensive. We need to be cautious about using rapid questioning with clients. This style of questioning can make clients feel interrogated instead of listened to.

MALE-FEMALE CULTURES

There is another kind of cultural difference that needs to be considered: male-female cultural differences. Ivey (1998) says that men tend to ask more questions than women. This gender difference has been interpreted as an indication that men may use questions to control their conversations. Tannen (2001) says that women tend to speak and hear a language of connection and intimacy, while men tend to speak and hear a language of status and independence. Such cross-cultural communication may affect the way men and women conduct interviews and the way male or female clients interpret them. In general, clinicians need to be aware of their choice of words, tone of voice, facial expressions, and body language when asking questions. Rapid-fire questioning with an intense facial expression and a closed body posture can sound and appear harsh and threatening during an interview. However, more relaxed questioning with a friendly facial expression and open body posture may sound and appear softer and more inviting.

Some female clients may perceive male clinicians, with their style of communicating competence and professionalism, as intimidating and insensitive. On the other hand, a female clinician who is striving to sound sensitive to a male client may be perceived as less competent than a female clinician who communicates in a more assertive manner. We do not want to ask questions of our clients as though we are walking on eggshells. Inexperienced clinicians often overestimate how fragile or vulnerable clients are, whereas clients often respect clinicians who are more direct and honest with them.

CHILDREN'S CULTURES

We may consider children as from a different culture and modify how we interview and counsel with them (Morrison & Anders, 1999). With children, a naturally warm, talkative clinician who likes and accepts them will be able to elicit more information more easily than a rather cold, reserved clinician who does not particularly enjoy children and their characteristic behaviors. (It is helpful to observe successful preschool and elementary school teachers' interactions with children to see how naturally they interact with, question, and instruct children.) The clinician should avoid looking down at children and talk to them as nearly as reasonable at their level—eye to eye. This may mean getting down on one or both knees, or sitting children in a higher chair than the one you sit in (try not to have children's feet dangling because that can be uncomfortable for them after a while).

It often helps to begin an interview or evaluation session with children by sharing something fun and interesting, such as games or toys. Children usually like to do something with their hands while talking, and having them draw a picture during the conversation can often be useful to therapists and may reveal salient events or feelings (Ivey, 1998). Clinicians should use short sentences, simple words, and a concrete style of language, avoiding abstractions. Use names rather than pronouns because children often get confused when under stress.

Closed Questions

Closed questions elicit a yes, no, or other very brief response and often include the words is, are, or do, for example, What *is* your name? How many children *do* you have? *Are* you able to be understood more easily now by your family? However, too many closed questions can seem like an interrogation to a person (Morrison, 1995). They also can inhibit the person from telling his story. We want to explore the person's experiences, not interrogate the person (Wachtel, 1993).

Open Questions (Probes)

Open questions are generally preferable to closed questions because they encourage longer and more expansive responses (Shipley & McAfee, 1998). Open questions do not elicit a particular response; that is, the SLP or audiologist cannot easily anticipate what the response will be. Open questions often use what are sometimes referred to as newspaper reporters questions, that is, who, what, when, where, and how. These are also referred to as "wh" questions. "Why" questions can be asked in a variety of ways without using the word "why," because that word often puts people on the defensive. Can, will, could and would questions are special types of open-ended questions.

Frequently the first word of an open-ended question helps direct the type of information that is sought. For example:

> *Who* questions provide information about people involved in a situation, e.g., "Who do you think is the easiest for you to talk to at home?" "Who do you think might be able to help you when you get home from the hospital?"

> *What* questions most often lead to factual information, for example, "What are some of your concerns about your speech?" "What did you do when the kids made fun of your speech?" "What happened next?" "What do you do when you can't understand your husband?"

When questions give information about time or sequences of events, for example, "When did you first notice your son's dysfluencies?" "When are you supposed to give your oral book report in front of the class?" "When is your appointment scheduled to see the ENT doctor?"

Where questions provide information about locations, for example, "Where does Hector spend most of his time when he is at home?" "Where do you sit in the classroom?" "Where in the hospital are you now?"

How questions often give "method" responses, that is, the client's thinking processes that illustrate his problem solving strategies, such as "How did you handle that situation with your teacher?" How questions also help us understand ways in which people's communication problems are affecting their lives, such as "How is your speech (voice, hearing, etc.) problem affecting your job?"

Why questions lead to reasons or causes, for example, "Why do you feel you are having more difficulty talking today than usual?" "Why do you think you have more difficulty with chewy foods than other textures of foods?" The word *why* suggests interrogation and a sense of disapproval. Why questions often put people on the defensive and cause discomfort because they may feel they are being attacked or criticized. Why questions require people to justify their ideas, thoughts, opinions, or actions, with the uncertainty that their reasoning and justification will be satisfactory to the person asking why. We can avoid asking why by reframing the question. Often times what questions work well, for example, "You seem to be having a little extra trouble talking today. What do you think is going on for you?" "The exercises I gave you may have been a little too hard for you right now. What do you think made them so hard?" *What* questions are typically perceived as friendlier and less judgmental than *why* questions.

Wachtel (1993) discusses the "art of gentle inquiry," meaning the ability to inquire into aspects of the client's experience and motivations, and to do so in a way that is minimally accusatory, judgmental, or damaging to the client's self-esteem. An example of a less-than-gentle inquiry is for a clinician to ask a client, "Why didn't you call to cancel our appointment?" while a more gentle inquiry would be, "You must have had some good reason for not calling to cancel our appointment" (spoken with an empathic tone). This statement invites the client to describe what is going on in her life, without feeling pressured or accused.

During an interview you may ask each of the "wh" questions in a variety of ways to obtain information. For example, early in an interview you may ask who referred the client to you, and late in the interview you may ask who might be supportive of the client to help with the therapy exercises at home. You may use two "wh" questions within a single question, for example, "What do the other children do when you are stuttering?" or "When you are stuttering, what do the other children do?" You can also make a declarative statement rather than using an interrogative to obtain information. For example, rather than asking, "What kinds of speech problems does your child have?" you can say, "Please describe your child's speech problems for me," or rather than asking, "What kinds of swallowing problems are you having?" you can say, "Tell me about the swallowing problems you are having."

During an interview or evaluation we want to answer as many of the "wh" questions as possible (Ivey, 1998). For example, we want to learn:

- *Who* is the client? What is the client's background? Who may be part of the support system for the client?

- *What* are the client's problems? What happened or is happening to the client? What are the specific details of the client's problems? What helps or hurts the client?

- *When* do the problems occur? When did the problems first begin? What precedes or follows when the problems occur?

- *Where* do the problems occur? In what environments and situations do the problems occur?

- *How* does the client react to the problems? How does the client feel about his/her problems? How do family members feel about the client's problems?

- *Why* do the problems occur? Why is the client having problems with speech, language, cognition, and/or swallowing? (Once again, the *why* question is in the clinician's mind, but the question that is asked is *what*.)

When you have information from or about the client, patient or family that answers the "wh" questions, then you have acquired much valuable information to help you understand the hearing, speech, language, cognitive, and swallowing problems of the people you are trying to help.

COUNSELING SKILLS IN ACTION:

An Interview with Miguel's Mother and Father

Miguel is a seven-year-old boy whom his parents have brought to you to evaluate his speech and language. You can use open-ended questions during your interview with the parents to obtain important history that will help you understand Miguel and the direction you will take in your assessment of him. Some of the questions you may want to ask are listed below (not necessarily in the order you may ask).

Please describe Miguel's speech for me.

What are some of the concerns you have about his speech?

When did you first become concerned about his speech development?

Continues on next page

Continued from previous page

Who first noticed or became concerned about Miguel's speech?

Has he been evaluated by another SLP?

Who evaluated him?

When did the evaluation take place?

What did you learn about the test results?

How long was Miguel seen by the other SLP?

What changes did you see in his speech while he was receiving therapy?

Who referred Miguel to this clinic?

What language is primarily spoken in the home?

How has his speech changed over time?

When does he have the most difficulty being understood?

In your family, whom do you think is easiest for Miguel to talk to?

Whom do you think is hardest for him to talk to?

In your family, who understands Miguel best?

Who has the most difficulty understanding him?

What do his brothers and sisters do when they cannot understand Miguel?

Where does Miguel like to spend his time when he is at home?

Where does he like to spend his time when he is not at school or home?

What have you tried to do at home to help Miguel improve his speech?

What do you hope will come out of my evaluation of Miguel?

(*Note*: Various questions about the child's language, educational experience, etc. would also be asked.)

During your interview and evaluation of Miguel you also ask many open-ended questions to better understand how he understands and views his speech problem. When interviewing children the questions are often interspersed throughout the evaluation and not necessarily in a formal interview format. Some of the questions you may want to ask are listed below (not necessarily in the order you may ask).

Miguel, what do you think is the reason your parents brought you here today?

What kinds of problems do you think you might have when talking?

In your family, who is most concerned about your speech?

Continues on next page

Continued from previous page

Who talks to you the most about your speech?

Tell me about what the other speech therapist did when she was working with you.

What language do you speak most often when you are at home?

Who at your home has the most difficulty understanding you?

Who understands you the best?

Where do you like to spend your time when you are at home?

What do your brothers and sisters do when they can't understand you?

Who do you like to play with the most when you are home?

Who are your best friends when you play in your neighborhood?

Where do you like to spend your time when you are not at home or school?

What does your teacher do if she can't understand you?

What do the other kids at school do when they can't understand you?

What do you think has helped you most with your speech?

What would you like me to do to help you?

Can, will, could and *would* questions are regarded as the most open-ended kind of questions because they may be considered by the person being questioned as either a closed question or a very open question. Because clients can respond either way they are sometimes called "swing questions" (Sommers-Flanagan & Sommers-Flanagan, 1993). Can and could actually ask if the person has the ability to do something, although both the person asking the question and the person answering the question usually interpret it as a choice question, much like will or would. For example, "Could you tell me about the problems you are having with your speech?" (A male therapist may want to ask, "Could you tell me a little about . . .?" The "a little" is intended to soften the request and is less threatening than asking the person to tell you "(all) about" the problems. "Can you say more about that? "Could you tell me (a little) about how people are responding to your new esophageal voice?" or "Would you tell me (a little) about how the kids at school are responding to your new hearing aids?" Depending on whether you are a female or male clinician, you may want to calibrate your style of questioning. Male clinicians may want to temper their questions to sound more gentle and less intimidating, while female clinicians may want to focus on being more direct and assertive.

As a closed question a client may respond to a can, will, could or would question with a "No, I don't want to talk about that." The better the rapport though, the more likely the client will respond as if it were an open question and present a narrative or elaboration of his or her experiences.

However, can, will, could or would may also be used as an open question to obtain specific or concrete information, for example, "Can you give me a specific example of . . .?" "Would you show me exactly what you do with your mouth when . . ."?

We can use open questions about content (e.g., experiences) to understand the client's meanings. For example:

"What does that mean to you?"

"What sense do you make of it?"

"That sounds very important to you. Can you tell me about that?"

"What are some reasons you think that may be happening?"

Children may have difficulty with general open questions such as, "Could you tell me about your speech?" or "What do you think is causing your difficulty talking?" It is helpful to break down such abstract questions into concrete and situational language using a mix of closed and open questions, for example, "When you are talking to your teacher, is your stuttering worse or better than when you are talking to other adults?" "Do some of the kids at school tease you about the way you talk?" "What do you tell the other kids about why you can't yell on the playground like you used to?"

Open questions can be rephrased in a manner that produces a closed question (Sommers-Flanagan & Sommers-Flanagan, 1993). However, when using an open question as a closed question it can sound confrontational (Burnard, 1999). Compare the four sets of questions below:

A. "How are you feeling about the therapy for your stuttering?"

B. "Are you feeling all right about the therapy for your stuttering?"

A. "What did you do when the kids made fun of your speech?"

B. "Did you get angry or embarrassed when the kids made fun of your speech?"

A. "What was it like to use your new lower voice pitch after having the falsetto voice for so long?"

B. "Did you feel more like a young man with your new lower voice pitch after having a falsetto voice for so long?"

A. "How do you feel?"

B. "Do you feel angry?"

With some clients, a closed question may facilitate a dialogue or their recollections of an experience. In other situations clients may feel it is a forced-choice question and may be reluctant to respond, or respond with the answer they think we want to hear. For example, if a SLP asks a client whether the exercises are improving his or her speech, the client may feel compelled to answer in the affirmative to please the therapist and perhaps convey that the SLP is doing a good job. If the SLP senses that the client's response represents an effort to please, she may inquire further and ask for elaboration on the changes or improvements that the client is seeing.

Other questions may be used in order to encourage the client to think about the future and its possibilities. These questions can result in clients beginning to make changes that will help them with their communication problems. The "miracle question" or "The question" is one example of a question used by counselors (Mosak & Maniacci, 1998), and it can be phrased many ways. For example, "Imagine that you wake up one morning and a miracle has happened; you no longer stutter. What would you do differently with your life if that happened?" "Pretend that I could wave a magic wand and make a miracle happen; your cleft lip is perfectly formed and your speech is perfect. How would your life be different?" The purpose of the miracle question is to see how the person would think, feel, or act if there were no problem. A follow-up question after the person has described how life would be if the "miracle" happened might be the following, "What can you do to start doing or getting some of those things to make your life different?" The purpose of the follow-up question is to help the person focus on what he or she can begin to do that will make the differences happen, whether or not the problem is completely resolved.

The "What would you do if . . .?" question is similar to the miracle question in that it attempts to have the client project, hypothetically, what he would do differently if circumstances were different or a particular situation arose. The question should be used to encourage the client to consider life if his symptoms were diminished or eliminated. This may plant a seed of hope or motivation to work on the current therapeutic tasks. For example, the following questions may help the client reflect on the current situation and how it may affect the future: "What will you do differently in your life once your stuttering is diminished?" "What would you do if your child was not able to function successfully in a regular classroom environment?" "What would you do if you were not able to return to your previous line of work?"

It is helpful with some clients, patients, or family members to ask, "What wouldn't you change about yourself or the situation? What would you want to keep the same because you are happy with it?" Such questions help people focus upon the positives in their lives. There is also a subtle secondary implication, that is, they *are* going to change. They are in control of what they want to work on and, we are hopeful, will change (Mosak & Maniacci, 1998).

Funneling Questions

Funneling refers to using questions to guide the conversation from general to specific. The conversation starts with broad, open questions and then, slowly, more specific questions are asked to focus the discussion. Open questions may be used throughout, but the content is increasingly narrowed (funneled). Funneling questions are particularly helpful during an interview. For example,

> Clinician: "How can I help you?"
>
> Client: "I'm having trouble with my speech."
>
> Clinician: "What kind of trouble are you having?"
>
> Client: "My boss thinks I get tangled up with my words sometimes."

Clinician: "What do you mean by tangled up?"

Client: "I'm having more trouble talking to customers on the phone than I used to."

Clinician: "What happens when you have trouble talking on the phone?"

Client: "I have a hard time getting my words started."

Clinician: "Can you show me what you do when you have a hard time getting your words started?"

Funneling questions can be used at any time in therapy to better understand specifics about a client's experience. For example, a fourth grade child who stutters:

Clinician: "You seem a little upset at the moment. Can you tell me what's happening?

Client: "My teacher?"

Clinician: "What about your teacher?"

Client: "She made me read in front of the class again."

Clinician: "How did you feel about that?"

Client: "Embarrassed."

Clinician: "Do you think working on your reading some in here will help so you are not so embarrassed in front of the class?

Client: "If you think it'll help."

Clinician: "It could."

Another example, an elderly patient in a convalescent hospital:

Clinician: "Mr. Williams, you seem a little upset today. Can you tell me what's happening?

Client: "My family."

Clinician: "What about your family?"

Patient: "I feel like they have abandoned me."

Therapist: "How often are they visiting you now?"

Patient: "Just a couple of times a month."

Therapist: "What do you think might be causing them to visit you less often?"

Patient: "I don't think they like seeing me getting old."

Funneling questions can help the clinician and the client focus on specific problems rather than broad generalities. Counselors and psychotherapists sometimes use the concept of the abstraction ladder (Ivey, 1998). If you or the client are too high on the abstraction ladder, there is more difficulty finding solutions to problems. The funneling or narrowing of the focus can often help clients recognize that their communication problem is comprised of several or many smaller problems, and the smaller problems are less overwhelming and more manageable than a global problem. Funneling questions also allow the clinician to determine specific needs of the client and ways to provide therapy and measure progress using functional goals.

Requests for Clarification (Checking for Understanding)

Sometimes a client or family member sounds a little confused and the clinician is left wondering just what the person is trying to say. It can be very important to ask for clarification at these times rather than guessing or making erroneous assumptions. Requesting clarification or checking for understanding involves either 1) asking the client if you understood him or her correctly, or 2) occasionally summarizing the conversation in order to clarify or confirm what has been said. It is wiser for a clinician to ask the client for clarification than to be confused or misinterpret the client's messages. The request for clarification asks the client to repeat or rephrase what she or he has said. For example:

"Let me try to clarify. You're saying that . . ."

"Could you try to describe what happened again? I'm not sure I'm understanding."

"When you say that your throat feels funny, what does that mean?"

"I think I got lost in that. Could you go through the sequence of events again?"

"Let me see if I can sum up what we have talked about so far."

After you have summarized what you think the client has said, it is helpful to ask the client if what you have said is accurate.

Requests for clarification help the clinician increase his or her accuracy of information and understanding. If a clinician is not attending and verbally tracking the client well, requests for clarification will need to be more frequent. However, if requests for clarification occur too frequently, the client may sense that the clinician is not attending to what he or she is saying or is not particularly interested in the client's information.

Comparison Questions

When clients complain about symptoms (e.g., vocal hoarseness, dysfluency, difficulty being understood, swallowing, etc.), the clinician typically needs more specifics about times and conditions when the symptoms occur. Comparison questions can be very useful to discover the factors that either exacerbate or alleviate the client's symptoms. Comparison questions tend to use phrases such as better or worse, more or less, hardest and easiest, this situation or that situation, with this person or that person. The clinician is presenting forced-choice polarities that can, over time, be further refined. Obtaining this information can help the clinician discover the patterns of symptoms and behaviors and develop an appropriate therapy strategy, including a hierarchy of difficulty.

Some examples of comparison questions:

"Is your speech more nasal when you are rested or when you are tired?"

"Is it easier to talk to your mother or your father?"

"Is your voice more hoarse in the morning or the afternoon?"

"Do you choke more on regular foods or ground-up foods?

Comparison questions are much like what an optometrist or ophthalmologist uses during an eye examination when he asks, "Can you see better with A or B?" There is a refining of information to determine as closely as possible the client's experience. Ultimately, the comparison questions are trying to answer more specifically the "wh" questions of who, what, when, where, and how.

Counterquestions

When someone asks us a question, we are conditioned to answer it. However, in counseling it is often more revealing if we ask a question in return. Luterman (2001) says that clients sometimes seek confirmation of a position or a decision they have already made, or they ask the clinician questions for which they already know the answers. The counterquestion allows the client to reveal his position or decision so that the clinician does not have to agree or disagree with him. Illuminating the client's thoughts and feelings is more productive and therapeutic than the clinician's sharing of opinions. For example:

Client: (mother of an 8-year-old child): Michael is starting to have a lot of trouble in school because the kids can't understand him. I'm not sure if talking to his teacher would help. What do you think?"

Clinician: "What are your thoughts about approaching his teacher?" (The mother's "hidden agenda" was to have the therapist talk to her son's teacher.)

Another example:

Adult voice client: "I am trying to decide how much longer I should continue therapy. What do you think?"

Clinician: "How much longer would you like to continue therapy?" (The client clearly had some idea about when she wanted to terminate therapy.)

Counterquestions are important tools to understand a client's thoughts and feelings, and for the clinician to avoid being hooked into answering a question the client may already have made a decision about. Counterquestions, however, if used too frequently can become frustrating to a client and the clinician may appear to be playing therapy games, that is, trying to play the role of a counselor or psychologist who avoids answering questions directly.

Keep in mind that clients may ask counterquestion themselves, and one we need to be particularly prepared for is, "Why did you ask that question?" or "Why do you need that information?"

Clinicians' questions about client relationships (e.g., parenting styles and a child's dysfluency, or coworkers and a client's voice disorder) may elicit a counterquestion from a client. The client may not understand the relevance of certain questions and the clinician needs to be prepared to explain the relevance in a calm, nondefensive manner. For example,

> Client: "Why are you asking me about my relationships at work?"
>
> Clinician: "I'm wondering when you are more stressed and if you notice a change in your voice at those times."

Counterquestions from a client may surprise an SLP and sound suspicious of the clinician's need to know certain information. Once again, responding in a calm, nondefensive manner to a client's counterquestion may not only provide the clinician with the information she is looking for, but may also strengthen the client/clinician relationship.

Counseling Counselors

On several occasions over the past 25-plus years in private practice I have had clients who themselves have been counselors, psychologists, or Marriage-Family-Child Counselors, or had a parent who was one of these professionals. During interviews and therapy with these professionals, or the children of these professionals, counterquestions from the client appeared to occur more frequently than with other clients. It was particularly important for me to maintain a nondefensive stance when responding to their questions.

Broken Record

Broken record is a technique of repeating a word or statement until you get the person's attention, or asking the same question over (and over) again with the same loudness and voice tone until the person answers that question. (Young children learn to use this technique automatically, like a four-year-old who says, "Mommy [pause] mommy [pause] mommy," and the mother says, "Huh? Did you say something?") Clinicians may use this technique when a client does not respond to a question that the clinician feels is important, for example:

> Clinician: "When are you going to schedule an appointment with the ENT doctor?"
>
> Client: "I'm really busy at work and have a lot of projects going."
>
> Clinician: "When are you going to schedule an appointment with the ENT doctor?"
>
> Client: "I can call this afternoon and try to get an appointment this week."

Broken record questions do not let the client off the hook until the clinician is satisfied with his response. This technique also may be useful if the client loses attention, concentration, and focus easily.

ACCURATE OBSERVATIONS AND LISTENING

In addition to asking questions, clinicians may also employ other useful techniques in order to ensure that they have understood their clients and their families. These techniques include: paraphrasing, reflections, and the appropriate use of silence. These techniques can help clients to feel that you are interested in them, want to better understand their difficulties, and are treating them as individuals rather than as symptom or disease categories. They are particularly useful in encouraging the client to expand their "story."

Paraphrasing

The primary purpose of paraphrasing is to assure clients that you have accurately heard the central meaning of their messages, and secondarily to allow clients to hear how someone else perceives them (Sommers-Flanagan & Sommers-Flanagan, 1993). Paraphrasing may also be used in an effort to keep clients focused on a particular content area. The clinician attempts to accurately and briefly reflect or rephrase the essence of what the client has said. It does not mean the SLP or audiologist tries to change, modify, or add to what the client has said. Clients typically perceive paraphrases or reflections as empathic responses to their communications. Once clients feel they have been heard, they are often able to expand on the experience they are describing or to move on to new topics.

Sommers-Flanagan & Sommers-Flanagan (1993) discuss several types of paraphrases, including generic, sensory-based, and metaphorical.

GENERIC PARAPHRASES

Generic paraphrases simply rephrase, reword, and reflect what the client just said. For example:

Client (8-year-old child with articulation problems): "I really love my teacher because she is always so nice to me and never teases me about my speech."
Clinician: "You're really fond of her and it's nice to know some people who don't tease you about the way you talk."

Client (10-year-old child with auditory processing problems): "I just hate my classroom because the teacher doesn't keep the kids quiet, and I can't understand what she's talking about!"
Clinician: "The classroom is noisy and that makes it really hard for you to understand what your teacher is saying."

Client (27-year-old TBI patient): "I can't pay attention to my work like I used to, and using machinist tools is dangerous."

Clinician: "Paying close attention to your tools is important for your safety on the job, and that's more difficult for you now."

The generic paraphrase retains the essence of what was said and does not include an evaluation from the clinician (e.g., opinion, reaction, or commentary, whether positive or negative).

SENSORY-BASED PARAPHRASES

Sensory-based paraphrases require the SLP or audiologist to be aware of the client's preferred sensory system to perceive the world (visual, auditory, or kinesthetic). The concept of individual verbal style is based on educational theory that posits that children have different learning styles (Ivey, 1998; Taylor, 2001). Some children learn best visually, others auditorally, and others tactile or kinesthetically. Apparently these learning styles continue through adult life and are illustrated by individual language usage. Some examples of sensory-based words are shown in Table 4-1.

TABLE 4-1	SENSORY-BASED WORDS	
VISUAL	**AUDITORY**	**KINESTHETIC**
see	hear	feel
looks	sounds	touches
visualize	in tune	in touch
imagine	rings a bell	handle that
sunny	quiet	warm

By listening closely to the words clients use to describe their experiences you will notice that some clients rely primarily on visually oriented words (such as, "I see what you're saying", "It looks like", or "I can see that"). Some clients rely on auditory words (e.g., "I hear what you're saying" or "it sounded like"), and others on kinesthetic words (e.g., "I feel" or "It really touched me").

Many of the idioms in our language have a sensory system reference, particularly tactile sensory, for example, ahead of the game, his bark is worse than his bite, beat around the bush, he'll come around, drop out, fall through, feel like a million, gain ground, hammer away, hit the ceiling, in the running, join forces, keep your chin up, labor of love, off balance, out of place, pass the buck, pitch in, pull through, ride it out, scratch the surface, shot in the arm, a throw away remark, tie down, up in the air, wear thin, you said it, and so forth. By being aware of and using clients' preferred sensory systems when paraphrasing or giving feedback, greater rapport may be established and maintained because clients may feel that you are tuned in to them. For example:

Client (18-year-old patient with a TBI): "I *feel* like I can never do anything again. Going to college now is going to be really *tough*. I *feel* lost."

Clinician: "I can understand why you *feel* that way. Yes, college could be *tough*, but with extra help and taking it slow, I expect you will be able to *work your way through*."

Client (42-year-old woman with vocal nodules): "I can almost *hear* what people in the office are *saying* behind my back about my hoarse voice now. And the subtle messages I get from my boss *sound* to me like if I can't have a normal voice with customers, he is going to put me in the back office."

Clinician: "It *sounds* like there is a lot of pressure on your job to get your voice better pretty fast."

Client (72-year-old wife of a patient with a CVA): "I can't *see* how all this work on George's memory is going to help him remember the things he needs to at home."

Clinician: "It is difficult to *see* sometimes how working on some things in therapy will have a direct affect on what you *see* George doing at home."

Clinicians need to be aware of their own preferred sensory modality and not to limit their sensory-based paraphrases to the modality that they favor. To make your counseling as meaningful as possible, it is helpful to use all sensory modalities and not limit yourself to just the primary modality the client tends to use. For example, "Can you *picture* yourself talking easily? How would it *feel*? What would it *sound* like?"

METAPHORICAL PARAPHRASES

Metaphorical paraphrases are language that refers to visual, auditory, or tactile experiences or feelings that have an implied comparison to something else. Metaphors can help establish a relationship between the client's somewhat abstract feelings or experiences and more concrete images. An accurate metaphor may also be a vivid reminder and motivator the next time the client is in a similar situation. Metaphorical paraphrases may require some creativity on the part of SLPs and audiologists. Some clients use rather colorful metaphors to describe their problems.

Using Metaphors in Therapy

A 43-year-old woman I worked with was diagnosed by an otolaryngologist as having muscular tension dysphonia. She tended to change subjects very rapidly in her conversation and was very animated, but she described herself as "like a turtle in mud." She responded well to metaphors that were both visual and tactile, one of which was that she reminded me of a

Continues on next page

Continued from previous page

racehorse rider who kept changing horses in the middle of a race, and each horse rode a little differently, but she never stayed on one horse long enough to get a real feel for it. The client liked this metaphor and thought about it frequently in her conversations outside of therapy. As therapy progressed she recognized that she was "staying on one horse longer" in a conversation, and eventually "rode one horse all the way to the finish (the end of a topic of conversation)." She also had decreased her overall tension and had a more relaxed sounding voice.

Another client I saw related to the classic metaphor of how we all wear different hats depending on where we are and what we are doing. However, I added to the metaphor by saying that the hats all have brims and the brims on our hats overlap with other brims, meaning that even though we wear different hats part of us is still interconnected with everything else we do in life.

Some classic metaphors therapists have used include: "Therapy is a tough row to hoe." "We can't expect smooth sailing all the time." "Everybody in your family says they are going to pitch in to help you." "In therapy I am going to be your coach, but you have to run the plays." "The ball is in your court now. You need to decide what you are going to do." It is important to notice which metaphors resonate with a client, and not to continue with a metaphor the client does not find useful. For example, a woman may not respond to a sport or military metaphor, and a man may not respond to a cooking metaphor. Clinicians, however, need to be aware of not stereotyping male or female clients by the metaphors they use or choose not to use in therapy.

A metaphor borrowed from Family Therapy (Brock and Barnard, 1992) that helps family members understand how changes in one family member affect in some way other family members is the use of a mobile. The therapist may hold up a mobile with various figures hanging from it. The therapist might say that families are like a mobile because everyone is connected, and when someone in a family changes, everyone else adjusts or changes too, with some members changing more than others. This particular metaphor (with or without the mobile in hand) is useful when counseling the parents of a child who stutters. The parents get the clear message that changes they make in their attitudes and behaviors toward their child can have a significant and positive affect on his dysfluency.

Reflection ("Echoing")

Reflection is the process of reflecting back the last few words the client has said in order to encourage her or him to say more (Burnard, 1999). It is as though the clinician is echoing the client's thoughts and the echoing serves as a prompt. The clinician should not be deterred from using occasional reflections for fear of being impolite by "talking over" or interrupting the person. The reflection should not turn into a question, and this can be avoided by making the repetition in much the same tone of voice as the client used, for example,

> Wife of a patient: "My husband was doing fine after the stroke, until our oldest son moved back home with us . . . "
>
> Clinician: "He moved back home . . . "
>
> Wife: "Yes. My husband and our oldest son have never gotten along well, and then when he moved back home last month after he lost his job, it just brought back all the old bad stuff and my husband started being angry a lot again."
>
> Clinician: "Your husband is angry recently . . . "
>
> Wife: "Yes, when he gets angry now he has a lot harder time talking than he did before the stroke."

Reflections serve to help the client say more, to develop the story. However, reflections need to be unobtrusive to the client and sound much like normal conversational interaction. If reflections are overused or used awkwardly, they can be noticeable to the client or sound stilted.

Selective Reflection (Restatement)

Selective reflection is repeating back to the client a part of something she or he said that was emphasized or seemed to be emotionally charged. Selective reflection may draw from the middle of the person's statement and not from the end. The use of selective reflection allows the clinician to develop further an idea that was embedded in the client's statement. Often these phrases have some important substance that can help the clinician better understand what is going on. However, if the clinician uses too many selective reflections there is a "parrot-like" effect that can be very annoying to the client. For example:

> Mother of an 8-year-old boy: "Jerome's stuttering had been getting better for the last few months, then something happened at school with his teacher and his stuttering started getting worse again."
>
> Clinician: "Something happened at school with his teacher . . ."
>
> Mother: "Yes. I never felt that the teacher really liked Jerome, and then when he got in some trouble it just gave her the chance to really come down on him."

The clinician needs to be willing to interject a selective reflection at the moment it appears most valuable and not wait until there is a break or lull in the conversation, because by that time the reflection may seem untimely or irrelevant.

Reflection of Feeling

Reflection of feeling is a paraphrased response of a feeling communicated by the client either verbally or nonverbally. When you reflect feelings, you add to the paraphrase those affective or feeling words that are in tune with the client's emotional experience. The clinician is making a statement to the client that indicates that he or she has understood the feeling the client is experiencing. Burnard (1999) refers to this as "empathy building." In reflecting feelings, the clinician must be alert to the affective state of the client regardless of the words being spoken. A certain intuitive ability is needed with reflection of feeling because these clinician observations and interpretations often refer to what is implied rather than what is overtly stated by the client (Scheuerle, 1992).

The phrasing for reflection of feelings is important. Certain phrases have been so overused that clients who hear them from therapists (or actors playing therapists on television) may think them comical stereotypes, for example, "I hear you saying . . . " "It feels like . . . " To effectively use reflection of feeling it is helpful to include the client's name and the pronoun *you* to soften and personalize the reflection (an empathic tone of voice is, of course, crucial as well), for example, "*Carlos*, it looks like *you* are . . ." Using the present tense tends to be more helpful than reflection using the past tense, for example, "Carlos, it looks like you *are* . . . " Providing a feeling or emotion word gives a term the client may be able to identify with, for example, "Carlos, it looks like you are *happy* about . . . " Presenting a context for the feeling provides a reference for your reflection, for example, "Carlos, it looks like you are happy *now about getting* the 's' sound." Finally, checking out your observation and reflection lets you know if you are accurate, for example, "Carlos, it looks like you are happy now about getting the 's' sound. *What do you think?*" A different kind of example could be, "*Monique, you look* a little *discouraged* about *therapy. Am I reading that right?*"

Other examples of a reflection of feeling:

> An adult patient with apraxia : "I never used to swear at all before my stroke, and now I swear all the $&! #@%! time. But it really bothers me most in front of women, so I avoid them."
>
> Clinician: "Frank, you are particularly uncomfortable around women for fear of swearing, and you're afraid that both you and they will be embarrassed. Is that about right?"
>
> Patient: #@%! straight!

Another example:

> Child with a repaired cleft lip and palate: "Kids still tease me at school about how I look and my speech, so I just avoid everybody and play by myself."
>
> Clinician: "Michelle, you have been hurt a lot by kids and are trying to avoid getting hurt any more. Is that what's happening?"
>
> Child: "Yeah. It just isn't worth trying to talk and have them make fun of me."

When reflecting a client's feelings, clinicians should attempt to understand not only their feelings but also whether the feelings are positive or negative and the strength of the feelings, for example, "Jose, you look *really* excited about the field trip! Are you?" "Mr. Perez, you look *very* worried about how your wife is going to do in therapy. Can you tell me about your concerns?" English

(2002b) and Schow and Nerbonne (2002) say that reflecting feelings can be particularly important with children with hearing losses because they often lack the practice in labeling a feeling with a word. Children with impaired hearing often have weaker vocabularies than other children, including words to describe feelings. Therefore, the audiologist or SLP can be helpful to the child by providing a word that can be used to describe the child's feelings. An audiologist might say, for example, "You look frustrated. Are you having some difficulty understanding your teacher?" or, "You sound kind of confused about whether or not you want to wear your new hearing aids to school."

It is important to remember that not all people will appreciate or welcome your noting their feelings. Clients tend to disclose feelings only after rapport and trust have been developed. Less verbal clients may find reflection puzzling at times or may say, for instance, "Of course, I'm angry! How do you think I would feel?" If the clinician does not know or understand the client well, she runs the risk of reflecting back feelings that are not actually the client's. For example,

> Clinician: "Mr. Herrera, you seem to be holding up well managing the children at home since your wife's accident."
>
> Mr. Herrera: "I am *not* doing nearly as well as you think I am."

Such inaccurate reflection may affect how sensitive or tuned in the client or family member feels the clinician is about the problems they are facing.

Clinicians also need to be cautious about not projecting their own feelings into the situation and reflecting those to the client (Ivey, 1998). In other words, your reflection should be based upon your attempt to read the client's body language or facial expression. Your reflection should not simply represent what your reaction would be to a similar event. For example, "Mr. Washington, I'm sorry about your father's stroke. I know how you feel. I went through the same thing with my father recently." or "Mrs. Schwartz, I know how I would feel if my daughter were injured like that, and I'm sure you feel the same way too." These responses are problematic because the clinicians are assuming that the clients' emotional responses are similar to their own.

Silence

Silence is an important component of any therapeutic relationship. The primary function of silence as an interviewer or therapist response is to encourage the client to talk or to have time to reflect about what has just been discussed (Hackney & Cormier, 1999; Ivey, 1998; Sommers-Flanagan & Sommers-Flanagan, 1993). Silence enables the person to "hear" what has been said, to hear the deeper meaning beyond the words. Silence enables the client to make associations and connections, and to engage in self-evaluation and problem solving. It is important that the clinician not interfere with this reflection time by being uncomfortable and speaking. Clinicians often have to work on their ability to tolerate silence.

Many clinicians are initially uncomfortable with silence during an interview or therapy, thinking that it requires an ongoing flow of speech from either the client or the clinician. Clients themselves are often uncomfortable with silence as well. Sometimes the clinician does not know what to say to the client and an awkward silence occurs (most experienced therapists will admit that they do not always know what to say to a client either). It takes some confidence to sit in silence for a few moments. The silence can give both parties a chance to digest what has been discussed or to formulate ideas for further discussion.

A Long Silence

I had worked a few sessions with a 19-year-old young man who was severely dysfluent. I met with him in my home on a once-a-week basis and his father, a plastic surgeon, often attended the sessions. The client sat to my left in a comfortable chair and the father sat to my right out of view from his son when the young fellow was looking at me. The client tended to have very long silent "blocks", and he used a variety of secondary behaviors to eventually end the silent periods. He had been working on improving his eye contact during his stuttering moments and was getting quite adept at this. Part of the therapy focused on learning to not use his secondary behaviors and to stay with the moment of stuttering. On one occasion the client began a statement and moved quickly into a tense, silent block. I felt this was going to be a long silent period, quickly noted the time, and sat perfectly still, maintaining eye contact with him, rarely blinking. He did the same with his eyes. Ten minutes later, without using any secondary behaviors, the client said the word he wanted. He was very proud of himself and this was a turning point in his therapy. The father later told me how uncomfortable and anxious he was during his son's long silent block, but that he also was proud of him for not using his old stuttering behaviors.

When supervising students in diagnostic and clinical practica, emphasis is placed on learning to ask a question during an interview or therapy session and then sitting quietly and waiting for a response, and after the client or family member has finished responding, to wait a moment longer before speaking again. This extra moment often gives the client or family member time to add information that would not have been included had the student made too quick an interjection.

Silence from the audiologist or SLP after a client or family member makes a statement or observation can encourage the person to voluntarily say more without the need for a question or request for more information. Looking expectantly but calmly at the client will likely encourage him or her to fill in the silence with words—frequently valuable words. What could be a constructive silence is easily ruined by too quick of a verbal (or even nonverbal) response from the clinician. Sometimes just a shift of your posture or an inadvertent cough can interfere with the moment.

If, however, the clinician feels the client's silence is a form of resistance and a game to see if he can outlast the clinician, it may be appropriate to ask the client what he is doing or thinking. If the client is not forthcoming, the clinician may wonder aloud if they have touched on a topic that makes the client feel uncomfortable. For example, "I'm wondering if talking about friendships is an uncomfortable topic for you." or "I'm wondering if some of the difficulty on your job that you mentioned is becoming too uncomfortable to talk about."

SELECTIVE FEEDBACK

Providing selective feedback is a more advanced interviewing skill which involves the clinician's attempt to influence how the client views himself, his problem, or his circumstances. Here, the clinician does not simply rely upon the client's viewpoint or appraisal of the situation but tries to introduce a new, more positive interpretation that will potentially lead to positive feelings and actions on the part of the client. Misuse of these techniques, however, can sound as though the clinician is minimizing the client's problems. Clinicians need to gauge carefully what feedback a particular client is ready to hear. Types of selective feedback include: reframing or relabeling, normalizing, suggestion, and confronting.

Reframing or Relabeling

Reframing or relabeling (Hoffman, 1981 & 2002; Watzlawick, Weakland, & Fisch, 1974) is a technique that presents the client with a new frame of reference through which to view the problem and, we hope, better understand and manage the situation or problem. The facts of the situation or problem may be unchangeable (e.g., the head injury did happen), but how the person perceives the facts and talks about them to him or herself and others influences the person's feelings, thoughts and behaviors. Clients have a choice of how they view themselves. By focusing upon the negative they discourage themselves; by focusing on the positive and considering failure a part of life, they can encourage themselves. One has the choice to learn from failure or to suffer from it (Mosak & Maniacci, 1998, p. 77).

Relabeling a behavior or situation means putting it into a new, more positive perspective, for example, a resistant child is an independent child; a stubborn child is a determined child; an angry person is a fearful person; a rigid person is a structured person; a difficult situation is a situation that may have some potent lessons. By changing the label of some key words, clients and families may begin to change their attitudes and feelings about a person or situation. The clinician may introduce the new descriptor, but the client or family members must begin to use it to incorporate it into their way of talking (and eventually thinking) about a person or problem. However, the clinician needs to be cautious not to sound like a Pollyanna or trivialize the problems. The word "challenge" is now often substituted for the words problems, difficulties, impairments, handicaps, disorders, and disabilities. Some clients, patients, and family members may feel that the word challenge to describe their situation or hardship indicates that the clinician is minimizing or unaware of the complexities or magnitude of the hardships they are facing. Such feelings may negatively affect the client-clinician relationship. In addition, clinicians who use reframing and relabeling too frequently or inappropriately may be seen as using a sophisticated form of invalidating a person's thoughts, ideas, opinions, feelings, or knowledge.

Family counselors sometimes use the concept of "bad—sad" (Brock and Barnard, 1992). If a family member identifies another member's problem behavior in terms that might be called "bad," for example, resistant, angry, unmotivated, lazy, and so forth, the clinician might reframe the behavior as possibly being the result of "sad" feelings, for example, fearful, lonely, isolated, or depressed. This shift in the family's perceptions of the problem behavior may be valuable for introducing greater flexibility in thinking about the behavior and increased empathy toward the person.

Reframing or relabeling may follow a 1-2-3 pattern of attending carefully to the client's frame of reference, providing the reframing/relabeling, and then checking out the client's reactions to the new frame of reference (e.g., "How does that idea sound to you?"). If the client does not agree or like the reframing/relabeling, the clinician can use this feedback from the client to develop another, more meaningful response. Reframes may be met initially with denial, but the process of having clients view their problems in a new or different way may promote flexibility in their perceptions or actions (Sommers-Flanagan & Sommers-Flanagan, 1993). Luterman (2001), for example, likes to reframe mistakes as "nuggets of gold" where the person learned something valuable (p. 95).

Some examples of reframing or relabeling are as follows:

> Client (18-year-old girl with hypernasal speech and a repaired bilateral cleft lip and palate): "The doctors told me that I will always have scars on my lip. I have never had a date and no one thinks I'm pretty."
>
> Clinician: "It will be very important for you to find somebody special and when you do you will know he loves you for who you really are."
>
> Client (45-year-old man with a CVA): "I never liked the work I used to do, and now I can't even do that."
>
> Clinician: "This might be an opportunity to find a different kind of work that you like better. (Pause.) How does that idea sound to you?"

Clinicians may want to experiment with reframing and relabeling "challenges" in their own lives to get a sense of how this technique can affect their thinking and approaches to viewing and solving professional or personal problems. For example, a difficult supervisor may be one from whom you can learn some important lessons, even lessons about how *not* to do some things. A family crisis may become the impetus to make some changes in the way things are done at home.

Normalizing

Normalizing is a special form of reframing or relabeling. It is an attempt to help people recognize and accept that however they are feeling about whatever has happened is *normal*. Normalizing helps decrease guilt toward themselves and resentment toward others so they can better manage the tasks they have in front of them. For example, "It's normal to feel overwhelmed with all the information that has been given to you about your child." "It's normal to be angry about having a child with a severe hearing loss." "It's normal to be confused about how to handle this kind of situation." "It's normal to feel angry when a husband has a stroke, and you feel that you can't cope with everything left for you to do."

Another phrase that helps people feel normal is, "It's understandable." For example, "It's understandable that you would want to hurt the driver who hit your son." "It's understandable to be discouraged when progress in therapy is so slow after your accident." Other words and phrases may be used as well, for example, "It's common that . . . " or "It frequently happens that . . ." or "I have seen this occur other times." Helping people feel that their worst thoughts and feelings are normal and understandable allows them to begin accepting and managing their thoughts and feelings, rather than being embarrassed about them as though they are unspeakable and reflect a possible flaw in their character.

Interpretations (Linking Statements)

Interpretations go beyond merely paraphrasing clients' statements, and may be presenting new information to them. Interpretations are an attempt by the audiologist or SLP to understand a person's thoughts, feelings, and experiences, and to relay the interpretation back to the person. Interpretations are observations voiced by the clinician which make a connection between things expressed by the client during the therapy. The goal of an interpretation is insight or increased client self-awareness and self-understanding. Clients sometimes report their stories as meaningless or confusing narratives, and one of the clinician's tasks is to remember statements, note significant themes, and reflect these back to clients for their consideration. Interpretations work best when we have correctly gauged the client's readiness to hear them. It is sometimes helpful to use an introductory phrase such as, "I wonder if . . . " "Is this a fair statement?" "Is it fair to say that . . . " "The way I see it is . . . " Some examples of interpretations include:

> Client (adolescent boy who is dysfluent and mentions occasionally in various therapy sessions his tendency not to talk to girls): "Usually I don't talk much to girls; I would just rather hang out with the guys."
>
> Clinician: "I wonder if your stuttering is one of the reasons you choose not to talk to girls."
>
> Client (adult woman with vocal nodules): "I get so angry with myself at work because my voice is so weak that it makes me sound like I'm uncertain of what I'm saying."
>
> Clinician: "Is it fair to say that you are concerned about how your coworkers are perceiving you because of your voice?"

Interpretations require clinicians to be attentive to clients' comments and to hold them in mind, sometimes for days or weeks, to be able to later link together their thoughts, feelings, and experiences. Brief therapy notes about key points made by clients may help clinicians see trends in statements made by clients that may later be interpreted and reflected back to the client.

The Beanie Baby Boy

I worked in the home of a six-year-old boy who stuttered. The boy had an extensive collection of Beanie Babies that he was very proud of and enjoyed showing them to me. After spending about half an hour with the boy in his room, I spent the rest of the time with the parents around the dining room table. Both parents were rather high powered no-nonsense business people. The mother began complaining about her son being "obsessed" with his Beanie Babies. I said that most everyone is obsessed with something and asked what she might be a little obsessed with. She said emphatically that she was an administrator of a residential care facility and had 200 elderly people she was responsible for. I said calmly, "Oh, you have 200 Beanie Babies." (Fortunately, in this case I had accurately gauged the mother's capacity to reflect on her own obsessive behavior.)

We, as SLPs and audiologists, need to be extremely cautious about using interpretations and playing the role of armchair psychologists and attempting to go beyond our boundaries or training with psychological interpretations of clients' affects, cognitions, and behaviors. Shipley (1997) cautions that interpretations can have powerful and sometimes negative effects on the clinician-client relationship, regardless of whether an interpretation is correct or incorrect. They may have negative effects because the client may not be ready to hear this information and may be upset or insulted by it. If the clinician's interpretation is incorrect or goes too far beyond the client's current understanding, he may feel as though the clinician has not understood him.

Suggestion versus Direction/Instruction

Suggestion is a way of helping people see new ways of looking at old problems (Ivey, 1998; Mosak & Maniacci, 1998; Sommers-Flanagan & Sommers-Flanagan, 1993; Wachtel, 1993). Suggestions are not designed to be manipulative, but to open the person to possibilities she or he may have not fully considered, or may have been on the brink of considering but needed a little support from the clinician to know that it is all right to think about it. However, suggestion is an intervention that makes some clinicians uneasy because it raises concerns about the client's autonomy and the danger of the clinician imposing her values on the client. Providing a suggestion does not mean being authoritarian (Wachtel, 1993).

A suggestion may be given to the client when the clinician wants to enhance the likelihood of maximum change or to encourage further change, especially when she notices a small amount of change that she wants to promote. Suggestion may also be used when the clinician notices inappropriate behavior to which she does not want to draw attention, and at the same time attend to or reinforce positive behavior.

The client may already have tacit inclinations that parallel the suggestion. Suggestion can be viewed as a way of initiating a process, and the process then gets maintained by its effectiveness (the suggestion "works" for the person). However, a suggestion only works if it is within the person's frame of reference (almost a tip-of-the tongue experience), where the person may have come up with the thought on his own (a tacit inclination), but needed a little help. In a way, the clinician gives voice to a thought or solution that the client has already considered or may eventually consider without the help of the clinician. A suggestion only works if it "rings true" to the person, that is, the client can imagine that it could occur or work in his ife.

Suggestions can be used to encourage compliance with an exercise or therapy procedure that we introduce to the client. For example, "When you use the chin-tuck technique, you will find that you don't choke as much when you are eating." "When you improve your articulation of words, you will find that your speech does not sound as hypernasal." Suggestion should *never* be used as a veiled form of advice to encourage clients to take action in other parts of their lives, for example, work or family life, even if we think those areas of their lives have an impact on their speech symptoms. There is an important distinction between a suggestion or advice on how a client's life should be lived, and instruction about specific aspects of the therapeutic process. If we suggest or advise a client to take some action on an area outside of our expertise and scope of practice, we have set the client up for potential failure and ourselves up for potential professional and legal entanglements if the client takes our suggestion or advice and it does not work out. Such suggestions step beyond our professional boundaries and could backfire if the outcome is not as positive as we expected. If, for example, an SLP suggests that a client's current line of work is causing excessive stress that is affecting his voice, and the client quits his job and then has difficulty finding new employment, the client could potentially blame (or sue) the SLP because he followed the "suggestion."

Some people can become very dependent very quickly on a clinician for advice on not only communication problems, but other personal problems as well. It is best to avoid the words suggest and suggestion, advise and advice. However, we can introduce thoughts and possible solutions without ever using these words. We can ask questions such as, "Have you considered . . .?" "Have you ever thought of . . . " "What do you think would happen if . . .?" "What do you think are the possibilities of . . . " "It's possible that . . . could work (happen). What do you think?" "I wonder how it would be if . . . What do you think?"

Another form of suggestion that is used by counselors and psychologists frequently incorporates the phrase ". . . as you are . . . " For example, to increase a positive behavior, the clinician might say, "It is very important for your child to feel she is listened to, and *as you are* listening to her more and more, you will probably find that . . . " Another example: "Using the chin-tuck position will help decrease your coughing and choking, and *as you are* using the chin-tuck position you will find that you will enjoy your meals more."

However, as SLPs and audiologists we do evaluations and therapy, which means we must try to help people change behaviors for their own benefit (much like physical therapists and occupational therapists). We know that not all clients, patients, and families willingly do what will help them with their hearing, speech, language, cognitive, or swallowing problems. An important challenge for us is shifting from focusing on therapy skills one moment to focusing on counseling skills the next moment. Therapy involves giving directions and instructions to help clients, patients, or families make changes in their current behaviors to improve hearing, communication, or swallowing problems. Counseling involves helping clients, patients, or families to understand hearing, communication, or swallowing problems, and ways of preventing, managing, adjusting to, or coping with these problems. Therapy skills and counseling skills are intertwined.

As clinicians we typically must be direct and very clear about the exercises and tasks we want clients to do. We do not want clients to have ambiguity or uncertainty about what we feel will help them. Because of this we must be explicit and sometimes adamant about what we want clients to do. A suggestion would not have the impact we feel is necessary to have the client follow through with an important behavior. For example, asking a seven-year old child, "Have you considered starting to wear your hearing aids in the classroom?" may not be as therapeutic initially as instructing the child to start wearing hearing aids in the classroom. Asking a child, "What do you think would happen if you stop yelling on the playground?" may not help him follow through with the behavioral changes needed. For children in particular, we often are initially direct about our instructions, expecting (hoping) the child will follow them. However, if we find that a child is not following our instructions, we may begin to inquire about his thoughts and feelings about our instructions to better understand why he is not following them.

The same is true with many of our adult clients and patients. To initially ask a patient, "What do you think would happen if you use the chin-tuck technique when swallowing?" is not as effective as being direct with our instructions for the client to use the technique during all swallows. If the patient does not choose to use the technique, then we need to better understand the patient's thoughts and feelings about using the technique during meals.

Confronting

In common usage, confrontation is often seen as hostile or punitive. In counseling, confrontation is considered an advanced microskill and is discussed by Evans, Hearn, Uhlemann, and Ivey (1993), George and Cristiani (1995), Ivey (1998), and Nystul (1999), among others. Confrontation may be briefly defined as noting discrepancies, incongruities, or mixed or conflicting messages in the client and presenting them back to the person.

Confrontations can be used to facilitate change, and it is confrontation of discrepancies that may be the catalyst to change for some clients. Often clients are stuck, experiencing internal conflict and their impasses may involve discrepancies of which they are unaware. Confrontation of a client can spur change because the clinician's observations of the client's thoughts and behaviors are presented back to the client for him or her to reassess. The confrontation should invite the client to further explore thoughts and behaviors, and to go beyond current ways of thinking. Confronting a person is a delicate procedure requiring both a sense of timing and a sensitivity and awareness of the client's receptivity (George & Cristiani, 1995).

In counseling, confrontation is *not* a direct, harsh challenge, but rather a gentle skill that involves listening to clients carefully and respectfully, and then attempting to help them examine a situation or their own thoughts, feelings, or actions. Confrontations should not include accusations, evaluations, or solutions to problems. Confrontation is not going against clients, it is going with them, seeking clarification and the possibility of a new resolution for their problems (Ivey, 1998). Confrontation should be tentative and nonjudgmental, encouraging the client to explore the discrepancy. Tentative confrontations often begin with such phrases as "Could it be" or "You tend to."

Often, if the clinician notices discrepancies but does nothing about them, the therapy remains stuck at an impasse and the clinician's frustration over the situation builds. Discrepancies are fairly common in our work with clients and families, and there are several types of discrepancies that may be seen, for example (Ivey, 1998):

■ Discrepancies between what is said and what is done: A parent may say how important her child's speech therapy is, but frequently cancels or is a no-show. Possible therapeutic confrontation: "You have mentioned how important your child's speech therapy is, yet there seems to be difficulty getting him to therapy on a consistent basis." Or, a child who says she has difficulty hearing in class but frequently does not wear her hearing aids: "You have said a few times that you can't hear your teacher very well in class but you seem to avoid wearing your hearing aids."

■ Discrepancies between two or more statements: "I agree with what you are saying, but I still think that telling my son to stop stuttering is just fine." Possible therapeutic confrontation: "You say you agree with what I'm saying, yet it doesn't seem to affect the way you talk to your son about his stuttering."

■ Discrepancies between verbal and nonverbal behaviors: The patient says that his drooping mouth from the stroke does not bother him, but he often covers his mouth with his hand when speaking. A possible therapeutic confrontation: "You mentioned that the way your mouth droops doesn't really bother you, but I notice that you frequently cover it with your hand when talking."

■ Discrepancies between nonverbal behaviors: The client may display a pleasant "no problem" type of smile along with a furrowed, tensed forehead or clenched fists. A possible therapeutic confrontation: "You tend to give two messages with your facial expressions and body language. You have a smile that says everything is OK, but at the same time your tense forehead and clenched fists tell me that everything isn't OK. Would you tell me your thoughts and feelings about what we have been talking about?"

■ Discrepancies between the views of different people. Parents disagree on the need for speech therapy for their daughter. A possible therapeutic confrontation: Mr. Ferrero, you feel that speech therapy for your daughter's attending and auditory processing problems isn't really necessary because you had problems like those when you were young and that you are very successful now, yet both you and Mrs. Ferrero indicated that you struggled quite a bit in school and your struggles were caused by attending and processing problems that are similar to your daughter's" (Adapted from Ivey, 1998).

To help clients, patients and family members resolve their incongruities or discrepancies, Ivey (1998) says the following may be helpful.

1. An increased ability to identify incongruities, discrepancies, or mixed messages in behaviors, thoughts and feelings.

2. An ability to increase a client's willingness to discuss and possibly resolve discrepancies.

3. An ability to utilize confrontation skills as part of mediation and conflict resolution.

Confronting a client, patient or family member is likely to be uncomfortable to most clinicians perhaps because of the negative connotation of the word itself, as well as the delicate nature of the technique. Confronting requires, like interpretations and linking statements, recalling what has been said or done in the past by the client that had some important discrepancies and then presenting them back to the person. Clinicians need to choose carefully those issues that may benefit from confrontation. Not every discrepancy or incongruity of a client or family member warrants confrontation, and, like our clients, patients, and their families, we may also present mixed or conflicting messages in our conversations and discussions with the people we are trying to help. Few clients and family members challenge our inconsistent messages, perhaps out of respect for us as professionals, or perhaps out of concern that we may react negatively to such a confrontation, and thus alter our care and treatment of a client.

CONCLUDING COMMENTS

This chapter provides a discussion of the numerous microskills used by professional counselors during interviews and therapy. When audiologists and SLPs have a variety of ways of eliciting information, thoughts, and feelings from clients and family members, a better understanding of the problems and the way they are being experienced is possible. Many of the microskills presented may seem artificial or unnatural when first attempted, but with use clinicians develop comfort and proficiency with them.

Discussion Questions

1. Discuss why microskills are transtheoretical.

2. What verbal encouragers do you tend to use in conversations with friends? With clients?

3. What "therapist noises" do you tend to use with clients?

4. Discuss male-female cultural differences in the ways they communicate with one another.

5. Discuss how you feel when you are asked "why" questions by a professor or supervisor.

6. If you have ever been interviewed, how did you feel about the experience? What made it comfortable or uncomfortable?

7. How do you normally check for understanding in a social conversation? When talking with a client?

8. What sensory system (auditory, visual, or kinesthetic) to you tend to prefer? What are some of the words you might use when describing something that reflects that sensory system?

9. Think of some idioms that involve the auditory system. The visual system. The kinesthetic system.

10. Discuss a metaphor you used with a client that helped the client better understand a concept you were trying to explain.

11. What are some examples of reframing "bad" behaviors to "sad" feelings?

12. Discuss how you felt when someone told you that something you had thought, felt, or did was normal or understandable.

13. Discuss an experience when you thought a friend was playing armchair psychologist. When you were playing armchair psychologist.

14. Discuss a time when you had a long silence in therapy? What were you thinking about? How were you feeling about the silence?

PART II

The Therapeutic Process with Challenging Situations and Behaviors

Beyond providing foundational information about counseling skills for speech-language pathologists (SLPs) and audiologists, this section emphasizes addressing the inevitable challenging situations and behaviors which our clients, patients, and families sometimes present. Our evaluations and therapy for children and adults, and our interactions with their family members inevitably involve complex emotional reactions and needs. In pragmatic terms, clinicians work with hearing, speech, language, cognitive, and swallowing disorders of clients and patients of all ages; however, skills and strategies for interacting that lessen their anxiety can help the therapy process go more smoothly. Clinicians' sensitivity and understanding can do much to relieve anxiety and emotional distress. Understanding and communicating with people about sensitive issues can enhance therapy, and ultimately help clinicians be more effective.

Some client, patient, or family behavior may trigger strong emotional responses on the part of the clinician. This part of the text will help you better understand the people you are working with and how to respond with more empathy and remain cool when surface behaviors appear to be defensive, resistant, self-defeating, or counterproductive. Different counseling issues and situations tend to occur depending on the setting you are working in and the stage of therapy. However, issues of most any kind may surface at unexpected times and places. Issues are not just dependent on the work setting or stage of therapy, but also the client and family's personality styles and their interactions with the clinician. Their responses to certain situations may represent their predominant style (e.g., defenses) or may occur in a general sequence (e.g., responses to loss), or in combination of these.

CHAPTER 5

Defense Mechanisms Relevant to Speech-Language Pathologists and Audiologists

CHAPTER OUTLINE

- Introduction
- Defense Mechanisms
- Concluding Comments
- For Discussion

INTRODUCTION

Defense mechanisms (ego-defense mechanisms) are automatic mental processes that people use as protective responses to stresses, threats and anxiety (*Diagnostic and Statistical Manual of Mental Disorders-IV TR*, 2000). The concept of defense mechanisms has its origins in Freud's psychoanalytic therapy (Corey, 2001; Freud, 1949). Individuals are often unaware of these processes as they operate. In addition, certain defenses are central to certain personality styles (Horowitz et al., 1984). Defense mechanisms protect a person from being overwhelmed by anxiety through adaptation to situations through distortion or denial of events or facts. Defense mechanisms are essential for helping people cope with failure and to maintain a positive self-image (George & Christiani, 1995; Gladding, 2000). They are used to combat the anxiety generated by everyday stresses as well as the overwhelming angst caused by significant losses. As Comer (1999) says, "The defense never rests."

Defense mechanisms serve a person's emotional and psychological survival (e.g., children with traumatic experiences often repress many of them; veterans who have seen combat often repress many of those memories). In other instances, however, they can interfere with personal growth, such as when a person's excessive rationalization interferes with taking responsibility for his or her own behavior. It is important to remember that everybody uses defense mechanisms; however, some are healthier than others. Defense mechanisms can be considered to exist along a continuum from those that are relatively healthy (i.e., help the person cope without significant distortion of reality) to those that are unhealthy (i.e., help the person cope but with significant distortion of reality) (George & Christiani, 1995). Although people may use a variety of defense mechanisms, they tend to have a preferred defensive style; that is, they may tend to use the same relatively healthy two or three defenses in most situations where defenses are necessary to cope. However, under extremely stressful conditions, people may use less healthy defenses that are not characteristic of their normal, everyday coping styles. We need to consider that in much of our work, particularly with children and adults who have significant impairments, the clients, patients, and family members are likely to view the situation as extremely stressful and, therefore, may temporarily use less healthy defenses than they otherwise might. It is important, then, to recognize and to respect our clients' needs for defenses to shield them from overwhelming experiences of threat, loss, and emotional or physical trauma.

As long as people employ relatively healthy defenses to assist them in coping with the stresses of hearing loss, communication delays, disorders, injury, illness, treatment, recovery, or death, their defensive styles often do not come to the attention of clinicians or interfere with therapy. For example, a person may use humor, laughing at the amusing aspects of his current medical condition or treatment to diffuse the anxiety he feels. Another person may use self-assertion, appropriately expressing the limits of tolerance for multiple appointments and demands in a single day. A third person may deal with stressors, such as receiving news about a poor prognosis by affiliation, appropriately turning to others to share feelings and to receive support to avoid intense feelings of anxiety.

In contrast, when clients use less healthy forms of defenses, they can create obstacles to forming or maintaining a therapeutic relationship and may, therefore, interfere with the professional's attempts to work on therapy goals. This chapter provides illustrations of these situations and some clinician responses that may be used to keep the therapy on track.

There are a few general guidelines that should be considered when deciding whether or not to address a person's defenses. First, one should not interfere with a person's defenses unless they persist in posing obstacles to therapy. Many times an individual's defenses occur briefly and help the person to register the challenging situation or crisis at his or her own pace. If, on the other hand, a person's defenses persist and interfere with therapy, your job is not to attempt to remove the defenses or to criticize them, but to respond in a respectful way that tries to re-establish the treatment process and empower the person. Clients', patients', and families' defensive strategies, however, can put clinicians to the test. Because, on the surface, defenses often seem like illogical responses, SLPs and audiologists may grow impatient, frustrated, or angry. They may even take personally the person's defensive actions. It is easy to get "hooked" into these negative interactions with people. However, another rule of thumb is to maintain a calm, professional demeanor and to avoid the power struggles in which you may feel pulled.

Although the *DSM-IV TR* (2000) discusses 27 different defense mechanisms (acting out, affiliation, altruism, anticipation, autistic fantasy, denial, devaluation, displacement, dissociation, help-rejecting complaining, humor, idealization, intellectualization, isolation of affect, omnipotence, passive aggression, projection, projective identification, rationalization, reaction formation, repression, self-assertion, self-observation, splitting, sublimation, suppression, and undoing), not all are typically relevant to the work of SLPs and audiologists. Some of the defenses are more commonly associated with severe psychological problems. The following are discussions of defense mechanisms that our professions may likely encounter and therapeutic responses to them.

DEFENSE MECHANISMS

Acting Out

When a child or adult is **acting out**, the individual is dealing with emotional conflicts or internal or external stressors by actions rather than reflections or feelings. In stressful or challenging situations, some individuals deal with their anxiety and external demands by responding in inappropriate ways. For example, a child with a hearing impairment who is teased or taunted by classmates may act or strike out at his tormentors, or a child who has reading problems who must read in front of the class may act out by throwing his book to avoid reading, or an elderly patient having to eat pureed food he or she detests may push the tray off the table. It is important to note that not all forms of a child or adult's bad behavior can properly be considered acting out. Acting out pertains only to behavior that is prompted by emotional conflict or stress. Acting out refers to a person acting out his or her feelings rather than talking about them. Children, in particular, have difficulty understanding and talking about their anxieties and fears and the demands being placed on them at school and home. They may use acting out behaviors (e.g., cursing, slamming books down, yelling at an adult, or disrupting therapy) as ways to express their feelings.

It is important to determine if a child's behavior is typical, age-related behavior (e.g., the result of boredom) or acting out, because that judgment will determine what response will be most therapeutic. If, for example, a child in group therapy begins disrupting the therapy by talking or playing, you may determine that the behavior is not the result of the child experiencing anxiety or stress, and manage the behavior using a behavioral approach such as rewarding more appropriate behavior. However, if you determine the child's disruptive behavior is the result of anxiety or stress that may be caused by his speech or language problems, then addressing his feelings (e.g., "It looks like you don't want to be here right now." or "It looks like some things are bothering you. Would you like to talk about them for a little while?") may be more helpful. When possible, spend a few minutes with the child alone to talk about any feelings she or he may have that are contributing to the acting out behavior, for example, embarrassment and frustration.

COUNSELING SKILLS IN ACTION:

Acting Out ... or Not?

The examples below contrast situations where children are acting out versus situations where they are not.

Continues on next page

Continued from previous page

Acting Out: Sanjoy is a moderately dysfluent 12-year-old and he is anxious about his upcoming oral book report. During recess he instigates a fight with another boy and gets sent to the principal's office for the afternoon, thereby missing his oral book report presentation.

Acting Out: Rochelle is extremely anxious about her parents' frequent arguments and fears her dad will leave home. At school she yells at her male SLP and calls him a jerk.

Not Acting Out: Leslie is participating in a speech group therapy session, but she continues to play with the board game pieces after the SLP has asked her to stop. She is not anxious, but is simply captivated by the novelty of the new game.

Not Acting Out: Joey is bored by his teacher's lesson. He understands the teacher's lessons and has mastered the current academic material. He pesters the girl next to him and makes paper airplanes and throws them across the room.

The clinician needs to make distinctions between acting out and mischievous behavior or misbehavior. When acting out behavior occurs, the clinician needs to address the feelings or the motivations behind the behavior rather than simply trying to eliminate (extinguish) it.

In medical settings you cannot always predict which patients will act out and when; therefore, it is best to take steps to try to prevent these episodes from occurring rather than simply dealing with the aftermath. Some individuals, particularly TBI patients at Levels 4 (Confused-Agitated) and 5 (Confused, Inappropriate, Non-Agitated) on the Rancho Levels of Cognitive Functioning (Hagen, 1998; Hagen, Malkmus, & Stenderup-Bowman, 1973), because of their neurologic impairments, exhibit disruptive behaviors. These patients have heightened states of activity, purposeful attempts to remove restraints or tubes, may crawl out of bed, and may exhibit aggressive or flight behaviors. Patients with TBI often are able to cope with minimal auditory, visual, and tactile stimuli (external stressors). These stimuli cause internal stress and may reach a level beyond what patients can tolerate, at which time they are likely to demonstrate acting out behaviors. These patients are also responding to internal stimuli such as pain or discomfort and a general sense of confusion about where they are, how they got there, and why they are in the hospital.

It is helpful to obtain information from family members about the patient's premorbid coping skills. Prior to a TBI, some patients may have had tendencies to be aggressive or abusive, and the TBI results in diminished capacity for self-control. In addition, some patients may view us as persecutors and punishers because of impairments in their cognitive functioning. It is important to keep in mind that the patient is doing the best he or she can and that acting out behaviors are not under cognitive control. The clinician needs to keep in mind that no matter what the Confused-

Working with Acting Out Behaviors

While working in acute care hospitals I have seen many TBI patients of all ages demonstrate acting out behaviors such as cursing and even striking out at rehabilitation therapists (PTs, OTs, and ST) and nurses. The acting out behaviors typically occur when patients feel stresses from the demands of rehabilitation programs. Clinicians must adjust the complexity, amount, rate, and/or duration of the therapy tasks to accommodate each patient's levels of tolerance to decrease internal and external stresses. That is, the rehabilitation therapist may choose to simplify a complex task, decrease the amount of stimuli presented or number of repetitions of a task, slow the rate of presentation of the stimuli or requested rate of the patient's responses to the stimuli, and/or decrease the length of time the patient is performing a task or in a therapy session. (See Chapter 8, Working with Resistance and Anger, for further discussion.)

Agitated patient says or does (including swearing, striking out, etc.) not to take it personally, but to maintain an empathic stance with acceptance of the patient's emotional, cognitive, and physical conditions. Clinicians should treat the patient with respect and dignity, and give the patient personal space (Kriege, 1993).

Speaking to patients in gentle, respectful, and nonthreatening tones may help to keep the therapy on an even keel. Initially, this may involve avoiding startling the patient by approaching the patient from the front, slowing down your pace, and maintaining a calm, self-controlled demeanor. Setting aside your agenda or therapy plan and simply "being with the patient" can be soothing. The payoff may be the prevention of time-consuming conflicts and explosions as well as possible physical injury to you. Also, keep in mind that patients who are prone to aggressive behaviors or acting out episodes may try to push you into a demanding or threatening posture which then serves as a trigger (or excuse) for them to blow up.

When other acting out episodes occur, polite but direct confrontation and limit-setting may be warranted in order to inform the patient of guidelines for appropriate behavior during therapy. It may also be important to give the patient specific examples of permissible behavior, keeping in mind the limited amount of information the patient can process. For example, you might say "Mr. D., please do not swear at me. You can tell me that you are angry and what you want; but do not swear at me." If you think a patient cannot process that much information, then simply saying "Swearing at me is not appropriate." may be the best method to set limits. Your tone of voice is important; it should not sound harsh. It is better to emphasize and reinforce appropriate behavior rather than confront inappropriate behavior. For example, you might say, "Thank you for waiting patiently the last few minutes." or "I appreciate it when you speak softly."

We need to keep in mind that acting out behavior means that the person, child or adult, is dealing with emotional conflicts and stressors that the person cannot manage in a more socially appropriate manner. If we can determine the conflicts or the stressors that are precipitating the acting out behaviors, we may be able to prevent or deter the behaviors. Determining the conflicts or stressors requires that the clinician: 1) listen to the patient for clues about anxieties and fears, and 2) try to behave in ways that help to calm the patient or de-escalate the situation.

Altruism

SLPs and audiologists may occasionally recognize **altruism** in the behavior of family members. Normally, altruism is not a significant concern to clinicians; however, we need to be aware of altruism when it interferes with family functioning and negatively affects our work with a child or adult. In many cases, altruistic behavior, where the individual becomes focused on meeting the needs of others, is considered a healthy response to stressful situations. Family members are often anxious and fearful about the well-being and future of their family members. In essence, individuals distract themselves from their own guilt or anxiety by performing helpful deeds for others. These deeds or acts may be gratifying in themselves or may elicit gratitude from others. In either case, internal anxiety is channeled into creating a positive interpersonal experience (DSM-IV TR, 2000).

In some cases, family members may make healthy adjustments to a disability or illness situation by engaging in altruistic behavior. For example, a mother who took drugs during her pregnancy may take on a second or third job to pay for extra services her child needs to maximize the child's potential. A husband may take on a caregiver role when his mate develops multiple sclerosis. Another example may involve a young adult who has a TBI while living independently, and his parents may act altruistically by having the adult son move back into the family home in order for them to become his caregivers. Frequently, adult children bring their elderly parents into the home to live with them. This can create additional family stress and what is commonly known as the sandwich generation where a couple are raising their own children and at the same time having one or more grandparents in the home or nearby and caring for them. (This latter situation may also have advantages because the grandparent may be able to help care for or monitor the grandchildren, and a strong grandparent-grandchildren relationship may develop.) Unfortunately, an increasingly common example of altruism involves grandparents who take in and care for one or more grandchildren when neither of the parents can or will care for their children.

In some cases, altruism may become problematic if it results in neglect of important areas of the person's life. A mother who focuses altruistically on her disabled child may neglect self-care, her other children's needs, or her marriage. This example illustrates that altruistic behavior towards one person may cause a disruption or damage to other family relationships. Despite this mother's positive intentions, she and her family may need brief counseling from a professional counselor to recognize imbalances in the family and reorganize family roles. In these examples it is important to note that the individuals who are behaving altruistically are not simply acting responsibly, but are using this strategy to channel their own anxiety into productive action.

In general, as clinicians our primary responses to an altruistic family member might be: 1) acknowledgement and validation in order to show empathy for the family member's focus on the person with the acute or chronic disorder; or 2) if the clinician feels the altruism is causing neglect of other important areas of the family member's life, a referral to a counselor or psychologist may be appropriate. The psychologist may proceed by inquiring about the neglected aspects of the family member's life, and by helping the person find solutions that respect the family member's need to behave in an altruistic manner.

Denial

In response to news or information that is overwhelming, some people respond with the basic defense known as **denial**. The DSM-IV TR (2000) defines denial as an emotional conflict or internal or external stressors that the individual deals with by refusing to acknowledge some painful aspect of external reality or subjective experience that would be apparent to others. In some cases, denial is a coping strategy that reflects feelings of inadequacy which are triggered by significant losses, injury, or impairment. The person may admit that the problem exists, but is not engaged emotionally. Even well adjusted people may initially employ denial to protect themselves from overwhelming anxiety (Gladding, 2000). Short-lived denial is a common response to receiving news of a diagnosis of a disability (e.g., hearing loss, ADD, CAPD, learning disability), or a serious illness or injury (e.g., laryngeal cancer, CVA, TBI, or spinal cord damage). The client, patient, or family member may protest, "No, I don't!" or "No, it can't be true!" This form of denial appears, on the surface, to be a distortion of reality. However, in many cases, it is a short-lived response that suggests that the person (or loved one) must make a radical adjustment to his or her self-image and expectations as this new information is processed. The diagnosis itself may be upsetting, but it also requires the person to revise assumptions about him or herself and the future. Thus, denial is a barrier that many people temporarily erect as they try to adjust to a profound change in their lives. It provides people with time to gradually register the new information and its ramifications for their lives.

Shipley (1997) points out that clinicians need to realize that even if clients or family members are denying something (e.g., a diagnosis), they may privately be contemplating whether the information is true and the clinician's descriptions are accurate. Minimizing, making a problem out to be less than it is, is another form of denial. The person recognizes a problem exists, but does not acknowledge the severity of it (Rolland, 1994). Also, some clients may respond with claims of omnipotence where they claim to have better judgment, wisdom, or ability than the clinician. The person's defensive omnipotence involves a kind of denial of vulnerability and, in its place, the fantasy that the person is invulnerable. A patient with dysphagia may say, for example, "I never choke no matter how fast I eat or how big a bite I take! I can eat whatever I want the way I want!"

In most cases, denial gives people time to process bad news. During this time, they may appear preoccupied with their thoughts and unable to respond to additional information or to collaborate in decision making and treatment planning. This is a sign that they are attempting to process or make sense of this new information. Typically, people cannot be rushed through this process.

Attempts to urge someone to face the truth or to make treatment decisions during this time may be met with withdrawal, resistance, or agitation. Therefore, except in emergency or crisis situations where an immediate medical decision is necessary, it is best to allow individuals the time to process the new information. Most people will discard this defense (denial) by themselves, that is, without any special interventions designed to address the denial.

In some cases, denial may persist or may emerge later in therapy. While denial at the time of diagnosis is often related to trying to limit the impact of shocking news, denial that persists later in the therapy process is likely to reflect shame or feelings of vulnerability that individuals experience regarding their disability or impairment (Rolland, 1994). A therapeutic response to this form of denial is to: 1) express acceptance of the person's present condition and respect for her or him as a person, and 2) if still needed, gently point out the discrepancy between your observations of the impairments and the person's denial of the problem. For example, "Kim, I see that you are having difficulty (because of severe articulation and phonological delays) being understood by your teacher and friends, but you are saying you don't have any problems with your speech and don't want to come to therapy. It must be frustrating when other people can't understand you. Would you be willing to come and visit me in one of my groups this afternoon?" This points out the discrepancy between what the clinician and others see as a problem and the child's denial, and provides a gentle invitation to visit the therapy group. It is important that this statement is communicated in a caring fashion that invites dialogue and exploration of the child's thoughts. It should not sound critical or as if you are simply interested in catching the child in an inconsistency (see the discussion on confrontation in Chapter 4). Another option in response to a person's denial is to assume that the person really does have a good handle on reality and to make an empathic statement such as, "It is difficult to come to grips with this condition, isn't it." This statement validates the person's current struggle and may provide the support needed to move beyond the defensive posture.

Denial is perhaps the defense SLPs and audiologists may encounter more often than any other defense mechanism. It is important to keep in mind the purpose denial serves for our clients, patients, and their families, and how we can manage or cope with this behavior. We can also consider the ways we have used denial in our own lives, how it may have helped us cope with information we were not yet ready to accept, and how we eventually worked through that denial. With this self-awareness we can be more empathic toward the people we are trying to help.

Displacement

Displacement refers to a process of transferring feelings about one object or person onto someone else who is perceived as less threatening (DSM-IV TR, 2000). The classic illustration of displacement is the employee who gets angry with the boss but fears expressing this directly and so goes home where he yells at his wife, or the parent who has a frustrating day at work and yells at her children when she gets home. The central idea is that the individual vents anxiety and/or anger toward a target that is less powerful and threatening than the original source of anger (Comer, 1996). For this reason, the recipient of displaced anger is often surprised or confused (e.g., responding with, "What did I do to deserve that?") and feels unfairly treated.

Clients or family members may displace anger regarding a diagnosis or treatment progress onto a clinician. We become the lightning rods that receive the jolts. In this case, the clinician is perceived as less threatening than the diagnosis or disorder itself. For example, a parent may become angry and hostile toward the audiologist who diagnoses a hearing loss in her child. On the other hand, some clients or family members may fear the audiologist's disapproving response to angry words and, therefore, channel anger toward a teacher, aide, or other person who is perceived as having less authority, status, or control over the child's or adult's treatment. For example, a patient with dysphagia may be angry with the SLP who has ordered a mechanical soft diet and nectar-consistency liquids for all meals, plus the use of specific safe swallowing maneuvers for each bite. The patient may show irritation by displacing it onto a Certified Nursing Assistant (CNA) who is trying to feed the patient and requiring her to use the safe swallowing maneuvers.

Displacement is a common defense strategy, and it is important to keep in mind that the individual employing this defense probably is not aware of it at the time. Thus, attempts to make the person aware of the displaced anger shortly after its occurrence are not likely to be met with a positive response. Instead, maintaining a professional stance and trying to recapture the person's attention and cooperation with the task at hand is advisable. For example, "Let's see, Mr. Phan, how about just three more attempts today with the injection method to see if you get some esophageal voice." The underlying idea is that if the client's anger is displaced, the clinician should avoid experiencing this as a personal attack and, instead, should attempt to redirect the client's energy to productive tasks.

Alternatively, validating the client's anger toward likely sources such as the illness or frustration with the lengthy course of treatment may also help. This response expresses empathy without criticizing the maladaptive nature of the displacement defense. An example of this might be, "I don't blame you for being frustrated with learning esophageal speech. It is difficult for most new laryngectomies." or, "Mrs. Green, I don't blame you for being angry about the delayed recognition and diagnosis of your child's developmental apraxia." However, the clinician should not attempt to tell a person what he is *really* angry about (Wachtel, 1993). Thus, saying, "Mr. Phan, I don't like your irritable tone with me. What you are really angry about is the problem you are having learning esophageal speech." This type of response is not advisable because it invalidates the person's emotional experience and criticizes him at a time when he is already feeling vulnerable.

Displacement is a defense mechanism that we are likely to see in most settings in which we work. Typically we may think that adults are the individuals who may use this defense, but children who are frustrated with their difficulty communicating, or even angry with a teacher may show some displacement toward the SLP or audiologist. We need to recognize that such anger directed toward us likely is not about us and, therefore, we should try not to take it personally or be offended. As with any defense mechanism used by a child or adult, an empathic understanding of the behavior and an appreciation of what is motivating the defense can assist us in managing the issue.

Help-Rejecting Complaining

Help-rejecting complaining behavior involves a person's repetitive complaints (e.g., "Nothing we are doing is helping." or "I don't know how this is going to help my swallowing." or "No matter what we do with my hearing aids, they never feel comfortable!"). While the clinician explains the therapy rationales or procedures, or devises new or different exercises for the client, the client continues to reject the information or suggestions from the clinician. In this defensive style, the client assumes a passive stance and appears to rely on the therapist's authority, wisdom, and expertise when, in fact, the client is experiencing hostility toward the clinician or another professional (displacement) (DSM-IV TR, 2000). Thus, the client's repetitive statements serve to disguise angry feelings and the forthcoming professional advice is quickly discounted or discarded. This pattern typically leads to exasperation on the part of the clinician. Some clients are experts at this process and are able to convince clinicians that they are genuine in their requests for help. The client's flattering but superficial acquiescence to the clinician's expertise can be effective in eliciting ongoing attempts to help the client solve his or her problems.

Evidence of help-rejecting complaining is often found in the clinician's response to this behavior. After being pulled into this futile pattern, a clinician typically feels frustrated, helpless, or even "used" by the client. The clinician may feel as though "It's no use trying to help Mrs. Rasmussen; she doesn't accept anything I suggest will help her." Clinicians who unwittingly succumb to these interactions may even develop anger toward help-rejecting patients.

Establishing and maintaining a collaborative style of communication with the person may help to prevent this maladaptive pattern from occurring. Even if a help-rejecting complaining pattern emerges, shifting to a more collaborative style may disrupt and positively alter this pattern of communication and interaction. In other words, when the person complains, engage the client in a mutual search for a solution rather than dictate the solution to the client. As long as the clinician plays the role of the authority, the client will reject all solutions. On the other hand, if the solutions come from the client or there is collaboration in the search for solutions, then it will be more difficult (or at least, it will no longer serve the hostile purpose) for the client to reject them. Therefore, the clinician may ask probing questions such as "What do you think you could do to help your Natasha be more fluent?" "When are the best times for you to work on your speech?" "What has worked best for you before?" "What diet texture do you seem to have the least amount of trouble with coughing and choking? Which one of the safe-swallowing maneuvers we worked on do you feel is most helpful?" As well as avoiding becoming hooked into a futile process power struggle, these responses empower the client to join with the clinician in finding the best solutions for the problems rather than allowing the client to be a passive recipient of therapy.

Intellectualization

With **intellectualization**, the client uses detached, logical, or abstract thinking to avoid a conflict or painful feelings (DSM-IV TR, 2000). This defensive strategy may be more common among people who possess high verbal skills and have a repertoire of abstract principles or linguistic skills upon which to draw. In this way, clients may provide a seemingly logical explanation why they cannot or should not do particular therapy tasks. Sheehan (1970) discusses intellectualization as a common strategy adults who stutter use to avoid working directly on their stuttering behaviors. Intellectualizing helps clients achieve emotional distance from their problems because talking about their problems is often easier than working on them directly.

Combating Intellectualization

While working at the University of California, Los Angeles (UCLA) Adult Stuttering Clinic with Dr. Joseph and Vivian Sheehan in the early 1970s, I worked with many clients who were very bright students or professionals, including physicians and attorneys. Although many of the clients stuttered severely, they often presented long and convoluted intellectualizations about their stuttering. Sheehan's therapy approach for stuttering emphasized that a person is changed not by what he thinks about his stuttering, but by what he does about it. Intellectualizing about stuttering was not as beneficial as working on it, that is, changing behaviors.

Intellectualization is often a relatively healthy response to illness or adversity that may help patients or family members feel that there is some meaning associated with the difficult, if not tragic experiences they are having. Trying to make sense of an adversity by intellectualizing or philosophizing about it helps to protect people psychologically from personal events that are destructive and beyond their control. Responses that reflect intellectualization are often easily identified because they express well-known principles such as, "Everything happens for a reason," "God has a plan for me," or "This illness has given me an opportunity to slow down, 'smell the roses', and recognize what is precious in my life." Intellectualization is often used in the service of accepting what we cannot change (e.g., a diagnosis of cancer or disfigurement as the result of a car accident). In some cases this defensive strategy may help the patient or family keep an intellectual distance from painful realities until they are emotionally prepared to further process what has happened to them. Here, intellectualization may reflect a stage in the patient's or and family's process of grieving the loss of their former health, functioning, or loved one.

Because intellectualization and philosophizing help people find meaning in adversity, it generally should be supported and respected. Clinicians should not try to contradict the person's intellectualizing or philosophical statements even if they do not share the beliefs held by the person. It is important for the clinician not to be distracted by the client's intellectualizing and philosophizing, and be drawn into an extended discussion or politics, religion, metaphysics, or the meaning of life.

In addition, people from different cultural backgrounds may hold beliefs that are foreign to us but common or encouraged in their communities.

Passive-Aggressive Behavior

The concept of **passive-aggression** is often misunderstood or the term is used to criticize clients who do not do what we want. In passive-aggressive behavior, the individual deals with emotional conflict, stressors, or demands placed upon her by indirectly and unassertively expressing aggression towards others (DSM-IV TR, 2000). Meanwhile, the person presents a façade of friendliness, compliance, or agreement. For example, the client may "forget" about his therapy appointment or forget about doing his exercises. This "forgetting" may be motivated by negative feelings toward the clinician or mistrust of the clinician's goals or procedures. The person has a conflict between hostile or mistrustful feelings and a desire to not disrupt the relationship too severely. The passive-aggressive behavior then represents a compromise between those opposing feelings. This behavioral style may reflect a person's general style of relating to others or it could occur only in situations where the person experiences being in a subordinate or helpless position relative to the professionals trying to help him. In the latter case, a person may feel fearful of expressing himself directly to someone whom he perceives as an authority. Other examples of passive aggression may include a parent who presents with a sweet, polite façade toward the clinician but then privately does not support the recommended exercises for her or his child. Excessive procrastination may also reflect negative feelings toward a task or person, with the procrastination carrying the not-so-subtle message that the task is not worth doing.

Some cultures place a priority, however, on polite behavior and harmonious interactions with others. Thus, people from these cultures may appear to understand and agree with a professional's recommendations, but then fail to follow through with these suggestions. These situations should not be considered examples of passive-aggressive behavior. This response is culturally learned and sanctioned; it does not necessarily reflect an individual's defensive strategies. This individual is not necessarily motivated by a desire to conceal aggression but only to maintain smooth social interactions.

In passive-aggressive behavior, on the other hand, the individual is motivated by hostile feelings, and a desire for approval or, at least, to avoid disruption of an important relationship (in this case, client-clinician). These contrary feelings pose a conflict for the individual. Thus, the individual's passive-aggressive behavior becomes a maladaptive way of responding to this internal polarity or conflict. The recipient may feel as if the person is saying "yes," but his actions are saying "no." This type of behavior often makes the recipient of the passive-aggression feel angry, lied to, or manipulated.

As mentioned above, however, clinicians may sometimes label certain clients as passive-aggressive when they fail to do what the clinician wants. This use of the term is usually a signal that the SLP or audiologist is frustrated with the client and using psychological jargon (perhaps incorrectly) to make a thinly veiled criticism. Often, the clinician needs to examine the situation further to see whether the client's behavior was passive-aggressive or whether there was simply a failure in communication. That is, either the client did not understand the clinician's instructions (and therefore did not comply with them), or the clinician did not hear or understand the client's concerns or reservations.

Whether the client is behaving passive-aggressively or the clinician wants to explore recent interactions to see whether a misunderstanding occurred, it is best to speak openly with the client and invite him to share his point of view. For example, "Mr. Engel, your assignment (exercise) was to do … this week and I see that you had some difficulty doing it. What made this assignment particularly difficult for you? What can we do to make this assignment more workable for you?" The first part of the response confronts the discrepancy between the SLP's assignment and the client's behavior. This statement should be clear and firm but should not sound irritated or angry. If it does, the client will likely respond defensively and the impasse will not be resolved. The second part of the statement encourages review of the assignment, the client's reluctance to complete it, and the possibility of revising it collaboratively.

If the clinician feels strongly that she is caught in a vicious cycle where the client is resisting her recommendations (while agreeing to them) and they are at an emotional and behavioral impasse, then it may help to simply admit that. "Mr. Engel, we've talked a little about some of the reasons for the assignment and some of challenges doing it, but it still seems to be rather difficult. I wouldn't blame you if you find yourself getting irritated or annoyed with all the demands that are being placed on you. I know that this must be a difficult time for you. What can we do to help make your assignments work better for you?" This response to the client admits that the client is struggling with the clinician's assignments but does so in a nonaccusatory way. It also gives the client permission to admit to feeling overwhelmed, irritated, or annoyed with the clinician who gave him such a difficult assignment.

Probably the most succinct and straightforward response to a client's passive-aggressive behavior is to first confront the discrepancy between the client's words and action and then honor the client's feelings. "Mr. Engel, each week we decide on your exercises to try to reach your goals. Some of the exercises turned out to be more difficult than we expected. Let's see what happened and then see what we can do to make this week's exercises more successful for you." In this way, you "join" with the client and avoid an escalating power struggle or heightening of his or her hostility. An empathic tone and using mild humor (depending upon the appropriateness with the particular client) can enhance this strategy. Probing questions (what, when, where, how) can help you better understand a person's thoughts and feelings about your working relationship. You may ask, for example, "I have the feeling that you are having some difficulty working with me. What are your thoughts about that?" "When is it most difficult for you to come to therapy?" "Where do you feel the therapy is headed and what are your concerns?" "How do you think we can work together more easily?" By asking such questions you are modeling direct, honest communication and encouraging the client to respond in this manner.

A client's or family member's passive-aggressive behavior can be challenging for clinicians in any setting. If we keep in mind that it reflects the person's fear or anxiety about opposing us directly, we can attempt to deal with this challenging behavior in a productive manner that enhances the client's positive feelings toward us and facilitates therapy. We should avoid becoming angry, sarcastic, or hostile toward the client or family member who is behaving in a passive-aggressive manner toward us.

Rationalization

Rationalization as a defensive strategy, at first glance, appears similar to intellectualization. Both use a kind of logic or explanation to avoid dealing with conflict or painful feelings. Intellectualization is often used to accept a situation that cannot be changed; however, rationalization is more likely to be used to justify a person's maladaptive or noncompliant behavior. In other words, rationalization uses self-serving but incorrect explanations to explain an action or the failure to take action (DSM-IV TR, 2000). It bends or stretches the truth and represents a type of faulty reasoning. Rationalizing can be annoying to clinicians because the pseudologic can be apparent to us but not to the client.

Illustrations of rationalization might include statements such as, "I know I didn't do the exercises you told me to do, but how do we know that those exercises will help me? A friend of mine who stutters tried the same kind of things and they didn't help him." "It doesn't matter what my wife says, I can still hear as well as I could when I was 40!" Typically, the pseudologic used in rationalizations is designed to help the person avoid the immediate discomfort or difficulty of working directly on the communication problem. In this way, rationalization is self-deceptive and may be self-destructive (e.g., the patient with dysphagia who says he can eat anything without choking, or the wife who says her husband with swallowing problems can eat the food she cooks and brings to the hospital because it is home cooked and is his favorite food). Clinicians who encounter these rationalizing maneuvers by clients, patients, and family members may find themselves feeling irritated with them. However, it is important not to show anger or engage in a power struggle because this may only provide the person with another excuse to rationalize more noncompliant behavior. For example, a patient may respond, "I'll be darned if I'm going to eat the kind of food the SLP told me I have to eat." The faulty logic here is that the patient is acting as though his cooperation is for the SLP's benefit rather than his or her own, and that noncompliance will punish him or her. One strategy for responding to a client's rationalizations is to assume that the client knows the logic she or he is using is faulty. We may remark to the client, "I'm sure you know that these exercises will be helpful for you" or "I realize it is hard on you to restrict how you normally cook and care for your husband." Avoid debating with a client or family member's rationalizations and focus on being empathic with what is difficult for them.

Despite the fact that client rationalizations may be irritating to us, we should strive to respond in a calm manner. Confrontation may only cause the client to dig in his or her heels regarding any illogical statements. Good-humored empathic responses may be helpful such as, "Mr. Jefferson, I know that you don't like these exercises, but you know that there is a much better chance for your recovery if you do them." The goal here is to join with the client in a good-natured way while expressing that *we know that they know* that they are deceiving themselves with their rationalizing statements. An alternative response to a client's rationalizing statements is to talk with the client about short-term discomfort versus long-term benefits. For example, "Mr. Fernandez, I know that what I am asking you to do is difficult and that it is going to take a while before you really see significant benefits, but in the long run these exercises will help you get home and back to work much sooner."

Splitting and Devaluation

Splitting and **devaluation** are often defensive strategies that are used together, and are often encountered when working with more difficult clients. Splitting represents a coping strategy in which a person deals with emotional conflict or internal or external stressors by compartmentalizing opposite affective states. The person fails to integrate the positive and negative qualities of the other person or, in some cases, him or herself. Devaluation occurs when an individual deals with emotional conflict or internal or external stressors by attributing exaggerated negative attributes to others or even the person him- or herself. The person who engages in splitting tends to have images of another person (or him or herself) that alternate between polar opposites such as all good–all bad, ecstatic–miserable, pleased–enraged, idealized–worthless, euphoric–devastated, loving–hateful (DSM-IV TR, 2000). Splitting involves dichotomous thinking and feeling about oneself, others, or life in general. There is no middle ground or consideration of multiple aspects of a person or situation. These extreme reactions may be distributed among different people, for example, "I love my SLP, but I hate my physical therapist," or the person's reactions may fluctuate so that the he declares one day that he has "the best SLP in the world" while the next day expressing the opposite view, "She is the worst SLP I've ever met." Labile or quickly changing moods are likely to accompany these shifting perceptions. Parents, for example, may express their anger toward school staff and talk as though they and the school staff are on opposing teams. In contrast, the parents may view the SLP as the "good" team and attempt to triangulate the SLP by recruiting her as a third party against the school staff, administrators, or even other clinicians.

COUNSELING SKILLS IN ACTION:

The Importance of Meeting as a Team

A single mother whose 6-year-old daughter had speech and behavioral problems complained bitterly to the psychologist about the school staff's incompetence and impatient approach to her daughter's symptoms. She also suggested that she and the psychologist might go out for a cup of coffee to discuss her daughter further. Then, in the business office where she paid her bills for the psychologist's services, she complained to the financial advisor about her relationship with the psychologist. Each professional was beginning to think that there was a problem with the other. The problematic perceptions were resolved once there was a team meeting between the mother and all her daughter's academic and treatment personnel.

Common signs that a person is engaged in splitting and devaluation are hearing extreme pronouncements, as illustrated above, and experiencing major discrepancies among different professionals when describing a particular child, client, or patient. For example, the audiologist describes a client or family members as sweet and easy to work with while another professional experiences the same client as hostile, demanding, and explosive. These polar opposite reports may reflect the fact that the person is splitting these professionals. When this happens, the client or family member may become invested in telling stories about the "bad" professional to the "good" professional. The latter professional may be enticed into accepting the person's perceptions since they flatter and elevate her in comparison to her coworkers. Meanwhile, the client who engages in splitting creates external conflicts between professionals instead of working through his or her internal negative feelings in a healthier manner.

Therapeutically, it is important to recognize the person's splitting and devaluing maneuvers rather than to overreact to them. Individuals who rely on splitting and devaluing as defenses against anxiety typically come from troubled homes and have low frustration tolerance. Paradoxically, however, their splitting and devaluing maintains and even creates conflict rather than solving it. It is essential for members of a multidisciplinary team, including school staff and administrators, to work collaboratively with one another especially when they recognize that a particular person is prone to splitting. This collaboration and team approach will help to prevent the person from creating conflict and confusion among the various professionals.

In terms of working with clients who engage in splitting, it is important to provide as much consistency as possible (e.g., regular daily appointment times for speech therapy) so that they do not become further stressed. It is also important to validate how they are feeling (although not with their split perceptions) and to encourage them to speak to the other professional directly about how they are feeling. For example, you might say, "It sounds like you have had a difficult experience with your teacher (physical therapist, nurse, etc.). Have you talked to him or her about how you feel? " Any evidence, however small, of their increasing ability to perceive shades of gray should be reinforced. For example, in response to a patient's statement that acknowledges positive qualities of a previously devalued professional you might say, "You're right, the PT does work hard to help you walk again," or in response to a parent you might say, "Yes, Jeremy's teacher really does care a lot about him."

Splitting and devaluation are difficult behaviors to deal with because they may go on for some time before they are recognized and considerable turmoil may develop between professionals before there is an understanding of what is occurring. We, as SLPs and audiologists, may be on either side of the splitting, either idealized or villified. Our self-image and self-esteem (as well as our professional reputation) may be elevated or damaged when we hear what a client or family member has said about us. Also, as professionals, we inevitably hear clients and family members discuss and/or evaluate other professionals (including children talking about their teachers). We take at face value every negative comment that is made about another professional. However, when working as a team with other professionals, including teachers, administrators, rehabilitation specialists, and supervisors, it is prudent to confer privately with the professional who has been negatively described by a client or family member to share experiences both of you are having with that particular person. This can help to sort out any problematic treatment issues and to maintain a strong collegial relationship and treatment team.

Coping Strategies

Coping strategies differ from defense mechanisms in that coping strategies are not automatic mental processes, but are more deliberately used behaviors or mental activities we employ to reduce or alleviate stress or anxiety. Coping strategies are learned and not necessarily intimately tied to personality style. Most people have learned a variety of coping strategies to take care of themselves, for example, talking with family or friends, going for a walk, exercising, shopping ("retail therapy"), eating comfort foods, sleeping, praying, going to a movie, listening to relaxing music, reading a book, or playing with a pet. Coping strategies help people refuel and nurture themselves. We may want to ask clients or family members how they take care of themselves when under stress, and encourage them to use those methods during this particularly stressful time. Coping strategies may be expanded as people learn new behaviors that help deal with stressful situations and environments, and we may even want to suggest new coping strategies. A more relaxed client and family will experience increased benefits from therapy and may find the therapy process less cumbersome or aversive.

COUNSELING SKILLS IN ACTION:

Helping Clients Identify Personal Coping Strategies

Typically, SLPs and audiologists see clients and patients when they are experiencing a new (or newly diagnosed) communication problem. Although most people have developed a variety of coping skills for many of their life problems, a clinical communication problem is not usually in the realm of their previous life experiences. Inquiring about how the person has managed common communication problems in the past may help the person recognize that she or he has already discovered ways of coping before the clinical communication problem developed. Common communication problems that are in most people's experience include not being understood by a young child or an elderly person, or not being able to hear in a noisy environment.

CONCLUDING COMMENTS

Everyone uses defenses; therefore, the task is not to eliminate them but to understand what stressful situations have triggered them so that a therapeutic response can be offered. Defense mechanisms can be considered to exist along a continuum from those that are relatively healthy (i.e., help the person cope without significant distortion of reality) to those that are unhealthy (i.e., help the person cope but with significant distortion of reality). Understanding defenses (our clients' and our own) can help us to respond in appropriate ways rather than triggering our own frustration, irritation, and defenses. Confronting a client's or family member's defensive style is rarely effective, can damage the therapeutic relationship, and may cause escalation in the person's defenses. Responding empathically is more useful and helps maintain the therapeutic rapport that is necessary in order to collaborate with the client on essential tasks.

Clients and patients who use defenses can be frustrating to therapists, particularly for clinicians who are very goal-oriented. We need to keep in mind that all the defensive maneuvers we see in clients, patients, and family members may be similar to ones we have used in our own lives under different circumstances. A quick, "I have *never* done *that*!" may be seen by people who know us well as the denial defense. In view of the fact that everyone uses defenses, and that these defenses may change under very stressful circumstances, SLPs and audiologists can be understanding and empathic with individuals who present challenging defensive styles.

Discussion Questions

1. Which defense mechanisms do you tend to use when you encounter everyday stressful situations?

2. During a time of high stress, what defense strategies do you use to help cope with the situation (or person)?

3. What coping strategies do you tend to use in stressful situations? What coping strategies might you add to your repertoire in the future?

4. Why is it important to respect a person's need for defenses?

5. What are some examples in which a person's defenses may become an obstacle in therapy?

6. When a person's defenses become an obstacle, what are some principles for addressing the defenses?

7. What are some of the internal and external stressors that may result in acting out behavior in a preschool child; an early elementary age child; a middle school age child; a high school age child; a young adult; an older adult; an elderly adult?

8. How can you determine if a child is demonstrating misbehavior versus acting out behavior?

9. Describe a situation in which you acted altruistically. What anxieties were you avoiding?

10. Describe an occasion when you felt a client or family member used denial as a defensive strategy. How did you feel about the person at the time? How did you respond? What would you do differently now? What do you think helped the person progress from denial to acceptance?

11. Describe an occasion in which you used denial. What feelings were you avoiding (e.g., loss, inadequacy, vulnerability)?

12. Describe an occasion in which someone exhibited displacement toward you. Who or what do you think was the source of the person's anxiety? How did you feel about the person when you were the recipient of the displacement? How did you handle the situation? How would you handle it differently now?

13. Describe an occasion when you demonstrated displacement toward someone else. What do you think was motivating this defense strategy? What would have been a healthier response?

14. Describe an occasion in which you felt a client demonstrated help-rejecting complaining. How did you feel about this behavior? What did you do? What would you do differently now?

15. Describe an occasion in which a client or family member used intellectualization or rationalization. How did you respond? What would you do differently now?

16. Describe an occasion in which you used intellectualization to cope with a significant change or loss in your family. What philosophical or spiritual beliefs formed the basis of your intellectualizing statements? How did this help you cope?

17. Describe an occasion in which a client or family member demonstrated passive-aggressive behavior toward you. What conflict do you think motivated this behavior? How did the experience make you feel? How would you handle this behavior differently now?

18. Describe an occasion in which you may have used passive-aggressive behavior toward someone. What was your motivation? How did that affect your relationship with that person? What could you have done differently to express your feelings more directly?

19. Describe an occasion in which a client or family member was using rationalization as a defensive maneuver. How did you feel about the person during this time? Was there any carry-over of your feelings to the person in later work with him or her?

20. Describe an occasion in which a person (client or other person) engaged in splitting or devaluation. What side were you placed on, that is, were you idealized or denigrated? How did you feel about the experience? How did you handle it?

21. Describe an occasion in which you may have been engaged in splitting. What was your motivation? How could you have handled it differently now?

CHAPTER 6

Working with Challenging and Difficult Emotional States

CHAPTER OUTLINE

- Introduction
- Anxiety and Fear
- Depression
- Grief
- Guilt and Shame
- Concluding Comments
- For Discussion

INTRODUCTION

Speech-language pathologists (SLPs) and audiologists commonly work with children and adults who present various challenging and difficult emotional states, some of which may be enigmas to us. It is important to remember that clients and patients are experiencing disabilities with one of the most important and fundamental human skills—the ability to communicate. Therefore it is natural that a considerable amount of emotion often surrounds these impairments (Shipley, 1997). Besides our clients and patients, family members frequently experience strong emotional reactions to the challenges they are confronted with when a loved one has a significant communication impairment. Viewing the people we attempt to help holistically allows us to work with more than just the speech, language, cognitive, or swallowing problems they present (Gravell and France, 1992; Shames, 2000). Holistic therapy involves focusing on the whole person (mind, body, and spirit), and the goal is the growth of the whole person (Bourne, 2000; Gladding, 2000; Nystul, 1999).

As SLPs and audiologists our responsibility is not to "cure" the negative emotional states or possible emotional disorders that may be presented by the individuals we are trying to help. Our responsibility is to work with each individual in such ways that his or her emotional states do not interfere or significantly hinder therapy progress. We can explore through various microskills (see Chapter 4) the negative feelings the client, patient, or family members are experiencing and attempt to understand them. In some cases our understanding will lead to a reduction in the individual's negative emotional states or the development of better coping abilities to manage their emotional states.

We need to be careful not to move out of our scope of practice when dealing with challenging emotions and behaviors, but we also need not be afraid to work within our scope of practice. As discussed in Chapter 3, we need to avoid "pathologizing" clients, patients, or family members by saying they are paranoid, depressed, schizophrenic, a hypochondriac, a kleptomaniac, have a dependent personality disorder, a mood disorder, or an obsessive-compulsive disorder. However, some aspects of what we see may need to be included in our description of individuals. In such cases it is best to use descriptions of behaviors that reflect our observations rather than global pathologizing terms. We can describe situation-specific behaviors but not label or diagnose the individual's general emotional state or disorder. Even though a client has a certain set of behaviors that we see in a particular situation, does not mean these are typical of the person. SLPs and audiologists need to make judgments as to whether behaviors, characteristics, or symptoms are understandable reactions to a particular experience, or whether the experience may be causing impairment in the client's functioning. In general, we can describe emotional or psychological symptoms but not specify an emotional or psychological disorder or diagnosis.

ANXIETY AND FEAR

Anxiety is an inevitable part of life. It is important to appreciate that there are many situations that occur in everyday life in which it is appropriate and reasonable to react with some anxiety. A lack of feeling of any anxiety in response to potential loss or failure would be abnormal. Anxiety is a distressing feeling of uneasiness, apprehension, or dread. The anxiety may be rational and based on actual events, or irrational and based on anticipated events that likely would not occur. Anxiety occurs in children and adolescents as well as adults. Children may have separation anxiety from their parents (we sometimes see this during initial evaluations of young children in clinical practicum), or anxiety about being abandoned or sent away from home. A main source of anxiety for both children and adults is the fear of being separated from other people who are felt to provide security, either physical or emotional, or both. However, when an individual's anxiety is chronic and not traceable to any specific cause, or when it interferes with normal activity, the individual may need professional help (Stewart, 1997). SLPs and audiologists need to avoid pathologizing a person's emotional response to a situation by labeling it an anxiety disorder. Anxiety disorder refers to a group of disorders that includes acute stress disorder, generalized anxiety disorder, panic attack, social phobia, and others (DSM-IV TR, 2000). Only appropriate mental health professionals can diagnose such disorders.

Anxiety and Communication Disorders

Anxiety is a common component of many communication disorders (Andrews & Summers, 1988; Bloodstein, 1995; Crowe, 1997; Ferrand & Bloom, 1997; Luterman, 2001; Parker, 1990; Shipley, 1997; Sohlberg & Mateer, 1989; Tanner, 1999). For example, SLPs and audiologists work with individuals and families who are confronted with acute anxiety, social anxiety, and panic attacks. In some cases, clients' anxiety may interfere with their performance on some language and cognitive assessments. For example, a child who is anxious during an evaluation may respond with a shorter mean-length of utterance during a language-sampling task than he would in a situation in which he felt more comfortable. Also, because of anxiety, a child may respond with less than complete answers to problem-solving assessments, which may be reflected in raw and scale scores. Some sources of anxiety for children, adults, and their family members are reflected in the questions they ask. Figure 6-1 lists some of these types of questions.

Anxiety serves an important function by providing a state of tension that can motivate individuals to action. Anxiety can be viewed from a time perspective, that is, acute versus chronic (Rolland, 1994). There are acute and chronic anxiety states. The acute states have a sudden onset occurring perhaps as a reaction to severe external stress and tend to be relatively brief in nature (e.g., receiving a diagnosis of a CVA). Chronic anxiety, however, runs a prolonged course and may not be associated with particular stressful events. Individuals with chronic anxiety often worry excessively and tend to respond to many situations with undeserved anxiety and trepidation. Anxiety can appear at different levels of intensity, from mild feelings of uneasiness to panic attacks (Bourne, 2000; Gravell and France, 1992).

A different way of viewing anxiety is to analyze it in terms of its triggers and causes. Situational anxiety (situation-dependent) refers to anxiety that tends to occur in relatively limited situations and times, for example, just before an examination or just before a job interview. Situational anxiety is the most common form of anxiety individuals with communication disorders experience (e.g., being understood in front of the class, a boy who stutters when talking to a girl, a job being in jeopardy because of apraxia after a stroke). Free-floating anxiety is a condition of persistently anxious mood in which the cause of the condition is unknown, and a variety of thoughts and events can trigger it.

Anxiety frequently manifests itself as the result of opposing or conflicting wishes, desires (e.g., wanting to stay home and be with the children and also wanting to be working outside the home), beliefs (e.g., believing that the work environment should always run smoothly but experiencing conflict between coworkers), life events (e.g., serious illness of a loved one), or stress resulting from conflict between roles (e.g., being a parent and a professional). The more difficult the decision between two opposing drives or pressures, the more severe the anxiety. When people cannot deal with anxiety through appropriate rational methods, they often resort to ego-defense mechanisms (see Chapter 5). The defense mechanism may operate until the person is better able to confront or manage the situation and stressors. This is a normal process that all people employ. Defense mechanisms do not extinguish anxiety; they try to bind or keep it from awareness (Stewart, 1997).

The distinction between anxiety and fear is not always clear. Lang (1985) and Craighead et al. (1994) consider anxiety and fear as being on a continuum. However, anxiety may be distinguished from fear in several ways. When people experience anxiety they often cannot specify what it is they are anxious about. On the other hand, individuals often misidentify the cause of the anxiety; for example, being anxious about traffic on the freeway when the underlying anxiety is about their supervisor's approval or their job performance. The focus of the anxiety is frequently more internal

"Will cochlear implants help my child?"

"Can my mouth be fixed so I don't sound like I'm talking through my nose?"

"Will my baby's cleft lip and palate affect the way he talks?"

"Do you think my child's frequent ear infections have affected his speech?"

"Do you think tubes (pressure-equalizing tubes) will help my child's hearing?"

"Can cytomegalovirus cause hearing problems in my baby?"

"My daughter had meningitis when she was three years old. Can that cause hearing problems?"

Do you think that all the antibiotics my son was on for such a long time could have affected his hearing?"

"Will hearing aids help my daughter? How much will they cost?"

"How much do you think hearing aids will help me?

"Will my child's Down's syndrome interfere with his language development and learning?"

"Will my son grow out of his stuttering?"

"Can I learn to talk without stuttering?"

"Will he ever learn to make his /s/ and /r/ right?"

"Can I someday make my /s/ and /r/ right?"

"Can I ever learn how to read?"

"Will his CAPD (or ADD) affect his school work? His social development?"

"How much will my son's head injury affect the way he talks? Will he be able to do well in school again?"

"Do you think I can do okay in school after I had the accident?"

"Will my voice get any better with therapy?"

"Do you think my husband will have another stroke?"

"Can I ever get back to work after my stroke?"

"Will my Meniere's disease get worse?

"Is presbycusis curable?"

"What are we going to do in therapy?"

"Will I ever be able to take care of myself?"

"Will I be a burden to my family?"

"Are you a really good audiologist/SLP?"

"How much will all this cost?"

Figure 6-1 Questions that reflect anxieties for counseling

than external and is a response to a vague, distant, or even unrecognized danger such as losing control, feeling that something bad is going to happen, or threats to self-esteem (Bourne, 2000). However, when people are experiencing fear, it is usually directed toward some concrete, external object or situation. Fear is an innate, primitive alarm response that is often accompanied by manifestations of fight or flight (Craighead et al., 1994; De Becker, 1997). The event that is feared is usually within the realm of possibility, for example, not getting a report completed on time, not doing well on an examination, possible loss of employment, being unable to pay bills, being rejected by someone who is seen as important, or the threat of emotional or physical harm.

PSYCHOLOGICAL, PHYSIOLOGICAL, AND BEHAVIORAL EFFECTS OF ANXIETY AND FEAR

Anxiety and fear affect people simultaneously in three ways: psychologically, physiologically, and behaviorally. Psychologically, anxiety is a subjective state of apprehension and uneasiness. Other mental symptoms may include irritability, poor concentration, mental tension, fear of losing control, fear of impending disaster, and worrying. There may be a reduction in awareness of the environment and surroundings, with the person appearing disoriented to person, place, time, and purpose (disoriented X 4). However, some individuals may become hypervigilant regarding the source of apprehension or fear (i.e., becoming excessively watchful and alert to danger). Individuals may have a decrease in emotional responsiveness, often finding it difficult to experience pleasure in previously enjoyable activities. Depressive symptoms are frequent for people with chronic anxiety (Bourne, 2000; DSM-IV TR, 2000; Gravell & France, 1992; Morrison, 1995).

On a physiological level, anxiety and fear may cause tightness in the chest and throat, respiratory distress, shaky or tremulous voice, queasiness in the abdomen, dizziness or feelings of light headedness, skin pallor, dry mouth, difficulty swallowing, increased pulse rate, urinary frequency, mild exertion producing undue increase in heart rate, muscle tension, headaches, sweating, flushing, or chills, and an exaggerated startle response. Sleep may be disturbed with difficulty falling or staying asleep, restlessness, or unpleasant dreams. Newly hospitalized patients may be given sedatives to help decrease their anxiety during the day and allow them to sleep better at night. Behaviorally, the appearance of anxiety may include a strained-looking face, furrowed brow, tense posture, clenched fists, restlessness, and pale skin (Craighead et al., 1994). Anxiety may cause people to speak rapidly and somewhat incoherently. Their voice volume (often decreased or erratic), pitch (unusually high because of tense vocal folds), and quality (strained, hoarseness) may be affected by anxiety (Boone & McFarland, 2000).

There may be several contributors to anxiety, including heredity, biology, family background and upbringing, recent stressors, self-talk and personal belief systems, ability to express feelings, and conditioning. A single-cause theory of anxiety overlooks the often-necessary combinations of contributors that may occur for any one person in any single circumstance.

Heredity is a possible contributor to some individuals so that they are predisposed to excessive anxiety. Some individuals may inherit anxious, inhibited temperaments that predispose them to strong reactions to relatively mildly threatening stimuli. Childhood circumstances may also contribute to childhood, adolescent, and adult tendencies toward anxiety. For example, parents who communicate an overly cautious or fearful view of the world, or parents who are overly critical with excessively high standards may contribute to individuals becoming excessively anxious or fearful. Children who experience neglect, rejection, abandonment through divorce or death, emotional, physical, or sexual abuse may develop emotional insecurity and dependency that form a background for anxiety reactions to stresses in later life (Bourne, 2000; Canino & Spurlock, 2000). Elective or selective mutism is an extreme example of the partial or complete withholding of vocal communication caused by severe psychological distress (Kolvin & Fundudis, 1981). Children who are physiologically capable of vocalization but deliberately refuse to speak at school are thought to be reflecting severe family conflicts (Andrews, 1999). Adults may develop long-term or permanent functional aphonia (elective mutism, Andrews, 1999) after events of acute stress (Boone & McFarlane, 2000).

STRESSORS AND ANXIETY

Short-term stressors may precipitate or trigger anxiety, such as a significant personal loss (loss of a job, loss of a loved one). However, cumulative stress over time may be a significant contributor to anxiety (e.g., health impairments, marital problems, employment uncertainty, or long-term impairment of communication abilities secondary to CVA). Cumulative stress producing anxiety is more enduring and less easily managed than short-term stress producing anxiety. In other cases anxiety may be the result of accumulation of several life events, that is, events that change the course of a person's life and that require adjustment and reordering of priorities. While one or two events each year are common and manageable for most people, a series of many life events over a one to two-year period can lead to chronic stress. Holmes and Rahe (1967) developed the *Life Events Survey* (also known as *The Social Readjustment Scale*) to assess the number and severity of life events that occur in a two-year period, and may be used as a general measure of cumulative stress (Bourne, 2000). Over time, stress can affect the neuroendocrine regulatory systems of the brain, which are important in mood and anxiety (Bear, Connors, & Paradiso, 2001). Biological causes of anxiety refer to physiological imbalances in the body or brain that are associated with anxiety, which may be the result of specific hereditary vulnerability and/or cumulative stress over time.

There are many possible factors that can contribute to an individual's level of anxiety: hereditary/temperamental factors, childhood history, cumulative stresses, or biological/medical factors. It is important to keep in mind that even positive events such as marriage, the birth of a child, a move to a new location, or a new job can be stressful. Therefore, avoiding being judgmental and focusing on an empathic approach to the person who is demonstrating anxiety will be beneficial to the therapeutic relationship.

Social Anxiety

Social anxiety involves fear of embarrassment or humiliation in situations where a person is exposed to the scrutiny of others. The anxiety may be at the level of fear depending on a variety of possibilities such as to whom the person is talking, how many people are listening or watching, their ages, their social status, and so forth. The anxiety or fear may be strong enough to cause individuals to avoid situations. Severe levels of social anxiety may be diagnosed by a psychologist or psychiatrist as social phobia and treated by individuals in those professions. A diagnosis of social phobia includes avoidance that interferes with work, social activities, or important relationships (DSM-IV TR, 2000).

Children and adults who stutter frequently have high levels of social anxiety when talking in front of a classroom, at meetings, or in front of groups. Talking to individual people, particularly those who are perceived as having a higher status, can create significant anxiety. For individuals who stutter, one of the highest levels of anxiety occurs when attempting to talk openly about their stuttering (Bloodstein, 1995; Sheehan, 1970; St. Louis, 2001).

Coping Through Avoidance

While working at the University of California, Los Angeles (UCLA) adult stuttering clinic, a man in his late 20s was in one of my small groups (3–5 people). The man stuttered severely and had decided to confront his problem and work to improve his fluency. He told the group that he had avoided people most of his life, going so far as to spend two years working on a military base on Wake Island in the Pacific Ocean where there were fewer than a hundred people. I asked the man what made him decide to come back to "civilization" and he answered, "I got tired of just having monkeys as friends." This man coped with his stuttering through extreme avoidance of human social interaction.

Some children with moderate to severe articulation or phonological disorders may demonstrate symptoms of social anxiety in their avoidance of interacting with other children or talking to adults because of fear of not being understood and fear of embarrassment. Children with repaired cleft lips and/or hypernasality may avoid speaking to others and may be considered shy by other children or teachers. When coerced to speak in front of a group, for example, giving a required speech or oral book report, these children may have panic attacks that are related to being embarrassed or humiliated. Adults with neurological impairments resulting in moderate to severe apraxia, dysarthria, aphasia, or cognitive disorders may avoid social settings or work environments in which they had been very comfortable and successful for decades. These adults may choose to remain in their homes and seldom leave to avoid potential difficulty communicating in public and being embarrassed or humiliated. The adult with a neurogenic communication problem who chooses to avoid normal social contacts may cause stress within the family because of the limited activities he or she now enjoys. It is important for clinicians to appreciate that some of our patients may have had significant social anxiety prior to their neurologic damage, and the neuropathology exacerbates their social anxiety to the level that it becomes a social phobia.

GENERAL APPROACHES TO HELP SOCIAL ANXIETY

General approaches that may be helpful for clients and patients who are experiencing social anxiety related to their communication disorders include: hierarchy analysis, relaxation training, cognitive therapy, and group therapy (Avent, 1997 & 2002; Boone & McFarlane, 2000; Bourne, 2000; Craighead et al., 1994; George & Cristiani, 1995; Gladding, 2000; Nystul, 1999). These approaches are discussed in the following sections.

HIERARCHY ANALYSIS

Many clients with voice disorders or fluency disorders benefit from hierarchy analysis in which the person is asked to list various situations in his or her life that ordinarily produce some anxiety. The person is then asked to arrange those situations in a sequential order from the least to the most anxiety-provoking. Wolpe (1987) developed this systematic desensitization approach in which a person is taught relaxed responses to anxiety-evoking situations. In a step-wise fashion the person learns to approach and master one anxiety provoking situation after another (Feldman, 2002). Boone & McFarlane (2000) provide details of this approach.

RELAXATION TRAINING

Many clients with voice disorders and some clients with fluency disorders benefit from relaxation training; however, most people with normal stresses in their lives may also benefit from this approach. Since people often cannot change their worlds, they need to learn to change their responses to it (Elliot, 1994). Regardless of who we are or what we do, good things, bad things, and tragedies are going to occur in our lives. Learning relaxation responses to stressful situations can help people maintain their emotional equilibrium so they can better maintain their ability to function satisfactorily in their work life, home life, and social life (Craighead et al., 1994; Bourne, 2000). Essentially, relaxation training helps people become more aware of their physiologic state of tension and then provides ways to manage it better. Boone and McFarlane (2000) provide specifics about the relaxation approach.

COGNITIVE THERAPY

The process of change in cognitive therapy initially involves the use of behavioral strategies to increase activities, especially those that give the person a sense of mastery and pleasure. The following procedures are also used: 1) identification of dysfunctional and distorted cognitions and realization that they produce negative feelings and maladaptive behaviors; 2) self-monitoring of negative thoughts or self-talk; 3) identification of the relationships of thoughts to underlying beliefs and feelings; 4) identification of alternative and more productive thinking patterns; and 5) hypothesis testing regarding the validity of the person's basic assumptions about him or herself, the world, and the future (Craighead et al, 1994; George & Cristiani, 1995; Prochaska & Norcross, 2003). Overall, the intention of cognitive therapy is to help the person change the way he thinks about a situation, which in turn will help him change the way he feels about the situation. (See Chapter 2 for more details and applications of cognitive therapy.)

GROUP THERAPY

Group speech therapy is commonly used in public schools in order to manage large caseloads of children. However, group therapy also provides benefits for children who have anxiety about their communication problems. Learning to speak openly in small groups can help them gain confidence and prepare them to speak in larger groups, such as in front of a class. Group therapy has long been used with individuals who stutter (Bloodstein, 1995; Sheehan, 1970; Stromsta, 1986; Van Riper, 1953). Sheehan felt that stuttering was a social problem and, therefore, was best worked with in a social (i.e., group therapy) environment. Group therapy and support groups for individuals with neurological disorders have been incorporated into hospital programs for many years. University clinics have many strong group therapy and support groups for clients with neurological disorders. (Avent, 1997, 2002, discusses a very successful group therapy program established at California State University, Hayward). Laryngectomy support groups have been established in some university programs. Support groups have been very helpful for many parents of children who are deaf or hard-of-hearing, providing the opportunity for parents to meet and interact with others who are in a similar situation (see Chapter 7 for information on group therapy for hearing impairment).

Acute Stress Response

Acute stress response (which may evolve into an Acute Stress Disorder) involves development of anxiety and possible disabling symptoms after a traumatic event, and may be considered a response to a crisis event (see Chapter 9). The initial trauma involves exposure to an event that carries the threat of death or serious injury. In an acute stress response the symptoms subside in less than one month; however, if the symptoms last beyond one month a psychologist may change the diagnosis from acute stress disorder to posttraumatic stress disorder (see Chapter 9). Causes of acute stress responses in individuals SLPs and audiologists may see include CVAs, TBIs, or sudden loss of hearing, and other causes of rapid or abrupt onset of communication disorders. These individuals may have a subjective sense of emotional numbing (being out of touch with feelings), feelings of detachment or estrangement from others, absence of emotional responsiveness, loss of interest in activities that used to be pleasurable, reduction of awareness of surroundings and environment (i.e., not being oriented to person, place, time and purpose; being in a daze), or derealization (feeling the experience was not real). The symptoms cause significant distress and interfere with normal functioning (Bourne, 2000; DSM-IV TR, 2000).

Individuals with acute stress responses also may have symptoms of despair and hopelessness that may be sufficiently severe and persistent to be diagnosed as a major depressive episode by a psychologist. Some patients may be the survivors of traumas in which other people were killed or injured (e.g., motor vehicle accidents, terrorist attacks, etc.) and the survivors may feel guilt about having remained alive or about not providing enough help to others who were injured or died. These individuals often perceive themselves to have greater responsibility for the consequences of the trauma than is warranted (Bourne, 2000; DSM-IV TR, 2000).

Panic Attacks (Panic Reactions)

Panic is an extreme level of an alarm reaction a person has in response to a perceived threat, whether physical or psychologic. In some cases there may be no perceived threat and the panic attack may emerge out of the blue, without any noticeable provocation, out of context, and without apparent reason. Physiologically, during a panic attack the autonomic (involuntary) nervous system's sympathetic branch (sympathetic nervous system) mobilizes several different bodily reactions rapidly and intensely. The adrenal glands release a large amount of adrenaline, causing a sudden surge or jolt, often accompanied by a feeling of dread or terror. Within seconds the extra adrenaline causes several reactions: 1) heart rate significantly increases, 2) shallow and rapid respiration, 3) profuse sweating, 4) trembling and shaking, and 5) cold hands and feet. Muscles throughout the body contract and in extreme cases a person may be too scared to move (compare the-deer-in-the-headlights phenomenon). Muscles in the chest and throat contract making it difficult to breathe or make any sound. An excess of stomach acid is released and there may be nausea; there is a release of red blood cells by the spleen and release of stored up glucose by the liver. There is an increase in metabolic rate and dilation of the pupils (Bear, Connors, & Paradiso 2001). Each physiologic reaction during a panic attack is the result of the fight or flight response. Panic attacks tend to last about 30 minutes during which time the kidneys and liver reabsorb the adrenaline that was released. Individuals who have recurrent panic attacks may have a panic disorder and should be evaluated by a psychologist or psychiatrist.

Some children who stutter may experience panic attacks when they are told they must speak in front of the class, and may exhibit a flight response by not attending school that day, or avoiding the experience any way they can. Children with other communication disorders such as hypernasality secondary to a cleft palate or significant articulation or phonological disorders may panic at the thought of speaking in front of the class. Avoidance of an anxious or fearful situation is one of the most common defenses used by children and adults with communication disorders. Avoidance may be accomplished by delaying the fearful communication situation or refusing to perform or communicate. Avoidance provides relief from threats to self-esteem caused by fears of communicating inadequately. Whereas avoidance prevents the fearful experience from occurring, escape provides immediate and effective relief from the feared situation at hand (Tanner, 1999). Escape may be used when postponements or refusals (i.e., attempts at avoidance) are not successful. People with severe communication disorders, such as severe apraxia, dysarthria, or aphasia may not be able to verbalize their anxiety and fears, but observations of their facial expressions and body language, and attempts to understand their limited verbal communications can help you appreciate the intensity of their feelings. Some hospitalized patients leave the hospital (escape it) by checking out against medical advice (AMA), that is, without the approval of their physicians. Patients may be escaping anxieties or fears of further invasive medical procedures, perceived isolation, or uncomfortable or painful rehabilitation procedures. This can have serious medical consequences, but it may provide patients with immediate (albeit temporary) relief from the fearful situation.

Anxiety Related to Places and Situations

Some individuals have significant anxiety or fear of being in places or situations from which escape might be difficult, or in which help may not be available in the event of a panic reaction. The anxiety may lead to pervasive avoidance of a variety of situations such as being home alone or being alone outside the home, being in a crowd of people, or traveling in a car or airplane. Psychologists use the term agoraphobia for this disorder, with the essence of agoraphobia being fear of panic attacks. These individuals not only fear panic attacks, but what other people will think of them should they be seen having a panic attack (Bourne, 2000).

Although SLPs and audiologists cannot diagnose or treat agoraphobia, we may see the problem in some individuals with whom we work. For example, individuals with cerebral palsy, CVAs, or TBIs may avoid going out in public for fear of being embarrassed by their handicaps, or becoming lost if they go too far from home. It is as though they are under a self-imposed house arrest. Likewise, some patients in skilled nursing facilities may refuse assistance from OTs or CNAs to get out of bed and into their wheelchairs so they can spend time in the day room or dining room.

Working with a Client with Agoraphobia

I worked with a patient with dysphagia in a skilled nursing facility. She had been an elementary schoolteacher for over 30 years before she retired. Her husband had died and her adult children lived in other states. The patient had made a comfortable little nest with her bed and side table. She had stacks of magazines, material for her needlework, a radio, and telephone. She was always happy to see me and did the necessary therapy tasks to improve her swallowing to be a safe independent eater. However, she chose to have all her meals in bed and refused assistance from anyone to get out of either her bed or the room. I discussed this with the nursing staff who said that she was probably afraid to leave her room and that she had become quite comfortable with her limited surroundings. Encouragement or coaxing did not help her get out of the room and extend her world. Sometimes all we can do is support and encourage; ultimately it is the person's choice where they want to live their life.

Cooccurrence of Anxiety Responses

Since the mid-1990s there has been increasing recognition that many people have more than one anxiety trigger, response, and/or disorder. For example, individuals with social phobias may also have panic attacks, and people with panic attacks may also have agoraphobia (Bourne, 2000; George & Cristiani, 1995). This is important for SLPs and audiologists to appreciate because some of our clients and patients may have experienced some type of anxiety symptoms prior to the current health-related anxiety responses. Individuals who previously experienced social anxiety may now be experiencing an acute stress response because of a hearing loss or aphasia. The communication impairment may exacerbate their previous social anxiety.

Summary

Some level of anxiety is normal for most children and adults who have their hearing, speech, language, cognition, or swallowing evaluated. The anxiety may also carryover into the initial stages of management by an audiologist or SLP. In most cases, we are seeing individuals who are trying to cope with their situational anxiety, which may not be reflective of their general manner of managing and coping with other areas of their lives. However, when an individual's anxiety interferes with the evaluation process we must consider whether the test results are valid. Also, when anxiety interferes with therapy, the client may benefit from the incorporation of anxiety management techniques into the therapy. We are not attempting to manage an anxiety disorder (the purview of psychologists and counselors), but we may be helping individuals learn and develop ways of recognizing, managing, and coping with the anxiety that is preventing or at least interfering with their gains in using hearing aid devices, or improving their speech, language, cognitive, or swallowing abilities.

DEPRESSION

Many people feel depressed during some point in their lives, but their symptoms may not warrant a clinical diagnosis of depression, particularly when grieving after a significant loss (see discussion of the stages of grief in this chapter). Other people suffer from more severe symptoms that together constitute a clinically diagnosed disorder, that is, depression. As SLPs and audiologists are not qualified to diagnose depression, we are primarily concerned with depressive symptoms and, in this text, will refer to depressive symptoms as depression.

Depression is a common response to a significant loss of hearing, speech, language, cognition, or swallowing abilities (Crowe, 1997; Schow & Nerbonne, 2002). Depression is the most common psychological reaction to stroke-related communication disorders, particularly aphasia (Tanner, 1999). However, young children with hearing loss or developmental communication delays or disorders may experience some depression if they sense disapproval or rejection from their peers or parents. The parents of these children may also experience some level of depression (along with guilt) from fears of possibly causing the delays or disorders (e.g., the mother's abuse of drugs or alcohol during the pregnancy). The parents may also experience depression if they feel they did not recognize and have the hearing or communication problem evaluated earlier and follow the recommended course of therapy (Alpiner & McCarthy, 1993; Schow & Nerbonne, 2002).

The DSM-IV TR (2000) discusses symptoms of individuals with depression. These symptoms may include individuals describing themselves as being sad, depressed, hopeless, discouraged, angry, having a loss of interest or pleasure in activities that were previously enjoyable, difficulty sleeping, loss of appetite, or possible food cravings. Many individuals with symptoms of depression report impaired ability to think, concentrate, or make decisions. They may appear easily distracted or complain of memory difficulties. In children, a precipitous drop in grades may reflect poor concentration caused by depression. In elderly people, memory difficulties may be the chief complaint and may be mistaken for early signs of dementia ("pseudodementia"). You may observe psychomotor behaviors including agitation (e.g., hand wringing, pacing, pulling or rubbing the skin) or psychomotor retardation (e.g., slowed speech, thinking, and body movements, low voice volume, little or absent voice inflection, or functional aphonia). Individuals often describe or demonstrate decreased energy, tiredness, and generalized fatigue, with even the smallest tasks requiring substantial effort. A sense of worthlessness or guilt may be associated with depression, with ruminations over minor past failings. Frequent thoughts of death or suicide ideation may occur.

In general, depressed mood reveals itself as sadness; depressed cognition is seen as a negative evaluation of one's self, the world, or the future, or impoverished thought (i.e., minimal thought processes with decreased ability to provide elaboration); and depressed behavior may include lethargy, isolation, disturbed eating and sleeping patterns (Craighead et al, 1994; Nystul, 1999). Our goal is to recognize the signs and symptoms of depression in order to make the appropriate referral to a professional who can manage the problem. However, whether or not a counselor, psychologist, or psychiatrist becomes involved with our clients and patients, audiologists and SLPs must provide therapy in our areas of expertise.

Some individuals prior to a hearing or communication disorder may have experienced depression, and their new communication disorder may exacerbate their depressive symptoms. Individuals with chronic, low-level symptoms of depression may be experiencing "dysthymia" (much like Eeyor in *Winnie the Pooh*). Also, family members may have chronic, low-level symptoms of depression prior to their loved one's communication impairment, and have surprising difficulty finding the energy or motivation we might expect of them to help the patient.

Interviewing

When interviewing clients or patients it is appropriate to ask about medications they are taking. In medical settings information about psychotropic drugs is available in medical charts, which should be reviewed prior to first seeing patients. Psychotropic drugs affect the psychological function, behavior, or experience of a person (Anderson, Keith, & Novak, 2002). Although we may ask clients in general terms about medications, we do not specifically ask if they are taking antianxiety or antidepression medications. Clients may not feel the need for the SLP or audiologist to know that information, and therefore may deny the use of medications or report taking some medications but not others. If, during the interview and evaluation of the client, we see signs and the person reports symptoms of depression, we may choose not to comment on it at that time, but to take note of our observations and be alert to them in future contacts with the person. Symptoms of depression may need to be evaluated by a psychologist, or the symptoms may be secondary to some other disorder, such as the hearing or communication disorder, which may also need evaluation and management by a mental health professional.

The challenge for audiologists and SLPs is to work with individuals who have symptoms of depression that may not be managed by the appropriate professionals, but which may interfere with therapy. A few approaches that are within our scope of practice may help improve the client's coping abilities and enhance the benefits of therapy.

General Approaches to Use with Symptoms of Depression

COGNITIVE-BEHAVIORAL APPROACH

There are several approaches clinicians can take to help clients with symptoms of depression, including the cognitive-behavioral approach, the humanistic approach, and the interpersonal approach. These approaches are discussed in more detail in Chapter 2. Cognitive-behavioral therapy (Beck, 1967; Beck, 1995) attempts to help individuals identify coping strategies, such as listening to uplifting music and reading positive books or other material. Clients can be encouraged to call or visit family and friends who are supportive and whom they enjoy spending time with. Speaking to people who have survived or worked through similar hearing or communication problems can help clients recognize that their goals in therapy are not insurmountable. Positive self-talk and affirmations can help change a client's negative view of themselves and rehabilitation potential. Clinicians may compliment the person when he or she is well dressed, neat, or looks nice. Reinforce smiles, jokes, and light-hearted conversation. The purpose of this is not to encourage the client to hide or mask his or her feelings, but to attempt to reinforce the person's more positive and upbeat behaviors which may influence the affective state (Craighead et al., 1994; Mosak & Maniacci, 1998). A client who is enjoying positive relationships and feedback is more likely to engage in and enjoy the tasks of therapy than a client who is focused on the negative side of life experiences.

HUMANISTIC APPROACH

Following the humanistic approach (Rogers 1951, 1957, 1961, 1980), the clinician will want to maintain genuineness, empathic understanding, unconditional positive regard, and acceptance of the client. Focus on "being with" the client rather than on what to say. Occasional reflections of feelings, such as "It looks like you are feeling a little low today" spoken in an accepting, empathic manner can help the client feel that you recognize his mood and understand him. This interaction can be very important to a depressed client who feels invalidated or ignored by others. It is often helpful to mirror the nonverbal language of the client (see Chapter 4, Interviewing and Therapy Microskills) who has symptoms of depression (e.g., speaking softly to match the client's voice, and moving slowly and gently in a manner that does not abruptly contrast with the client's). This mirroring can help the client feel that you are "in-tune" with him, which may help him be more responsive to you and the therapy (Corey, 2001; George & Cristiani, 1995; Prochaska & Norcross, 2003).

INTERPERSONAL APPROACH

Clients with symptoms of depression sometimes express themselves in ways that elicit negative responses from others (e.g., whining, moaning, complaining) (Sullivan, 1953, 1972). If we feel ourselves becoming irritated, the client is probably having a similar effect on other people too, including family and friends. We need to avoid responding in ways that the client has learned are predictable of other people, such as impatience, irritation, harshness, or anger. Responding in a predictably negative manner reinforces the vicious cycle that the client is already experiencing with others (Anchin & Kiesler, 1982; Klerman & Weissman, 1993). We need to be supportive and encouraging, not demanding. Our tone of voice and body language are as important as the specific words we say (Corey, 2001; Prochaska & Norcross, 2003; Wachtel, 1993).

Summary

Depression is a common response to a significant loss of hearing, speech, language, cognition, or swallowing abilities. Audiologists and SLPs need to be aware of the signs and symptoms of depression and make appropriate referrals to other mental health professionals when it appears that the symptoms are chronic and interfering with the person's life. We need to recognize when symptoms of depression are the likely result of the newly diagnosed or long-standing hearing or communication problem, and consider the client's affect as a part of the total person and his or her capacity to engage in the treatment process. Although we cannot diagnose or treat depression, there are approaches we can incorporate into our therapy that may improve our clients' coping abilities and enhance the benefits of therapy.

GRIEF

Loss is a natural consequence of living, as is grief (bereavement), the human reaction to loss. Loss is a fundamental aspect of any disability (including hearing, speech, language, cognition, and swallowing) which requires rehabilitation; the client or patient has lost a function, and family members have lost a loved one as the person they knew. Ultimately, the clinician's interaction with the grieving person can affect the overall prognosis for recovery of function (Alpiner & McCarthy, 1993; Rolland, 1994; Tanner, 1980, 1999).

Loss can have both real and symbolic meaning. Real loss involves loss of either a person (death or separation of a significant person), function (use of an arm), ability (hearing, speaking), or meaningful object (a prized possession). Symbolic loss includes a loss of either self-esteem, personal or professional standing, or the role a person plays in his or her family. A hearing loss or communication disorder can result in both real and symbolic losses (Tanner, 1980, 1999). Loss also involves an "intruder" (the impairment) coming into a person's life, much like an unwanted visitor who may stay forever.

The expression or outer manifestations of the inner grief experience can be quite varied. How individuals grieve is often influenced by their age and gender (Sanders, 1998). While gender differences before adolescence have not been studied, there are indications that early socialization has an effect on the way children respond to loss. The grieving behavior of a child will often be similar to that of the surviving parent of the same sex. For example, after his mother's death, a son may try to be stoic and "strong," much as he sees his father trying to be. While family and friends may say in an admiring way, "What a little man you are being!" or, "He is acting so grown up!" these comments tend to discourage the boy's important emotional expression.

Men and women tend to express their grief differently. Women who are grieving tend to have the following characteristics (Sanders, 1995, 1998),

1. Express anguish in tears and laments

2. Are not afraid to discuss grief

3. Seek support

4. Have difficulty expressing anger

5. Are prone to guilty feelings

6. Are caregivers to friends and family

7. Are keepers of the family circle

Martin and Doka (1996) and Sanders (1998) noted that men who are grieving can be described by the following generalizations,

1. Feelings are limited or toned down.

2. Thinking precedes and often dominates feelings.

3. The focus is on problem-solving rather than expression of feelings.

4. The outward expression of feelings often involves anger and/or guilt.

5. Internal adjustments to the loss are usually expressed through activity.

6. Intense feelings may only be expressed privately; there is a general reluctance to discuss feelings with others.

7. Intense grief is usually expressed immediately after the loss or postdeath rituals.

Sanders' (1998) grieving reactions may be viewed along an affective-cognitive continuum. Females tend to invest more energy toward the affective end of the continuum, while males tend to invest more energy towards the cognitive end. Perhaps because many women express grief in an emotionally expressive manner, caregivers tend to overlook much of the masculine (husband, father, son, grandfather, brother's) reactions to grief and focus instead on feminine (wife, mother, daughter, grandmother, sister's) reactions to grief (Martin & Doka, 1996). Although there are masculine and feminine cultural traditions of grieving, many men and women have surpassed them and, therefore, these stereotypes may not reflect a particular individual's processing of grief.

Stages of Grief

Elisabeth Kubler-Ross (1969) discussed the grieving process in her book, *On Death and Dying*. Our discussion of the grieving process expands Kubler-Ross's to grieving the loss of hearing, speech, language, cognitive, and swallowing functions, and, in a way, a loss of sense of self (Rolland, 1994). Grief is not considered a single reaction, but a complex progression involving many emotions and attempts to adjust and cope with loss. Kubler-Ross presents five stages in the grieving process: denial, anger, bargaining, depression, and acceptance. Parents of infants and children who are diagnosed as deaf or hearing impaired frequently go through the grieving process. Their child who looked so normal now may have a profound handicap that will affect all aspects of communication and many aspects of life. The parents may begin to envision possible restrictions and difficulties in their child's education, friendships and relationships, and eventual employment. The parents also will likely consider the challenges they will be facing in their parental roles and how the hearing impaired-child might cause limitations in the family's future plans. For example, the added expenses for hearing evaluations and hearing aids, and possibly special schooling for the hearing impaired child, may limit financial resources for other things the parents had hoped for.

It is helpful to keep in mind that patients and families may go through the stages more than once. For example, a child with a head injury and his parents may progress from denial to acceptance while in the hospital and rehabilitation settings, but when the child returns home and he and the family begin to recognize his severe limitations in that environment, they may have denial about new issues and eventually have to progress to acceptance again. Furthermore, when the child returns to school and is confronted with his severe losses by being moved to a lower grade level or into special education and adaptive physical education, and begins to see how his friends and teachers treat him differently, the child may again go through the stages from the beginning. For example, the child may experience denial (I don't need to be in special ed! I'm still smart!"); anger (I won't do this stupid work!"); bargaining ("If I do everything you want me to do, can I go back to my real classroom?"); depression ("I can't to this stuff like I used to. I'll never be smart again."); acceptance (I have to stay in this class, I guess, even if I don't like it.")

DENIAL

Denial has been discussed in some detail (see Chapter 5), but a few concepts may be reviewed. In response to news or information that is overwhelming, some people respond with the very basic defense known as denial. A person's first reaction may be a temporary state of shock from which she recuperates gradually (Kubler-Ross, 1969). Even well-adjusted people may initially employ denial during times of overwhelming anxiety (Gladding, 2000). Short-lived denial is a common response

196   ■ CHAPTER 6

to receiving news of a diagnosis of a disability or a serious illness or injury and is not considered an unhealthy response. The client, patient, or family member may protest, "No, I don't!" or "No, it can't be true!" This form of denial may be a relatively short-lived response when the person must make a radical adjustment to his or her self-image and expectations as this new information is processed. Denial is the barrier that many people temporarily erect as they try to adjust to a profound change in their lives. Denial becomes a concern when it persists for an extended period of time.

Some clients may need confirmation of a diagnosis (e.g., CAPD or dysphagia) and request a second opinion, particularly if the client does not understand the nature of the problem or is uncertain of the clinician's expertise. In many cases clients do not present a total denial of a diagnosis or the need for therapy, but a partial denial where they acknowledge some part of what is explained, but are not ready to accept all the diagnoses (e.g., hearing, phonological, and language impairments) or commit to a therapy regimen. Later, when the person has progressed to the stage of acceptance, there may be times when she reverts back to denial and again may need to work through the stages, although the progression is usually more rapid.

Parental denial of a child's hearing or communication problem can delay or even prevent the child from receiving much-needed help. In some cases, parents may admit a problem exists but not be sufficiently emotionally engaged to make the arrangements or carry out the needed management for the child (e.g., having the child's hearing tested by an audiologist, purchasing hearing aids, or enforcing the child's wearing of them). We need to keep in mind that denial is a plea for help and not a dereliction of duty on the parents' part (Luterman, 2001).

When a person denies or minimizes a communication problem for which he needs an evaluation and therapy, it is helpful to gently but clearly state the problems you see and the need for management. A strong statement about the need for therapy may result in stronger denial and resistance. Letting the person know that there is some urgency about beginning therapy and the reasons for the urgency may help the person accept therapy before he truly accepts the loss.

ANGER

Anger is discussed in some detail in Chapter 8, but a brief review of a few concepts may be helpful as they relate to grief. When the first stage of grief cannot be maintained any longer, it is replaced by feelings of anger and possible rage (Kubler-Ross, 1969; Rolland, 1994). The parents, child, or adult may ask aloud or to themselves, "Why me?" Although people do not wish hardships on someone else, they may be thinking, "Why couldn't it have been him?"

Anger in the grieving process can be very difficult to cope with because it may be displaced in all directions and projected onto the environment at times almost at random. Sometimes anger is projected onto people who have what the client has lost. For example, patients who must begin eating pureed meals with thickened liquids may become angry toward the therapist who ordered them, the individuals who deliver them, and even toward patients who have regular meals and thin liquids.

Clinicians need to keep in mind that the client or patient's anger is not a personal reaction to the clinician or the therapy program. The clinician needs to understand the anger and its source, and not judge it or automatically react to it. This perspective can be shared with family members who often have particular difficulty responding to a grieving person's anger. Family members may have a tendency to avoid or reject the person for angry behaviors. Helping the family understand the grieving process and the need for acceptance of the individual's moods and behaviors can help the grieving person feel accepted and loved.

Children and adults with severe communication problems often are not able to adequately express their feelings verbally, and may use angry behaviors to express the depth of pain they are experiencing. If reprimands are needed for physical displays of anger, they should be reserved for acts that are destructive or could harm the person or other individuals.

BARGAINING

In the first stage of grief the person is unable to accept the difficult facts of the diagnosis and the need for management, and in the second stage the person is angry with others, even God. In the third stage the person attempts to enter into an agreement which may postpone or reduce the effects of the loss. The bargaining stage, like denial and anger, is normal and helpful in the process of eventually achieving acceptance of loss. The person may bargain with whomever he feels may have some power or control over the loss: God, physicians, nurses, clinicians, or family. Some individuals even bargain with themselves saying, for example, "I will never take drugs again if I can just get my speech back." People often bargain for time or "one more chance;" however, when the bargained-for time has passed or one more chance is available, they bargain for more time and more chances. During the bargaining stage patients are often motivated and enthusiastic in therapy, which may be the result of hope for a rapid cure. Bargaining is about hope and/or trying to reverse the loss or change the outcome; however, when the hope for the ending or alleviation of the loss does not materialize through bargaining, the person will likely move to the fourth stage of grieving, depression.

DEPRESSION

Depression, discussed in some detail above, is discussed now in its relationship to the grieving process. When grieving people find that their denial does not make the problem go away, their anger does not frighten it away, and their bargaining does not gain them anything, they move into the fourth stage, depression. We need to keep in mind that people's loss of hearing and loss of communication abilities represent changes in their lives that can have profound effects. From these losses countless other losses may follow: loss of positive self-image, loss of self-esteem, loss of relationships as the person has known them, loss of employment with resulting loss of income and financial dependence, and many others.

As clinicians we may only see the tip of the iceberg of a person's loss. Our focus is on the hearing, speech, language, cognitive, and swallowing problems of the person. Although we try to view our clients, patients, and their families holistically, we can never imagine the total magnitude of losses they may be experiencing, or the depth of depression and despair they may be feeling. The cost of evaluations and therapy, hearing aids, and assistive devices can burden families so heavily that little luxuries may need to be dispensed with, and even household and family necessities re-evaluated and possibly eliminated. Financial burdens can weigh heavily on the individual and family, adding to their depression.

Friends or family may attempt to cheer up the grieving person; however, this response may reflect a lack of sensitivity and an implicit devaluing of a person's losses and need to grieve. The grieving person may try to smile or laugh to please or appease the individuals who are trying to be cheerful, but the person will likely revert back to grief when those people are gone. Grieving individuals should not be told to find the silver lining or to look at the brighter side of life. Such admonitions are usually for the benefit of the family or friends who make them; they are a reflection of their inability to tolerate another's sadness for an extended period of time. Rather than cajoling or attempting to cheer the grieving person, relatives and friends can be most helpful by being quietly present and not placing demands or having expectations of their conversations or interactions.

Some people may remain in the depression stage for only a few days, but for others it may last for a few months or longer. How long a person remains in this stage depends on a variety of factors, such as what was lost and how much was lost; the cognitive capacity of the person (severely brain-injured patients may not be aware of the extent of their losses); the pre-existing personality; and the support of family and friends. Brief episodes of depression can even be triggered by photographs of the person or family members, or other visual, auditory, or tactile sensations that remind the person of who or what the person was before the loss. Some people do not pass successfully through this stage but become fixated in the depression stage (Tanner, 1999).

Working with a Client Who Is Depressed

I supervised a man for several semesters who had been a successful automobile mechanic and taught automotive mechanics at a community college. He was also a stockcar race driver. He sustained a TBI in an accident during a practice run—the one time he did not wear his helmet. He was diagnosed with moderate to severe receptive and expressive aphasia, cognitive impairments, and apraxia. He often demonstrated depression when he attempted to speak about his former work, his racing, and his family (his wife left him and he had little, if any, contact with his young daughter). The students working with the client were encouraged to use strategies that were discussed earlier in this chapter under Depression. However, I felt that his depressive symptoms needed professional attention and referred him to the Counseling Psychology Clinic at the university.

People who are grieving and depressed often have difficulty attending and staying focused in therapy and may be generally unresponsive, lethargic, and pessimistic. There may be a significant change from the motivated and enthusiastic attitude the person had during the bargaining stage to an "It's no use" attitude during the depression stage. Individuals in this stage of grieving need to be monitored for signs of severe clinical depression, which may require mental health intervention. Our goal as audiologists and SLPs is not to eliminate the depression, but to show empathy and help the grieving person advance to the stage of acceptance.

ACCEPTANCE

Acceptance is an admission and acknowledgement of the truth: the loss did occur, denying it, being angry about it, bargaining over it, and being depressed about it will not change it. There is a resignation to the loss and the person is no longer resistant to it. The person may have consciously resolved to accept the way things are and to move on from there. In essence, the person has gone through each of the three ways people change: revolution (a significant event in the person's life has changed the way he or she thinks and believes); evolution (the person has progressed through the stages of grief); and resolution (the person has accepted things as they are and that he or she must move forward from there).

Summary

Although there is general agreement that grieving involves a dynamic process in which individuals progress through multiple stages, a particular stage model (such as Kubler-Ross's) may not apply to all individuals. The stages or phases of grief are not clear-cut and people may show evidence of signs of being in more than one stage at a time. Also, stages may recur: a person who appears to have advanced to the acceptance stage may suddenly appear to again be in the bargaining or depression stage.

Most of us have had a significant loss in our lives and know how it feels, although we may not have known or recognized various stages of our own grieving. In general, people tend to remember the last two stages, depression and acceptance because they are often more long-lasting than the denial, anger, and bargaining stages. However, as SLPs and audiologists, we may not see clients, patients, or family members progress through all the stages, particularly in acute care medical settings where patients are discharged after a few days to a few weeks. While in therapy in outpatient clinics and rehabilitation centers, clinicians may see patients and families work through the latter stages and arrive at some level of acceptance. In university clinics it is common for clients and families to have reached the acceptance stage and appreciate the continued therapy available to them.

GUILT AND SHAME

Guilt and shame are both negative emotions that often occur in the context of illness or injury. Although guilt and shame are distinct and different emotional experiences, they may coexist (George & Cristiani, 1995). Guilt is a feeling that frequently occurs when people believe that they may have in some way contributed to the cause of a loved one's problem (e.g., a mother and child are in a motor vehicle accident and the child is seriously injured), or that they have caused their own problem (e.g., not taking blood pressure medication and having a CVA). Parents (especially mothers) often feel some guilt for a child who has a congenital condition. Parents of hearing-impaired children often experience strong guilt feelings, manifested by overindulging the children or placing excessive demands on them (Schow & Nerbonne, 2002). Even when there is no direct cause, it is natural for parents to reflect upon what they could have done during the pregnancy that may have caused the problem to occur. An incessant search for a cause often reflects the desire to alleviate feelings of guilt (Luterman, 2001). Shame, on the other hand, is the result of not only believing that the person has *done* something bad, but that she or he *is* bad. Shame is reflected in low self-esteem, a sense of alienation, and disgust toward oneself. Individuals who feel shame may feel a need to punish themselves for their wrongdoing, or to compensate for their wrongdoing by engaging in overprotective or oversolicitous actions (George & Cristiani, 1995; Rolland, 1994).

A family's beliefs about the cause of a child's problem need to be explored because those beliefs often influence their actions and willingness to participate in the therapy process. During interviews with both parents, it is helpful to get each parent's explanation of what caused the child's communication problems. By asking each parent the same question in the same manner, the therapist communicates her or his respect for each parent's belief system and avoids the appearance of blaming either parent for the cause of the child's problems. The query can be framed in a curious, neutral manner that invites collaborative dialogue. For example, "All of us come up with reasons about how or why something happens, but do not always get an opportunity to share them. I'm interested in what each of you have thought about why Michael has a problem with stuttering." The responses from each parent provide insight into the understanding each parent has about the cause of stuttering in general, and each parent's view about the cause of the problem in that child (Rolland, 1994).

One or both parents may harbor a "guilty secret" in which they have a strong suspicion about the cause of their child's problems. For example, one or both parents may have been taking drugs or alcohol before or during the pregnancy and believe that the drugs or alcohol may have contributed to the child's speech and language delays. In some cases, a parent may share the secret during the initial interview by saying something to the effect, "I haven't really told this to anybody, but I think that . . . may have caused some of my child's problems." When interviewing only one parent and a secret is shared with you, it should remain confidential and not be shared with the other parent or included in a report.

Summary

Guilt and shame felt by clients, patients, or family members (particularly parents) may be effectively hidden from the therapist during the initial interview; however, with ongoing contact with the client and family, indications of guilt and shame may surface. If the clinician feels that other professional help is needed, appropriate referrals should be made.

COUNSELING SKILLS IN ACTION:

Parental Feelings of Shame

A mother in her mid-20s brought her four-year-old daughter into a clinic for a speech and language evaluation. The child had a very rare syndrome (only a few known cases in the world), and was part of a medical study of children with that syndrome. After the child was identified with the syndrome, the mother and father were also tested for it, and it was found that the mother was the carrier of the gene. The mother expressed considerable guilt about being the parent who passed on the genetic defect. She received genetic counseling and psychological counseling to help her examine and manage her feelings of guilt and shame.

CONCLUDING COMMENTS

The reality is that people do not experience just one negative emotion at a time, they may feel anxious, fearful, depressed, bereaved, guilty, shameful, and others simultaneously. Some clients come into therapy with a plethora of painful emotions that they have long had difficulty managing. The emotional responses to communication disorders compound their original distress. Some clients and patients are more resilient than others; some bounce back from emotionally difficult or traumatic experiences better than others. How well individuals cope with emotionally or medically challenging experiences reflects how they have coped with such experiences in the past. In addition, not all our clients, patients, or their family members may be emotionally stable prior to our involvement with them. Most of these individuals are not receiving professional assistance for their possible emotional difficulties and, therefore, their emotional difficulties may interfere with or complicate our evaluations and therapy.

Fortunately, most people have some methods of coping with anxiety, fear, and grief in their lives. Our task is to help people identify and draw upon their inner strengths and coping abilities to manage their emotional responses to their communication problems. In order to do this, we need to have knowledge of counseling skills and theories. When we feel that our education and training are not sufficient for this task, or that individuals have emotional difficulties that need other professional attention, proper referrals need to be made.

Discussion Questions

1. Have you ever had a hearing, speech, or language problem? What were your feelings about having the problem? How did it affect the way you thought about yourself? Did it influence your interest in becoming an SLP or audiologist?

2. Has anyone in your family had a hearing, speech, or language problem? What were (are) your feelings about how the problem has affected that person and other members of your family? Did it influence your interest in becoming an SLP or audiologist?

3. Anxiety is a part of everyone's life. What experiences, situations, or stressors cause anxiety for you? How does this relate to interactions with clients with communication disorders?

4. In your clinical work with children, adults, and their family members, what are some of the questions they have asked you that reflect some anxiety about the communication disorder they are experiencing?

5. Have you had an experience where you felt a client's anxiety affected the evaluation results? What were some of the behaviors the client was demonstrating that reflected anxiety? How were the test results affected? What did you do to try to reduce the anxiety?

6. How do you distinguish for yourself the difference between being anxious about an experience and being fearful about it?

7. Do you know anyone who you feel may have "free-floating" anxiety? How does their anxiety affect your interactions with them?

8. In what situations do you feel social anxiety? How do you handle that anxiety?

9. Have you ever had a client who appeared to have social anxiety? What were the signs and symptoms that you noted? Was the anxiety related to the communication problem?

10. Have you ever had an acute stress response to an experience? How did you manage your feelings in order to cope with the experience?

11. Has a client ever discussed an experience that may have caused him or her an acute stress response? What did he or she do to cope with the experience?

12. Have you ever had a panic attack? What was the situation and how did you manage your feelings?

13. Have you ever observed someone (not just a client) have a panic attack? What did the person do during the panic attack? How was the person eventually calmed?

14. What places and situations tend to cause anxiety for you? Do you avoid them sometimes? How do you manage your anxiety in those places and situations?

15. Have you had clients discuss places and situations that cause anxiety for them because of their hearing, speech, or language problem? What did you do in therapy to help them manage their anxiety in those places and situations?

16. Recall a time that you felt depressed. What were your thoughts (cognitions)? What were your symptoms (behaviors)? How long did the depression last? What did you do that helped? What did you do that did not help? What did people say that helped? What did people say that did not help?

17. Have you had a client who you felt had signs or symptoms of depression? What were they? How do you think the depression affected therapy? What did you do that may have helped the person with his or her depression? What did you do that was not helpful?

18. Of the various approaches discussed in this chapter that may help with symptoms of depression, what approach resonates with you the most? The least?

19. Recall a time of grief in your life. How did you express your grief? What did other people do or say that was helpful to you? What did they do or say that was not helpful? Recall how you progressed through some of the stages of grief discussed in the chapter. What stages were the most difficult for you? The least difficult? If you think deeply about the experience, do some of the feelings return? How do you manage those feelings now?

20. Recall a time when a friend was grieving. What did you do or say that you felt was helpful? What did you do or say that you felt was not helpful?

CHAPTER 7

Communicating Bad News and Working with Challenging Situations

CHAPTER OUTLINE

- Introduction
- Communicating (Giving, Sharing) Bad News
- Hidden Agendas
- Recurrent Themes
- Overly Verbal People
- Manipulative Behavior
- Emotional Lability
- Patients' Feelings of "Abandonment" After Discharge
- Repairing Counseling Errors
- Concluding Comments
- For Discussion

INTRODUCTION

Fortunately, most clients, patients and family members with whom we work are motivated to attend and work diligently in therapy, and they appreciate what we can do for them. The rewards of doing treatment are far beyond the monetary compensation we receive. Often the most important rewards are the intangibles of personal pleasure and professional gratification. However, even with "ideal" clients there can be challenging moments, and with some clients each encounter seems to present a different challenge that must be managed. The nature of being a speech-language pathologist (SLP) or audiologist involves working with challenging situations and difficult behaviors in ways that are therapeutically productive and, we hope, will even enhance the therapeutic relationship—or at least not lead to its deterioration.

This chapter and the following two chapters focus on challenging situations and difficult behaviors, and how to respond to them therapeutically. This chapter begins with communicating (giving) bad news, and is followed by other challenging situations. The next two chapters are organized to progress to increasingly challenging situations and difficult behaviors. However, it is recognized that for any clinician a particular situation or behavior may be especially challenging or difficult to manage.

COMMUNICATING (GIVING, SHARING) BAD NEWS

Buckman and Kason (1992), both physicians, state that most professionals in clinical practice have not been taught very much (if anything) about the technique of communicating bad news. Also, the psychologists and social scientists who carry out research on the subject do not have to perform this task in daily practice. The Buckman and Kason text is the only text known on this particular challenging subject. The nature of our work as SLPs and audiologists is that we must give "bad news" (usually the evaluation information) to individuals before we can begin to provide therapy (aural rehabilitation, speech, language, cognitive, or swallowing) or management techniques (hearing aids, assistive devices, etc.). Bad news may be defined in practical terms as any news or information that significantly or drastically negatively alters a person's view of him or herself and the future (Buckman & Kason, 1992). This definition implies that the "badness" of any bad news depends on what the person already knows or suspects about him or herself and the future, that is, the gap between the person's self-identity or future and the reality of the situation. In many cases we may consider the information we must share as difficult news rather than bad news.

Understanding principles of communicating (giving) bad (difficult) news can assist with future client-clinician interaction. Buckman and Kason (1992) and Banja (1999) say that if bad news is communicated poorly, our clients and patients may never forgive us. However, if bad news is communicated well, they may never forget us. Presenting bad news is a particular communication challenge that may be especially trying and possibly go poorly without sufficient understanding of several basic principles. Although audiologists and SLPs do not present the initial news to clients, patients, and family members about life and death issues or serious physical illnesses (e.g., cancer), the difficult information we must convey may be perceived by the receiver as more serious, profound, or life-changing than we might expect. How we share bad news can make an important difference as to how it is received and accepted. Also, if a person has received bad news from several other professionals in a short amount of time (e.g., a serious medical diagnosis, nursing concerns, physical therapy [PT] and occupational therapy [OT] diagnoses), our bad news may be the straw that breaks the camel's back, and the person may have an unexpected catastrophic reaction from feeling overwhelmed. This can occur in educational settings as well, for example, when parents attending an Individualized Educational Plan (IEP) meeting are presented discouraging information about their child from the school psychologist, the classroom teacher, the resource specialist, the audiologist, and the SLP.

Greenberg (1999) described a training program to help SLPs and educators increase their sensitivity about sharing bad news with parents. In the initial training she had participants recall an occasion when they received bad news about their own children, another family member, or themselves. Responses typically were sadness, shock, anger, disbelief, fear, anxiety, guilt, or despair. The memories of these occasions were also vivid in how they were told the bad news, and typically the memories were not positive. The same group was then asked to recall a time when they had to share bad news and how they felt. The participants described a variety of fears associated with giving the news, including fear of causing pain, being blamed, feeling they had failed, and losing control of their own emotions. This exercise may be helpful for other professionals to increase their understanding and empathy when sharing disappointing or bad news with a parent, child, client, patient, or other family member. The following is a discussion of six principles from Buckman and Kason (1992) and Banja (1999) that are helpful when giving bad news.

The Physical Environment and Presentation of Yourself

If possible, take the client, patient, or family members to a quiet room, which may require "the long walk." You may want to give an explanation such as, "I know that it's a bit of a walk, but it'll be much easier to talk if we can sit down" or "You'll find it easier to ask questions if we find somewhere quiet and private." If you will be talking to an inpatient in a hospital, draw the curtains (which gives an illusion of privacy and makes neighboring patients or visitors aware that they should not be listening, although they likely will be). Before clients, patients, and families hear what you will share they are often sensitive to your body movements, such as haste or composure, tension or comfort.

Walk into the room at a normal or slightly slower pace. Avoid a fast pace that may give the impression that you are in a hurry. Shake each person's hand, the client's or patient's hand first, then other family members, or individuals invited by the family. Shaking the client's or patient's hand first demonstrates that the client or patient comes first and is the focus of the time together. Buckman and Kason (1992) recommend that the client or patient be touched at least once during the meeting to reduce perceived emotional separation between you and the other person, and that the initial handshake may be the best time for an initial touch. A handshake at the end of the meeting or a brief touch of the arm may confirm to the client, patient, or relative the connectedness we hope they felt earlier.

The worse the news is, the more private the environment should be. A relatively small, quiet room feels more intimate and confidential than a large open, noisy room. There should be few or no distracting noises such as telephones ringing or fax machines whirring. There should not be potential for intruders who could walk in at the moment you are disclosing the bad news, during the time the individual(s) is trying to process the information, or during the time of emotional reaction to the news. The only people who should be present are the ones who are directly involved with the situation. There should not be any curious bystanders or noninterested people. If appropriate, introduce yourself again and your professional title because the person may have heard numerous names and titles already that day. All people should be sitting down because the reaction of the person receiving the information may cause a loss of strength in the legs or a loss of balance. The worse the news that must be presented the more time should be devoted to the person for processing and reacting to it. Some people, however, may have very strong emotional reactions to information you may feel is not particularly serious. Plan ahead so that you can avoid giving the bad news and then rushing off to another appointment. Even though you may not do or say very much after you have shared the information, your presence will likely be appreciated. However, if you are asked to leave after you have disclosed the difficult information so the person can be alone, honor the request.

Ideally, a desk or table should not be positioned between you and the receiver of the bad news. However, sitting at a table or desk at right angles facing one another with just the corner between you and the other person can facilitate a sense of openness as well as connectedness. The desk or table should have an area cleared of clutter so the person receiving the information has some place to rest her hands and arms, and possibly even her head if weeping occurs. Cups or glasses of water on the table for each person present, including yourself, are a thoughtful gesture. An emotional situation can cause people to have dry mouths, which can make talking more difficult. A box of tissues should be within easy reach of both you and the other person so that you can hand the person a tissue or she can get one for herself. Sitting within arms' reach of the person receiving the news gives a feeling of interconnectedness and allows the person to take your hand if she feels the need, or for you to touch the person's hand if you feel it is appropriate and helpful. Your body posture is important. You should sit in a relaxed posture (a rigid posture increases both your tension and the other person's), but not too relaxed because that degrades the importance of what you are saying. Use open body language (legs uncrossed, arms uncrossed, hands open) and lean forward slightly. Your facial expressions should be of concern and empathy, not strained or stressed. Maintain eye contact with the person as best you can without appearing as though you are staring, waiting for the person to react to what you are saying.

Use a gentle but not faltering tone of voice with moderate loudness so the person will hear you and not have to ask you to repeat because your volume was too soft. If the person asks you to repeat because she cannot believe what was just heard, repeat the same information in as close to the same words and tone as you just said. This allows the person to confirm that she heard you correctly, without having to compare new words or word order. Speak slowly, and pause after each important statement to allow the person to ask a question. Use as few technical words as possible. Speak in layman's terms. Professional and medical jargon "distance" you from the person and make it more difficult for the person to process both the bad news and the jargon. The therapeutic goal is to assist the person in processing what will likely be unsettling information.

What Does the Person Already Know

If appropriate, ask the person what he or she knows about the problem, or what the family knows about the client's problem. For example, "Mr. Farris, I'd like to know what you understand about your hearing problem." or "Mrs. Adams, what do you understand about your husband's stroke?" or "What did the doctor (nurse) tell you about your stroke (hearing problem, swallowing problem)?" This gives you the opportunity to assess the accuracy of the person's understanding and gives you a chance to hear the level of sophistication of communication the person has, which allows you to adjust your level of communication so you are not speaking too much above or below the person's language abilities. If the person says that no information has been given, consider that the person may have received the information and may be in denial, or possibly is wanting to see if you will tell the same story as was presented earlier by the other professional. Do not say anything negative about the person who should have (or did) give the bad news to the person, such as, "That doctor often doesn't take time to explain things to patients or families." It may not be true.

Communicating the News (Sharing the Information)

Reinforce the accurate information the client or patient knows about his or her problems, using the person's words if possible. This helps give the person confidence that what he or she said was heard and is being taking seriously. Educate the person about the delays, disorders, or disabilities as you understand them, which may be the presentation of new information or correction of information that had been previously misunderstood. Disclosing the bad news may only take a moment or there may be a number of areas that must be covered, for example, the person's hearing ability, speech systems (respiratory, phonatory, resonatory, articulatory), speech intelligibility, receptive language, expressive language, cognition, and swallowing. It is possible that the person has significant impairments in each of these areas, therefore some information may not be particularly bad while other information may be very serious. If there are a few areas with serious impairments, it may help the person process the information if you have a momentary pause after you present the information to allow the person to consider what you said and to ask a question for clarification about each impairment. Asking yes-no questions may help you recognize whether the person is understanding you well, for example, "Am I making sense?" "Do you follow what I'm saying?" "Does this seem sensible to you?" "This might be somewhat bewildering, but do you follow roughly what I'm saying?" "Do you see what I mean?" Such questions demonstrate that it matters to you that they understand what you are saying; the questions allow each person to feel encouraged to speak; they allow the client or family to feel an element of control over the meeting; and they validate the feelings of each person by making those feelings legitimate subjects for discussion.

It is helpful to alert the person that something serious is coming, that is, preface the disturbing information by saying something like, "Mr. and Mrs. Mehta, the evaluation results on Jenna indicate she is having problems in several areas." or "Mr. O'Hara, the hearing evaluation results revealed some significant problems." or "Ms. Childers, there are some problems with your swallowing beyond what we initially thought." Then tell the client or family the news straightforwardly and objectively. It is helpful to imagine yourself in the person's situation and consider how you would want to receive such information. Avoid being judgmental or accusatory with your tone of voice, facial expressions, and choice of words. Be careful not to make any innuendo that implies the person could have prevented this difficulty. The person may already have a strong sense of guilt and any negative insinuation you convey may unnecessarily add to the person's burden (e.g., a mother who was on drugs during her pregnancy and now has a seriously handicapped child).

Do not assume that the person will feel the same way you would if you received that particular information. The person may process the information in a different way than you. Perhaps the person anticipated the news all along and became mentally and emotionally prepared for it. Based upon your previous interactions with the person, you may anticipate how the person may likely respond to the information and then fashion your presentation accordingly. After you have shared the news, an empathic response is always appropriate when a person is trying to process disturbing information, for example, "This must be very upsetting for you." Do not say, "I know how upsetting this is to you" because you do not really know. You may also want to say, "This is a lot of difficult information to receive at one time." or "You have heard a lot of people talking about your child's problems today. It can be very overwhelming to hear so much all at once." Overall, during this difficult time of communication we need to be able to manage our own feelings so they do not interfere with the client and family managing theirs.

Reactions to the Bad News

Reactions to the bad news may range from nothing apparent or stoic resignation to a wide range of emotions and behaviors. Tears and crying are perhaps one of the more difficult responses we must be ready to see. Crying is not an emotion, it is a symptom. It can be a symptom of several emotions: fear, pain, frustration, anger, rage, despair, depression, and even joy, love, and humor (laughing so hard you cry), and others. Some people are moved to tears easily and will cry when almost any emotion reaches what may be considered a moderate level of intensity, while other people do not cry even when passionately moved.

Most people (including SLPs and audiologists) are not comfortable with the tears of people they do not know well. As clinicians, we are often uncertain how or whether to give comfort. Buckman and Kason (1992) suggest practical steps for professionals to use when a person cries.

MOVE CLOSER TO THE PERSON

Most people feel very vulnerable when crying, and feel even worse if they are rejected or perceive disapproval of their crying. Depending on what you feel is the person's comfort level, you may lean forward in your chair toward the person or move a little closer, but at least do not move away. Maintain eye contact with the person; this helps convey interest and empathy for the person's suffering. In contrast, looking away when a person cries may convey discomfort, criticism, or disapproval.

OFFER A TISSUE

Make certain that there are tissues available in the room where you are meeting with the client or family. If none are available and the person begins to cry, go get several or, ideally, a box of tissues. Providing tissues does several things: it gives the person permission to cry; it gives the person a means to restore his or her face (it is difficult to talk normally if your nose is running and your eyes are wet with tears); it gives the person an opportunity to hide his or her face; it brings you into closer proximity with the person; and offering them gives you something to do that is positive and helpful.

TOUCH THE PERSON

If you feel that both you and the person crying will be comfortable with contact, a light and brief touch of the person's hand or arm may show comforting support. The clinician needs to be alert to the person's response to this gesture and be prepared to withdraw the hand and refrain from further touch. Do not encourage a person to cry on your shoulder because this can easily be misconstrued by other people, including colleagues.

TRY TO IDENTIFY THE EMOTION THAT IS CAUSING THE TEARS

The cause may be obvious, in which case you can use an empathic response (e.g., "It's understandable that you would be very upset with this news."). If the cause is not obvious, a question may help you understand the source of the tears (e.g., "Can you tell me what is upsetting you at the moment?").

STAY WITH THE PERSON UNTIL HE OR SHE IS A LITTLE CALMER

By planning ahead you may have the time to be present during the acute reaction to the bad news. If you cannot remain with the person, try to find someone else who can be with the person for a while (e.g., a relative or coworker). If the person asks to be left alone, honor the request.

Buckman and Kason (1992) say that crying as an acute reaction to bad news is normal. However, prolonged, uncontrollable, and unstoppable crying is rarer and more serious. If the person frequently cries during other meetings or sessions with you, a referral to a counselor or psychologist may be appropriate.

Planning and Follow Through

Clients and families typically feel very alone and isolated immediately after they receive discomforting news. If the professional who presents the bad news does not have any follow-through plan, then the client or family will feel even more isolated and in a quandary. It is important for the bearer of bad news to also be the bearer of directions for support. By having a plan for help you are therapeutically responding to the isolation the person or family might be experiencing by emphasizing that support is available to them (recall the discussions in Chapter 2 on existential uncertainty, existential meaninglessness, and existential isolation). Try to get a sense of the client's or family's priorities and mesh the planning with those priorities. If what you feel is important is not quite what the client or family feels is important, the wrong kinds of plans may be made. In order to get a sense of the client's or family's priorities you may want to ask them what is important to them at this time. This helps the client or family feel somewhat in control of the situation, which is a perception that is therapeutic when there is an overall feeling of loss of control of one's life.

The clinician needs to identify the client's and family's coping strategies and sources of support and work with them. Most people have some kind of support network such as family, close friends, church, or coworkers. These will be the pillars on which people lean during difficult times. This is a time most people feel a pressing need for relationships. However, many people, particularly the elderly, have few if anyone they can call upon and expect support. Most of their family may be at a great distance or deceased, and friends may be too frail or have their own burdens that prevent them from providing the support they would like to give. There are no easy solutions for situations in which a person does not have family or community support.

Usually when audiologists or SLPs are presenting evaluation results something positive can be pointed out to the client or family. It may not balance the unsettling information but it may help provide some hope to the client and family. Providing the more positive information after the disturbing information may help the client and family recognize that the client is doing well, or at least better in some areas. Audiologists and SLPs sometimes feel a need to cheer people up even when it may be inappropriate. This is not a time to introduce levity or cheeriness to help decrease your own discomfort and anxiety. Maintaining an earnest manner provides respect for the significant changes that are likely to occur in the client's and family's lives and the adjustments they will need to make.

After the information has been shared and the client and family have processed it, at some point everyone must depart. Maintaining an attitude of sensitivity, compassion, and professionalism can help the client and family leave with the sense that you are someone they can rely on to be a part of their support system. If they do not already have your business card or telephone number, provide it with the encouragement to call you if they have any questions. Often after individuals have processed disturbing news they begin to have numerous questions they could not pose at the time they first learned it.

Communicating Bad News to Children

Audiologists and SLPs frequently have to give potentially upsetting information to children about their hearing, speech and language, and sometimes their swallowing. Buckman and Kason (1992) provide guidelines for communicating bad news to children.

HAVE A CLOSE ADULT RELATIVE PRESENT IF AT ALL POSSIBLE

If at all possible, talk to the adult first and agree on the manner in which the information will be shared with the child. The adult may want to participate (which you should welcome) and may have valuable insights into what will be the most difficult areas for the child. If the adult has no particular suggestions, describe how you will share the bad news with the child and ask the adult for his or her impressions.

CHECK YOUR COMMUNICATION LEVEL FREQUENTLY

With children of all ages it is difficult to be certain of their developmental level of understanding. Check your communication level frequently to determine if the information you are providing aligns with the understanding of the child. Answer the child's questions with the words and language level he or she will likely understand.

BE READY TO REPEAT WHAT YOU HAVE SAID

Children often require repetition of information, usually to be reassured that they have understood correctly. Be patient if the child asks the same questions several times or in different ways. This may be the child's way of assuring him or herself that you really mean what you say.

UNDERSTAND "MAGICAL THINKING"

Magical thinking refers to children's beliefs that their thoughts or actions can magically cause negative events to happen in their world. Magical thinking attributes unrealistic power to a child's thoughts and ascribes a cause-and-effect relationship to unrelated thoughts and actions. The young sister of an ill or injured boy may feel guilty and believe that her wishing that her brother was dead caused her brother's illness or accident. The injured child may also engage in magical thinking and imagine that his illness or accident are punishment for "bad thoughts" about a sibling or parent. Although children are not likely to express their magical thinking directly, it is important to make clear to children that the illness or injury is nobody's fault ("Your mother's illness [stroke] is not her fault, or your daddy's fault, or your brother's fault, and definitely is not *your* fault.").

GET PROFESSIONAL HELP IF YOU FEEL THE CHILD WOULD BENEFIT

Children who are seriously ill or injured often have difficulty communicating their thoughts and feelings to their families, and families often do not know what to say to their children. In addition to the ill or injured child, siblings may also be struggling emotionally as they try to understand the illness or injury and its causes. Professional counselors or psychologists may help these children communicate their thoughts and feelings, and help the parents as well as the other professionals better understand how these children are processing the bad news.

Summary

Sharing bad news is a part of our professional tasks no matter what setting we are in. It is never easy telling parents about serious hearing, speech, language, cognitive, or swallowing problems of their children, and often it is not any easier when sharing such information with an adult and their family members. Sharing bad news with children may be some of the most sensitive and challenging work we do. We sometimes work with the tragedies of life: TBI in children, unusual and severe syndromes, CVAs and other neurological impairments in adults of all ages. The list could go on and on. Our professional role requires us to maintain our poise and be as sensitive, insightful, and empathic as possible when sharing discomforting news to clients, patients, and their families.

HIDDEN AGENDAS

Hidden agendas are undeclared intentions of a person that may become evident during an interview or therapy session. Clients and family members usually have explicit concerns or goals that are shared with the clinician during an evaluation or family conference. Meanwhile, they may have concerns or goals that remain concealed, that is, implicit. When hidden agendas occur, there is usually some potential gain for the person that differs from the stated intentions or goals. When therapists suspect a person has a hidden agenda they may view the client or family member as indirect or manipulative, and may experience countertransference reactions or become irritated with the person. Clients and relatives may be reluctant to communicate directly about hidden agendas because of emotions such as anxiety, embarrassment, and shame. It is important to recognize their discomfort with expressing certain feelings, thoughts, or information and maintain an empathic view toward them.

The following situation has arisen many times in subacute hospitals and skilled nursing facilities. An elderly patient is approaching her or his maximum potential in therapy and is at a level where she or he can function with modified independence in a home environment. Early in the hospitalization and rehabilitation of the patient, the adult children were adamant about wanting their parent to live with one or the other of them. A discharge planning meeting with the family is scheduled and the director of nursing, discharge planner, and rehabilitation therapists (PT, OT, SLP) are present. Discussions about the needs of the patient are presented to the family. However, as the meeting progresses the team begins to suspect that the family has concerns about their parent being able to return to a home environment—at least *their* home environment (the implicit concern).

The family may be reluctant to be explicit about their concerns, perhaps out of embarrassment that they do not actually want their parent to live with them (the potential gain—home life as usual). The family's reluctance signals to the discharge planning team that this topic is very sensitive or taboo. This interaction may cause some team member's annoyance or irritation with the family. However, an alternative and more therapeutic response to what is suspected may be a hidden agenda is to show empathy and understanding for the family's concerns. The team may express the fact that many adult children understandably view such a move as a burden and that it can be very disruptive to already-busy households. Such a statement shows empathy and gives permission to the family members to talk about their previously unspoken concerns.

Hidden agendas may be common occurrences in cases where caregivers feel a reluctance to express their personal needs. Once permission is given for the person to talk about the issues, it may affect treatment and discharge plans of the patient. For example, in the above case, the patient may need to be discharged to an assisted-living facility, board-and-care home, or continuing-care retirement community.

When we recognize that a person has a hidden agenda during an evaluation, therapy session, or family conference, probing questions such as, "What other concerns do you have? or "Is there something you would like to talk about that we haven't discussed yet?" or "You seem to have something else on your mind. Would you like to talk about it?" can help the person more openly discuss a hidden agenda. Once the clinician recognizes the agenda she should explore what it is about and then help the person problem-solve the issues around the theme. We may need to deal with the hidden agenda as *the* issue, that is, the primary issue, regardless of what was anticipated to be the direction of the session. If the hidden agenda is not recognized and sufficiently managed, the issue may become a recurrent theme.

RECURRENT THEMES

Recurrent themes represent problems (issues) of particular concern which arise more than once that need to be addressed. As mentioned above, occasionally the recurrent theme may begin as a hidden agenda. Recurrent themes may involve most any issue, including a clinician's qualifications, the direction of therapy, or the cost of therapy. There is usually some level of anxiety the person has about the issue, and until the issue is addressed, anxiety may increase. The client may have difficulty focusing on therapy tasks until the recurrent theme is recognized and sufficiently discussed. If the issues are not addressed, a second issue emerges. The first issue is what the recurrent theme is about, and the second is the client's negative feelings about the clinician for not "picking up on" the issue (Shipley, 1997).

Clinicians can explore the recurrent theme using the open ended reporter's questions (what, when, who, and how) to gain general and specific information to help understand the client's concerns. Requests for clarification (asking the client if you understood him or her correctly, or summarizing the conversation in order to clarify or confirm what was said) can help the clinician discern the accuracy of understanding.

OVERLY VERBAL PEOPLE

Some clients and family members are overtalkative and do not give the clinician time to provide the information or deal with the issues she feels need to be addressed. New clinicians (and some experienced clinicians) often have considerable difficulty with such people trying to get a word in edgewise. The clinician may begin an interview or discussion using normal verbal encouragers (head nods, "um hums"), and then find that no encouragement is needed for the person to continue talking, ad nauseam. These individuals often talk rapidly and with somewhat of a monotone so that the listener does not get a cue as to the ending of a statement (a time to "jump in" to the conversation). They often use numerous "ands" as though each statement or topic is intimately related to the previous one. Their conversations may be rambling and convoluted, leaving the listener in a quandary about what the main topic of conversation is. These individuals may not be aware of or will ignore turn-taking pragmatics. Individuals with neurological disorders (particularly right hemisphere damage) may have "press of speech" and may not be aware of verbal or nonverbal cues from the listener that the listener wants to speak (Hartley, 1995; Tompkins, 1995; Worrall & Frattali, 2000).

When the clinician becomes aware of the person's overtalkative manner or the client's press of speech, in order to redirect and refocus the discussion the clinician may need to intentionally interrupt the person using vocal, nonverbal, or verbal interrupters. These are used to signal to the person that it is the clinician's turn to talk, or that some redirection is desired. Examples of vocal, nonverbal, and verbal interrupters include, clearing the throat, interjecting a short "ah," checking a clock or watch, raising a finger to indicate stop for a moment, getting a calendar to indicate you are scheduling another appointment, touching the person's hand or arm to get his or her attention, saying "Let me interrupt (stop, interject something, add something, etc.) for a moment." If the clinician feels the client's over verbalizations are the result of excessive anxiety or stress, friendly, reassuring or supportive comments about the client's fears and anxieties may reduce the tendency to oververbalize (Shipley, 1997).

MANIPULATIVE BEHAVIOR

Manipulation refers to behavior that covertly elicits desired responses from others, and implies an element of inauthenticity or deceit (Feltham & Dryden, 1993). However, perceptions of manipulation are in the eye of the beholder and may reflect how secure (or insecure) we are feeling with an individual. When clinicians feel tricked, fooled, or frustrated by a person, they often describe that person as manipulative. Clinicians do not like to think of themselves as gullible and easily manipulated, and sometimes clinicians deal with those feelings by blaming the client. However, when we are comfortable with our clinical skills and have an understanding of our client's motivations and typical interpersonal patterns, we are much less likely to pathologize the person's behavior and apply this derogatory term.

A child or adult who may be viewed as manipulative is probably trying to gain some measure of control and self-esteem in a situation where she or he feels vulnerable and does not currently possess better coping or interpersonal skills. Children may use manipulative behaviors when they avoid working directly on therapy tasks by distracting the clinician with playful and charming antics and conversation. These children may be attempting to avoid or postpone doing tasks that are difficult for them and threaten their self-esteem. In response to a child who is using such tactics, the SLP may respond with, "I know these exercises are difficult for you, but by doing them your speech will get better and I'm sure you will be happy about that." This response acknowledges the child's difficulty with the tasks and provides an opportunity for a nonthreatening discussion about the therapy.

In some situations, manipulative behavior occurs when a person has a sense that his or her goal is not socially acceptable. The classic example of manipulation in adults is the malingering patient. Malingering involves intentional simulation of an illness or disorder with a conscious motivation of external incentives or gains, for example, financial compensation from insurance or avoiding expectations of others, such as returning to gainful employment (Johnson & Jacobson, 1998). SLPs or audiologists may see patients who are malingering who have neurological damage but feign symptoms for compensation of more severe impairments than evaluation results indicate.

If a clinician experiences a person's behavior as manipulative, consider first the motivations and feelings of the person. Is he or she fearful or uncertain about what is being asked in therapy? The clinician can use a reflection of feeling to help identify and understand what the person is feeling. Confrontations are seldom effective or useful in these situations; they only cause the person to retreat or assume a defensive posture. In response to the patient who is suspected of malingering, the clinician may respond with, "I wonder if you are feeling uncertain or even a little fearful about your future and the possibility of returning to work." These reflections acknowledge the patient's struggles and convey an empathic, respectful tone.

Mr. M.

A patient (Mr. M.) in an acute-care hospital where I worked was receiving physical, occupational, and speech therapy following a mild stroke. After a few sessions with each of the rehabilitation team members we began to suspect the patient was malingering. Upon my initial evaluation, I noted specific receptive and expressive language problems; however, as Mr. M. had opportunities to observe other patients in their rehabilitation programs who had had strokes, he began to take on some of their impairments. He began to have more difficulty walking and using his right arm. I noticed inconsistent signs of dysarthria and apraxia, and his receptive and expressive language problems varied from day to day. Further brain imaging techniques conducted by the radiologist revealed no additional cerebral hemorrhages or other complications. I discussed with Mr. M. the possibility of him having concerns about returning to his former job and not performing at the level that was expected of him. I asked him if he was willing to meet with the social worker to discuss his concerns. He agreed and the referral was made. Mr. M. began making more rapid improvements in all areas of rehabilitation and eventually returned to his work, albeit at a lower level of expectations and performance.

When we have not fully explained or clients do not fully understand our therapy goals and strategies, they may view our therapeutic strategies and techniques as sophisticated forms of manipulation, and may understandably respond with resistance. Clients want to maintain control of their own lives, perhaps saying to themselves, "No one is going to get me to do something I don't want to do." If the clinician thinks this type of resistance is occurring, she may need to review the rationales for the therapy goals and strategies with the client, and encourage a collaborative process.

EMOTIONAL LABILITY

Emotional lability refers to uncontrolled and often rapidly changing expressions of emotions or mood swings (Feltham & Dryden, 1993), particularly secondary to neurological impairment (Brookshire, 2003). Situations in which emotional lability are likely are CVAs and TBIs, which may cause a loss of inhibitory control, and the patient's intense emotional responses to loss of abilities. The most common sign that the patient is emotionally labile is that he or she cries easily or appears overreactive to neutral situations or conversational topics. The patient's overreactivity may include other emotional expressions, inappropriate laughter in situations that are not humorous, or excessive laughter in response to mildly amusing stimuli. Emotional lability may also be seen as undue anger or rage. In some instances the lability may be a reflection of an emotionally significant thought or feeling (e.g., thoughts of family), but in other instances the lability may not have a significant emotional context (e.g., thoughts about breakfast). Some contexts or topics may understandably precipitate emotional reactions, but in other cases labile behaviors may reflect the neurological impairment.

Helping the Person Who Is Expressing Emotional Lability

Rollin (2000) makes several suggestions about helping patients who are emotionally labile. He suggests not bringing attention to the behavior if it is only a momentary lapse of emotional control, and to continue on with the planned therapy. "Normalizing" the behavior may also be helpful, for example, "What you are experiencing now is natural considering what you've been through," or "Because of your stroke, it's hard to control your feelings all the time," or "As you improve physically, you'll have better control of your crying" (p. 51). In some cases the clinician may choose to reflect the patient's feelings of sadness, uncertainty, or anxiety and provide empathy about the feelings and reactions. Gently acknowledging the patient's behavior and asking a probing question may help the clinician better understand what the patient is thinking and feeling, for example, "You are crying. Is there something we are talking about or doing that has upset you?" If the clinician feels a therapy task has precipitated the labile response, changing the task may help the patient regain his or her composure. Having tissues on the table or nearby can help the person manage tears. We need to remember that patients are often embarrassed about their crying and to reassure them occasionally that it is quite all right and understandable.

PATIENTS' FEELINGS OF "ABANDONMENT" AFTER DISCHARGE

Many patients, particularly those in convalescent hospitals, feel somewhat abandoned when discharged from therapy. Patients may develop some dependency on the audiologist or SLP, not only for rehabilitation, but also for companionship and a sense of nurturing and support. In convalescent hospitals it is often only the SLP who gives patients (residents) undivided attention, listening to every word, conversing with them at the level they understand, and showing enjoyment and caring during the time together. Most all the other care given to such patients reflects their physical needs such as bathing and toileting, eating and exercising, physical and occupational therapy. Patients in convalescent hospitals often become easily attached to their SLPs, sometimes viewing them as a favorite child.

Realizing Your Impact on Your Patients

I have spent many summers working in convalescent hospitals (skilled nursing facilities), and I particularly enjoy working with elderly people. Some patients have touched my heart and I miss them even now. I have given several patients little stuffed animals after discharging them from therapy, wanting them to have something to hold and cuddle during their lonely days. The stuffed animals became more important to some of them than I could have imagined. Some patients kept them with them all the time; beside their pillow at night, and holding them in their laps when in their wheelchairs. The family of one patient contacted me after I had returned to my fall semester teaching to inform me that their mother had died, and that they buried the little stuffed animal with her.

At some point we must end therapy with all clients and patients and discharge them from our services. Many, if not most, of them, we never see again, knowing that we have passed through their lives as they have passed through ours. If we are working in a long-term care facility it is considerate of us to take a few minutes each day and visit as many of the patients as possible for whom we have provided therapy. They recognize that we cannot spend half an hour or an hour with them as we did before, but the short visits can help them feel valued and allay their feelings of abandonment. The clinician may want to invite or encourage some clients or patients after discharge to contact him or her if they need further help, or if they just want to let the clinician know how they are doing.

REPAIRING COUNSELING ERRORS

We can assume that if we are working with people who have complex issues that affect their lives, we are going to make mistakes in what we say and how we say it. Our education and training provide the foundational skills for being SLPs or audiologists, but our advanced skills come from on-the-job-training (OJT). This is true not just for our profession but all professions. Clinicians have sometimes said, "Physicians bury their mistakes. Our mistakes live on to talk about us." The adage is still true; however, mistakes with dysphagia patients can be life-threatening as well. Most of our errors, though, are verbal and nonverbal; that is, not saying something in the best way or not being aware of the messages our body language may be projecting. Clients, patients, and family members may recognize our counseling errors more easily than we can. They know when we have said something in an insensitive manner and they can read our body language better than we can read our own.

During undergraduate and graduate clinical training, clients and their families are usually very tolerant of student mistakes. Clients may be bewildered and families may see humor in the errors student clinicians make. Ultimately, in the university setting the faculty supervisor must take responsibility for what is said and done by the student clinician. However, once students graduate, the professional responsibility is on their shoulders.

Most clinicians would likely agree that with each person they try to help, they make some error(s) in what they say or do. In *The Imperfect Therapist: Learning from Failure in Therapeutic Practice* (1989), Kottler and Blau reveal and discuss errors they and other highly regarded psychotherapists have made. In some cases, their counseling errors have had devastating consequences on people's lives.

Regardless of the attention and empathy we give to our clients, patients, and their family members, we are still going to make errors. How we repair our errors depends first on whether we are even aware of them. If we notice the client or family wincing from something we have said, we should quickly reflect whether our verbal and nonverbal messages were received in the way we had intended. Were we clear and accurate in what we said? Were we congruent? Were we sensitive and empathic? Did we say too much or too little? Did our statements sound critical or blaming? Was the information presented prematurely or in a harsh manner? It is important to ask these questions and, based upon our self-evaluation, determine what needs to be said or done to repair the error. Even when a person looks at us with a stoic expression we need to be asking ourselves these questions throughout a time of counseling. Individuals who have a stoic presentation and give little visual or verbal feedback are more difficult to work with than those who give us much feedback. We tend to misread or read into expressionless faces. Negative feedback is easier to work with than no feedback. We need to keep in mind that our neurologically impaired patients may have expressionless faces but may still be having intense feelings that they would like to reveal but cannot.

Pipes and Davenport (1998) and Morrison (1995) emphasize that the possibility of clinician error needs to be consistently acknowledged and that the clinician must be willing to listen to client feedback and change behavior or expectations to increase the clinician's credibility. When we realize that we have made an error, we have some options regarding how to manage it. The first possibility, of course, is an apology followed by a correction. Most people accept such apologies and recognize that everyone (including clinicians) makes mistakes, and that everyone has good days and bad days. Appropriate and timely apologies can enhance the clinician-client relationship. For example, if a clinician makes an error with the client's name, a rapid apology and saying the correct name is all that is needed. However, it is not necessary to provide personal reasons for the error, such as, "I'm sorry. I'm very tired. I didn't sleep well last night." Sometimes an apology may seem like an overstatement, and a brief revision or correction of what we said is sufficient. If the error is not corrected, the person may harbor some ill feelings about us and we may never really understand what caused the change in the person's attitude toward us. As clinicians, we tend to be sensitive to other people and recognize subtle changes in their behaviors toward us. If we feel that something is wrong, we may try to talk to the person about it, but we may not get open, honest responses. What is left unsaid by the client or by us may haunt us for a long time. At best, sometimes all we can do is learn from our mistakes and try to do better the next time. We will always remain imperfect clinicians.

CONCLUDING COMMENTS

The nature of our work is that we must give bad news to children, clients, patients, and families about the evaluation results. Although we try to sandwich it between good news about the child's hearing, speech, language or general behavior, or about the preserved abilities of an adult, usually some negative information needs to be presented. The setting and manner in which the information is presented can have important effects on how well it is received and accepted. Skills in presenting bad news are essential for our profession.

Some clients and family members have hidden agendas that may become evident during an interview or therapy session. Recognizing and appreciating the person's discomfort with expressing certain feelings, thoughts, or information helps us to respond in a therapeutic manner rather than allowing ourselves to feel the person is being manipulative and become irritated. Sometimes hidden agendas become recurrent themes if they are not recognized and openly discussed by the clinician. Recurrent themes are issues that present some level of anxiety for the person, and until the issue is recognized and sufficiently managed, the anxiety will likely continue and possibly escalate. Overly talkative people are a challenge for many clinicians. In therapy we listen when a client speaks, but when their verbalizations become increasingly tangential or they do not exercise the pragmatics of turn-taking in conversation, we may feel the session is out of our control and time is being wasted. Learning how to politely interrupt an overly talkative client can help the therapy progress and help the client make gains more quickly.

Emotional lability is fairly common in patients with neurological impairments and may become evident when patients cry easily and display overreactivity to minor events. The clinician's manner of responding to the lability can help patients accept and better manage the uncontrolled emotions. Some patients, particularly the elderly in convalescent hospitals, may feel abandoned when the SLP or audiologist discharges them from services. We need to appreciate that for many of these patients, our therapy means a significant amount of face-to-face contact with a person who is interested in them as people, presents a caring manner, is not typically physically invasive (other than with swallowing problems), and may remind patients of loved ones, such as children or grandchildren.

Whether we are new or experienced clinicians, we make mistakes in what we say and how we say it. The more complex and the more sensitive the issues, the greater the likelihood that something we say or do will not be received well by someone. We first may need to do some self-evaluation to recognize an error, and then consider options for ways to manage it. Appropriate and timely apologies can enhance the clinician-client interaction.

Discussion Questions

1. Remember a time when you were given some bad news, perhaps the death of a relative or friend. How was the information shared with you? How do you wish it had been shared?

2. Recall a time when you had to give a client or family member some bad news. What do you think you did well? What do you wish you had done differently?

3. What do you prefer people around you do when you are crying?

4. What do you do when you are trying to help someone who is crying?

5. Recall a situation in which you had a hidden agenda. Did you get your agenda out into the open? Until it was in the open, how were you feeling and what were you thinking about? How have you felt when you had a hidden agenda and it was not brought into the open?

6. Have you recognized when a client or family member had a hidden agenda? Discuss the situation.

7. What have you done when you felt that someone you were talking to missed a subtle but important point you wanted the person to understand?

8. Recall a time when you recognized a client's recurrent theme. How did you respond to it once you recognized that it was important to the client?

9. Do you have a friend whom you feel is overly verbal? What is it like having a conversation with that person? How do you get your points into the conversation?

10. If you have had a client or family member who was overly verbal, how did you manage the situation?

11. Have you had a client or family member who you felt was trying to manipulate you? What did the person do? How did you manage the situation?

12. Recall a situation in which you may have been manipulative. What were your motives? What was a better way to get what you wanted?

13. Have you had a client with emotionally labile behaviors? How did you manage the situation? What might you do differently now?

14. If you worked in a convalescent hospital, what are some things you could do to help patients (residents) not feel abandoned after you discharge them from therapy?

15. Recall a time when you made an error when counseling with a client or family member. Discuss the situation and how you handled it. How might you handle it differently or better now?

Working with Resistance and Anger

CHAPTER OUTLINE

- Introduction
- Resistant and Noncompliant Attitudes and Behaviors
- Angry or Hostile Attitudes and Behaviors
- Communicating and Responding to Angry Behavior
- Concluding Comments
- For Discussion

INTRODUCTION

This chapter presents situations and behaviors that are often difficult for clinicians to manage. The focus of this chapter is on resistant attitudes and behaviors, and angry or hostile attitudes and behaviors. Although these situations may not arise often, they can be particularly challenging to manage in a safe and therapeutic manner. In all cases, the clinician's safety is the first concern. However, by recognizing potentially escalating behaviors, the audiologist or SLP can often assuage potentially threatening situations.

RESISTANT AND NONCOMPLIANT ATTITUDES AND BEHAVIORS

Resistance and noncompliance are terms that are used loosely, often to describe what a client, patient, or family member does that makes the therapist feel inadequate (Morrison, 1995; Pipes & Davenport, 1998; Teyber, 2000). Although resistance and noncompliance are not synonyms, they are often used interchangeably by SLPs and audiologists (as well as physical therapists [PTs] and occupational therapists [OTs]). Resistance refers to ambivalence about doing what is asked or recommended in therapy. Meanwhile, noncompliance refers to failure to comply or follow through with what is asked or recommended and does not necessarily involve ambivalence. However, the clinician is seldom privy to all the thoughts and feelings of the person, and rarely knows whether ambivalence or refusal is at the heart of the matter. In view of this and the fact that the behaviors are similar for resistance and noncompliance, for this discussion we use the term resistance to include noncompliance.

Resistance (Freud, 1914) is a natural occurrence when people fear change or are uncertain about a new situation. The paradox is that many people who seek and are involved in therapy experience resistance to it (e.g., consider the person who stutters who wants to change but resists the therapy). People are likely to show resistance when they feel frightened or threatened. Resistance does not mean that people are being irresponsible or obstinate in order to make our work difficult. Resistance may be some people's life-long pattern of coping with anxiety-provoking feelings. Their resistance serves to protect them from giving up familiar patterns of behaviors (e.g., dysfluent speech). Resistance can also serve to protect people from facing a change in identity; that is, accepting therapy means accepting that something has changed (e.g., loss of ability to communicate because of a CVA) or needs to change (e.g., wearing hearing aids). Resistance is frequently the result of the fear of change. People change in essentially three ways.

1. *Evolution*: where a person slowly, sometimes almost imperceptibly, changes over time (e.g., normal maturation and growth, education, rehabilitation).

2. *Revolution*: where a significant event in a person's life changes the way he or she thinks, believes, or behaves (e.g., marriage, parenthood, a stroke or TBI).

3. *Resolution*: where a person decides that it is now time to change (e.g., going back to school; stopping drinking or taking drugs; or taking responsibility for improvement in therapy).

SLPs and audiologists work with individuals and families who are changing or have changed in each of these ways. Change through evolution is perhaps the easiest and least painful way people change in both positive and negative ways, and only after a significant amount of time do individuals, retrospectively, realize there is much change that has occurred. However, resistance may occur when a person is informed that a significant negative change has occurred over time and needs to be managed (e.g., hearing loss that has progressed to needing hearing aids, or a brain tumor that has developed sufficiently to cause obvious impairments in a person's communication abilities). In speech-language pathology and audiology, a revolutionary event for a person may be a CVA, TBI, or sudden hearing loss. A sudden loss of communication or hearing abilities may result in resistance to accepting the loss and the need for managing it because there was little or no adjustment time to the significant changes in the person's self-image. In both evolutionary and revolutionary changes, people often have little or no control to prevent the significant negative changes in their lives. Resolution is an important step in therapy for most individuals; that is, the person in therapy needs to resolve to cooperate with the therapist, attend sessions on a consistent basis, and do the tasks that are designed to be helpful. However, a client or patient who does not have this resolve may demonstrate resistance by sabotaging therapy by not attending consistently, refusing to do therapy tasks, or doing them in a perfunctory manner.

However, if we can view client or family resistance as a signal of fear that deserves our empathy and support rather than as an annoying obstacle, it becomes easier for us to maintain the therapeutic alliance and encourage the person to work to change. Our ability to offer the best of ourselves rather than withdrawing or becoming adversarial when we sense resistance is what inspires clients to persevere even when they are fearful.

In therapy we are likely to see resistance expressed by a variety of behaviors, e.g., passive-aggressive behaviors ("Oops! I forgot my appointment again!"), denial ("I don't think my son's speech problem is that bad."), shifting the focus of the conversation ("Have you ever had somebody in your family have a stroke?"), being late for therapy, canceling therapy, subtle or overt forms of inattention, disagreement with something we say, tense silence, wanting to end therapy sessions early, or not doing assignments or exercises. In medical settings, a patient who takes pride in his independence and self-sufficiency may appear resistant because his medical condition has deprived him of a former sense of self-control, and may have created a sense of shame for needing other people's assistance with self-care, including meals. The patient may be resisting being a patient. Coming to therapy may mean continually being forced to admit that he has disabilities. Therapy also can be very repetitive and clients may prefer to be resting or doing something more enjoyable. Sometimes a patient may fear the consequences of regaining certain abilities because it would mean losing emotional or financial support. Occasionally a patient may be malingering, that is, he pretends to have a more significant impairment than he actually does to receive some secondary gain (e.g., insurance or workman's compensation). Malingering patients may be resistant to performing exercises that are expected to lead to improvement of their feigned or exaggerated impairments (see Chapter 7 for further discussion of malingering).

Reluctance

Before considering resistance and noncompliance, its necessary to discuss a related process which is often mistaken for resistance; that is, *reluctance*. Reluctance, in contrast to resistance, has an interpersonal basis (Pipes & Davenport, 1998; Teyber, 2000). Reluctance arises out of interaction with the clinician, while resistance arises primarily out of ambivalence within the client. Reluctance is more the result of fear or mistrust of the clinician, while resistance is more a fear of change and growth. In both cases, the client hesitates or refuses to attend therapy or do certain therapeutic tasks, but the reasons behind the hesitations or refusals differ. The classic example of reluctance is a child's reluctance to come to the initial therapy session, but the reluctance is easily resolved once the child discovers the clinician is nonthreatening and friendly.

Clients may be reluctant (either temporarily or permanently) to perform recommended tasks or to continue therapy because the therapeutic alliance was insufficiently established or has deteriorated. Clients who feel unsupported or offended may show considerable reluctance to follow a clinician's goals or recommended exercises, at least with *that clinician*. The client is conveying that something about the clinician or something she or he has said or done is not acceptable or tolerable. It is the client's perception that matters, and until the client feels sufficiently reassured and supported, not much therapy can be accomplished.

The relationship we have with clients and family members is often what is most helpful to them. Many clients and family members agree to therapy or to do difficult assignments because they like and respect us and want to please us. However, individuals who feel slighted, not respected or appreciated, discounted, or emotionally wounded by a clinician are likely to be reluctant to interact with the clinician or to do what the client realizes would be helpful. Some clients and family members are reluctant to do what is suggested or recommended because of fear of control or intrusion by the therapist. Clients have both hopes and fears: hope that they can be helped by the SLP or audiologist, and fear that they may not be helped. When beginning therapy, to the client, the clinician is the unknown quantity. The client may know something about his own communication problem, but initially knows little about the clinician.

Working in the Client's Home

The mother of a six-year old boy called to ask if I could work with her son who stuttered. After she described some of the boy's speech problems and I felt that I could help the child and his parents, I agreed to see him for an evaluation and possible therapy. I informed the mother that much of the therapy would involve the parents having their own assignments, and that I viewed therapy for young children who stutter as a team approach which involves both parents. I prefer to see these children in their home environment rather than in a clinic or office. I asked the mother if she and her family would be comfortable with me coming to their home. She was rather surprised about this request and said she needed to talk it over with her husband. A couple of days later she called me again and said she had discussed it with her husband and he agreed for me to come to the house. The mother said that she also called an SLP in a nearby city and asked if she knew anything about me. The SLP apparently gave the mother a strong recommendation, which helped alleviate her concerns about my working with the family and coming to their home.

Clients sometimes are reluctant to share their problems with an SLP or audiologist out of concern that the clinician may develop some control over their lives. This is not altogether unreasonable. A child who stutters may be reluctant to come to therapy for fear that the SLP will ask him to do things that might embarrass him, or that the SLP and his parents are collaborating against him. A patient with dysphagia may be reluctant to be evaluated by an SLP because he knows that a roommate received a swallowing evaluation and was placed on pureed foods with thickened liquids. As SLPs and audiologists, we cannot assume that all our clients will immediately like or trust us and be willing to do the things we feel will help them.

Another reason clients or family members are reluctant to participate in therapy or do particular tasks is their lack of understanding of what our goals are, the rationales for our goals, and the connection between the therapy tasks and the goals. If an individual is not doing what we feel is helpful, we need to first be certain that she clearly knows what it is we want done and why. Second, we should not expect that one persuasive five-minute explanation will be sufficient for the client to understand and follow through with all our therapy suggestions. Reluctance can often be successfully resolved by adequately answering the client's questions and reassuring the client or the client's growing familiarity with the clinicain.

Poor Motivation versus Resistance

Resistance involves an internal conflict, that is, the client wants to improve but has some reasons for fearing change. In this case, the client's ambivalence or contradictory motivations should be examined. Poor motivation, however, does not involve internal conflict; that is, the client does not have the incentive or enthusiasm to improve and, therefore, chooses to only minimally or perfunctorily participate, or to discontinue therapy altogether. Many clients come to therapy because of external motivation or encouragement; that is, a family member (e.g., parents) may want therapy for their child, or an employer may tell an employee that if his or her speech (e.g., fluency or voice) does not improve significantly, the person's job may be in jeopardy. In such cases the client may agree to enter or continue therapy to please or meet the demands of another person. External motivation alone is not conducive to improvement in therapy. Clients may demonstrate considerable resistance to the clinician or therapy and may sabotage the therapeutic process. Internal motivation, however, refers to the client's desire to be in therapy and recognition of its benefits. Clients with strong internal motivation usually have the best chance for achieving their maximum potential in therapy. Often, however, there is a mixture of external and internal motivation. If a client's internal motivation wanes over time, the external motivators (parents, teachers, friends, colleagues, employers, etc.) may be sufficiently encouraging for the client to continue progressing in therapy.

There are other reasons besides coercion or duress from others to attend and participate in therapy that may result in poor motivation. For example, the client's and clinician's goals may not be in accord, which is likely the result of the therapeutic alliance not being initially well established. Trying to understand the client's goals and helping him or her understand ours may help increase the client's motivation. The effects of illness, injury, or medication can significantly affect a patient's motivation. Patients who are very ill, in pain, or sedated may not be sufficiently motivated to attend therapy or do therapy exercises. Patients with neurological disorders, particularly TBIs or CVAs with frontal lobe damage, may have significant cognitive impairments that affect their personality and character. Individuals who, prior to the neurological insult, were typically industrious, highly motivated people now may be apathetic, lethargic and not have the incentive to be in therapy or do therapeutic tasks (Parker, 1990; Solberg & Mateer, 1989; Tanner, 1999). This can be particularly frustrating to the patient's family and friends who knew him or her as a hard worker and willing to do what it takes.

In therapy we must do all that we can to stimulate, encourage and reinforce the patient's participation. We should persevere, exercise tolerance, and move at a pace that benefits the patient. These patients may not be able to comprehend long-term goals, so more immediate goals should be identified and emphasized. However, regretfully, as SLPs and audiologists we sometimes must discharge such patients from therapy because of lack of participation or frequent cancellations of therapy.

Responding to Resistance

Morrison (1995) and Teyber (2000) emphasize that the crucial ingredient for responding to resistance is to refuse to adopt an adversarial stance and instead to "join" with the client, thereby providing client support, lessening the client's fear, and encouraging discussion about what might be causing the resistance. This can be viewed as a three-part process. First, draw the client's attention to the resistant behaviors in as nonthreatening a manner as possible. For example, you might say in a noncritical tone, "You seem to be rather quiet today," or "These exercises seem to be more difficult for you than usual," or "For a while you were always on time for our appointments, but lately I notice that you've been five to ten minutes late." If you can show genuine interest in what the client is thinking and feeling rather than annoyance, it will be easier to convey warmth and support. However, empathizing with the client's feelings does not mean that you support the resistance.

The second step, which may be combined with the first step, is to identify the specific context in which the resistant behavior occurs. For example, you may note, "Just when we begin talking about how your stuttering is affecting your job, you change the subject," or "You seem reluctant to talk about how your voice sounds when talking to your father," or "The last time we met you looked rather angry, and then you cancelled the next appointment." The more sensitive, threatening, or fearful the issue is to the client, the more resistant or defensive he or she likely will be. Being quietly supportive rather than accusatory will help the client feel more free to share his thoughts and feelings.

The final step is to invite the client to explore what is going on for him. Approaching the exploration as though you are curious and interested can be helpful in conveying an open, noncritical attitude. Clinician congruence is essential during this process, that is, the clinician's thoughts, feelings and emotional tone should match her behavior. Steps one and two are intended to prepare the client for the third step, and all three steps may be taken in a single brief interaction. Probing questions can help obtain information from the client to understand his thoughts and feelings. You may merge the three steps in a statement such as, "You seem to be rather quiet today. The last time we met you appeared rather angry, and then you cancelled the next appointment. How have you been feeling about the therapy?" (or, "What are your feelings about what I have just said?") Other examples are, "You are generally very open when talking about your stuttering and how it affects different parts of your life, but now just when you begin to tell me about how your stuttering is affecting your job, you change the subject. I'm wondering if this subject is especially difficult to talk about. Would you tell me about what's going on?" or "For a while you were always on time for our appointments, but lately I notice that you've been five or ten minutes late. What do you think is going on for you?" or "These exercises seem to be more difficult for you than usual and you are having some trouble getting them done. What do you think makes these exercises more difficult than the ones you have done in the past?" or "You seem to be in a rush when we are meeting and not focusing on your voice when we're together. Your speech sounds more pressured than in the past. Can you help me understand what might be going on for you?"

Clients are not always immediately able to respond to these questions in a meaningful way. However, these questions may trigger the client's reflections and introspection, and open the door for further exploration at a later date. Essentially, these questions give the client permission to discuss difficult and negative feelings with the clinician.

When the SLP or audiologist invites such exploration she needs to be willing to hear anything the client says, even if it reflects the client's negative or hostile feelings toward the clinician and the therapeutic relationship. The invitation to explore is done supportively, unapologetically, and nondefensively. If in fact the clinician erred in some way, she needs to be able to acknowledge the error nondefensively. This can strengthen the therapeutic alliance by legitimizing the client's feelings and by showing respect. The clinician's apology also provides a good model for the client that being human and making mistakes does not have to destroy one's self-respect or a relationship (Morrison, 1995; Pipes & Davenport, 1990).

Summary

When dealing with reluctance or resistance, audiologists and SLPs need to avoid slipping into a defensive or adversarial mode that can jeopardize the therapeutic relationship and sabotage future progress in therapy. If clinicians can reframe to themselves the client's reluctance or resistance as a normal and expected component of therapy, they will find it easier to remain empathic while simultaneously encouraging the client to explore what he or she is thinking and feeling, and the fears the client may have about change.

ANGRY OR HOSTILE ATTITUDES AND BEHAVIORS

We have all experienced being angry or having someone's anger directed toward us. Anger is a normal human emotion. Whatever a person is angry about, that person likely feels strongly about. Ordinarily, people do not get angry about things they do not care about. When handled appropriately and expressed assertively (directly, without violating the rights of others or hurting oneself), anger can be a positive, creative communication that may lead to problem solving and productive change. However, when channeled inappropriately and expressed as verbal aggression (verbal attacks of others) or physical aggression, it can be a destructive and potentially life-threatening force (Keltner, Schwecke, & Bostrom, 1999).

Broadly speaking, anger is an affective response to frustration or perceived injustice and can encompass behavioral acts of hostility, self-defense, protection of others, and reactions against threats to our physical or emotional well-being (Feltham & Dryden, 1993). Hostility suggests a feeling of unfriendliness, animosity, or antagonism. Hostility may reveal itself in angry behavior. Controlled anger usually involves a person's attempt to regain some restraint of his or her anger in a socially appropriate manner. On the other hand, anger may be overcontrolled where the angry person is intent on not showing how she or he is feeling. The overcontrolled angry person may be tight-lipped and apparently passive, but may be storing up anger that may explode at a later time (Fein, 1993).

The Neurochemical and Neurophysiologic Basis of Anger

Anger and hostility, like all emotions, have a neurochemical and neurophysiological basis. An important trigger for anger is a feeling of frustration with the sense that obstacles have been imposed by others and the fear of not achieving one's objectives. Another important trigger is the perception of being threatened or endangered either physically or emotionally (e.g., our self-esteem or self-image), which creates fear. Goleman (1995) and Bear, Conners and Paradiso (2001) describe the neurophysiology of fear. Perceptions of threat or danger act as triggers for the hypothalamus and a surge in the limbic system. One part of the surge is a release of catecholamines (the neurotransmitters dopamine, norepinephrine, and epinephrine), which generate a burst of energy that lasts for a few to several minutes, which is sufficient time for fight or flight. Meanwhile, an amygdala-driven response through the adrenocortical branch of the nervous system creates a general background of action-readiness that lasts longer than the catecholamine energy surge. The generalized adrenocortical excitation can last for hours to days, keeping the emotions in readiness for arousal, and becoming a foundation on which subsequent reactions can rapidly build. This adrenocortical arousal process helps explain why people are more prone to anger if they have already been provoked or slightly irritated at something else. Stress of all kinds creates adrenocortical arousal, lowering the threshold for what provokes anger.

We usually visually discern people who are angry before we hear their angry remarks. Izard (1977), Fein (1993), and Burgoon et al. (1996) describe unique patterns of facial muscular contractions that are associated with primary emotions, including anger, and state that an angry face can be recognized by people around the world. Tense facial muscles are often the first indication that a person is angry. The muscles of the brow move inward and downward, creating a frown and a foreboding appearance about the eyes, which seem to be fixed in a hard stare toward the object of anger. The nostrils dilate and the nares of the nose flare out. The lips may be tightly pursed and the chin tightened, or the lips may be open and drawn back in a rectangle-like shape, revealing clenched teeth. Often the face flushes red because of a rapid increase in blood supply. The observer will likely get a clear message that the person is frustrated and is either holding back an angry response or about to have a display of anger. The angry facial features allow the listener (observer) to make some adjustments in what she or he is saying or doing to manage or quell the anger, and therefore avoid a verbal or physical attack. However, individuals who "telegraph" few or no visual signs of anger but simply lash out at a person are particularly dangerous because the listener has little time to adjust the communication or assuage the anger.

The Assault Cycle

Keltner, Schwecke, & Bostrom (1999) discuss Smith's stress model (1981) that includes the assault cycle with five phases of a predictable pattern or chain of aggressive responses to emotional or physical stress (see Figure 8-1). Assault is legally defined as any behavior that physically or verbally presents an immediate threat of physical injury to another individual (Garner, 2001). We as SLPs and audiologists are rarely confronted with assault (other than perhaps with TBI patients at Level IV of the Rancho Scales); however, the assault cycle model can help us understand an anger cycle.

The five-phase cycle adapted from Smith (1981) includes the following:

1. Triggering phase: the stress-producing event occurs, initiating the stress responses (e.g., in an IEP meeting a parent hears difficult information about her son from the classroom teacher, resource specialist, and SLP, or a patient in rehabilitation is in physical pain and the SLP asks him to work on tasks which he either feels are of questionable value or does not understand). Behaviors that may be observed include muscle tension, changes in voice quality, tapping of fingers, pacing, repeating statements with increasing intensity, restlessness, irritability, anxiety, perspiration, glaring, or changes in breathing (Keltner et al., 1999).

2. Escalation phase: responses represent escalating behaviors that indicate a movement toward the loss of control (e.g., the parent begins displaying defensive strategies such as denial and devaluing, or a patient starts refusing to do therapy tasks). Behaviors that may be observed include pale or flushed face, loud voice, swearing, agitation, threats, demands, loss of reasoning ability, or clenched fists (Keltner et al., 1999).

3. Crisis phase: a period of emotional and physical crisis in which loss of control occurs (e.g., the mother begins yelling, screaming, and cursing at the staff, or the patient begins to verbally and/or physically attack). Behaviors that may be seen include loss of control, swearing, fighting, hitting, kicking, scratching, and throwing things (Keltner et al., 1999).

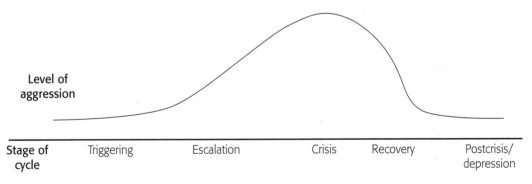

Figure 8–1 The assault cycle (Adapted from Smith, 1981).

4. Recovery phase: a period of "cooling down" in which the person slows down and returns to normal responses (e.g., the parent stops yelling and cursing the staff and sits with arms folded, or the patient lowers his voice and sits back in the chair with a defiant expression). Behaviors that may be seen include decreased body tension, mumbling accusations, and change in conversational content (Keltner et al., 1999).

5. Postcrisis depression phase: a period in which the person feels remorseful or contrite and attempts reconciliation with others (the parent feels embarrassed and apologizes for her outburst and asks forgiveness, or the patient rationalizes his explosive behavior and then asks to continue therapy). Behaviors that may be seen include apologies, crying, and reconciliatory interactions (Keltner et al., 1999)

Uncontrolled angry behavior may be considered a type of acting out behavior that is the result of emotional conflicts or internal or external stressors. The person who is angry may respond with verbally aggressive behavior and/or physically aggressive behavior. In either case, the person is acting out his or her feelings rather than talking about them in a more socially appropriate manner. The fundamental purpose of anger is to influence others, not to injure them (Fein, 1993). Angry behavior is a form of communication that the person is frustrated, threatened, or fearful. A healthy expression of anger may include expressing what one thinks and feels in a way that does not emotionally or physically harm others.

A key element in preventing and managing angry behavior is to understand the triggering phase, that is, the stress-producing event or events that initiate the stress response that lead to the angry behavior. Almost anyone experiencing significant or catastrophic change will experience some anger. Moreover, even though the person may not be aware of the anger or may be unable to express it, the anger is present nonetheless (Fein, 1993; Luterman, 2001; Rollin, 1994; Tanner, 1999). The person's anger may emerge or become apparent at a later date or unexpected time. Immediate and appropriate angry reactions are often considered healthy expressions and verbal signals to others. Visible angry behaviors span a continuum from mild irritation and arguing to verbal or physical abuse, to uncontrolled rage and violence (see Table 8-1). Expressions of anger may be viewed as behavior-toward-others or behavior-toward-self (Fein, 1993; Keltner et al., 1999).

Some people tend toward more internalizing styles and their anger is expressed predominantly in behaviors toward the self. Other individuals tend toward more externalizing styles and the predominant ways of expressing anger are in behaviors toward others. In some people, however, anger is expressed both toward self and others.

SLPs and audiologists may see anger or hostility in clients and family members for a variety of reasons. Clients may become angry when they receive a diagnosis of a serious hearing or communication problem, or when they receive bad news in an insensitive manner (see Chapter 7, Communicating Bad News and Working with Challenging Situations). Sometimes client or family anger is displaced onto the professional, and the professional can easily become the lightning rod for negative feelings. People sometimes "slay the messenger when they do not like the message" (Luterman, 2001). When disability in a family is present, life options are narrowed and people may

TABLE 8-1	EXPRESSIONS OF ANGER (NOT IN SEQUENTIAL ORDER)	
FEELINGS THAT MAY ACCOMPANY ANGER	**BEHAVIORS TOWARD OTHERS**	**BEHAVIORS TOWARD SELF**
Feeling upset	Irritation	Crying
Tension	Argumentiveness	Self-neglect (e.g., poor hygiene and nutrition)
Unhappiness	Swearing	Substance abuse (e.g., drugs or alcohol)
Feeling hurt	Hostility	Self-destructive behavior (e.g., reckless driving, binging or purging)
Feeling injustice	Contempt	Self-mutilation (e.g., cutting wrists, head-banging)
Disappointment	Clenched fists	Suicide
Guilt	Insulting remarks	
Feeling inferior	Intimidation	
Low self-esteem	Verbal abuse	
Sense of failure	Temper tantrums	
Humiliation	Maliciousness	
Feeling harassed	Violations of others' rights	
Envy	Screaming	
Feeling violated	Rage	
Feeling alienated	Defiance	
Feeling demoralized	Provoking behaviors	
Feeling depressed	Threats	
Resignation	Sadistic acts	
Powerlessness	Assault	
Helplessness		
Hopelessness		
Desperation		
Apathy		
Somatic symptoms (tension, headaches, stomachaches)		

become angry at these restrictions. Clients may become angry when they realize that they cannot be "cured" or the result of therapy was a less favorable outcome than predicted. Family members feel angry when someone (e.g., a drunk driver) physically hurts a loved one. Parents feel angry when their child is permanently injured because of a tragic accident. Sometimes family members even become angry with a spouse or parent who is seriously injured, disabled, or killed. The spouse or children may feel that the injured, disabled, or deceased person has abandoned them, and may say to themselves, "But you promised me you would always be there for me. Where are you now when I need you most?"

Once again, anger is a normal feeling and reaction to many disturbing situations; however, it is the manner in which the anger is expressed that becomes the challenge to therapists. Anger from clients and family members can provoke strong emotional responses in clinicians (including counteranger) and can test our patience and tolerance. We may not feel we are being treated with proper respect. We need to keep in mind that anger is likely the surface behavior that hides emotional or physical pain, anxiety, frustration (i.e., being thwarted from doing what one wants or being unable to stop something unwanted from happening), fear, and a sense of helplessness or hopelessness.

Despite the natural tendency to respond defensively when someone demonstrates anger toward us, it is important to reflect on our possible contributions to the person's feelings. For example, clients and family members may become angry with us if we are not communicating with them sufficiently to keep them abreast of progress; if we are late for appointments; if we are explaining information at too technical a level; or not truly understanding what they are telling us because of lack of careful listening (Wachtel, 1993; Shipley, 1997). By considering what we may have said or done to engender anger toward us we can decide if an apology or making amends is needed and thereby decrease or eliminate some or all of the frustration contributing to the person's anger.

The first goal as a clinician is to try to understand the person's motivation for the anger and the feelings that are being masked or overshadowed by the anger. Knowing the client's case history may help us understand whether the hearing, speech, language, cognitive, or swallowing problems may be perceived by the client and family as an acute threat to their emotional well-being. Also, it is helpful to understand whether the person is experiencing chronic emotional pain with feelings of frustration that further improvements have not been achieved and a sense of helplessness that little or nothing may ever change. By considering the feelings behind the feeling we are able to more easily respond in an empathic and therapeutic manner. We need to respond consciously and carefully to the person's angry behavior to maintain the therapeutic relationship. In responding to a person's anger, the first step is to try to hear the person's concerns while not becoming emotionally intimidated or retaliatory. It is important that our response instills trust rather than impairs it.

Some clients have difficulty expressing their anger appropriately, and may benefit from learning more appropriate cognitive, communication, and relaxation skills (Deffenbacher, 1999; Deffenbacher, Oetting, & DiGiuseppe, 2002; Novaco, 1976, 1983). The SLP may teach these skills to some children and adults (particularly those neurologically impaired) who have problems with the pragmatics of language and behavior when they are angry or upset. Learning how to express their anger can help clients maintain an amiable or respectful relationship with other people.

Mosak and Maniacci (1998) and Gordon (2000) distinguish between "You-messages" and "I-messages" and how they can be effective as a teaching device for clients. Clients frequently experience difficulty expressing anger and other emotions, particularly when they are upset, and teaching them how to use "I-messages" can help improve their communication skills. "I-messages" place the responsibility of the person's feeling on him or herself, not the other person. Three sentence stems are used: "When you . . . I feel . . . because . . . " For example, clients who are having difficulty communicating their anger can be taught to say, "*When yo*u don't understand what I'm saying, *I feel* angry *because* I don't think you are paying attention to me." The first part of the stem ("When you") describes the behavior that is producing the emotion. The second part ("I feel") names the emotion. The last part ("because") tells why the person feels that way. Through role-playing clients can practice these skills and learn to use them both within and outside the therapy environment. As clinicians we can use the same technique to communicate our feelings toward a client or family members. "I feel" statements allow us to help people understand how we are feeling about something they have said or done without sounding accusatory. Instead of saying "You did this . . . " or "You make me feel . . . " We are simply stating how we feel, for example, "When you talk to me in a loud voice, I feel attacked because your words and tone of voice sound rough and hostile."

If you are working in a medical setting where you see many TBI patients, it may be helpful to develop a behavioral management team where each team member agrees on specific management approaches to use with individuals displaying hostile, angry, or aggressive behavior. A one to ten scale may be used to measure an individual's anger or aggression, with one indicating very mild anger and ten indicating rage. Some patients can quickly escalate from one or two to eight, nine, or ten. The goal is to prevent the anger or aggression from escalating, and by not escalating, the anger has a better chance to subside. Reflections and probing questions may help reveal the source of the frustration, hostility, irritation, anger, or fear, for example,

"You seem a little annoyed with _____ ."

"You seemed to have had a difficult experience with _____ ."

"I sense that you're irritated about _____ ."

"You seem angry right now. Can you tell me what you are thinking about?"

"You seem a little more tense than when I saw you last time. Would you like to tell me what's going on?"

"You seem a little more tense today. I'm wondering if I have paced the exercises a little too fast. What do you think?"

"Therapy can be a little frightening because it is difficult to predict how much improvement may be made. Do you feel concerned about that sometimes?"

"Besides what we have been talking about, what other concerns do you have?"

Reflections and probes allow the person an opportunity to ventilate and express his thoughts and feelings and communicate to the person that his feelings are respected. The anger/aggression scale and therapeutic communication techniques should be taught to all staff working with these patients so they have consistent and predictable strategies to deal with problem behaviors.

COMMUNICATING AND RESPONDING TO ANGRY BEHAVIOR

Being Verbally "Attacked"

The following are a number of principles and strategies for dealing with angry behavior: 1) Respond with unconditional positive regard; 2) Maintain your poise; 3) Be aware of the person's defense mechanisms; 4) Maintain good eye contact and listen without interrupting; 5) Give the person time to blow off steam; 6) Pause briefly before responding; 7) Offer empathic statements or reflections of feelings; 8) Give the person the opportunity to respond more appropriately; 9) Provide opportunity for the person to save face; and 10) Help the person feel validated and important.

RESPOND WITH UNCONDITIONAL POSITIVE REGARD

The general approach is not to control or manage the person's anger, but rather to maintain and possibly even enhance the therapeutic relationship by responding to the person with unconditional positive regard (Rogers, 1951), that is, acceptance of the person without reservation. Consistently nonjudgmental responses can allow the person to feel accepted and, therefore, more relaxed. While it is important to accept the person, we do not necessarily have to accept all the person's behaviors. When people feel accepted, they feel less tense and more calm, which can defuse some of the angry feelings and diminish angry behaviors.

MAINTAIN YOUR POISE

When you do not get angry in return, the person does not have anything to "push against" and it destabilizes him, which allows him to try a different tactic or behavior other than anger. Maintaining your poise is the most important strategy you can use to ebb a person's anger.

BE AWARE OF THE PERSON'S DEFENSE MECHANISMS

Remember that the person is probably feeling overwhelming anxiety. He or she may be using defense mechanisms such as denial, displacement, passive-aggressive behavior, or devaluing to protect him or herself from anxiety or frustration (see Chapter 5, for more information on defense mechanisms). It is important that you not become defensive yourself in response to the person's defense mechanisms. You need to be aware of your own defensive tendencies and aggressive impulses, how you deal with your own anger, and how you can channel it into constructive, productive actions. You cannot defuse a person's anger or aggression when you are in a similar emotional state, and any retaliatory anger on your part will likely intensify or escalate the person's anger.

MAINTAIN GOOD EYE CONTACT AND LISTEN WITHOUT INTERRUPTING

If you must interrupt, do it politely. Listen intensely but not tensely; that is, try to appear calm, relaxed and in control of yourself so the person does not think he is getting to you. In a calm voice call the person by last name to show respect, for example, "Mr. Adams, I need to interrupt you." Being courteous and respectful may be surprising to the person and help defuse the anger.

GIVE THE PERSON TIME TO BLOW OFF STEAM

He may do it quickly or it may take a little while to get everything off his chest. If you feel it is in the best interest of the therapeutic relationship, you may choose to hear the person out. However, if you feel that the person's anger is escalating and that he may not be able to control himself, it is quite justifiable to tell the person that you will be happy to talk again when the person is less angry and can talk in a more appropriate manner, and then discontinue or postpone the rest of the session.

PAUSE BRIEFLY BEFORE RESPONDING

Your willingness to listen and a brief pause before you speak lets the person know that you are in control of yourself. A rapid response can escalate a feeling of threat to the person and his anger may intensify. Maintain good eye contact when you speak which can help the person feel that you are confident about what you are saying.

OFFER EMPATHIC STATEMENTS OR REFLECTIONS OF FEELINGS

A statement such as, "Mr. Adams, you are understandably upset" reflects empathy and being nonjudgmental. Do not tell the person, "I understand how upset you are" because you probably do not know the intensity of his feelings. Other empathic statements may be, "Mr. Adams, this must be hard for you" or "Mr. Adams, I know this situation is quite upsetting." A collaborative statement might be, "Mr. Adams, let's try to figure this out together."

GIVE THE PERSON THE OPPORTUNITY TO RESPOND MORE APPROPRIATELY

Can he calm down after he has blown off steam? Does the person look less tense? Is his voice softer? Are his words less harsh? Is his face less tense and his body more relaxed?

PROVIDE OPPORTUNITY FOR THE PERSON TO SAVE FACE

Many times people are embarrassed after they have displayed excessive anger. If the person wants to apologize for his angry outburst, allow it. However, do not say in response, "That's all right" because that may give the false impression that such behavior is acceptable. An empathic response such as "Your anger is understandable" may validate his feelings but not his behavior. Saying "Thank you" after an apology acknowledges that you have accepted it. Sometimes just nodding your head once slowly with a concerned facial expression is sufficient to acknowledge the acceptance of the apology. If the person does not spontaneously offer an apology, do not ask for one. This could set up more resistance and intensify the person's feelings that he again is being asked to do something he does not want to do.

HELP THE PERSON FEEL VALIDATED AND IMPORTANT

If you can return to therapeutic tasks, the tasks need to help the client feel some measure of success. Provide reinforcement for any behavior that is appropriate, but avoid sounding patronizing or condescending with your choice of words or tone of voice.

Various Therapeutic Approaches to Angry Behavior

The following illustrations provide some different approaches to dealing with angry behavior, including the behavioral approach, culture-sensitive approach, humanistic approach, and interpersonal approach. For further information, the reader is referred to Chapter 2, Theories of Counseling and How They Relate to Speech-Language Pathology and Audiology.

BEHAVIORAL APPROACH

If the person's anger is mildly inappropriate but transient (e.g., swearing at you), you may simply ignore the behavior and appear more attentive and engaged when the person expresses him or herself in a more rational and appropriate manner. You may attempt to "shape" appropriate behavior and extinguish inappropriate behavior. You do not want to reinforce inappropriate, angry behavior.

CULTURE-SENSITIVE APPROACH

Some cultures are socialized to express their emotions in an open, demonstrative (even dramatic) way. Be careful not to inaccurately label or overestimate the person's emotional reaction to the situation. Instead of interpreting the person's feelings (e.g., "Mr. Jones, you certainly seem angry."), it is better to inquire about his feelings (e.g., "That information got a strong response from you, Mr. Jones. How are you feeling about things right now?")

HUMANISTIC APPROACH

You can express empathy and acceptance of the person's angry feelings while encouraging the person to explore the feelings that may underlie the surface emotion (e.g., frustration, anxiety, fear, sense of helplessness). A therapeutic response might be, "It is understandable that you are quite upset (empathy). Would you like to say more about how you are feeling now (exploration)?"

INTERPERSONAL APPROACH

Avoid getting "hooked" by the person's anger. The person may have a history of eliciting defensive, angry, or retaliatory responses, and is demonstrating the same tactic with you. Resist the urge to respond with counterhostility and, instead, provide a response that reflects the person's feelings toward you at the moment, for example, "I can see that you're very upset that I don't have all the answers."

Rage or Potential Physical Abuse (Catastrophic Reactions)

Although audiologists and SLPs are unlikely to be confronted with a person's rage or potential physical abuse, it has occurred in a variety of settings. The most likely environment for such behaviors are medical settings with Level IV (Rancho Scales) TBI patients; however, patients with CVAs, particularly in the posterior left frontal lobe area (Tanner, 1999) are susceptible to catastrophic reactions. We need to keep in mind that when such patients have catastrophic reactions it is secondary to the nature of the neurological damage, and that the patients' behaviors are not completely under their cognitive control. As a result, the SLP working with these patients needs to take a significant amount of responsibility for managing the potentially dangerous behaviors until patients can manage their own anger and angry behaviors.

Catastrophic reactions may be seen as explosive outbursts by a patient with potentially uncontrolled rage (Brookshire, 2003). The causes of the reaction may be the same or similar to the anger or rage response, that is, frustration and fear. Some clinicians have been physically injured by patients, resulting in workman compensation claims and loss of work time needed for recovery. If a clinician injures a patient during an attempt to protect him or herself, legal involvement may be the result.

In a medical setting office where you are likely to work with patients who have had CVAs and TBIs, it is prudent to arrange your therapy table so that the patient and you both have the door to your sides rather than having the door behind you or in front of you. Having the door to your sides without any hindrance for either you or the patient may help both of you feel unimpeded if there is a need to quickly leave the room. If, for example, the table is arranged so that the patient is behind the table with his back to the far wall and he becomes agitated and wants to leave the room immediately, you may be blocking the exit (Figure 8-2A). On the other hand, if you are behind the table with your back to the far wall and the patient becomes agitated and possibly threatening, you may be trapped (Figure 8-2B). Your exit or the patient's can be expedited with the table arranged so that either you or the patient can simply turn and walk out of the room (Figure 8-2C).

Fein (1993) discusses methods for clinicians to manage client rage and potential physical abuse. He emphasizes that the clinician's safety is essential. The first priority for dealing with problem anger must be avoiding injury to yourself and others, and, secondarily, to the angry person. The best way to protect against problem anger is to perceive that it is coming. If frustration is what triggers a person's anger, if at all possible remove the cause of the frustration. Fein describes several ways this can be done.

A.   **B.**   **C.**

Wall   Wall   Wall

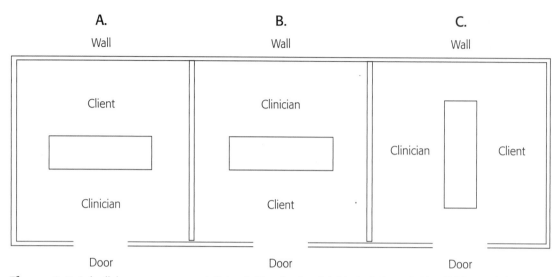

Door   Door   Door

Figure 8-2 Safe clinic room arrangement. Setup A: The client's exit is blocked; Setup B: The clinician's exit is blocked; Setup C: both client and clinician can easily exit the room if needed.

REMOVE THE INDIVIDUAL FROM THE SOURCE OF ANXIETY

It is prudent for clinicians to be aware of an expedient method to move a patient from one environment to another. This can prevent the patient from harming other staff or patients and can prevent an altercation between patients. Patients do not only strike out at staff but may attack other patients who cannot escape or defend themselves.

Removing a Patient from an Anxiety-Producing Environment

I was working in a skilled nursing facility during the summer. The social service director had arranged for an entertainer to come into the facility for an afternoon and the residents were encouraged to attend. Many of the staff, including me, assisted residents into the large room, and many of them were in wheelchairs. The room became crowded and personal space for some of the residents was violated. One man in a wheelchair who was surrounded by other residents became agitated. Before any of the staff could reach him, he began cursing at another resident and tried to hit him with his fists. A certified nursing assistant (CNA) who had earlier cared for the agitated resident quickly told the staff that she knew him well and could take care of the situation. She rushed to the resident and knelt down beside his wheelchair and in a soothing way tried to calm him; however, the resident struck out at her with his fist and hit her in the face. I reached the CNA and resident in an instant, helped the CNA

Continues on next page

Continued from previous page

off the floor, started moving other residents to clear a path for the agitated man, and quickly wheeled him out a side door and into an open courtyard to get him away from what precipitated his agitation—the violation of his personal space. Fortunately, the CNA was unhurt and realized the error she had made by placing her face within arm's reach of the resident.

MOVE THE SOURCE OF ANXIETY

For some patients a particular staff person may not be tolerated well and, for whatever reason, may precipitate or escalate a patient's uncontrolled anger. If a staff member recognizes that his or her presence is frustrating or agitating a patient, it is wise for the staff member to remain out of view and voice range of the patient.

COUNSELING SKILLS IN ACTION:

Keeping Distance from Agitated Patients

An elderly woman in a convalescent hospital who had cognitive impairments became convinced that the OT was having an affair with her husband. Although there was no rational basis for this belief, the elderly woman had no doubt about the OT's involvement with her husband. One day the elderly woman struck the OT with her fist, knocking her down. It became apparent to the rehabilitation team that there was no possibility of persuading this cognitively impaired patient that the OT was innocent of her allegations. The solution was to keep the OT at a distance from the patient so that she would no longer agitate her.

DISTRACT THE ANGRY PERSON FROM THE SOURCE OF ANXIETY

Directing the patient's attention and gaze to yourself or something more tolerable to the patient may briefly take his or her focus away from the offending person or situation. Distractions and diversions provide a more agreeable stimulus, which is incompatible with anxiety and anger. Having the patient focus on some interesting visual stimulus or initiating some casual and enjoyable conversation may be sufficient to divert the patient's attention away from the anger-producing person or situation.

INTERCEDE BETWEEN THE ANGRY PERSON AND THE SOURCE OF ANGER

When the angry person cannot physically reach the source of frustration or anxiety, a physical and psychological barrier allows the person to cool down. The time may allow the person to regroup and calm him or herself sufficiently to begin to manage the angry behaviors. This time also allows the clinician an opportunity to assess the situation and consider another, more permanent strategy to manage the person's aggressive anger. The clinician should keep in mind that it is not prudent to place himself between the angry person and the source of frustration without being at least a leg's distance from the person.

Calming Techniques

The eventual goal is for the patient to be able to calm himself and control his own anger. To do this the patient must recognize what triggers his anger and the signs that he is getting angry. The clinician may introduce calming techniques that may later become a part of the patient's behavioral repertoire for self-management. These coping strategies can help the person feel some control over stressful situations. Calming techniques may be implemented by the angry person himself or by those near by. When the person can implement them, he is in a better position to develop and maintain positive social interactions. Calming techniques include the use of safe places, safe persons, and safe activities (Fein, 1993).

SAFE PLACES

The purpose of a safe place is to remove an enraged person from a frustrating environment that may escalate the anger. Most people tend to calm down once they are no longer provoked. The person or situation causing the frustration is removed, or the angry person is moved to a more neutral location. The patient's antagonist is asked to leave the room or the patient may choose to leave. This reduces the patient's stress, frustration, or fear. If the SLP or audiologist has learned who or what may provoke a patient, that person or situation should be kept away from the patient. Most clinicians attempt to create a warm and inviting therapy area; however, in a busy hospital environment noise levels and visual distractions are often difficult to control, and make safe places a premium.

SAFE PERSONS

Patients typically relate better to some staff than others, and often the SLP is the person who is the least threatening or anger-provoking person in the patient's environment. Physical therapists (PTs), OTs, nurses, and physicians may be placing demands on patients or touching or prodding them in ways that are irritating. TBI patients may have catastrophic reactions when their threshold of tolerance is exceeded and more is asked of them than they can comfortably do. The SLP may be the professional who is most sensitive to subtle signs of frustration, anxiety, or irritability. The SLP may also be the person whom other staff members recognize as having the best rapport with a patient and range of abilities to communicate in a nonthreatening manner. Therefore, it is quite possible that for a particular patient with uncontrolled anger, the SLP may be the safe person, the person who can most easily calm and soothe the patient.

To calm or soothe a person, our voices should be reassuring and our demeanor nonthreatening. Our language should be easily understood with words of support and encouragement. Similarly, our body language should convey openness and comfort, with no obvious indication of being prepared to defend ourselves or to escape (although we must be ready to do either). The message safe people want to deliver is that they are not angry, frightened, or demanding and, therefore, have no reason to be frustrating or threatening to the patient. Successful calming depends upon trust, which the clinician must earn from the patient. The angry person can only be calmed if he feels safe with the person trying to calm him. The clinician needs to convey that she is on the side of the patient and must behave in a nonconfrontational and nondemanding manner. When talking to the aggressively angry person the clinician must be sincere and nonmanipulative, and not talk down to the person, be patronizing, or condescending. This may take considerable self-restraint on the part of the clinician. The SLP must recognize if on a given day in a particular situation that she has the resources to take on such a challenging task, and if not, she should defer the task to someone who may manage the situation better at that time.

SAFE ACTIVITIES

Frustration usually arises from not attaining what is urgently desired. Patients need a feeling of accomplishment and respect. They may also need a quiet, nonthreatening environment, people they enjoy, relief from pain, being able to stop an activity they cannot tolerate, or having the foods or food textures they like. If we can discern what the patient wants or needs that he is not getting and then, if possible, provide that, the anger may rapidly subside. However, if it cannot reasonably be provided, then a diversionary activity may help calm the person.

When an angry person shifts focus to another task, he may also shift immediate priorities. What the person no longer is focused on loses its importance and, therefore, its frustrating effects. For example, intensely angry people can be encouraged to take a walk with you, do some exercise, or work out in the gym. Physical activity requires concentration that can be drawn away from the frustrating person or situation. Physical activity also uses energy that can be dissipated toward healthier and safer pursuits. Fatigue produces a sense of tranquility. If, however, because of physical limitations the patient can do little or no physical activity that may be sufficiently distracting and/or fatiguing, the patient may be asked to do nothing at all, that is, to sit quietly during a brief time out. The person may be left alone (if you feel the person or your office will be safe), or may be placed in a quiet room with few distractions, not as a punishment but as an opportunity to try to settle himself. He may find this time peaceful and welcoming. He can also learn this as a strategy for managing himself when he is feeling intense anger in the future.

Cue Training

Cue training is a technique aimed at helping people induce self-control, based on the assumption that few people willingly lose control; their anger gets out of hand and they cannot restrain it. Once they become enraged, they cannot think clearly and are less likely to get their wants, needs, thoughts, and feelings understood and met. Cue training involves helping the patient become aware of escalating anger and the triggers for it. Increased self-awareness of escalating anger may involve reflection on one's moods, physiological responses (tense jaw, clenched fists, perspiration, etc.), and interpersonal behavior (raised voice, hostile language, impatience, etc.). In this way the person can recognize anger in an early stage and, we hope, prevent it from intensifying. Being more aware of these cues can help the person better manage him or herself by using such techniques as removing oneself from the frustrating or anxiety-provoking person or situation, asking the person to leave, finding a quiet, placid place to be alone for awhile, and so forth. The goal is to help the person learn to manage intense feelings as well as aggressive angry behavior. This allows the person to become more self-confident in social situations as well as in hospital or rehabilitation settings.

Summary

Angry or hostile attitudes and behaviors from clients, patients, or family members may be some of the greatest challenges SLPs and audiologists are confronted with in our work; such challenges may occur in any setting. It is important for us to appreciate that anger is a normal feeling and reaction to many disturbing situations. We also need to understand that a person's angry behavior is often a coarse and socially inappropriate manner of communicating a message, and that if a less drastic method of communicating had been successful, the angry behavior may not have been necessary. Behind angry or hostile behaviors there are usually feelings of frustration, threat, or fear. If SLPs and audiologists can recognize the feelings behind the feelings, they can better communicate with the person who is angry and diminish or allay the person's anger. Clinicians must also be aware of their own tendencies to become defensive or angry in response to another person's anger. There are numerous principles for communicating with a person who is angry and techniques for managing catastrophic reactions.

CONCLUDING COMMENTS

Resistance is a natural occurrence when people fear change or are uncertain about a situation. Some people who seek therapy are also resistant to it, particularly if they feel frightened or threatened by the challenges and tasks put before them. A sudden loss of hearing or communicative abilities may result in resistance to accepting the loss. Viewing an individual's resistance as a signal of fear that deserves our empathy and support can help us avoid responding in a defensive manner, and provide a better opportunity to maintain the client-clinician relationship.

Anger is an affective response to frustration or perceived injustice that can be recognized behaviorally in a variety of ways. Clinicians may become lightning rods when clients or families feel threatened by a diagnosis of a communication disorder, or therapy has not progressed as fast or as far as was hoped. We need to manage our natural tendency toward defensiveness and counteranger in order to respond in a therapeutic manner.

Discussion Questions

1. Think of a time when you were reluctant to do something asked of you. Why were you reluctant? Was there anything about the person that made you reluctant? Was there something about the request that made you reluctant?

2. Recall a situation in which you felt a client or family member might have been reluctant to do what you asked. What do you think was the source of that reluctance? How did you help the person go beyond the reluctance to do what you felt was therapeutic?

3. What do you see as the similarities and differences between resistance and noncompliance? Which is more difficult for you to work with?

4. Think of your own education and how you have changed through evolution, revolution, and resolution.

5. Discuss a client with whom you worked that you saw change through evolution; through revolution; through resolution.

6. What are some of the ways that you have seen resistance in clients or relatives?

7. What are your first reactions to a client or family member you feel is being resistant to you? How do your reactions affect the interaction with the person?

8. What do you see as similarities and differences between poor motivation and resistance? Do you feel that poor motivation or resistance has a greater effect on therapy? Why?

9. How might you view resistance differently now? How might you respond differently to perceived resistance of a client or relative?

10. What tends to make you irritated? Angry? Enraged? How do you express your anger? How do you keep from expressing it?

11. Recall Smith's assault cycle as it relates to your own anger. What triggers an angry outburst in you? What escalates it? What do you do when you have an angry outburst? How do you cool down? How do you feel afterwards?

12. Remember an incident when you saw someone have an angry outburst. What do you think triggered it? What escalated it? What did the person do during the outburst? What helped him cool down? How do you think he or she felt afterwards?

13. What are the behaviors you see that indicate a person is becoming angry?

14. How do you tend to react when someone becomes angry with you? What defenses might you use? What seems to help you respond in a helpful manner?

15. What are some reflections and probing questions you might ask a client that may help you understand his or her frustration, irritation, fear, or anger?

16. Which of the 10 principles and techniques for communicating and responding to angry behavior (being verbally attacked) do you feel the most comfortable using? The least comfortable using?

17. Have you ever observed a person who was enraged? What did the person do? How did other people protect themselves? How was the situation managed? What seemed to calm the person down?

18. Have you ever intervened to calm a very angry or enraged person? What did you do that helped calm the person? What did not help?

CHAPTER 9

Working with Crisis Situations

CHAPTER OUTLINE

- Introduction
- Managing a Crisis
- Threat of Suicide or Self-Harm
- Threat of Harm to Others
- Reporting Child or Elder Abuse/Neglect (Being a "Mandated Reporter")
- Children and Clients with Posttraumatic Stress Disorder
- Concluding Comments
- For Discussion

INTRODUCTION

This chapter discusses several of the most challenging situations and behaviors that may confront a speech-language pathologist or audiologist. Crisis situations can occur in any work environment at any time, and few if any clinicians who have worked for more than a few months or years have been able to avoid facing and dealing with them. The most serious crisis is threat of suicide. Fortunately, most clinicians can enjoy a long career without the challenge of a child or adult threatening suicide. However, the threat needs to be managed in a professional and legal manner that may ultimately save a person's life. Threat of harm to others is becoming an increasing possibility, particularly in public school environments. The speech-language pathologist (SLP) or audiologist may be the first adult to hear of a child's potential serious threat to other children, teachers, or administrators, or even to physical property. As professionals, we are mandated reporters of child and elder abuse or neglect, and need to know the proper procedures for such reporting.

MANAGING A CRISIS

Clinicians in all settings working with all ages, from infants to elderly, encounter crisis situations in their work. George and Cristiani (1995) and Nystul (1999) state that a crisis is characterized by

1) symptoms of significant psychological or physiological stress or discomfort, 2) an attitude of panic or defeat where the person feels overwhelmed by the situation and experiences both helplessness and hopelessness, but may exhibit either agitation or withdrawal, 3) a focus on relief from the crisis where the person wants, more than anything, relief from the feeling of being in crisis, 4) lowered efficiency in other areas of life apart from the crisis, for example, family life or employment, and 5) limited duration, that is, the experience is temporary, not chronic.

Crises may overload a person or family's coping abilities, making their usual problem-solving strategies unworkable and ineffective. A crisis, by definition, is a dangerous time; however, it may also represent an opportunity. A crisis creates a time of turmoil and transition which may bring about important changes in a person or family system by forcing one to adopt new perspectives or allowing role changes as a means of adapting to changing conditions (Goldenberg & Goldenberg, 2000).

It is important to keep in mind that the defining characteristic of a crisis is not the instigating event, but rather the client's difficulty in coping with the situation (Zaro et al., 1995). Although a crisis usually is the result of a catastrophic situation such as death of a family member, SLPs and audiologists are more likely to see clients or families in crisis from the survival of a catastrophic event, such as a stroke or traumatic brain injury (TBI). However, a series of apparently much more benign events may also precipitate a crisis. The severity of the crisis is based on the person's reaction to it, not the apparent seriousness of the instigating event. Psychologists may diagnose an individual in crisis as having an acute stress disorder which involves severe anxiety and other disabling symptoms after a traumatic event (Bourne, 2000; DSM-IV TR, 2000).

Common physiological responses to crisis include tense muscles, racing pulse, pounding heart, dry mouth, queasy stomach, and sweating. Some general responses of people who are in crisis include being noticeably anxious to being extremely upset or in a state of panic. The person may be visibly agitated, moving quickly and aimlessly. The person's speech may be rapid and pressed, that is, sounding as though he or she is unable to control how fast, how much, or what is being said. The person will likely be somewhat confused and have impaired judgment, with difficulty making even very simple decisions, and therefore want and need considerable direction from others. Some individuals, however, may become hypersensitive to the environment and other people, or withdrawn and uncommunicative (Baron, 1998). In contrast, some individuals seem to be able to rise to the occasion, muster their resources, and perform even better under very stressful conditions. In these situations people seem to be able to exercise an extraordinary degree of energy and focus to accomplish the task at hand. After such experiences, there is often a sense of accomplishment and self-discovery of personal resources they did not know they had.

There are many kinds of crises that occur in people's lives and one crisis may lead to another. For example, a motor vehicle accident resulting in TBI of a child creates a crisis around the child's neurological damage and the initial concern about his or her survival. Crises can have a cascading effect that are escalated from the parents' loss of time from work, expenses that are incurred that insurance will not cover, attempts to care for the other children at home, as well as numerous other "little crises" that arise, all of which can be magnified by the parents' loss of sleep. As SLPs and audiologists we can reasonably assume that a previously normally functioning individual who now has a moderate to

Turning Personal Crisis into an Opportunity for Professional Growth

Several years ago a graduate student's father died while she was in the middle of a semester. She, of course, flew home to attend the funeral. When she returned a few days later to resume her classes and clinical work, I felt that she was still in crisis and talked to her about possibly canceling therapy that week with her adult voice case. She assured me that she wanted to go ahead and see the client and that she would be all right. I observed her carefully during the next two sessions and noticed that her therapy was the best I had ever seen. She was tuned in to every nuance and emotion of the client. This actually was the beginning of significant clinical growth for the student. In some cases a crisis may interfere with a student or professional's work; in other cases a crisis may enhance the clinician's performance.

severe communicative or cognitive problem, is in crisis, and so is the family. Even seemingly mild problems can put some people into a crisis. Although we are not crisis counselors, we must work with clients, patients, and families who are in crisis. Understanding general principles of crisis management can help our clients and their families maximize the benefits they receive from therapy during the acute stage. Crisis management should be a team approach where all the professionals working with a person or family are following similar strategies to help them cope with the crisis as best they can.

Crisis situations can create an intense feeling of frustration, inadequacy and incompetence in clinicians. To some extent the clinician will experience many of the feelings of the person in crisis, for example, anxiety, uncertainty, and confusion. These reactions are natural and understandable, but the clinician must be in control of them when talking to the person in crisis. The clinician should convey an attitude of concern, but not alarm, and model a rational problem-solving approach to the situation. It is through education, training, and experience that SLPs and audiologists will be able to manage a crisis situation with some degree of confidence. However, some clinicians by their nature maintain an aura of calm even in very disturbing situations. Maintaining a sense of calmness allows a person to think more clearly and act more rationally.

Three-Stage Crisis Intervention Model

George and Cristiani (1995) present a three-stage crisis intervention model with emphasis in each stage on the special needs of the individuals in crisis. Burnard (1999) outlines crisis management principles and techniques that crisis teams use. The following is an integration of the George and Cristiani model and the Burnard principles. The model can be used whether the SLP or audiologist is working independently or as part of a crisis management team.

FIRST STAGE

During the first stage of this model (Burnard, 1999; George & Cristiani, 1995) the clinician attempts to establish that she has an understanding of what the individuals in crisis are going through—the fears, feelings, and confusion. This helps the clinician establish an alliance with the individuals in crisis and provides some confidence that she is able to be of assistance because of an ability to understand the situation. For example, the parents of a child newly diagnosed with a hearing loss, central auditory processing disorder (CAPD), or attention deficit disorder (ADD) may be in crisis because of the fear that the child has significant problems that may affect schooling, social interactions, and family life. The clinician needs to get a sense of the family's current abilities to cope with the crisis. In some cases, a support group may be helpful for family members to cope with the new diagnosis.

An example of a clinician working with a family in crisis concerns a young father with a TBI. Depending on what level he is in on the Rancho Scales (Hagen, 1998), he may have little or no awareness of his deficits. However, each family member is likely to experience his or her own crisis: the wife, the children, the man's parents, his siblings, and possibly others. As the patient progresses through the Rancho Levels and develops increasing recognition of his impairments, he may begin to go through the crisis stages. In some medical settings the SLP may be chosen to be a member of a behavioral or crisis management team. This is not surprising because of the areas of expertise of SLPs (e.g., neuropathologies) as well as having developed communication skills that are nonthreatening in challenging situations.

The two important processes of the first stage are establishing rapport and assessing the situation. To establish rapport, the clinician creates an environment that allows the person to discuss the crisis. The clinician's emphasis should be on communicating genuine warmth and empathic understanding. The manner in which a clinician talks with a person in crisis may either help de-escalate the sense of crisis or escalate it. Using a slower than normal rate of speech and calm tone of voice may help moderate the intensity of speech of the person in crisis. The clinician will need to make an assessment of the crisis situation, which involves getting a sense of how the individuals understand what has happened and the problems that are involved.

SECOND STAGE

The second stage of crisis management involves assessment of the client, and developing an understanding of the client or family's knowledge of the communicative disorders. This is followed by communicating a professional opinion in a way that is tailored to the client and family's knowledge and understanding. For example, during the interview of the parents whose child is newly diagnosed with CAPD and ADD, the clinician should learn what they know and understand about these problems. Only after evaluating the child's auditory processing, speech, language, and cognition can the clinician provide clarification about the areas that need attention from an SLP and/or audiologist. In a medical setting, the clinician may or may not meet with the family before she does her evaluation of the patient with the TBI. If she does meet with the family briefly before the evaluation, she may follow the processes of the first stage, that is, establish rapport and assess the situation. After the evaluation of the patient the clinician will provide information about the patient's speech, language, cognition, and swallowing to the family to clarify the problems that the patient has. During this time the clinician may want to help the person or family face the crisis. Encouraging recognition and understanding of the problems helps people accept the realities of the symptoms, illness, or injury. The clinician will want to avoid false reassurance and resist the temptation to prematurely assure the person or family in crisis that everything will be all right because it may *never* be all right, only tolerated or accepted.

The transition from the second stage to the third stage of crisis management can be made most smoothly if the clinician summarizes and reviews her evaluation and perceptions with the client and family. This serves two functions: 1) it reassures the client and family that the clinician has a good understanding of the client's problems and the crisis as the client and family perceive it, and 2) it helps the clinician recognize whether the client and family understand the need for therapy and the potential goals. Once the clinician, client, and family agree on the need and direction of therapy, they are ready for the third stage of the process in which a plan of action is determined.

THIRD STAGE

The purpose of the third stage of crisis management is to determine what the treatment goals are and possible therapy procedures. Although this may not appear different from the normal process we would follow of establishing rapport, assessing the situation, evaluating the client or patient, and then determining appropriate therapy goals and procedures, there are a few additional factors that need to be considered when the client, patient, or family is in crisis. Most people can deal with serious problems more easily if they are not overwhelmed by the magnitude of the situation; therefore, breaking up the crisis into manageable parts can be very helpful. Looking at individual potentially manageable parts of the crisis helps people feel less overburdened and frustrated. If one small part of a crisis can be managed, then another small part may also be manageable. Encouraging the individuals in crisis to help themselves by actively seeking help from family or friends can lessen their dependence on the clinician and allows more independent decision-making on their part. Once the immediate crisis has passed and individuals are more open and capable of learning new skills, the SLP or audiologist may want to teach a few strategies or coping skills to help them manage future stresses or crises. The next sections describe examples of coping skills SLPs and audiologists may teach your clients.

MONITORING SELF-TALK

Often times for people in crisis their distress is increased by the negative statements they make to themselves (e.g., "My daughter will never do well in school because of her language and learning problems." "I will never be able to work again because I can't talk after my stroke."). These negative statements also contribute to a sense of helplessness or hopelessness about a situation. Self-statements are often automatic and the person does not realize they are contributing to the distress.

Clinicians can have individuals in crisis monitor their "self-statements" (i.e., what they are saying to themselves when talking to themselves), and change negative statements to positive statements, such as "I can't cope with losing my hearing" to "I *can* cope with losing my hearing." "I don't know if I can make it through this time" to "I'm *going* to get through this time." "My speech is getting worse" to "My speech is getting *easier* and more fluent." "I can't cope with all of this" to "I *can* cope with this." The process of replacing negative appraisals of life events with more positive ones is sometimes referred to as cognitive restructuring and is a common technique used by cognitive-behavioral therapists (Baron, 1998; Meichenbaum, 1977; Zebrowski, 2002) (see Chapter 2, Theories of Counseling and How They Relate to Speech-Language Pathology and Audiology).

AFFIRMATIONS

An affirmation is a conscious, positive thought that helps change a particular image or belief a person has about him or herself. Affirmations begin with first person, present tense and may be helpful in times of crisis as well as times of relative calm. The purpose of affirmations is to focus on what is wanted, not what is unwanted. A metaphor may be helpful to understand focusing on what is wanted. When a horse that a person is riding begins to head in the wrong direction or toward a hazard (e.g., a cliff), the rider does not keep looking at the wrong direction the horse is going or the cliff he is headed for, the rider looks in the direction he wants the horse to go. The rider's body then automatically uses its muscles to move the horse in the right or safe direction. Affirmations help the mind stay focused on what the person wants, which allows it to begin finding ways to achieve its goals. By saying affirmations using the first person, present tense, it is as though what is desired is already acquired, as if it is spoken into existence. Examples of affirmations include, "I am speaking more fluently now." "I am using my esophageal speech easily." "I am using the chin-tuck position with every bite." Affirmations are powerful tools that many highly successful athletes use before and during competition.

VISUAL IMAGERY (VISUALIZATIONS)

Visual imagery is the deliberate exercise of imagining scenes designed to have helpful or therapeutic value (e.g., speaking confidently in front of a classroom, visualizing using safe-swallow techniques). The clinician can help the person in crisis practice, with eyes closed, to "see" successful completion of activities and tasks that meet the person's goals.

RELAXATION TECHNIQUES

Relaxation techniques, such as progressive relaxation, can be an effective tool to increase coping abilities (Wolpe, 1958, 1987). To use this technique, the person begins by alternately flexing and relaxing groups of muscles (e.g., the hands) to appreciate the difference between relaxed and tense muscles. The person can then move to other muscle groups such as the arms, shoulders, back, and so forth. Controlled breathing is also helpful, with slow, deep, relaxed breathing being most helpful.

PROBLEM-SOLVING SKILLS

Clinicians can teach problem-solving skills that may be helpful in managing the communication problem: for example, watching people's faces as they are talking, asking people to get the client's attention before they begin to speak, writing down information to not have to rely on auditory memory, having an electrolarynx by the bedroom telephone for a laryngectomee, or wearing a MedicAlert bracelet.

Another factor that may need to be explored in the third stage of crisis management are the resources and support immediately available to the client and family. For example, the child with CAPD and ADD may have a teacher or reading specialist who is very supportive of him, or the patient with a TBI may have family and friends who can take care of the other children while the patient is in the hospital and the spouse is visiting there. Note that there may be an overlap in the information the SLP and social service staff in the hospital obtain; however, this can help patient care conferences go more smoothly because there is a better general understanding of the family's support system. The client and family may need to be provided with information about support groups (e.g., ADD or stroke support groups) so they can become connected with other people who have had similar experiences and crises, and understand the problems the client and family may encounter in the future.

Limitations

Many people, particularly those in convalescent hospitals, do not have family or friends available for support. Many elderly people have outlived the rest of their family and are essentially alone in life. Regretfully, the hospital staff usually is a poor substitute for close family and friends during a time of crisis. During a summer when I was working in a convalescent hospital I had an elderly patient who had a stroke that resulted in aphasia, cognitive impairments, and dysphagia. Both the patient and his wife were in the hospital and were roommates. The hospital's staff had arranged the room so that it was like a small apartment and the couple was happy to be together. The wife was relatively healthy and able to watch over and take care of her husband in many ways. The couple had been together in this environment for many months when one of them died—the wife. The man was very confused and did not understand what happened to his wife, although it was explained to him many times. He wandered around the hospital in his wheelchair often searching for her. All the staff and rehabilitation team, as well as a psychologist who evaluated the patient, felt helpless in this situation. This vignette illustrates our limitations in helping some clients and patients who are in emotional distress.

The three crisis management stages may move along very quickly or they may take several meetings or sessions to work through; however, during this time you will have probably initiated therapy for the client or patient. As discussed above, one crisis may precipitate a cascade of other crises, some of which may not be discussed with the SLP or audiologist, and others that fall out of the scope of our expertise (e.g., financial matters). If a client or family appears to be advancing in coping skills and then experiences a sudden change in therapeutic progress or motivation, it may reflect that a new crisis has occurred which has not been shared with the clinician. In this case the clinician may empathically question the client and family about the changes noticed. If the changes in therapy progress reflect issues that are within the clinician's expertise, they can be addressed, otherwise the clinician may wish to refer the client or family to a counselor, psychologist, or social worker who can address these new crises. However, although the clinician may make such a referral, an appointment may never be made by the client or family and the clinician may be left to do the best she can with individuals who may be moving in and out of various crises. The clinician should follow up on a referral to a psychologist or counselor and provide support to the client or family to get them involved in such therapy.

Summary

Clinicians in all settings who are working with all ages encounter crisis situations. The defining characteristic of a crisis is not the instigating event, but rather the person's difficulty coping with the situation. Some crisis situations may cause cascading effects that make the initial crisis more difficult to manage. We can reasonably assume that a person who functioned normally all his or her life but now has a moderate to severe communication problem, is in crisis, and so is the family. Understanding general principles of crisis management can help clients and their families better cope with the crisis situation. A three-stage model for crisis management was presented; the first stage involves the clinician establishing an alliance with the client, patient, or family that helps them develop confidence in the clinician. The second stage involves clarifying the problems based on the clinician's assessment of the client. The third stage is to determine the treatment goals and possible procedures. Although these stages may appear routine to the clinician, additional factors may be involved to help the individuals in crisis manage their thoughts and feelings in productive ways to allow maximum gains from therapy.

THREAT OF SUICIDE OR SELF-HARM

Over 30,000 recorded suicides occur annually in the United States, ranking it as the eighth leading cause of death in this country. The incidence of suicide is increasing dramatically among all age groups, and especially among young people aged 15 to 24 where it has become the third most frequent cause of death after accidents and homicide (Maxmen & Ward, 1995; Morrison & Anders, 1999). Suicide is the second leading cause of death among college students, and their suicide rate is

50% higher than that of the general population (Gladding, 2000). In addition, approximately 10,000 people over age 60 kill themselves each year (Eliopoulos, 1996; Hooyman & Kiyak, 2001).

Suicide at any age is tragic, and it is even more so with children. Public school clinicians need to be alert to any indications of depression or hint of self-harm by a child of any age and make the appropriate referrals to the school counselor. However, not all schools have a counselor who is readily available. Even though a referral may be made, an appointment may not be immediately scheduled. The child may see the counselor for a relatively brief time and then must return to his or her classroom or home to face the painful emotional experiences that have precipitated the thoughts of self-harm. For many of these children, the language problems on which the SLP is working are also the language problems that interfere with the child explaining his or her thoughts, feelings, and experiences to the counselor. When time is of the essence, the counselor has the burden of attempting to communicate with a hearing-impaired, speech and/or language-impaired child in order to establish rapport and trust to talk about very sensitive issues. Many counselors are able to do this smoothly; however, not all children are willing to talk openly with a stranger about delicate topics such as family problems, anxieties, and fears. Counseling with a professional may not be as helpful as needed if a child cannot communicate effectively or is reluctant to talk to the counselor.

Children who have had a parent commit suicide will very likely be depressed and themselves at risk for suicide. These children need to be carefully monitored. Renwick (2002) described an experience where a father of three young children committed suicide by setting himself on fire in his home, which resulted in the house burning with all the children's possessions. Each child responded to the tragic experience in a different way. For example, the youngest child became very stoic and matter-of-fact when she mentioned the death of her father, apparently much as her mother reacted. She never spoke about the death of her father again while working with the speech clinician. The middle child (a girl) began dressing like a boy, including wearing a boy's haircut. In such situations it is difficult for an SLP or audiologist to know what to say or do, other than be empathic and make the appropriate referrals.

Stewart (1997) discusses classifications of suicide, including 1) *egoistic* suicide resulting from a deep sense of personal failure coupled with a lack of connection to other people; 2) *altruistic* suicide which is based on sacrificing oneself for the good of another with a strong sense of connection to others (e.g., a parent risking and sacrificing her or his life to save a child); and 3) *alienation* suicide based on the belief that life no longer has meaning and there is little or no connection with others. *Suicidal ideation* refers to thoughts of wanting to die, but do not necessarily signify suicidal intentions. *Parasuicide* indicates an action for which there is little or no intention that death should result (e.g., when a person overdoses on medication and then calls someone for help). In this case, the attempt is a cry for help. *Attempted suicide* signifies that an act that would have led to death has been prevented. A *suicide gesture* refers to an act that results in minor self-harm, such as taking a half-dozen aspirin tablets or scratching but not cutting the wrists. Regardless of the level of suicide ideation or attempt that is made, it should be taken seriously and all appropriate actions should be taken to determine the seriousness of the possibility of suicide or the direct prevention of a suicide.

A "Code 3" Call

During my years as an ambulance driver and attendant in Southern California, I had many emergency ("Code 3") calls where people had attempted or were successful in their attempts to commit suicide. Some people were very creative in their choices of ways to die. I had learned and later experienced that women often choose overdosing of medications for suicide, while men tend to choose more dramatic forms such as shooting themselves with a pistol or shotgun.

One evening my driver and I received a Code 3 call to a residence. When I entered the home two young boys, ages about five and eight, pointed to the garage and said "Mommy's in there!" When I opened the door from the house into the garage I saw an automobile running and a woman behind the wheel slumped over. I immediately opened the garage door to get fresh air inside and the carbon monoxide outside. I then shut off the engine of the car, pulled the woman out, put an oxygen mask over her face, and pumped oxygen into her. On the way to the hospital the boys rode in front with the driver while I continued pumping oxygen into their mother. She survived, although I have often wondered how much brain damage she may have had and whether she ever needed speech therapy. As SLPs in acute-care hospitals and rehabilitation centers we see patients a significant amount of time after they have been brought to the hospital's emergency room. Often the life-saving and "brain-saving" work has been done days before we see them as our patients.

Important Points About Suicide

Sommers-Flanagan and Sommers-Flanagan (1993) present several important points about suicide.

■ Twenty-five to 50% of people who commit suicide have previously attempted to do so (previous suicide attempts are one of the better predictors of future attempts).

■ People who eventually commit suicide often have tried to communicate their despair to others in a variety of ways. They also usually give clues or warnings either verbally or through their behavior that they are contemplating suicide; however, older people (60 years and above) tend to communicate their suicidal intentions less often than younger people.

■ Medical patients are often at risk for suicide if they are depressed and/or in extreme pain.

■ People who attempt suicide are more likely than other psychiatric patients to use disinhibiting substances (including alcohol) in the 24-hour period before the attempt.

The disinhibiting substances can help people get up the nerve to follow through on thoughts of killing themselves.

▪ Men are about three times more likely to complete suicide than women, while women are about three times more likely to attempt suicide than men (men's success with suicide may be partly the result of their more drastic and violent means).

▪ Almost all people in the pre-suicidal state experience ambivalent feelings. They want to die and also to be saved. They want to escape from an intolerable situation, and they also wish that the intolerable situation could be changed so that they could continue living.

Myths About Suicide

Numerous myths are associated with suicide (Nystul, 1999), including the following.

Myth: Suicide is only committed by people with severe psychologic problems.

Reality: Most individuals who commit suicide have not been diagnosed as having a psychologic disorder.

Myth: Suicide usually occurs without warning.

Reality: Most suicides are preceded by warning signs such as a sudden change of behavior, verbal threats of suicide, talk of hopelessness, and depression.

Myth: Discussing suicide may cause the person to carry out the act.

Reality: The opposite is true; talking with a caring person can often prevent suicide.

Myth: When a person has attempted suicide and pulls back from it, the danger is over.

Reality: Another period of danger may be during the upswing period, when the person becomes re-energized following a severe depression and has the energy to commit suicide.

Myth: People who are suicidal will always be prone to suicide.

Reality: Most people who become suicidal do not remain in that state through the rest of their lives. They may be struggling through a temporary personal crisis, and once they work through the crisis they may never be suicidal again.

Risk Factors

There are certain risk factors for suicide that clinicians should be aware of, although none can predict suicide behavior in a particular individual. SLPs and audiologists should never attempt to predict which clients or patients may be at risk for suicidal ideation. The relationship between depression and potential suicide is well-documented, with about 80% of suicide attempts being done by people of all ages who are depressed (Gladding 2000; Maxmen & Ward, 1995; Morrison & Anders, 1999; Sommers-Flanagan & Sommers-Flanagan, 1993; Roy, 1991). A strong sense of hopelessness is an important predictor of suicide. The risk of suicide escalates as the person's suicidal ideation (thoughts) intensify and become more frequent. Almost everyone has had fleeting suicidal thoughts; only the suicidal ruminate about it. It is more dangerous if the person has a plan, particularly a detailed plan. In general, the major risk factors for suicide are being male, older, unemployed, living alone, having a chronic illness, and being unmarried (single, never married individuals have a suicide rate of nearly double the rate of married individuals, with men over 70 years old having the highest suicide rate of any group). Other risks and indicators include financial loss, a lack of religious faith, a recent loss or death of a loved one, a family history of suicide, or suddenly giving away prized possessions (Maxmen & Ward, 1995). However, knowing these risk factors only tells the statistical risk of suicide; these factors cannot tell a clinician what the risk for a particular child or adult is.

The Speech-Language Pathologist and Audiologist's Role

SLPs may have long careers without having a child or adult verbalize suicidal ideation or intention. During informal surveys conducted by the author (P.T.F.) in cities around the country with SLPs, PTs, OTs, and audiologists (primarily those working in medical settings) who attended seminars on counseling skills, many indicated that they have had patients who either attempted or succeeded in committing suicide. The possibility is of increasing concern and we need to know how to respond to it. Recognition of suicidal tendencies and appropriate interventions by professionals and family members may save a person's life.

It is the mental health professionals' responsibility to conduct a systematic and thorough suicide evaluation. The SLP or audiologist, however, can provide critical information to these professionals that may facilitate their determination of the level of suicide risk for a particular person. In order to gather this critical information, the primary task of the clinician is to listen carefully and, perhaps, to ask the client to elaborate on his or her suicidal thoughts. In some cases, the SLP or audiologist may discern that the person has no intention of carrying out the suicidal thoughts. In other cases, the clinician may learn that the person has a general or specific plan for suicide. The clinician may ask general questions such as, "Tell me more about your thoughts about hurting yourself (committing suicide, taking your life)." Depending on what the person discloses, the clinician may ask specific questions (described in the following sections) about suicidal history, lethality, and specificity. However, it is important to remember at all times that the clinician should not attempt to conduct a suicide evaluation. This means that all disclosures of suicidal ideation must be reported immediately to a mental health professional, regardless of the clinician's impressions of the level of suicidal risk.

In most situations, if you plan to break confidentiality in order to ensure the client's safety, it is advisable to inform the client of your intention. This action may help preserve a trusting relationship between you and the client. For example, in response to a client's voicing self-destructive or suicidal thoughts, the clinician may say, "Mr. S., in order to ensure your safety, I feel it is necessary to

Obtaining Information from Clients Threatening Suicide

I was working in a convalescent hospital for several weeks during the summer and had a patient with cognitive impairments whom I was seeing on a daily basis. One day I wheeled him into the therapy room and after we worked for a few minutes, he told me he was going to kill himself. I talked to him about it at length because I felt we had a good working relationship and that he would share information with me that he might not easily share with others. As an SLP, I cannot do a suicide assessment, but I can obtain as much information as possible to share with the other professional staff. At the end of our therapy session I did not take him back to his room as I normally would, but wheeled him to the nurses' station where there were a variety of people to oversee him. I then told the charge nurse about the patient's suicidal ideation and followed up by informing the DON, social service director, and the administrator. Appropriate actions were taken and the patient was put on suicide watch where a staff member was with him 24 hours a day, observing him eat, sleep, and go to the bathroom. A review of his medical chart revealed that he had attempted suicide previously by setting himself on fire. A psychologist was called in for a suicide assessment who, after extensive interviewing and testing of the patient, decided the patient was not a risk to himself at this time. After approximately seven days, the patient was taken off suicide watch.

share this information with the nurse and your doctor (psychologist, etc.). They will be able to take the appropriate steps to make sure you do not harm yourself." If the client protests your disclosure of this confidential information, you may apologize for opposing the client on this matter while maintaining that your primary concern and responsibility at this time is for the client's safety.

Be prepared to write a detailed report on what the client says and does. Careful documentation is essential and must be immediate. Document what the client said verbatim as much as possible, being concrete and without drawing inferences or interpretations (these are left to the mental health professionals). Record what steps you took to alert other professionals of the client's suicidal thoughts. Report relevant details in the sequence or order they occurred so other professionals can evaluate and draw conclusions. It is also useful to report on any questions the client refused to answer, for example, "After declaring she wanted to end her life, the client refused to elaborate on whether she has a plan to do this."

The following sections describe signs and symptoms that SLPs and audiologists will want to be alert for when talking with individuals who express thoughts of self-harm. The information is summarized from several sources, including Burnard (1999), Gladding (2000); Maxmen and Ward (1995), Meir and Davis (2000), Morrison (1995), Renwick (2002), Sommers-Flanagan and Sommers-Flanagan (1993), Willams-Quinlan (2002), and Zaro et al. (1995).

LISTENING FOR SIGNS OF DEPRESSION

It is difficult to know how best to talk with a person who is expressing suicidal or self-destructive thoughts; however, there are guidelines that can be helpful. Listen closely to the person's thoughts and feelings. Throughout the conversation or interview, your tone of voice, facial expressions, and body language should convey warmth, caring, concern, and empathy. You may be the first person to whom the individual has ever voiced these thoughts and feelings. The person needs to feel that you hear accurately how miserable and desperate she or he is. Avoid expressions of shock or surprise when a person begins to talk about suicide. Responding to the person in a matter-of-fact manner suggests that you have dealt with such issues before and, therefore, that you are competent to listen and respond appropriately. Many of the suicidal individuals SLPs are likely to work with have some neurological damage from CVAs or TBIs, and, therefore, their speech, language, and cognitive functioning may be significantly impaired with resulting difficulty expressing their thoughts and feelings, which adds to their frustration and feelings of justification for wanting to end their lives. Some of these individuals may experience an impaired capacity for self-control, which may put them at higher risk for suicide.

Depression is implicated in many of the risk factors for suicide; therefore, one of the first questions you may reflect on is how the person is feeling. Sad? Depressed? Helpless? Hopeless? From the person's perspective, helplessness may indicate a feeling or belief that she is unable to make any changes necessary to feel better on her own. The person's feelings of helplessness may represent an indirect request for help from the clinician. She may believe that while unable to effect change in her own life, someone else might be able to do so for her. If the person feels hopeless regarding the possibility of positive changes and believes no one can help, she may make statements such as, "I don't see how things will ever be any different," or "I've felt like this for a long time and I'll probably always feel like this."

A common indication of depression is withdrawal from friends, family, and usual activities. Listen for indications that the person has lost some interest in activities she used to enjoy and people she used to enjoy being with. Depression is often accompanied by somatic changes such as loss of sleep or sleeping much more than usual, loss of appetite or an unusual amount of eating (particularly comfort foods). People who show signs of depression may have psychomotor retardation with an overall slowness of movement and speech. The converse of that may also occur, where the person may appear agitated and anxious, speak rapidly, pull on her hair or clothing, rub her hands together, or even pace back and forth. The agitation may indicate the person has the energy to commit suicide. Cognitive changes such as slowed thinking, difficulty remembering, inability to concentrate, and difficulty making decisions and solving problems may be present.

LISTENING FOR SUICIDAL IDEATION

When individuals make vague references to suicide (e.g., "I'm going to end it all." "Soon it will be over." "It doesn't matter anymore."), an SLP or audiologist may ask, "I'm wondering what you are thinking about doing (what your intentions or plans are)." If the client alludes to suicide, then the clinician may ask, "Are you thinking about harming yourself in some way?" The phrasing of this question is preferable to asking whether the client has "thought about" committing suicide. Asking the client whether or not she has thought about committing suicide could be misinterpreted by some clients as offering a solution or giving advice (see Chapter 4, Microskills, where questions may be used as suggestions to encourage a client's action). In a similar vein, when a client has confided to a professional (psychologist, minister, etc.) misery in her or his marital situation, and is asked, "Have you thought about leaving your spouse?" the client may easily interpret the professional to be making a suggestion.

If the person answers "yes" to any of the questions about suicidal ideation or intent, open-ended follow-up questions may help get more specific information, for example, "Could you tell me more about your thoughts?" Most suicidal people will admit self-destructive thoughts when asked about them. The clinician can normalize the situation by talking about how natural it is for people who are very sad, or who have long-term illnesses or recent significant losses to *think* about ending their lives. This response can help the person feel that it is okay to admit and talk about such thoughts. Williams-Quinlan (2002), Director of the Counseling Center at the University of the Pacific, advises that the clinician's questions convey empathy and help the person feel understood. Asking the person questions reflects that the clinician is interested and concerned about the person's thoughts and feelings. The person needs to tell someone about the suicidal thoughts, and the fact that she has voiced them to the SLP or audiologist indicates that the clinician has been chosen.

LISTENING FOR SUICIDE PLANS (SLAP-I)

The acronym "SLAP-I" refers to various areas that need careful listening from a clinician, that is, Specificity of the plan, Lethality, Availability, Proximity, and Intent. These areas can provide a framework for listening to or teasing out important information embedded in the sometimes rambling or disjointed information a cognitively impaired or depressed patient may provide. The clinician can then report essential information to the mental health professional in an organized manner. This information may be obtained by listening to the client or by asking questions. The questions should be kept open-ended so that the clinician's questions are not perceived as suggestions. SLPs and audiologists need not try to make judgments about the client's level of suicide risk, but simply be responsible for reporting the information as quickly and accurately as possible.

SPECIFICITY OF THE PLAN

Specificity refers to the details the person has thought through about how she would carry out suicide. The more specific the plan, the higher the risk. You may ask about the person's plans, for example, "Do you have a plan about how you would kill yourself?" At this point the person may assure you that she really does not have a plan and does not intend to kill herself even though she has thought about it. The person may give reasons why she would not carry it out, such as religious beliefs, children, or other family members. If the person assures you that she or he will not commit suicide and gives reasons why not, do not continue pursuing questions about a plan. However, if the person describes some planning to carry out the suicide, further questions are needed.

When a child mentions to an SLP or audiologist that he or she is thinking about suicide, the clinician may learn about the specificity, lethality, availability, proximity, and intent by using a therapy task the child is familiar with. Many children receiving speech-language therapy are taught how to answer "wh-" questions. Renwick (2002) says that the clinician can have the child practice answering these questions around the theme of suicide or self-harm. For example, "Who wants to kill herself?" "What are the reasons you want to kill yourself?" "When do you plan to do it?" "Why do it then?" "Where would you do it?" "Why do it there?" "How would you try to do it?" Tape recording or writing the child's words as close to verbatim as possible will help analyze the child's words and tone of voice. A child's drawings may also reveal his or her thoughts and intentions, such as self-harm or harm to others. The purpose of gathering this information is to share it with the school counselor or psychologist.

LETHALITY

Lethality refers to how quickly or effectively the person's method of attempt could cause death. The greater the lethality, the higher the suicide risk; for example, firearms, overdose of medications, or driving a car off of a bridge have different levels of lethality. If the person has already indicated she has a specific plan to commit suicide, you may ask a "how" question in order to gauge the level of lethality, for example, "How are you thinking about carrying out your plan?" A client may report a plan to take an overdose of aspirin, which may not be as lethal as an overdose of sleeping pills, or may describe a plan to drive off a low bridge into a shallow stream, which may not be as lethal as driving off a high bridge into a rocky ravine.

AVAILABILITY

Availability refers to how quickly a person could potentially carry out the suicide plan. Does the person actually have the means to implement the plan? An elderly person in a convalescent hospital may talk about driving a car off a bridge, but if unable to ambulate or drive and there is no bridge in the vicinity, the plan would be thwarted. However, this does not mean the person is any less serious about a suicide attempt, but it may indicate that he or she does not have the cognitive capacity to have a workable plan. Many people have sufficient medication in their home medicine cabinets to achieve a lethal overdose. The immediacy of the availability is also important; for example, there is a difference between a person who says, "I'm going to go out and buy a gun," and the person who says, "I have a loaded gun in the car." Therefore, the clinician who hears that the client wants to shoot himself may want to ask, "Do you have a gun?" In most cases, considering the availability of a suicide method is important in determining suicide risk and whether or not immediate intervention (e.g., hospitalization and suicide watch) is needed.

PROXIMITY

Proximity refers to how near helping resources are to the person who is planning to attempt suicide, that is, other individuals who could intervene and rescue the person if an attempt is made. Does the person live alone or with family or friends? Are there neighbors nearby who know and look after the person? Never let a potentially suicidal person leave alone. Call a relative or friend of the person to drive the person home and do what you can to have someone with the person at all times or to check in on the person frequently. Nighttime is usually the worst time for someone who is suicidal, and many people have been discovered by family or friends the next morning.

LISTEN FOR INTENT

Intent refers to how determined the person is to carry out the suicide. Some people are resolute in their seeking self-destruction and, short of hospitalization or incarceration, it may be nearly impossible to prevent them from killing themselves. Asking the person to rate her or himself on a 1 to 10 scale, with 1 being no intent and 10 being total intent, can provide a good indication of the person's determination. A rating scale that provides the terms absent (1—no intent), low (2–3), moderate (4–6), and high (7–10) provides terms that reflect the numbers of the scale.

IDENTIFYING ALTERNATIVES TO SUICIDE

The thought process accompanying suicidal ideation is a pathological narrowing of the mind's focus, called constriction, which takes the form of seeing only two choices; either continuing life that is painfully unsatisfactory or cessation of life (Nystul, 1999; Shneidman, 1984). Rather than debating with a suicidal person about whether or not the person should kill herself, it is better to identify options to suicide, that death is not the only way to handle the problems. Even asking the person, "Why commit suicide now?" may open the person's thinking to an alternative time. This, of course, is a therapeutic strategy to "buy time" to get other professionals involved and to organize the person's support system to have care when she is away from the hospital or therapy environment. The person may realize that suicide can be committed later, after other life options are explored. The next task is to help the person become involved with life, which may provide the rewards and gratification that reduce or eliminate the desire to commit suicide and thereby end life. Brainstorming with the person for options to suicide and writing them down provides a visible means for the person to see and review these at other times. Also, brainstorming for alternatives to managing general and specific problems in the person's life that seem overwhelming can help open thinking to solutions the person had not considered. After alternatives are listed, the person can be asked to rank them in order of preference.

SUICIDE-PREVENTION CONTRACTS

Suicide-prevention contracts may be either verbal or written, and sealed with a handshake. Many suicidal people will honor such a contract, which also buys time for you to contact other professionals and family members. A contract may be as simple as having the person agree not to kill herself until after she or he has seen you for another appointment. Becuase it may be too easy for the person to say, "Sure, I won't do anything until I see you again" it may be better to give the person the option of declining the contract offer by saying, "I only want you to agree to this contract if you really believe you can follow through with it." Suicide-prevention contracts also help assess a person's self-control and intent. If a person is willing to agree to a suicide prevention contract, the person is probably in some control and may have only low to moderate intent. However, a person with low self-control or high intent usually will not agree to a suicide contract. Asking the person to call you at your office or at home is not necessarily the best approach because you may not be available or at home. The person may also call you just to say "Good-bye." Providing the person with telephone numbers of local suicide hotlines constitutes a lifeline that the person can use 24 hours a day and speak with people who are well-trained and experienced to deal with such a life-threatening crisis. Above all, you should recognize that if you are engaged in such a discussion with a client, you need to document the discussion and make a referral to a mental health professional immediately.

A TEAM APPROACH

A mental health professional must become involved in the care and management of a suicidal person. However, even though such a professional may quickly establish a therapeutic alliance, the professional will likely recognize and appreciate the relationship you have already established with the person (which is probably the reason the suicidal ideation was disclosed). Therefore, the mental health professional may encourage you to continue seeing the person to use a team approach to help manage the suicidal risks. Careful documentation of each session is essential and discussing each session with the mental health professional can help you and the team of professionals work for the best interest of the person.

5150 AND 5250 CODES

The 5150 Code (California Welfare and Institution Code, 2002) may be initiated when a person is a danger to himself or herself, or to others. (*Note*: other states may designate a different code number. To obtain this information contact the local mental health professional board.) The person may be taken into protective custody (involuntary detention) and placed in a mental health facility designated by the county and approved by the state department of mental health for up to 72 hours for evaluation and treatment. Two professionals must certify the person placed in involuntary detention. Both must be physicians (board-certified psychiatrists) or licensed psychologists who have doctorates in psychology and at least five years of postgraduate experience in the diagnosis and treatment of emotional and mental disorders. In some cases, a registered nurse or a licensed case social worker who participated in the evaluation may sign the notice of certification.

Code 5250 allows the person to remain in a facility for not more than 14 days of intensive treatment related to the mental disorder certified during the Code 5150 evaluation. If the individual is a danger to himself (suicidal), he may be recertified and held for a second 14-day period, but not longer. The total amount of time a person may be hospitalized in protective custody is 31 days, after which he or she must be released unless reclassified as a danger to others. If an individual is certified as a danger to others, he or she can be held for an additional 180-day period.

Summary

A person's threat of suicide can be a very unsettling experience for SLPs and audiologists, and when it occurs it *cannot* be ignored. We are mandated reporters and, therefore, the concern for breaking professional confidentiality is secondary to the responsibility of preventing harm to self and others. SLPs or audiologists may be the professionals to whom clients or patients first voice their suicidal ideation because of the close therapeutic alliance we have established, with our emphasis on helping people communicate their wants, needs, thoughts, and feelings. We are often the only professionals whom clients or patients see who give them undivided attention for half an hour to an hour each day. The consistency of seeing them on a regular basis for several days, weeks, or sometimes months, and the close working relationships we develop may encourage them to share thoughts and feelings with us that they have not disclosed to others. Our initial and primary goal is to help ensure the client's safety. By understanding risk factors for suicide and our professional role within the suicide prevention team, we may make an important difference in a person's life.

THREAT OF HARM TO OTHERS

SLPs and audiologists must be aware of and willing to appropriately respond to new and frightening crisis situations that were unheard of and perhaps unthinkable several years ago. Because of our close interaction with children and adults of all ages, when working with their communication and cognitive skills, we are in a position to hear individuals vent frustration and sometimes make threats toward parents, teachers, other children, doctors, nurses, other professionals, and even random others. At one time we may have been naïve, thinking that such comments were idle threats. However, we cannot ignore such comments and assume that the person will not act on his or her thoughts.

Tarasoff Versus the Board of Regents

A legal precedent for counselors and psychologists to take decisive action to protect human life was set in the landmark case of Tarasoff versus the Board of Regents of the University of California (1974, 1976). The case involved a psychologist who provided counseling services to a student. After the student threatened to kill his girlfriend, Tarasoff, the psychologist, failed to warn the woman of the threat. Two months later the young man killed his girlfriend. Her parents filed suit against the university and won on the basis that the psychologist had been irresponsible by not alerting the young woman or the proper authorities about the man's threats.

The Speech-Language Pathologist and Audiologist's Role

Although the Tarasoff versus the Board of Regents ruling may seem like a case unrelated to anything that may occur in our professions of speech-language pathology and audiology, we need to keep in mind the tragic school shootings around the nation over the past several years. In the United States between 1997 and 2001 there were 11 school shootings, resulting in the deaths of 28 children and the wounding of 70 other children, from middle school age to high school age. Four teachers and one principal were killed in those numerous incidents. It is not known whether any of the children who committed those shootings had received or were receiving speech therapy or audiological services in their schools or privately. Had a child informed an SLP or audiologist working in one of the schools or working privately with one of the children that such events might occur, and the clinician failed to inform the school administrator and psychologist, the clinician may have acted irresponsibly and with professional negligence. The question of whether the clinician could be subject to legal action in such a situation may depend on individual state laws.

As extreme as these incidents are, they are now within the realm of possibility of any school-based SLP or audiologist. It is possible for a child to disclose to a clinician that he or she has heard of or knows that another student is thinking about or planning to harm another child, a teacher, administrator, parent, or others. The clinician may, in a nonthreatening manner, talk to the child about the situation. As mentioned above, many children receiving speech-language therapy are taught how to answer "wh-" questions, and the clinician may obtain information by having the child practice answering questions around the theme of another child's possible harm to other children, adults, and/or the school. For example, "Who wants to hurt a teacher (or children)?" "Who is the teacher (or children) that is going to be hurt?" When does the student plan to do this?" "Where is the student going to do it?" "How is the student going to hurt the teacher (or children)?" Once again, tape recording or writing the child's words as close to verbatim as possible will help analyze the child's words and tone of voice. A child's drawings may also reveal his or her thoughts and intentions. The purpose of gathering this information is to immediately share it with the school counselor or psychologist, administrators, and law enforcement agencies.

As mandated reporters, we legally and ethically must inform the proper supervisors, administrators, or authorities about the child's statements or threats. The same responsibility is present if an SLP or audiologists hears or learns of a child's intent to damage property: the SLP or audiologist should immediately inform the school principal or administrator. Whether it is a threat to a person or property, the clinician or audiologist should obtain a verbal commitment from the principal/administrator that the school psychologist will be contacted immediately. The psychologist is then mandated to take immediate, decisive action to evaluate the child, inform individuals who may be threatened, and contact law enforcement authorities if needed. The SLP or audiologist must carefully document all that was said by the child and the clinician's contact with the school principal/administrator about the incident.

Although it is unlikely, it is possible that an SLP or audiologist working in a medical setting or in home health may hear a client suggest that he or she is thinking about harming another individual or damaging property. It behooves the professional to act responsibly by inquiring in a nonthreatening manner about such intentions. By obtaining what information the person is willing or able to share, the professional can then document what was disclosed and present it to the proper administrator or authorities.

Summary

SLPs and audiologists are mandated reporters for threats of harm to people or property. The concern for breaking professional confidentiality is secondary to the responsibility of preventing harm to others. Although it is extremely unlikely that any one SLP or audiologist will have to respond to such threats, it is possible. In order to prevent any unnecessary and tragic loss of life or injury to others, we must be alert to such threats and take immediate action by informing the proper individuals.

REPORTING CHILD OR ELDER ABUSE/NEGLECT (BEING A "MANDATED REPORTER")

Child Abuse or Neglect

All states have laws related to child abuse, and most require teachers, counselors, psychologists, physicians, nurses, SLPs and audiologists, as well as other professionals to report suspected abuse, neglect, or mental suffering; that is, these professionals are mandated reporters.

Although children have been neglected and abused throughout history, it was not until the early 1960s that counselors recognized child abuse and neglect as social problems that require comprehensive assessment and treatment. The incidence of child abuse and neglect in the United States is estimated to be approximately two million children a year, with many of these children having been sexually abused. In addition, psychological abuse may be the most prevalent and destructive form of child abuse (George & Cristiani, 1995; Nystul, 1999). Child Protective Services (CPS) is the state or county service system that becomes involved in instances of abuse or neglect.

Nystul (1999) identifies the following warning signs of the various forms of child abuse and neglect.

- Physical abuse: signs of bruises, burns, and broken bones
- Child neglect: poor health and hygiene and excessive school absenteeism
- Sexual abuse: use of sexually explicit terminology, nightmares, genital injury, and sexually transmitted disease
- Psychologic (emotional) abuse: depression, self-deprecation, somatic (bodily) complaints such as headaches or stomachaches, and fear of adults

SLPs and audiologists may become suspicious or aware of possible child abuse or neglect when working in any setting, but particularly in schools because of the large caseloads of children of all ages. According to state law, "Reasonable suspicion" means that it is "objectively reasonable for a person to entertain a suspicion, based upon facts that could cause a reasonable person in a like position, drawing when appropriate, on his or her training and experience, to suspect child abuse" (Section 11166 of the State of California Penal Code, 2002). A Child Protective Services (CPS) agency must be notified immediately or as soon as possible by telephone and a written report received within 36 hours of the incident. In California, failure to comply with the requirements of Section 11166 is a misdemeanor, punishable by up to six months in jail, by a fine of $1,000.00, or both.

The following information should be included in a telephone report to CPS:

- the name of the person making the report
- the name of the child
- the present location of the child
- the nature and extent of the injury
- any other information that led the person to suspect child abuse

The identity of all persons who report suspected child abuse or neglect will be confidential and disclosed only between CPS agencies, to legal counsel representing a CPS agency, or to the district attorney in a criminal prosecution. No CPS agency may disclose the identity of any person who reports suspected child abuse or neglect to the person's employer, except with the employee's consent or by court order. Also, no supervisor or administrator may impede or inhibit the reporting duties and no person making such a report shall be subject to any sanction for making the report. The individual reporting the possible child abuse or neglect has immunity from criminal and civil liability.

The assessment of child abuse and neglect by a psychologist or counselor is a multistage process, beginning with impressionistic information from the reporting and referral source (Morrison & Anders, 1999; Nystul, 1999). That stage is followed by a refinement of information during interviews with parents and the child, with various assessment instruments used by the examiner to survey the attitudes of parents on topics relating to marriage and the family, and familial patterns associated with child abuse. Assessment of the child may include measures of the degree of positive and negative influences in the home. After an investigation, CPS may determine the report is "unfounded" (i.e., determined to be false, inherently improbable, involve an accidental injury, or not to constitute child abuse), "substantiated" (i.e., determined, based upon credible evidence, to constitute child abuse or neglect), or "unsubstantiated" (i.e., determined not to be unfounded, but in which findings are inconclusive and there is insufficient evidence to determine whether child abuse or neglect has occurred).

Sroufe and Cooper (1996) describe a common profile of parents at high risk for child abuse. They tend to be young, poorly educated, single, living in poverty, socially isolated, and feel little support from a significant other. Abusive mothers tend to have a negative attitude toward their pregnancy. Compared to nonabusive parents, they are less prone to plan for pregnancy, do not attend childbirth classes, have less understanding of what is involved in caring for an infant, do not have special living space for the baby to sleep, and have unrealistic expectations about raising an infant.

Once again, SLPs and audiologists are mandated reporters of suspected child abuse and neglect. This is, of course, an extremely delicate, awkward, and uncomfortable aspect of our professional responsibilities. However, reporting suspected child abuse or neglect is not a personal choice and we cannot shirk this responsibility.

Dependent-Adult and Elder Abuse or Neglect

Dependent adults are developmentally delayed or physically handicapped individuals of all ages (18–64) who are dependent on others for their daily care. Elders are individuals 65 years of age or older. Elder abuse or neglect is estimated to occur in 5% of the elderly population, and most of the abuse is committed by a close family member (Springhouse Corporation, 1997). Elder abuse can occur in all kinds of families, regardless of social, financial, or ethnic background. Frail, older people who live alone are particularly vulnerable to self-neglect, and those who become dependent on others for care are at higher risk for abuse by either a family member or caregiver who is under intense strain. Elderly females are more likely to be abused than elderly men (Springhouse Corporation, 1997). In addition to cases of abuse and neglect, elderly and dependent adults may receive inadequate care because of inadequate information about how to care for an elderly and/or disabled person, lack of financial resources, and lack of access to care.

Definitions and categories of dependent adult and elder abuse vary from state to state and among agencies. The U.S. Department of Health and Human Services (DHHS) (1989) defines abuse and neglect as "the willful infliction of injury, unreasonable confinement, intimidation, or punishment with resulting physical harm or pain or mental anguish, or deprivation by an individual, including a caretaker, or goods or services that are necessary to attain or maintain physical, mental, and psychological well-being." Psychological abuse, psychological neglect, and financial exploitation are often difficult to document.

Staab and Hodges (1996), and Weinrich (2002) present commonly defined types of maltreatment or abuse of the elderly, which may also apply to dependent adults.

- Physical abuse: bodily force that has a deleterious effect on an older person's body evident by malnutrition or injuries such as bruises, welts, sprains, dislocations, abrasions, lacerations, burns, and internal injuries (victims are often dependent on the abuser for care).

- Sexual abuse: nonconsensual sexual contact of any kind (those suffering from dementia or who are nonverbal are particularly vulnerable).

- Psychological abuse: willful infliction of mental or emotional anguish by threat, humiliation, or other abusive conduct such as verbal assault, fear, or isolation (elderly people often accept such abuse as a way of life).

- ▧ Medical abuse: withholding or improper administration of needed medications, or withholding of aids such as dentures, glasses, or hearing aids.

- ▧ Financial abuse or exploitation: theft from the person, illegal or improper use of an older person's assets or resources for another person's profit or advantage (the most common form of elder abuse).

- ▧ Active neglect: willful failure of a caregiver to fulfill caregiving responsibilities.

- ▧ Passive neglect: nonwillful failure of a caregiver to fulfill caregiving responsibilities.

- ▧ Self-neglect: inability or refusal to provide for one's own essential needs; it may be associated with mental or physical impairment (the most difficult form of neglect to investigate and prove).

Additional warning signs of abuse or neglect may be: depression, hesitation to speak freely, implausible explanations for events or behaviors, personality changes, isolation from family or friends, changes to documents such as wills, lack of affordable amenities, unpaid utility bills, and unusual banking and ATM activity (e.g., withdrawing large amounts of money).

The Speech-Language Pathologist and Audiologist's Role

SLPs or audiologists may become suspicious or aware of possible elder/dependent-adult abuse or neglect, or self-neglect when working in various settings, including home health, acute-care and long-term care hospitals. As in the case of suspected child abuse or neglect, the clinician is bound by all laws of the state to report dependent-adult and elder abuse. The clinician should immediately discuss her or his observations and impressions with a supervisor and/or administrator. Careful and detailed written documentation will be needed. A careful evaluation of the dependent adult or elderly person, including interviewing and physical examination, will likely be performed by a qualified person. The possible perpetrator of the abuse or neglect will also likely be interviewed. If there appears to be sufficient cause for intervention, the local Adult Protective Services (APS) or other appropriate agencies will be notified. APS or other agencies may interview the SLP or audiologist. Keep in mind that the individual reporting the possible elder/dependent-adult abuse or neglect has immunity from criminal and civil liability. The individual or individuals reporting the abuse are guaranteed anonymity, that is, neither the abused person nor the abuser can obtain information that identifies the reporter (Weinrich, 2002).

The following information should be reported when there is suspicion of elder or dependent-adult abuse or neglect (Weinrich, 2002):

- ▧ The person's name, address, date of birth, and gender
- ▧ A description of the incident
- ▧ Name, address, phone number, and relationship of the alleged abuser
- ▧ Name and relationship of person(s) with whom the person resides, if any

■ Any other information that may establish the cause or manner in which abuse has been or is occurring.

By providing pertinent information about the suspected abuse, the SLP or audiologist can assist the appropriate investigating agencies to expedite and complete their inquiry.

Summary

As professionals working with children and adults, we are mandated reporters of suspected abuse and neglect. This can be one of the most challenging situations SLPs and audiologists are confronted with in their professional careers because of the numerous ethical and legal ramifications. Our responsibility is not to make inferences or accusations, but to report our observations and information to supervisors or administrators, and, in some cases directly to CPS or APS.

CHILDREN AND CLIENTS WITH POSTTRAUMATIC STRESS DISORDER

The concept of posttraumatic stress disorder (PTSD) has existed since World War I when soldiers were observed to suffer chronic anxiety, nightmares, and flashbacks for weeks, months, or even years following combat. At that time the condition was known as shell shock. Since then it has been recognized that all wars and combat experiences can result in posttraumatic stress disorders for the men and women involved.

Beyond war experiences, posttraumatic stress disorder can occur in anyone following a severe trauma outside the normal range of human experience. These are traumas that would produce intense fear, terror, and feelings of helplessness in anyone, and include natural disasters such as earthquakes or tornadoes, motor vehicle accidents or plane crashes, rape, assault, or other violent crimes against oneself or loved ones (Bourne, 2000), and more recently, terrorist attacks (Pyszczynski, Solomon, & Greenberg, 2003). The frequency of PTSD may be increasing in children and adolescents, especially those who live in the inner city, where stressors are numerous. Juvenile PTSD may be among the most underrecognized of mental health disorders (Morrison & Anders, 1999).

It is important to note that not all people who experience severe trauma develop PTSD. There are a number of factors that may operate as either protective or risk factors in a particular individual (Pynoos et al., 1987; Morrison & Anders, 1999), including the following.

■ Duration and severity of the stress and the duration of the evoked terror

■ Proximity to the traumatic event

■ The emotional stability of the child, adolescent or adult

■ Reactions shown by parents and other family members

■ The community's social network

■ Cultural and political factors (e.g., national tragedies)

After the Oklahoma City bombing on April 19, 1995 and the September 11, 2001, terrorist attacks on New York City and Washington, D.C., some children and adults needed audiological services because of sustaining hearing losses, while others needed speech therapy after suffering traumatic brain injuries or damage to the oral cavity or larynx. In many cases, these individuals also suffered from posttraumatic stress disorders. In addition to the children and adults at those sites, there likely were many children in speech therapy or receiving audiological services in their communities who lost a parent, relative, or friend during those tragedies. Clinicians had to be prepared and willing to listen and help these children as best they could.

Experiencing Traumatic Events

An earlier tragedy hit closer to home for me. On February 17, 1989, at Cleveland Elementary School in Stockton, California, one of the nation's first schoolyard multiple shootings occurred. During the school's late-morning recess for first, second, and third graders, Patrick Purdy—who himself attended those grades at Cleveland Elementary some 20 years earlier—stood at the playground's edge, and with a semiautomatic rifle fired scores of 7.22 mm bullets at over 100 children at play. He continued shooting into the playground for seven minutes, then put a pistol to his head and shot himself. When the police arrived they found five children dying and 29 wounded (Goleman, 1995). A teacher was wounded in the leg.

The school and entire community were in shock and posttraumatic stress disorder was the aftermath for many of the children, teachers, and staff. Many children became hypervigilant, as though continually on guard against a repetition of the terror. During recess, some children hovered next to the classroom door, afraid to venture out onto the playground. Other children played in small groups, posting a designated child as lookout. Many continued for months to avoid the "evil" areas where children had died (Goleman, 1995).

The Cleveland Elementary School SLP is a former student of mine, and was at the school at the time of the shooting. She allowed me to interview her about the traumatic experience. Mrs. Sue Ulmer, M.A., CCC-SLP, has provided speech therapy at Cleveland Elementary School since 1984. On that morning she had just stepped outside her therapy room and into a hall to watch for a boy who was a little late for therapy. As Mrs. Ulmer stated, when the shooting began it sounded like a jackhammer—rapid and sharp (jackhammer sounds bother her still). She could tell the direction of the shots from the playground. Children began running up to her and she told them to go into a classroom. One child who was shot was scheduled to be in therapy later that day. Mrs. Ulmer saw an injured girl, picked her up, and carried her to the school office. The girl had a hole in her foot the size of a quarter. Other injured children were brought to the office, many shot in the stomach, arms, and legs. The kindergartners saw much of the worst of the trauma because of the location of their classroom.

Continues on next page

Continued from previous page

Mrs. Ulmer spent the next hours in the school office taking phone calls from parents and other people. While attending the phones in the office, she received a call from a radio station in Australia that had heard about the tragedy. When the paramedics arrived only minutes after the shooting began, they triaged the children in front of the school. For a few hours the school staff did not know for certain that Patrick Purdy had killed himself. They learned about it on the news.

That night every effort was made to clean up the blood and other matter, patch the bullet holes in the playground blacktop and walls of the buildings, and paint over the areas that were repaired. Cleveland School chose to be open the following day, not for academic work but for grief and trauma counseling. Not all children returned the next day: some were too afraid to return and some parents chose to keep their children home. Psychologists and counselors were brought to the school from throughout the Stockton Unified School District. They talked to the children in groups, primarily to help them feel they were not alone. Mental health professionals continued working with the children at the school daily for about two weeks, and then were called when help was needed for individual children. Well-wishes and donations came to the school from throughout the city, state, nation, and other countries. Cards, drawings, and posters from children and adults from Stockton and throughout the world covered the walls of the school.

During the early weeks after the shooting, Mrs. Ulmer was kept busy doing tasks other than therapy. When she resumed seeing children in the speech room many of them shared their experiences. The older children who had been kept in their classrooms and told to hide under their desks during the shooting had worried about their little brothers and sisters who were on the playground. Mrs. Ulmer assured the children that the school was doing things to keep them safe.

The staff and faculty of the Cleveland School had individual counseling available to them, but it is not known how many made use of the service. Mrs. Ulmer chose not to receive counseling. She felt that being with the other staff daily and supporting one another was more helpful. She said that she tries not to think about the experience, although on anniversary dates of the shooting it always comes to mind. Cleveland Elementary School was one of the first schools in this country to have such a tragedy, and because of that incident, schools around the United States began requiring all visitors to sign in and sign out when visiting.

As discussed earlier, between 1997 and 2001 there were 11 school shootings, resulting in the deaths of 28 children, the wounding of 70 other children, and deaths of four teachers and one principal. In those incidents, it was schoolchildren shooting other schoolchildren and teachers. It is possible that one or more of the children killed or wounded were in speech therapy during those shootings (no information is available on this). Certainly, some friends of the children who were killed were receiving speech therapy. Counseling services were provided for the children. However, the SLPs continued with their caseloads while still in shock. Children typically talk uninhibitedly about what they are thinking and feeling, and what they have recently experienced. The SLPs, no doubt, listened attentively and empathically, while sometimes having difficulty staying focused, attempting to sort out their own feelings, and make sense of senseless acts. (The SLPs' emotional needs are discussed further in Chapter 10.)

SLPs and audiologists never know all the emotional and/or physical traumas a child has experienced. It is important for clinicians to be aware of the symptoms of PTSD in order to make needed referrals for counseling, which may be the first counseling a child has received. Likewise, adults may have experienced emotional and/or physical traumas that have long-term effects on their cognitive and emotional responses to the environment. The following are symptoms of posttraumatic stress syndrome described in the DSM-IV TR (2000).

Symptoms of Posttraumatic Stress Disorder

- Repetitive, distressing thoughts about the event
- Nightmares related to the event
- Flashbacks so intense that the person feels or acts as though the trauma were occurring all over again
- An attempt to avoid thoughts or feelings associated with the trauma
- An attempt to avoid activities or situations associated with the trauma
- Avoidance of social settings or situations related to or reminiscent of the trauma
- Emotional numbness—being out of touch with feelings
- Restricted range of affect
- Inability to recall important aspects of the trauma
- Feelings of detachment or estrangement from others
- Losing interest in activities that used to give pleasure
- Persistent symptoms of increased anxiety, such as falling asleep, difficulty concentrating, startling easily, or irritability and outbursts of anger
- Symptoms of depression
- Symptoms of guilt
- Fear of being hurt (again) or of dying soon

In addition to these symptoms, children with PTSD may also exhibit separation anxiety, regressive behavior, and re-enactment of the event (Fletcher, 1996; La Greca, Silverman, Vernberg, & Roberts, 2002).

Our purpose is not to diagnose posttraumatic stress disorder, but to recognize it in the children, clients, patients, and families we work with (as well as our colleagues and coworkers), and to make the appropriate referrals to mental health professionals.

CONCLUDING COMMENTS

Crisis situations may occur in any setting at any time; however, what defines a crisis is the combination of an unusually threatening or dangerous situation and a person's difficulty coping with that situation. Some crises may cause cascading effects that make the initial crisis more difficult to manage. People in crisis may have intense feelings of frustration, inadequacy, and incompetence. Helping clients cope with a crisis and find their inner resources can help them develop problem-solving skills and self-confidence, and allow them to maximize gains from therapy.

Threat of suicide or self-harm is one of the most difficult experiences a clinician may be confronted with, and every threat must be taken seriously. Many people who threaten or attempt suicide have signs and symptoms of depression. Although SLPs and audiologists are not able to perform suicide assessments, the fact that a client or patient has disclosed self-destructive thoughts or intentions to us indicates some level of trust. Clinicians can listen for both direct and indirect suicidal references and share those with the appropriate administrative and mental health professionals. A team approach with a mental health professional may be used where the clinician continues working with the client, and meanwhile monitors the client's thoughts and feelings about suicide.

Clinicians cannot ignore threats of harm to others, because we are mandated reporters. Ethical and legal issues for the clinician may be consequences of not reporting such a threat. Knowledge of suspected child, dependent-adult, or elder abuse or neglect requires clinicians to report the information to appropriate administrative and/or legal authorities. Careful and detailed documentation are needed.

Posttraumatic stress disorder (PTSD) is an increasing experience for children who have experienced shootings in their schools or national crises such as terrorist attacks. Such traumatic events can have similar effects on people of all ages. Other personal and domestic physical and emotional traumas may cause PTSD in both children and adults. Our goal is to recognize the signs and symptoms of the disorder and make appropriate referrals to mental health professionals.

Discussion Questions

1. Recall a crisis situation that occurred in your personal life. What psychological or physiological symptoms or discomfort did you experience? What feelings of panic, defeat, helplessness, or hopelessness did you feel? What did you want most during the crisis? How did it affect your life outside the specific crisis situation? How long did the crisis last? What did you learn from the crisis?

2. Have you had a child or adult client who experienced a crisis while in therapy with you? What was the crisis? How did the crisis affect your client? How did it affect your therapy? What did you do or say that you felt was helpful? What did you do or say that was not helpful?

3. How have you been of assistance to people in crisis? What was the situation and what did you do?

4. What coping skills have you used to manage crises in your life?

5. What coping skills might you teach to a client in crisis?

6. Have you known a person who threatened suicide? What did you do? What did other people do?

7. What do you feel is the role of the speech-language pathologist or audiologist with children or adults who threaten self-harm or suicide?

8. What are the equivalent 5150 and 5250 codes in your state?

9. What would you do if a child you were working with told you he knew someone at school who was going to shoot some kids?

10. What would you do if you suspected a child you were working with was being abused or neglected?

11. What would you do if you suspected an elderly patient at a convalescent hospital where you were working was being abused?

12. Have you worked with a child whom you felt might be suffering from posttraumatic stress disorder? What were the indications?

13. Have you had an adult client who discussed a crisis or threatening situation that resulted in posttraumatic stress symptoms? What was the client's experience? What were the symptoms? How did the symptoms contribute to the client's hearing, speech, language, or cognitive problems?

Taking Care of Ourselves

CHAPTER OUTLINE

INTRODUCTION

Speech-language pathologists (SLPs) and audiologists must learn how to take care of themselves emotionally, physically, socially, recreationally, and spiritually in order to best help others. One source of emotional fatigue may come from our ongoing emotional involvement with our clients and the challenges they present. Another source of professional stress can come from our own appraisals of our work and our shortcomings or imperfections. Strong negative emotions can influence our clinical perceptions, decisions, and treatment approaches. When we feel burdened by our errors and failures, suffer from posttraumatic stress, are grieving for patients who have died, or are experiencing professional burnout, we cannot provide the best care that our clients, patients, and their families deserve. Taking care of ourselves, which may include seeking professional help, reflects our personal responsibility and commitment to ourselves, the people with whom we work, and our professions. In this chapter, we discuss some of the sources of professional stress and some ways that clinicians can take care of themselves. Ultimately, if we do not take care of ourselves, symptoms of stress or professional burnout may be the result.

Most clinicians are reluctant to discuss their insecurities and/or therapeutic failures. Even experienced clinicians may still wonder with each new client or patient, "Will the person like me? What if he has a problem I don't know very much about? Will this be the one who discovers my weaknesses? What if I fail and the person tells his family or friends that I am incompetent, or worse, tells my colleagues?" With every client we are putting ourselves on the line, bringing all our knowledge and skills to bear. We take risks with every person we try to help: Will we be the right clinician at the right time with the right approach for this person? Although we may perceive the failure as ours, in reality, the client is the one who has the most to lose. The client's improvement may be delayed or, even worse, the client may not have the chance for therapeutic success again. Many children and adults who stutter have worked with only one SLP in their lives, and if that SLP was not able to successfully manage their stuttering, no other SLP was given the opportunity to try.

THERAPEUTIC FAILURES

Chapter 7, Communicating Bad News and Working with Challenging Situations, discussed repairing counseling errors and the fact that it is inevitable that we are going to make errors in our interactions with clients and their families. Beyond making specific errors, we also may experience therapeutic failures in which a child or adult does not make the improvements in hearing, speech, language, cognition, or swallowing that they and we would like. Clinical failures may be the result of making a variety of errors, and in some cases, perhaps, only a single fateful error (e.g., with dysphagia patients). Failures can also be the result of factors outside of our control, such as when clients or patients have physical or emotional illnesses that prevent them from receiving maximum benefit from therapy, or when they move or terminate therapy early. Errors and failures are not synonymous, and we need to recognize that we can make a variety of errors and still have a successful outcome.

There are countless client and family variables that interact to determine the outcome of therapy, such as the age and motivation of the client, the nature and severity of the problem, multiple communication problems, support of the family and other professionals, medical complications (e.g., syndromes or diabetes mellitus), and intellectual and cognitive impairments of the client. Clinician variables also play a part in the success of therapy, such as the clinician's education and training, professional experience, therapeutic skills, up-to-date information on disorders and management approaches, and availability to provide consistent and ongoing therapy.

Therapeutic failures are seldom discussed in either the SLP or psychology literature. Most clinicians do not want to admit or make public their failures. Professional journals rarely publish treatment outcome research with nonsignificant results (it would be interesting to see a monthly journal filled with such studies, and their results could be very enlightening). Professors and supervisors prefer to discuss their successes and seldom present their therapeutic failures, favoring students' perceptions that professors rarely, if ever, have failures. These failures can become private experiences that haunt us and contribute to professional stress and burnout, but this experience can be turned around.

Failures are often our best learning experiences because we need to evaluate and re-evaluate what we did that worked and did not work. We tend to remember our failures more clearly than our successes, and sometime dwell on them to the detriment of our self-confidence. When we have a failure, we are sometimes reluctant to take on a similar case because we may not be certain that we, or the client, will do better than the last time. Kottler and Blau (1989) point out that psychologists and counselors teach their clients to forgive themselves (and others), to accept themselves as they are, to view their weaknesses as aspects of their uniqueness, and to welcome their failures as opportunities for learning. However, psychotherapists (as well as SLPs and audiologists) do not easily apply this valuable wisdom to themselves.

Sometimes an initial error can lead to a cascade of errors, and result in therapeutic failure. For example, if a child or adult is misdiagnosed and the therapy is focused on the presumed impairment, then little if any success will result. There are consequences for diagnoses which represent either false positives or false negatives. For example, if a client is diagnosed with a problem that he does not have (a false positive) and therapy is designed to remediate a problem that in fact does not exist, therapeutic failure is certain (e.g., a misdiagnosis of apraxia). Likewise, if a diagnosis is overlooked (a false negative), then therapy may not be made available (e.g., a cognitive impairment or swallowing disorder is missed).

Judging whether or not treatment has been successful can depend upon the goals or criteria the SLP or audiologist and client have established. We tend to think in terms of improvement, while clients and patients often think in terms of cure. "Cure," however, is not a word we typically use in our professional vocabulary. It tends to be reserved and more appropriate for the medical profession. Some illnesses and diseases can be cured. The cause or causes of communication problems may include physiological, cognitive, affective, social, and behavioral factors; therefore a single cause may never be identified or eliminated (Shames, 2000). Our clients and patients "improve," "make significant gains," "reach their therapy goals," or "reach their rehabilitation potential." We write functional goals which identify a practical outcome. We write measurable goals so that we can quantify the degree of success—or lack of success. In order to be considered a good or at least competent clinician, we need to have successful outcomes far more often than unsuccessful ones.

Benefits of Therapeutic Failures

Although none of us wishes or intends to have therapeutic failures, there are lessons that can be learned from these experiences. Kottler and Blau (1989) discuss the benefits of therapeutic failures in psychotherapy. Many of these points are applicable to SLPs and audiologists.

Failure is a signal that something has not worked in the way it was intended. It is part of a feedback loop that provides information on the effects of our therapy, which allows us to make adjustments in our behavior so that we have better (or at least different) results the next time. If we can appreciate failure as much as we appreciate success, it becomes a valuable source of information for us to improve our skills.

Failure teaches us to be persistent. If we fail once, it does not mean we will be successful the next time; but we persist in learning and trying new techniques and approaches until we have successful results with our clients. Every client is a single-subject research design where the final conclusion in the discussion is "Further research is needed." Even though we may have a successful outcome with a client, could we have had the same outcome with a different approach? Could our therapy have been more efficient, with more expeditious success? Which aspect of the therapy was problematic?

Failure is a stimulus. Because we do not have all the answers for any of the disorders we work with (the data are *never* all in), our clinical failures stimulate research and experimentation on new or better techniques.

Failure makes us introspective. More self-reflection likely takes place after a failure than after a success. After a success we quickly move on to the next client, but after a failure we ruminate and consider what went wrong. We learn our limits from our failures. If we have success after success, we may begin to see ourselves as omnipotent; "Who could have done a better job with that client?" "I am such a good clinician!" When an inevitable failure occurs, it shakes us enough to keep our egos in check and have more appreciation of other clinicians who also experience failures.

In time, we learn to tolerate some failures; that is, to fail, accept them, learn from them, and move on to the next challenge. We have the choice to pat ourselves on the back for what we learned or to beat ourselves up for what we failed to do well. We need to avoid making excuses for our failures (most experienced clinicians can see through such excuses). When we make excuses, we are not taking responsibility and are learning fewer of the lessons the experience has to offer. In short, a healthy stance for clinicians is to be nondefensive about the errors they have made and failures they have had, and be willing to reflect on them. In contrast, clinicians who have not learned from their errors, tend to externalize blame, that is, they tend to blame others for what has not gone well. As mentioned earlier, we will always be imperfect clinicians.

ON DEATH OF PATIENTS

Over the years of supervising graduate students during their internships at various hospitals throughout California, several students have had patients who died (fortunately, not during therapy sessions). In a current and ongoing study, one author of this text (P.T.F.) is investigating students' reactions to the experience of the death of a patient. The students are writing detailed narratives of their reactions to their patients' deaths. They also are writing about how they were informed of the deaths, what support (if any) was provided for the students by on-site hospital supervisors, and what the students felt was most helpful to them to cope with the loss. (*Note:* students or new professionals who experience the death of a patient or client are encouraged to contact me for inclusion in the study.)

Preliminary results of the study may be helpful for student interns and supervisors in hospitals who are processing the death of a patient. One graduate student (Carley—name used with permission) wrote, "My experience of the loss of a patient was quite remarkable. I don't think I will ever forget that day." Carley remembered talking to her patient about five minutes before he passed away. She had left the room for a few minutes to allow another rehabilitation therapist to fit the patient's prosthesis and was about to return to finish her therapy when over the hospital's intercom system she heard "STAT, STAT" and the room number of her patient. When she arrived at her patient's room, the door was closed and the person fitting the prosthesis was standing outside. He told Carley that the patient was not doing well. At the nurses' station, Carley overheard a nurse calling the patient's wife, telling her that her husband had another stroke and for her to come to the hospital. Carley's SLP supervisor was with her by this time and was the one who told Carley that her patient was "gone." "It was almost a surreal experience. I said 'What?' in disbelief and with the attitude of, 'That couldn't have happened. I just talked with him.' The next moment it hit me that it was the truth, the patient had died. My eyes immediately filled with tears. I couldn't hold back my emotions. My supervisor comforted me, telling the other staff that were around, 'Oh, it's her first one.' " Carley's supervisors were very caring and allowed time for her to "gather" herself. She chose to stay at the hospital the rest of the day and found it helpful to talk with other SLPs about similar experiences they had had and how they had coped with the loss. Later that day, Carley saw the wife of her patient crying and, "Again the tears filled my eyes and my heart went out to her." Carley felt fortunate that she was surrounded that day by other supportive staff.

Another student's experience (Katina—name used with permission) is also enlightening. She had begun an evaluation of an 81-year-old male patient who had dysphagia and was nonverbal secondary to a CVA. After completing a portion of her evaluation, a nurse told Katina that the patient needed his shower. Katina finished what she was working on and as she was about to leave the room the patient "grabbed my hand and squeezed it. I patted him on the shoulder and I can't remember my last words to him, however, I was thinking 'you are a sweet man.' " Later she heard over the hospital's intercom "Code Blue East 5, Code Blue East 5." Katina distinctly remembers her knees getting weak, feeling that the code was for her patient. Her stomach started to "feel funny, and a million thoughts were running through my head: Did I accidentally unplug his oxygen when I was moving the table or lowering the bed? No! I had to reassure myself that he wasn't receiving any oxygen. Did I do something wrong? I continued to reassure myself that I didn't do anything wrong, but I wasn't convinced."

As soon as she was able, she went to the patient's room where she saw numerous hospital personnel standing inside and outside her patient's room. "My stomach sank. I went to the nurses' station where I saw my supervisor who said, 'Mr. P. coded.' " Katina watched the Code Team working on him. "I couldn't see his face, just his body, and I was drawn in. From what I could tell, they got him back." Katina asked her supervisor if the patient had his shower, "Partially because I wanted to know what happened and mostly I wanted to know if I was the last person to see him. I really needed some reassurance that I didn't do something to cause all this." Katina thought about the patient all night, and when she got to the hospital the next day her supervisor told her that Mr. P. had died. "I was told by my supervisor and the head of the department that people on rehab don't often code and the last one was probably ten years ago. I really needed to hear that this was not my fault but I didn't in so many words from any of the people I work with. I just don't think it occurred to them that I needed reassurance even though I felt I was hinting at it."

A week later Katina was talking to a friend of hers, a fourth year medical student at the University of California, San Francisco, explaining the experience to her when "In the middle of my story she stopped me and said, 'Katina, his death was not your fault.' I kind of laughed but felt sort of relieved and said, 'I know.' She said something along the lines of 'I just felt that I had to say that to reassure you because sometimes it is just good to hear it. Instantly I felt better and it is amazing how good that feels."

Some Lessons for Students

There are some lessons to be learned from these students' experiences: 1) Do not be afraid to show your emotions, although it is more appropriate to restrain them until you are away from the family. Other staff may have strong reactions as well, depending upon how closely they worked with that patient. 2) Seek support from other staff members immediately after the incident. Staying at the hospital to be around coworkers may be better than leaving for the day and returning to an empty apartment or house. 3) If reassurance that the death was not your fault is not explicitly provided by your supervisor or other rehabilitation or nursing staff members, specifically ask for that information/reassurance. 4) Discuss the experience with your university supervisor if you feel that would be helpful to you. 5) Seek help from the hospital psychologist, counseling, or chaplain service if you feel the need.

Some Lessons for Supervisors and Staff

Lessons from these students' experiences for hospital supervisors and staff include: 1) Try to respond empathically. Even if you respond less emotionally, consider that the student or young professional is reacting in a normal, expected manner to loss. 2) Provide immediate reassurance in explicit language that the student was not the cause of the death—that she was not at fault. The student may need to hear that reassurance more than once. If the student brings up the incident hours, days, or even weeks later, consider it an indication that she may again need reassurance or someone to help her process the series of events and her role in them. 3) Encourage the student to remain at the hospital for the rest of the day so that she can be around other supportive people who understand and can help the student process the experience. 4) Spend time with the student over a cup of coffee or lunch to allow the student to process the experience in a comfortable environment. 5) Avoid explaining to other staff the student's reaction to the death by saying, "Oh, it's her first one." This can sound demeaning and patronizing. 6) If the student insists on leaving the hospital for the day, ask if there will be someone at home when she gets there. It will likely be better for the student not to feel alone for a while. 7) Realize that the death of the patient may cause the student to reflect on the death of a friend or family member. The student's reaction may be compounded by other losses. 8) Consider that the student may process the experience by moving through stages of grief; perhaps not going through each stage, but a few of them such as denial, depression, and acceptance.

Over time, many hospital-based clinicians develop self-protective strategies so that they can continue to function effectively in spite of the death of patients. However, for clinicians as well as other health care workers, the loss of patients near their own age and especially children may cause strong emotional reactions and long-term (sometimes life-long) memories of the experience regardless of their professional maturity. A registered nurse shared an experience that she had when she worked in emergency rooms. After a two-year-old girl died, the child's mother held her daughter and said, "Talk to me. Talk to me." The experience occurred over 35 years ago and it still brought tears to the eyes of the nurse. Sometimes it may not be the death of a patient that touches us, but the reactions and grief of the family that we remember most.

SYMPTOMS OF POSTTRAUMATIC STRESS DISORDER IN CLINICIANS

Posttraumatic stress disorder (PTSD) and how it can affect children and adults was discussed in Chapter 9, Working with Crisis Situations. SLPs and audiologists also may experience PTSD. They may be exposed to tragic situations directly or they may empathically experience a client's pain and tragedy. SLPs in public schools where tragedies have occurred most likely spent many hours trying to assist children, parents, and school personnel in any way possible to cope with their physical and emotional traumas. How much and what kind of professional help the SLPs received to manage their own stress is unknown. In addition to being on the site of a school tragedy, many individuals (including clinicians) may experience trauma symptoms at various levels of intensity as a result of other local and national tragedies, such as terrorist attacks, or natural disasters. Clinicians who have worked with children or adult clients who were injured or killed in such disasters may respond with anxiety and other strong feelings. Psychologists (Figley, 2002) have recognized that professionals who absorb their clients' emotional pain may suffer from "compassion fatigue" as they experience their clients' emotional roller coasters themselves.

COUNSELING SKILLS IN ACTION:

Resiliency in the Face of Tragedy

On September 11, 2001, Jacqueline Gavagan, an SLP, lost her husband, Donald, as well as several close friends in the New York World Trade Center. At the time of the national tragedy, Mrs. Gavagan had two young children and a third child due in seven weeks. As part of her healing process, at her husband's memorial service she asked people to contribute to a fund that might save a child's life. Surgeons at NYU Medical Center had successfully repaired her own toddler's defective heart earlier that year, and Mrs. Gavagan wanted to sponsor the surgery for a child whose family could not afford it. Thus far, she has raised sufficient funds for the surgery of two children (Cowley & Underwood, 2002). This vignette illustrates that some individuals who suffer acute stress in reaction to a tragedy or significant loss may have emotional resources and resiliency that enable them to find meaning in loss and a way of helping others as well as themselves after a personal tragedy.

After directly experiencing (i.e., being injured or physically present during a traumatic experience) or indirectly experiencing (learning about a traumatic event but not being physically injured or present at the scene), clinicians may initially react with acute stress from anxiety and fear. Unless mental health professionals evaluate clinicians, a diagnosis of acute stress disorder cannot be made, although it may exist. The DSM-IV TR (2000) lists the symptoms of acute stress, including a subjective sense of numbness; detachment; or absence of emotional responsiveness; a reduction in awareness of surroundings; derealization (subjective sense of the world being unreal); depersonalization (loss of the sense of being the person one usually is; a feeling of being outside oneself in the role of an onlooker); and dissociative amnesia (inability to recall important personal information, usually related to a traumatic or stressful experience that is too extensive to be explained by normal forgetfulness). Following the trauma, the traumatic event is persistently re-experienced, and the person has a marked avoidance of stimuli that may arouse recollections of the event. For example, a person who was injured in a motor vehicle accident may become fearful of driving. The symptoms typically last for at least two days but do not persist beyond four weeks after the traumatic event. When symptoms last beyond four weeks, PTSD is considered.

Beyond the above symptoms, the DSM-IV TR (2000) uses the following diagnostic criteria for PTSD: the person has been exposed to a traumatic event in which both of the following were present: 1) the person experienced, witnessed, or was confronted with an event or events that involved actual or threatened death or serious injury, or a threat of physical harm to self or others, and 2) the person's response involved intense fear, helplessness, or horror. The traumatic event is persistently experienced in one or more of the following ways: 1) recurrent and intrusive distressing recollections of the event, including images, thoughts, or perceptions; 2) recurrent distressing dreams of the event; 3) acting or feeling as if the traumatic event were recurring, including a sense of reliving the experience, illusions, and dissociative flashback episodes; 4) intense psychological distress at exposure to internal or external cues that symbolize or resemble an aspect of the traumatic event; and 5) physiological reactions (e.g., shaking or a "chill") on exposure to internal or external cues that symbolize or resemble an aspect of the traumatic event. Other symptoms of PTSD may include difficulty falling asleep or staying asleep, irritability or outbursts of anger, difficulty concentrating, hypervigilance, and exaggerated startle response.

Acute PTSD is considered to last less than three months, and chronic PTSD has a duration of more than three months. Delayed onset of symptoms is considered when symptoms begin to emerge at least six months (and in some cases, many years) after the traumatic event. Awareness of the phenomenon of delayed onset of symptoms began in the mid 1970s with Vietnam veterans who began experiencing signs and symptoms of the disorder approximately 10 years after being in that war. We need to be aware that even though we may appear to be coping well with a traumatic event, it may take several months or longer before symptoms begin to emerge, at which time the individual may have difficulty recognizing the original source of the symptoms.

It is important to recognize that while many therapists may not have the breadth and severity of symptoms necessary to be diagnosed with either PTSD or acute stress disorder, they may suffer some of these symptoms. Figley (2002) notes that compassionate therapists (i.e., those vulnerable to "compassion fatigue") should be alert for signs of stress, such as:

- withdrawal from family or friends
- emotional numbing or hyperalertness
- anhedonia (a loss of interest in everyday pleasures)
- a preoccupation with clients' problems
- physical symptoms, such as headaches and muscle tension
- insomnia

All clinicians should become aware of their responses to stress, regularly assess themselves, and take steps to rebalance their lives when necessary.

Treatment for Posttraumatic Stress Disorder

Psychological treatment for posttraumatic stress disorder is complex and multifaceted (Bourne, 2000). Many of the strategies used for other anxiety disorders are helpful (e.g., hierarchy analysis, relaxation training, and cognitive-behavioral therapy), but additional techniques may be used as well. *Exposure therapy* involves helping the individual confront fearful situations. In some cases, the work is begun with imaginal exposure where the person working with a mental health professional repeatedly reviews fearful memories of events, objects, or persons associated with the original trauma. With real-life (in vivo) exposure, the person returns to the actual situation where the trauma occurred. Repeated exposure helps the person realize that the fearful situation is no longer dangerous. *Support groups* help individuals understand that they are not alone and that other people are having similar reactions to the traumatic experience. *Family therapy* may be needed to help educate family members about how to understand and support the person who is experiencing posttraumatic stress disorder. *Medication* may be helpful, especially when the symptoms are severe and long-lasting.

PEER COUNSELING

Fortunately, most SLPs and audiologists have coworkers and friends in their profession. It often takes someone in the same profession to understand and appreciate the trials and tribulations of our work. We can be the first line of comfort and support for one another by relating and empathizing with another clinician's experiences and feelings. We can recognize when clinicians become frustrated with clients or family members. We also can recognize when clinicians become frustrated with supervisors, administrators, or "the system." We can often detect interpersonal difficulties among coworkers (and sometimes we may be the ones having the difficulties). We can frequently recognize that external pressures are affecting our own or a coworker's performance.

With a trusted coworker, you may be able to share some of your "challenges" (insecurities, errors, failures, frustrations, etc.). In turn, coworkers may place confidence in you when they share their experiences and feelings. We need to be careful not to break that confidence or use it perniciously. In many cases, just listening to a coworker relate an experience or feeling is sufficient, and there may be no need to try to help the person work through it. When a problem is severe or chronic, mentioning the value of additional (professional) help may be appropriate.

PROFESSIONAL COUNSELING FOR THE CLINICIAN

As students you may experience many of the same emotions as your clients and their families. It is normal to feel anxious and even some fear when seeing a client for the first time, or working with a disorder with which you have no experience and little or no course work. Report writing can be both mentally and emotionally draining. No matter how much education and training you have, you will feel anxious, fearful, and insecure during a clinical internship at a hospital, during your Clinical Fellowship Year, and on your first job when you are expected to know what you are doing. There are three absolutes for all clinicians: 1) you are going to make mistakes, 2) you are going to get tired, and 3) you are never going to know enough.

As a professional, you may feel guilty that you did not try to learn more in your classes or attend a workshop or seminar that could have helped you learn how to better manage a particular client or patient. You may feel vulnerable that a client or family will too easily recognize your weaknesses and insecurities. You may feel resentment that you have to work late when you would really rather be at home. You may occasionally feel resentment or anger that you have to spend your time dealing with other people's problems when you have your own "crisis" at home that needs your attention. You may be fearful that your report writing and documentation may not be adequate for your supervisors, Medicare, insurance companies, or HMOs. You may feel vulnerable that the kinds of tragedies that befall your clients or patients could happen just as easily to you or someone you love, and say to yourself, "There, but for the grace of God, go I."

We need to find ways to take care of our own stresses and negative emotions. The information and strategies for helping our clients, patients, and family members with their challenging and difficult emotions can also be strategies we can use to help ourselves. The principle for helping others: "First, do no harm" applies to ourselves as well. We need to take care of ourselves emotionally, physically, socially, recreationally, and spiritually to be balanced enough and strong enough to help others and still have reserve to enjoy the other aspects of our lives.

Counseling and therapy are very personal experiences that not only change the client but also change the clinician. SLPs and audiologists tend to present a professional façade and appear rather stoic about their own emotional struggles, and may not acknowledge when they need professional help. We can appear very secure and emotionally stable most of the time, and then experience an emotional crisis or shock that puts us in a tailspin. We are all vulnerable to such reactions. We need to recognize whether we have enough personal resources to get us through a crisis, or whether we need professional help. Do not think that it is a personal or professional stigma or failure to seek professional help. It may be the best thing we can do to help ourselves. Most health care and mental health professionals would benefit from professional help at some time in their lives. A basic principle of survival is: Take care of yourself so you can take care of others.

PROFESSIONAL BURNOUT

Professional burnout is a serious concern for people in the helping professions (Blood, Thomas, Ridenour, Qualls & Hammer, 2002; Corey, 2001; Gladding, 2000; Lubinski & Frattali, 2001; Luterman, 2001). Burnout is usually attributed to chronic stress; over time clinicians are worn down (or out) by repeated stress. Even though job satisfaction tends to be high for our professions of speech-language pathology and audiology, stress can take its toll on our feelings about our work and job performance. Burnout may occur even with the strongest personalities when stresses are prolonged, intense, or unresolved (Lubinski & Frattali, 2001). Burnout is insidious and may take years to be recognized by a clinician, and by that time the clinician may not have the motivation or energy to reverse the process.

Sources of Burnout

A multitude of factors can contribute to burnout. Lubinski & Frattali (2001) discussed sources of burnout that were adapted from Macinick and Macinick (1990), Maslach (1982), Scheller (1990), and Tschudin (1990). There are three primary factors that are sources of burnout: client factors, professional situation factors, and personal factors.

CLIENT FACTORS

Client factors, such as age of clients and medical complications, can vary depending on the settings in which therapists work. Because therapy is performance driven, clinicians must demonstrate (often in a relatively short amount of time) clinical success. When client or patient improvement is slow or is less than hoped for, increasing demands are often placed on clinicians. Even when there are good results, client or family appreciation may be modest.

PROFESSIONAL SITUATION FACTORS

Professional situation factors that contribute to burnout for SLPs and audiologists are numerous in all work settings. Blood et al. (2002) discuss several factors that contribute to stress and burnout for public school clinicians, including the rise in technology assistance for children with communication disorders, new legal mandates requiring additional paperwork and meetings, new competencies in literacy, larger caseloads, and uncertainty in role identification and expectations. In some environments job security is relatively high, while in others such as medical settings there are many fewer salaried positions and more contracted and hourly arrangements, which results in clinicians being sent home if their caseload is down; consequently monthly income may not be consistent. There is always someone, some institution, or some organization or agency that oversees our work. We are never totally autonomous, even in private practice. Salaries may be inadequate with little potential for significant increases, and create financial stresses on clinicians and feelings of being underappreciated and undercompensated for their education, training, and quality of work. Documentation is a burden both in time and energy in all work settings. Most clinicians feel they could provide more and better therapy if they did not have to spend so many hours filling in forms, documenting results, and writing reports. However, the paperwork is needed for the "bottom line" of our employers, that is, financing our time and work and the institution. Even where the overall physical work environment is adequate or good, the space, equipment, and materials for SLPs and audiologists may be grossly inadequate. There are still clinicians in the public schools who are working out of converted custodian closets and even restrooms. In many hospitals, there is not an office or room dedicated to speech therapy or audiology, which leaves the SLP or audiologist to share counter space with other rehabilitation team members. Treatment rooms may have physical and/or occupational therapy tables and equipment filling the space.

Although we recognize the importance of our work, administrators, teachers and other school personnel may not fully appreciate it (Blood et al., 2002). In medical settings, physicians and nurses commonly understand the goals of physical and occupational therapists more easily than they understand our goals to improve patients' speech, language, cognition, and sometimes even hearing. Swallowing disorders may be in the forefront of physician and nursing referrals partly because those professionals recognize the physical consequences of dysphagia more easily than they recognize the impairments of mild to moderate hearing loss, apraxia, dysarthria, aphasia, and cognitive impairments.

PERSONAL FACTORS

Personal factors of individual SLPs and audiologists can be a source of burnout. Although many SLPs and audiologists appear to be generally well-adjusted individuals, they often have perfectionistic tendencies that create self-imposed stress. We care deeply about the individuals we try to help and frequently go "above and beyond the call of duty" to provide the best therapy we can. When we feel children or clients have not improved to our (or their) levels of expectation, we often place the culpability on ourselves, feeling that we have failed them *and* ourselves.

Many clinicians tend to have high energy levels and are quick to please others, which means that additional tasks and responsibilities are added to our daily workload. Because of good people skills and communication abilities, clinicians are often asked to be on time-consuming committees. Clinicians often have difficulty saying "no," which may reflect the need for approval from others rather than a genuine desire to accept more responsibilities. Accepting more tasks results in clinicians having more to do with less time and energy, which may cause the quality of their therapy to suffer, creating guilt for not doing their best at what they most enjoy. SLPs and audiologists tend to be remarkably patient and tolerant people with everyone *except* themselves. We tolerate weaknesses and foibles in others that we do not tolerate in ourselves. We strive to be better clinicians and people, and never quite live up to our own expectations. Like other professionals, we also have family pressures and competing demands for our time. We feel the need to give 100% on the job and 100% at home. We sometimes feel that we have joined the army, trying to "be all we can be!" We have learned how to take care of others, but not sufficiently how to take care of ourselves.

Stages of Burnout

The process of burnout may take one, two, or more decades; however, for some clinicians it may begin just a few years after beginning professional employment. Most new professionals in speech-language pathology and audiology have strong commitments to their chosen professions. On the other hand, some individuals may not have a particularly strong commitment and their initial enthusiasm for the day-to-day work of a clinician may quickly wane. They may become disenchanted with their work and "burnout" in a relatively short amount of time. Cherniss (1980) in Lubinski & Frattali (2001) describes a three-stage process of burnout for people in helping professions, while Baron (1998) describe a four-stage process. The following is an integration of the two models.

STAGE ONE

In stage one, there is an imbalance between the demands and resources to deal with job stress, with too few personal or institutional resources to equalize the increasing demands. New therapists often feel overwhelmed on their first job for the first several months. They realize that in many instances the "buck" stops with them. They must make the final decisions about diagnoses and treatment strategies. As they become increasingly proficient in their work and well-known in their work setting, additional demands are placed on them. At the same time, marriage and/or children may increasingly complicate their personal lives. Home and job demands and stresses collide.

STAGE TWO

Clinicians (as well as other professionals) react to the stress and strain with feelings of anxiety, tension, cynicism, and negative views of others and their own work. They find it increasingly difficult to enjoy their coworkers and their own work. They begin to see their therapy as less pleasurable and more of a burden. They become impatient with others and wonder why the children or adults they are trying to help do not improve more rapidly. The negative attitudes may carry over into the home causing family discord.

STAGE THREE

Emotional exhaustion develops and defensive mechanisms may emerge such as displacement (showing anger at home rather than on the job), help-rejecting complaining (complaining about stresses but rejecting coworkers', family and friends' helpful suggestions), and passive-aggressive behavior (dealing with emotional conflict, stressors, or demands by indirectly and unassertively expressing aggression toward others). Clinicians may become emotionally detached from coworkers and withdraw, spending less time in their company and possibly alone, brooding.

STAGE FOUR

Clinicians become physically exhausted and increasingly fatigued from a day of work. More sick days are taken, some because of increasing amounts of illness and others as a take-care-of-myself-day. They have less energy for family activities in the evenings, often just wanting to rest. Marital conflict and family disharmony may be reflections of clinicians' dissatisfaction with their job or work environment. Getting up in the mornings and getting to work on time becomes more difficult. Weekends and vacations do not replenish and renew the energy and "spirit" needed to perform well on the job.

Preventing Burnout

Baron (1998), Corey (2001), Lubinski & Frattali (2001), and Blood et al. (2002) discuss strategies for preventing professional burnout. The emphasis is on clinicians' self-awareness and retaining or regaining control of their lives. The following is an integration of those strategies.

KNOW YOUR STRENGTHS AND WEAKNESSES, PREFERENCES, AND DISLIKES

As clinician we know the importance of working with clients' strengths in order to improve their weaknesses. Self-reflection helps us identify our own strengths, and we need to play to those. For example, if your strength and preference is working with children, then working in a setting where you see primarily children would be better than working in a setting (e.g., hospital) where you may see relatively few children. Conversely, if you prefer to work with adults, the public schools may not be the best job placement for you even if the salary is somewhat higher. If, after you have had some experience with dysphagia patients, you find that swallowing disorders are not an area you enjoy, find a setting where you can work with the age population you prefer and where dysphagia is not a significant part of your therapy duties.

Other strengths that are helpful for us to be aware of are our emotional strengths (e.g., being patient), character strengths (e.g., honesty), intellectual abilities, family support, friends and social connections, and spirituality. No one is equally strong and balanced in all areas of their lives, but recognizing what internal and external resources we can draw upon helps us feel self-confident, and that we do not have to manage all our work challenges and life's vicissitudes alone.

BE IN CONTROL OF YOUR OWN LIFE

When people feel that someone or something (particularly an impersonal institution or agency) is in control of their lives, they feel threatened, weakened, and impotent. Emotional and physical tension are associated with feeling a lack of control, with fear that someone with power over us will say or do something that might harm us professionally or personally. Recognizing that we, as individuals, are responsible for the quality of our own lives places the burden of our happiness and success on our own shoulders.

An important principle of preventing burnout is to avoid managing other people's lives. Some people have a tendency to meddle and act as though they have all the answers for what other people need to do to improve their lives, but have difficulty effectively managing their own lives. By our nature as clinicians we are helpers, but we need to avoid being rescuers in both our professional and personal lives.

FIND OTHER INTERESTS BESIDES YOUR WORK

Although we may enjoy our work and be happy to spend many hours involved in it, if the majority of our off-duty hours are consumed with thoughts of work, our minds do not have an opportunity to be renewed with other (perhaps more pleasant) diversions. We need to consider our motivations for being totally absorbed in our work. What do we want that we are not getting from a relatively normal amount of work involvement? Whom are we trying to please (or appease)? What rewards are we looking for? We may need to answer these questions before we can let go of our work and develop other interests and other aspects of ourselves.

THINK OF WAYS TO BRING VARIETY INTO YOUR WORK

Boredom is an important cause of dissatisfaction with our work and a strong contributor to burnout. Doing essentially the same therapy year after year, where the only real changes are in the faces and names of the children and adults we are working with, means we have lost our creativity and intellectual stimulation. Challenging ourselves to learn new therapy approaches or working to develop a new area of expertise can be professionally invigorating.

We are fortunate in our professions to have a wide variety of work settings in which to practice and age ranges of individuals in which to specialize. For example, we can work in preschool programs; public schools with kindergarten through high school levels; provide services for special programs in community colleges; a variety of hospital settings, including acute, subacute, and long-term care, inpatient and outpatient services; residential health care facilities, physicians' offices such as otolaryngologists; industrial settings for audiologists to administer hearing conservation programs; various clinics such as Easter Seals; home health agencies; private practice; and universities as instructors, professors, and clinical supervisors (Gelfer, 1996; Hegde, 1995; Johnson & Jacobson, 1998).

With these diverse areas of employment opportunities, SLPs and audiologists have options that perhaps few other professionals have. If a clinician begins to burn out working in one setting, he or she has opportunities to work in others without having to relocate to another town or city. Clinicians also have the option of leaving the profession for a number of years and returning later. Leaving the profession permanently is not the only solution to burnout.

MONITOR YOUR PHYSICAL HEALTH

Like most professions, speech-language pathology and audiology are stress-producing. Having your blood pressure checked annually can forewarn you of your body's reaction to stress. Essential hypertension may be hereditary and/or stress related (Keltner et al., 1999; Komaroff, 1999). Illness caused by stress increases the difficulty of managing the stress. Most people know the importance of healthy diets and lifestyles, but for many professionals it becomes increasingly difficult to eat regular, healthy meals, exercise a few times a week, and get seven to eight hours of sleep a night.

Clinicians approaching middle age need to be particularly aware of their physical health. It is during this time that some of the greatest demands are placed on us personally and professionally. Professionally, many middle-aged clinicians have advanced to administrative positions or have additional work-related demands on their time. Personally, they may have added domestic stressors, such as adolescent children. They also may be in the "sandwich generation" (Hooyman & Kiyak, 1993; Shadden & Toner, 1997) where they are still raising their children and, in addition, are the primary caregiver for one or both elderly parents. (Our professional training lends itself for us to be the caregiver for parents.) The burnout may reflect personal as well as professional stresses.

WORK SMARTER, NOT JUST HARDER

Clinicians often feel that if they work harder and put more time and energy into their work, they will be more successful (and please more people). Working smarter includes knowing what is expected of you on the job, and knowing what is not expected. Knowing who will be evaluating you and the criteria for evaluations can help you know what your supervisor is looking for. On any new job, seek out a mentor to help you "learn the ropes" and "navigate the landmines." Procedures that you have learned in your academic training will not likely be the same that are used in any particular job setting. Also, on every job there are certain situations and/or people that tend to be challenging to work with—or around. Blood et al. (2002) found that one of the more effective strategies for managing stress is obtaining social support from family, friends, coworkers, and supervisors.

Summary

SLPs and audiologists need to be aware of the possibilities for professional stress and burnout from their earliest years of professional work. Successful students have found ways to cope with and manage educational burnout in order to complete their graduate studies. Some of the strategies they have used as students may help them during their professional careers. Being aware of the numerous sources of professional burnout, the stages of burnout, and ways to prevent burnout can help lead to longer and more enjoyable careers in the satisfying professions of speech-language pathology and audiology.

Maintaining Enthusiasm for Your Profession

At the beginning of each academic year, I tell the graduate students in my Neuropathologies of Adults course the following story.

In the Ancient Olympics in Greece there was a race in which every runner had to carry a lighted torch. The winner was not the person who was the fastest, but the person who finished the race first with his torch still lit. The challenge for students is to finish their graduate work with their torch still lit with enthusiasm for learning and the profession.

CONCLUDING COMMENTS

Helpers and caregivers (including SLPs and audiologists, mental health professionals, medical professionals, and others) sometimes are more conscientious about the care they provide for those who need their skills than the care they provide for themselves. If we do not take adequate care of ourselves, we will have less mental and physical energy to help our clients and patients who depend on us. Our inevitable therapy errors and failures need to be accepted and their lessons learned so that we can provide better therapy to others. Following personal or professional traumas, we need to reflect on our symptoms of stress, self-care strategies, and the possible need for professional help. The death of clients and patients can affect us intensely, and we need to know what to ask for and from whom in order to maintain or regain our emotional equilibrium. Professional burnout is a very real problem, which may be the reason most SLPs at state and national conventions appear to be in their 20s or 30s, with fewer in their 40s, fewer yet in their 50s, and primarily only those in academia in their 60s. If we are aware of the professional and personal factors that are contributing to our burnout, we may be able to take steps to prevent them, or at least slow the process.

 Discussion Questions

1. Have you experienced a therapeutic failure in which a client did not make the improvements in hearing, speech, language, cognition, or swallowing that either the client or you have would liked? What were some of the errors you may have made that resulted in less than an optimal outcome? How did you explain the lack of progress to

the client? How did you feel about the experience? How did you "talk to yourself" about it? What did you learn from the experience?

2. Have you ever experienced symptoms of posttraumatic stress disorder? What was the experience? What were your symptoms? How long did the symptoms last? What helped you resolve them? Have you experienced any residual symptoms, such as continuing to avoid certain situations?

3. Have you had a relative or friend who died? How were you told about the death? How do you wish you had been told? What support did you have immediately after you learned of the death? What support do you wish you had?

4. Have you had a client or patient in your training who died? How were you told about the death? How do you wish you had been told? What support did you have immediately after you learned of the death? What support do you wish you had?

5. Do you have one or more classmates with whom you can discuss class work, and share clinic challenges confidences? How would you feel if you did not have anyone to share those experiences and feelings? How much do you share your clinic challenges with your supervisor?

6. What do you do to be a person with whom classmates and friends feel comfortable sharing confidences and challenges in their lives?

7. Assume that you are seeking help from a psychologist or professional counselor about a problem in your personal or family life. Write down 10 qualities or characteristics of the person you would want to be your counselor. Which of these characteristics also describe you?

8. You have survived as a student through the rigors of undergraduate and much of graduate school. What have you done to prevent educational burnout?

9. If a student just beginning in the major or just beginning graduate work asked you what you would suggest to prevent educational burnout, what would you tell the student?

EPILOGUE

Tying It All Together

Congratulations on having read the information in this book on counseling skills for speech-language pathologists (SLPs) and audiologists. We hope it will not be the only book you ever read on this important topic. Counseling skills are a relatively new area in our professional literature; however, we expect that more will be written in the upcoming years that underscores the need for SLPs and audiologists to possess a basic fund of knowledge in this area. Other recent texts written by SLPs and audiologists on counseling for our professions have much to offer from a variety of perspectives. This epilogue recaps and highlight the basic concepts and principles of this text in the order of the chapters written.

Our approach to counseling emphasizes that there is always a relationship between the people involved, the helper and the "helpee," and that this relationship is never static; it is always changing. We believe that this relationship is often the fulcrum upon which change occurs. We can often affect our clients' motivation and enthusiasm for change. Further, when clients present themselves for speech, language, cognitive, or swallowing therapy, or need audiological intervention and aural rehabilitation, they bring all the emotional experiences surrounding those losses or deficits in their ability to communicate. Sometimes, however, the issues that arise during counseling and therapy move beyond our professional scope of practice, training, and skill levels. We need to be aware of when those issues arise and be careful not to assume the role of psychotherapist or counselor when we do not have the proper credentials. Our discussions of various therapy scenarios try to address the strategies that can enhance the SLP and audiologists' work and the professional limits and boundaries that are encountered.

Although there are numerous counseling therapeutic approaches in the psychotherapy literature, about a half dozen approaches are particularly applicable to speech-language pathology and audiology (although many more theories potentially have important contributions they could make). Humanistic therapy, also know as person-centered therapy, (Gladding, 2000; Prochaska & Norcross, 2003; Rogers, 1951, 1957, 1961, 1980), with its emphasis on promoting the individual's natural positive striving and growth, encourages the therapist to be nondirective and supportive when responding to clients' emotional struggles. Person-centered therapy also focuses on the therapist characteristics that are necessary for therapeutic change in clients. Interpersonal therapy (Anchin & Kiesler, 1982; Gladding, 2000; Prochaska & Norcross, 2003; Sullivan, 1953, 1972; Teyber, 2000) focuses on interpersonal interactions, styles of communication, and self-defeating patterns of communication and behavior. With humanistic and interpersonal theoretical foundations, clinicians are better equipped to interact with clients in a positive way and to avoid negative interactional patterns.

Behavioral therapy (Craighead et al., 1994; Gladding, 2000; Prochaska & Norcross, 2003; Skinner, 1953; 1974; Wolpe, 1958, 1987) provides systematic assessment and treatment to help clients make changes in their behaviors. Identifying systematic links between stimuli in the environment and symptoms can help provide a framework for recommended changes. Behavioral therapy, which draws upon learning theory, is applicable to much of our therapy and counseling work with clients. Meanwhile, family systems therapy (Gladding, 2000; Goldenberg & Goldenberg, 2000; Hoffman, 1981; Prochaska & Norcross, 2003; Rolland, 1994; Satir, 1964, 1976, 1983) underscores that individuals live and are influenced by a family context. Individual client behaviors are often affected by their family roles, communications, and interactions; therefore, clients need to be viewed as a part of a family system. Working effectively with family systems is often necessary to achieve positive changes.

Existential therapy (Gladding, 2000; Nystul, 1999; Prochaska & Norcross, 2003; Yalom, 1980) provides a philosophic framework for thinking about how people respond to uncertainty, loss, and death in their lives. Existential writings address the meanings that people create in order to tolerate the existential conditions inherent in life. When we work with clients who are elderly or have experienced substantial losses, they are always dealing with these issues in one way or another. How we view our lives and the world in general is also strongly influenced by our culture. Multicultural theory and the role culture plays in our work as SLPs and audiologists is becoming increasingly clear (Battle, 2002; Roseberry-McKibbin, 2002; Salas-Provance et al., 2002), and clinicians must practice in a manner that is sensitive and respectful of all people.

We have also addressed the basics of good counseling skills, regardless of the clinician's theoretical affiliation or affinity. Technical expertise is necessary but not sufficient to be a competent clinician. Our task is to enter the client's world and develop a positive therapeutic relationship. Attending and listening to clients are the foundation for helping them. Empathy is important to communicate to clients in order for them to feel understood and that we are accurately weighing all the factors facing them. In all of our work, from our first "Hello" to our final "Good-bye," we are using counseling skills with our facial expressions, body language, choice of words, and tone of voice.

When working with clients we need to carefully consider what we say and how we say it; that is, to be intentional (Ivey, 1998). Microskills form the foundation of interviewing and obtaining information throughout our interactions with clients and their families. There are a variety of types of questions and responses we can use to elicit important information that may assist us in being better helpers, and these take time and practice to use in a natural way.

Although we may be empathic and effectively use microskills, clients and family members may react defensively, that is, have automatic psychological processes that operate to protect against unbearable anxiety and dealing with stressors. We need to appreciate that defense mechanisms are natural responses and that our task is not to eliminate them but to understand what stressful situations have triggered them. As clinicians, we also need to be aware of our own tendencies to use defenses and not let them interfere with the therapeutic relationship.

Being a clinician includes working with challenging and difficult emotional states. Our clients and patients are experiencing difficulties with the most important and fundamental human skill—communicating. The families of these individuals also frequently have strong emotional responses that reflect their caring, concern, and frustration with their loved one. It is not sufficient for us to merely recognize the emotional states of the individuals with whom we work; we also need strategies to help them manage or cope with emotions that are intertwined with their communication disorders. Our professional responsibility is to work with individuals in ways so that their emotional states do not interfere or significantly hinder therapy progress. We also need to be aware when an individual's emotional state transcends our scope of practice and warrants referral to a mental health professional.

In our professional work, a wide range of challenging situations and behaviors cause apprehension, especially if we are uncertain how to best respond. We may think of such situations and behaviors as being on a continuum, much like levels of severity of communication disorders; that is, minimal, mild, moderate, severe, or profound. For one clinician what may be a "severe" challenge may be only a "moderate" one for another. Knowledge, experience, and skills help decrease anxiety and uncertainty when working with challenging situations and behaviors. Often the first significant challenge with a client or family is disclosing and explaining the hearing, speech, language, cognitive, or swallowing problems the person presents. Sharing this information may require giving (breaking) bad news to the individuals involved. The manner in which the information is presented by the therapist can have a significant effect on the way it is received and accepted by the client and family. During evaluations and therapy a variety of challenging situations and behaviors may emerge, such as resistance and anger or hostility. How the clinician responds to such situations and behaviors may enhance or impair the therapeutic relationship. Crises may occur in therapy in numerous forms and clinicians need to be able to manage them in a therapeutic manner.

SLPs and audiologists must learn how to take care of themselves mentally, physically, socially, recreationally, and spiritually. We need to learn from our failures and not let them burden us; to empathize with our clients' losses but not feel irreversibly drained by them; and to develop our own healthy coping strategies to prevent professional burnout; and to find meaning and renewal in the rich experiences and interactions with our clients.

GLOSSARY

acculturation The process of learning, incorporating, and adopting values, customs, and beliefs of a dominant culture.

acting out A defense mechanism in which the person deals with emotional conflicts by acting in inappropriate ways rather than by reflecting or talking about one's feelings.

action language Language that describes the client's specific behaviors and does not make inferences, pathologize, or label the client.

altruism A defense mechanism in which the person deals with emotional conflicts (e.g., involving guilt and anger) by performing helpful deeds for others.

bicultural adjustment Refers to a positive state of psychosocial adjustment in which an individual feels comfortable in both the dominant and her or his ethnic society, and has friends and interests in both cultures.

boundaries Refers to the demarcation or differentiation between family members or family subsystems. Healthy boundaries enable appropriate levels of privacy (e.g., between parents and children), identity, and role differentiation.

catastrophizing Faulty thinking that involves an exaggerated, negative view of the future (i.e., thinking that a catastrophe will occur).

classical conditioning A learning process in which a neutral stimulus (e.g., a nurse's presence) is repeatedly combined with another stimulus which elicits a physiologic reaction (e.g., a painful injection). Over time, the person develops a physiologic reaction to the neutral stimulus, in this case, growing fearful or anxious every time a particular nurse appears. The behaviorist Joseph Wolpe used this model to show how anxiety to any (neutral) stimulus can be learned.

cognitive distortions From a cognitive therapy viewpoint, these are various types of erroneous or faulty thinking that contribute to a person's fears, pessimism, and maladaptive behaviors. These include catastrophizing, "I should" statements, and dichotomous thinking.

complex interpersonal message Communications that carry two, often contradictory, messages. On one level, the communication may sound benign or simply express a factual request (e.g., "When did you get your degree?"). On the second level, there is often a negative interpersonal message, for example, communicating doubt that the therapist has enough experience to help the client. Dysfunctional families are sometimes characterized by giving frequent complex interpersonal messages to each other.

congruence Refers to the consistency between one's feelings and one's behaviors. According to humanistic therapists, healthy personality development occurs when a child repeatedly receives the clear message (congruence) that she will be accepted even when she expresses her true feelings and experiences. Likewise, clinicians must demonstrate congruence in order to gain their clients' trust and confidence.

countertransference The therapist's perceptions, beliefs, wishes, and responses to the client which are influenced both by the client's characteristics and behaviors and by the therapist's past experiences.

culture Any group of people who associate with one another on the basis of a common purpose, need, or background. The group often has shared beliefs, traditions, and values.

defense mechanisms Automatic mental processes that people use to protect themselves from intolerable levels of anxiety and internal conflict.

denial A defense mechanism in which the person deals with emotional conflicts by refusing to acknowledge some painful aspect of reality (e.g., the presence of a disorder or the severity of impairment) or a subjective experience (e.g., sadness and lethargy) that is apparent to others.

devaluation A defense mechanism in which the person deals with emotional conflict or stressors by attributing extreme, negative qualities to another person or object (e.g., the treatment). Devaluation may occur in the context of another defense mechanism, splitting, and may represent the "all bad" pole of the person's split perceptions.

dichotomous thinking Faulty thinking that tends to inaccurately divide all situations and people into "good" and "bad" categories rather than perceiving more subtle nuances or "shades of gray."

disengagement A family that has minimal contact, structure, order, or authority. Family members feel disconnected and unrelated to one another.

displacement A defense mechanism in which the person transfers feelings about one person, object, or event onto someone else who is perceived as less threatening and/or less powerful.

empathy An attitude of entering the client's world as if it were our own, allowing ourselves to feel what the client is feeling, and communicating this to the client. Empathy is a key element in developing a positive therapeutic relationship with clients.

enmeshed (families) These families have weak boundaries and insufficient differentiation of roles and identity. To others, they may appear "too close" and unable to tolerate healthy levels of autonomy among themselves.

existential isolation Our ultimate aloneness in the world—as we can never totally understand each other and our growth may lead others to reject us. This is a condition of life that produces anxiety according to James Bugental.

existential meaninglessness The lack of an inherent meaning in life. The questions we ask about the significance of our existence highlight how tenuous our meanings are and how easily they can be changed or obliterated.

existential nonbeing The existential conditions of life such as uncertainty, meaninglessness, and isolation. In healthy personality functioning, the person grasps, admits, and grapples with these aspects of life.

existential uncertainty The uncertainty that we experience in our lives even as we take reasonable steps to shape, control, and predict it. This inescapable uncertainty is a source of anxiety in our lives according to existential writers.

generalize The process of expanding newly learned skills from one environment to another.

help-rejecting complaining A defense mechanism in which the person expresses repetitive complaints or pleas for assistance but then systematically rejects all suggestions and recommendations that are offered. In this way, the client "defeats" the professional who is trying to help her or him.

hierarchy This refers to the hierarchical organization considered to be central to healthy family functioning. At the top of the hierarchy is usually the marital subsystem which takes charge of the child or sibling subsystem.

homeostasis The balance of roles and functions that is maintained in a family. A family's homeostatic functioning may be deemed as either healthy or unhealthy.

"I should" statements Faulty thinking that involves a moralistic or perfectionistic self-statement and an intolerance of personal flaws. Examples are: "I should always think of others first," "I should be able to control myself," and " I should always be organized."

intellectualization A defense mechanism in which the person uses detached, logical, or abstract thinking in order to avoid a conflict or painful feelings.

intermittent reinforcement schedule A pattern of providing a reward on only some of the occasions when the desired behavior occurs.

interpersonal style Recurrent patterns of relating to others; a learned style of communication and interaction. Examples of interpersonal styles can include friendly-dependent, hostile-suspicious, and controlling-devaluing.

metacommunication In interpersonal psychology, metacommunication refers to dialogue which focuses on the immediate interpersonal process occurring between the clinician and client. For example, the client may be talking about topics unrelated to the therapy. The clnician may metacommunicate by asking the client whether he or she is having difficulty or experiencing anxiety about talking about his or her hearing impairment.

microskills Specific communication skills that enhance therapists interactions with clients. Microskills include open-ended questions, nonverbal encouragers, paraphrasing, and reflections.

negative reinforcement The removal of an unpleasant or aversive stimulus which increases the frequency of a certain behavior. A client's cries or screams which halt an important but painful medical procedure may be negatively reinforcing to the client.

nondirective The therapist role advocated by humanistic therapists. These therapists are nondirective, and allow clients to direct the flow of conversation in sessions.

observational learning A process of learning through others who provide a model for certain behaviors (e.g., correct speech articulation).

operant conditioning Learning that occurs as a function of its consequences (e.g., rewards or punishments). Behavioral therapists have developed the notion of using operant techniques to modify a person's problematic behaviors.

overgeneralizations Faulty thinking that involves making incorrect inferences or "leaps in logic" from one situation to other situations that may not be related.

passive-aggression A defense mechanism in which the person presents a façade of friendliness, compliance, or agreement while indirectly and unassertively expressing aggression or hostility. "Forgetting" and procrastination are classic examples of passive-aggressive behavior.

positive reinforcement Desirable consequences of a behavior that increase the frequency of that behavior.

rationalization A defense mechanism in which the person uses self-serving and incorrect logic to explain her or his maladaptive behavior.

reinforcement contingencies The system of consequences associated with a person's behavior. Behavioral treatment plans typically develop a new system of reward contingencies to modify a person's behavior.

reinforcement schedule The frequency or consistency of applying a particular reward or reinforcement after a certain behavior has occurred. Reinforcement schedules can be altered to increase the likelihood of desired behaviors.

scapegoat A person who is blamed for the family's unhappiness. Often this is a child whose misbehavior becomes the family's focus so that other problems/conflicts can be avoided.

secondary reinforcers Consequences of a behavior that did not serve as the initial reinforcement, but help to maintain a desired behavior. Often they are not as powerful as the original rewards or else they are considered somewhat hidden from view. Following a period of formal rewards, a teacher's smiles and nods may become secondary reinforcers to a child, or a person who dislikes his job may find that his disability payments become secondary reinforcers for maintaining illness behavior.

self-actualization A concept central to humanistic therapy. Self-actualization refers to the inherent human tendency to strive towards positive growth and emotional development.

social learning theory A perspective adopted by many behaviorists such as Bandura which posits that most of human learning occurs through a process of observing and imitating others.

splitting A defense mechanism in which the person perceives others or situations in "black and white" or "good and bad" terms. By engaging in this dichotomous thinking, the person eliminates the challenge of confronting ambiguity and complexity in her or himself and others.

stimulus-response chains A pattern of behaviors and consequences (e.g., a child's stuttering behavior and the parent's subsequent taking over the conversation for her or him may develop into a predictable, stimulus-response chain).

structural family therapy A school of family therapy developed by Salvador Minuchin in the 1960s to 1970s. This therapy focuses on understanding and changing the unhealthy family structure and organization that maintains psychological symptoms in a family member.

successive approximations Clients behaviors that gradually approach (i.e., approximate) the desired behavior. From a behaviorist viewpoint, it is generally advisable to provide reinforcement for the client's successive approximations so that they will continue to make progress toward a goal.

systematic desensitization A behavioral approach for treating learned anxiety responses and phobias that was developed by Joseph Wolpe. In this treatment method, a person learns to gradually approach a frightening situation (e.g., a dog or a medical procedure) while practicing a relaxation response. In this way, an anxiety response or phobia is unlearned.

technical eclecticism This refers to the practice of borrowing therapy techniques which appear to work from various theoretical perspectives, without necessarily embracing the theories in which the techniques are embedded.

theoretical integration The development of a cohesive conceptual or theoretical framework which blends ideas from two or more theoretical approaches.

therapeutic alliance This refers to the professional and working relationship between the clinician and the client. Core elements of the therapeutic alliance include the client's trust in the clinician motivation to overcome his or her symptoms or disorder, and willingness to follow the clinician's instructions.

therapeutic distance This term suggests that there is an ideal or optimal distance to maintain in the therapeutic relationship with the client. Maintaining a therapeutic distance involves empathy and attention to the client's needs, while neither detachment nor overinvolvement in the client's life.

transference The client's perceptions of the clinician which are influenced by past relationship experiences and certain unconscious elements as well as by the clinician's real qualities.

triangulation A process where two family members recruit a third family member into an unhealthy alliance, often to avoid conflict with one another. Often, in unhealthy family functioning, children are triangulated into family interactions to avoid marital conflict.

unconditional positive regard A key characteristic of therapists that was first described by Carl Rogers. According to Rogers, therapists must show unconditional caring for their clients and positive regard for their inherent worth. Only by showing this consistent and unwavering positive regard can clients feel free to show and to accept themselves.

world view An individual's assumptions and perceptions of the world from a moral, social, ethical, and philosophical perspective.

REFERENCES

Ackerman, N. (1984). A theory of family systems. In I. Goldenberg & H. Goldenberg (Eds.), *Family therapy, an overview* (4th ed.). Pacific Grove, CA: Brooks-Cole Pub. 2002.

Adams, P. (1993). *Gesundheit!: Bringing good health to you, the medical system, and society through physician service, complementary therapies, humor, and joy.* Rochester, Vermont: Healing Arts Press.

Adler, A. (1956). *The individual psychology of Alfred Adler.* H. L. Ansbacher & R. R. Ansbacher (Eds.). New York: Harper & Row.

Alpiner, J., & McCarthy, P. (1987). *Rehabilitative audiology: Children and adults.* Baltimore: Williams & Wilkins.

Alpiner, J., & McCarthy, P. (1993). *Rehabilitative audiology: Children and adults* (2nd ed.). Baltimore: Williams & Wilkins.

Alpiner, J., & McCarthy, P. (2000). *Rehabilitative audiology: Children and adults* (3rd ed.). Baltimore: Williams & Wilkins.

American Psychiatric Association. (2000). *Diagnostic and statistical manual of mental disorders* (4th ed., Rev.). Washington, DC: Author.

Anchin, J., & Kiesler, D. (1982). *Handbook of interpersonal psychotherapy.* Elmsford, NY: Pergamon Press.

Anderson, D., Keith, J., & Novak, P. (2002). *Mosby's Medical Nursing & Allied Health Dictionary.* St. Louis: Mosby, Harcourt Health Sciences Company.

Andrews, M. (1986). Application of family therapy techniques to the treatment of language disorders. *Seminar in Speech and Language, 7,* 347–358.

Andrews, M. L. (1999). *Manual of voice treatment: Pediatrics through geriatrics* (2nd ed.). San Diego, CA: Singular Publishing Group.

Andrews, J., & Andrews, M. (1990). *Family based treatment in communicative disorders: A systematic approach.* Sandwich, IL: Janelle Publications.

Andrews, M., & Andrews, J. (1993). Family-centered techniques: Integrating enablement into the IFSP process. *Journal of Childhood Communication Disorders, 15*(1), 41–46.

Andrews, M., & Summers, A. (1988). *Voice therapy for adolescents.* Boston: College-Hill Publication.

Arkowitz, H. (1997). Integrative theories of therapy. In P. Wachtel & S. Messer (Eds.), *Theories of psychotherapy: Origins and evolution* (pp. 227–288). Washington, DC: American Psychological Association.

Avent, J. (1997). *Manual of cooperative group treatment for aphasia.* Boston: Butterworth-Heinemann.

Avent, J. (2002, June). *Aphasia group treatment.* Presentation at the Department of Speech-Language Pathology 32nd Annual Summer Colloquium, University of the Pacific, Stockton, California.

Bandura, A. (1968). A social learning interpretation of psychological dysfunctions. In P. London & D. Rosenhan (Eds.), *Foundations of abnormal psychology*. New York: Holt, Rinehart & Winston.

Bandura, A. (1969). *Principles of behavior modification*. New York: Holt, Rinehart & Winston.

Banja, J. (1999). Breaking bad news. *The Journal of Care Management. 5* (4), 72–85.

Barkley, R. (1998) *Attention-deficit hyperactive disorder: A handbook for diagnosis and treatment* (2nd ed.). New York: Guilford Press.

Baron, R.A. (1998). *Psychology* (4th ed.). Boston: Allyn and Bacon.

Bateson, G. Jackson, D. D., Haley, J., & Weakland, J. (1956). Toward a theory of schizophrenia. *Behavioral Science, 1*, 251–264.

Battle, D. (2002). *Communication disorders in multicultural populations* (3rd ed.). Boston: Butterworth-Heinemann.

Bear, M. Connors, B., & Paradiso, M. (2001). *Neuroscience, exploring the brain* (2nd ed.). Baltimore: Lippincott Williams & Wilkins.

Beck, A. (1995). *Cognitive therapy: Basics and beyond*. New York: The Guilford Press.

Beck, A. T. (1967). *Depression: Causes and treatment*. Philadelphia: University of Pennsylvania Press.

Beck, A. T. (1970). Cognitive therapy: Nature and relation to behavior therapy. *Behavior Therapy 1*, 184–200.

Beck, A. T. (1976). *Cognitive therapy and the emotional disorders*. New York: International University Press.

Beck, A. T., Rush, A, Shaw, B., & Emery, G. (1979). *Cognitive therapy of depression: A treatment manual*. New York: Guilford Press.

Bellack, A.S., Hersen, M., & Kazdin, A. E. (Eds.). (1982). *International handbook of behavior modification and therapy*. New York: Plenum.

Bellis, T. J. (1996). *Assessment and management of central auditory processing disorders in the educational setting*. San Diego, CA: Singular Publishing Group.

Benjamin, L. S. (1993). *Interpersonal diagnosis and treatment of personality disorders*. New York: Guilford Press.

Bishop, A., & Scudder, J. (1990). *The practical, moral, and personal sense of nursing*. New York: University of New York Press.

Blood, G. W., Thomas, E. A., Ridenour, J. S., Qualls, C. D., & Hammer, C. S. (2002). Job stress in speech-language pathology working in rural, suburban, and urban schools: Social support and frequency of interactions. *Contemporary Issues in Communication Sciences and Disorders, 29*, 132–140.

Bloodstein, O. (1995). *A handbook on stuttering* (5th ed.). San Diego, CA: Singular Publishing Group.

Boles, L. (2002). *Counseling elders with communication disorders, their families and related professionals: Multicultural populations*. Institute Course, American Speech-Language Hearing Association Convention, November 23, Atlanta, GA.

Boone, D., & McFarlane, S. (2000). *The voice and voice therapy* (6th ed.). Boston: Allyn and Bacon.

Boss, M. (1963). *Daseinanalysis and psychoanalysis*. New York: Basic Books.

Bourne, E. (2000). *The anxiety and phobia workbook* (3rd ed.). Oakland, CA: New Harbinger Publications, Inc.

Bowen, M. (1978). *Family therapy in clinical practice*. New York: Jason Aronson.

Brammer, L. M. & MacDonald, G. (1999). *The helping relationship, process and skills*. Boston: Allyn and Bacon.

Brock, G., & Barnard, C. (1992). *Procedures in marriage and family therapy* (2nd ed.). Boston: Allyn and Bacon.

Brookshire, R. (2003). *Introduction to neurogenic communication disorders* (6th ed.). St. Louis: Mosby.

Buckman, R., & Kason, Y. (1992). *How to break bad news: A guide for health care professionals.* Baltimore: Johns Hopkins University Press.

Bugenthal, J. F. T. (1965). *The search for authenticity: An existential-analytic approach to psychotherapy.* New York: Holt, Rinehart & Winston.

Burgoon, J., Buller, D., & Woodall, W. (1996). *Nonverbal communication, the unspoken dialogue* (2nd ed.). New York: McGraw-Hill.

Burnard, P. (1999). *Counseling skills for health professionals* (2nd ed.). New York: Chapman and Hall.

Butler, S. F., Flasher, L. V., & Strupp. H. H. (1993). Countertransference and qualities of the psychotherapist. In N. E. Miller, L. Luborsky, J. P. Barber, & J. P. Docherty (Eds.), *Psychodynamic treatment research.* New York: Basic Books.

California Penal Code, Section 11166. (2002).

California Welfare and Institution Code, Section 5150. (2002).

Canino, I. & Spurlock, J. (2000). *Culturally diverse children and adolescence: Assessment, diagnosis, and treatment.* New York: Guilford Press.

Caporael, L. R. (1981). The paralanguage of caregiving: Baby talk to the institutionalized aged. *Journal of Personality and Social Psychology, 40,* 876–884.

Capuzzi, D., & Gross, D. R. (1995). *Counseling and psychotherapy theories and interventions.* Englewood Cliffs, NJ: Prentice Hall.

Carleson, J. & Ardell, D. (1988). Physical fitness as a pathway to wellness and effective counseling. In R. Hayes & R. Aubrey (Eds.), *New directions for counseling and human development.* Denver: Love Publishing.

Cassell, E. (1996). *Talking with patients.* Cambridge, Massachusetts: The MIT Press.

Cautela, J. R. (1977). *Behavioral analysis forms for clinical intervention.* Champaign, IL: Research Press.

Chapey, R. (Ed.). (2001). *Language intervention strategies in aphasia and related neurogenic communication disorders* (4th ed.). Philadelphia: Lippincott Williams & Wilkins.

Cherniss, C. (1980). *Staff burnout job stress in the human services.* Beverly Hills, CA: Sage Publications.

Chermak, G. & Musiek, F. (1997). *Central auditory processing disorders: New perspectives.* San Diego, CA: Singular Punlishing Group.

Ciminero, A. R., Calhoun, K. S., & Adams, H. E. (Eds.). (1977). *Handbook of behavioral assessment.* New York: Wiley.

Clark, J., & Martin, F. (1995). *Effective counseling in audiology.* Englewood Cliffs, NJ: Allyn and Bacon.

Cohen, M. (2002, March). *Communicate, Advocate and Negotiate.* Paper presented at the California Speech-Language Pathology and Audiology Annual Convention, Los Angeles.

Cohen, G. & Faulkner, D. (1986). Does "elderspeak" work? The effect of intonation and stress on comprehension and recall of spoken discourse in old age. *Language and Communication, 6,* 91–98.

Comer, R. (1999). *Fundamentals of abnormal psychology.* New York: Freeman.

Conture, E. (2001). *Stuttering, its nature, diagnosis, and treatment.* Boston: Allyn and Bacon.

Corey, G. (2001). *Theory and practice of counseling and psychotherapy* (6th ed.). Belmont, CA: Brooks/Cole, Thomson Learning.

Corsini, R. J, Wedding, D. (Eds.). (2000). *Current psychotherapies* (6th ed.). Itasca, IL: F.E. Peacock Publishers.

Cowley, G., & Underwood, A. (2002, September 16). The science of happiness. *Newsweek*, p. 46–48.

Craighead, L., Craighead, W., Kazdin, A., & Mahoney, M. (1994). *Cognitive behavioral interventions: An empirical approach to mental health problems.* Boston: Allyn & Bacon.

Crowe, T. (Ed.). (1997). *Applications of counseling in speech-language pathology and audiology.* Baltimore: Williams and Wilkins.

Culpepper, B., Mendell, L, & McCarthy, P. (1994). Counseling experience and training offered by ESB-accredited programs. *ASHA, 36*, 55–57.

De Becker, G. (1997). *The gift of fear: Survival signals that protect us from violence.* New York: Little, Brown and Co.

Deffenbacher, J. L. (1999). Cognitive-behavioral conceptualization and treatment of anger. *Journal of Clinical Psychology, 55*, 295–309.

Deffenbacher, J. L., Oetting, E. R., & DiGiuseppe, R. A. (2002). Principles of empirically supported interventions applied to anger management. *Counseling Psychologist, 30*, 262–280.

DeJong, P., & Berg, I. (1998). *Interviewing for solutions.* Pacific Grove, CA: Brooks/Cole, Thomson Learning.

Department of Health and Human Services. (1989). Medicare and Medicaid: Regulations for long-term care facilities. *Federal Register, 54*, 5322.

Dollard, J., & Miller, N. E. (1950). *Personality and psychotherapy.* New York: McGraw-Hill.

Eliopoulos, C. (1996). *Gerontological nursing* (4th ed.). Philadelphia: Lippincott.

Elliot, R. (1994). *From stress to strength: How to lighten your load.* New York: Chelsea House.

Ellis, A., & Grieger, R. (Eds.) (1986). *Handbook of rational-emotive theory*, (Vols. 1-2). New York: Springer.

English, K. (2002a). *Counseling children with hearing impairment and their families.* Boston: Allyn & Bacon.

English, K. (2002b). Psychosocial aspects of hearing impairment. In R. Schow and M. Nerbonne (Eds.), *Introduction to audiologic rehabilitation* (4th ed., pp. 225–246). Boston: Allyn and Bacon.

Evens, D., Hearn, M., Uhlemann, M., & Ivey, A. (1993). *Essential interviewing: A programmed approach to effective communication.* Pacific Grove, CA: Brooks/Cole.

Faber, A., & Mazlish, E. (1980). *How to talk so kids will listen & listen so kids will talk.* New York: Avon Books, the Hearst Corp.

Fein, M. (1993). *Integrated anger management: A common sense guide to coping with anger.* Westport, CT: Praeger.

Feldman, R. (2002). *Essentials of understanding psychology* (3rd ed.). New York: McGraw-Hill.

Feltham, C. & Dryden, W. (2002). *Dictionary of counseling.* London: Whurr Publishers Ltd.

Ferrand, C., & Bloom, R. (1997). *Introduction to organic and neurogenic disorders of communication.* Boston: Allyn and Bacon.

Figley, C. (2002). *Treating compassion fatigue.* New York: Brunner-Rutledge.

Fisher, R., & Ury, W. (1991). *Getting to yes.* New York: Penguin Books.

Flarey, D. (2001). *Legal and ethical issues in counseling, social work and mental health.* New York: Heritage Professional Education.

Fletcher, K. (1996). Childhood posttraumatic stress disorder. In E. Mash, & R. Barkley (Eds.). *Child psychopathology*. New York: Guilford Press.

Fogle, P. (1978, November). *A study of perceptions of parental attitudes and behaviors compared with how the parents believe their children perceive them*. Paper presented at the American Speech-Language Hearing Association Convention, San Francisco, CA.

Fogle, P. (2000). Forensic speech-language pathology: Testifying as an expert witness. *Advance for Speech-Language Pathologists and Audiologists*. King of Prussia, PA: Merion Publications.

Fogle, P. (2001). Professors in private practice: Rediscovering the joy of therapy. *Advance for Speech-Language Pathologists and Audiologists*. King of Prussia, PA: Merion Publications.

Frank, A. (1991). *At the will of the body: Reflections on illness*. Boston: Houghton Miffin Company.

Frank, J. (1973). *Persuasion and healing*. Baltimore: Johns Hopkins University Press.

Frank, J. (1979). The present status of outcome studies. *Journal of Consulting and Clinical Psychology, 47*, 310–316.

Frank, J. (1982). Therapeutic components shared by all psychotherapies. In J. H. Harvy and M. M. Parks (Eds.), *Psychotherapy research and behavior change*. Washington DC: American Psychological Association.

Frankl, V. (1959). *Man's search for meaning*. In R. George & T. Cristiani (Eds.), (4th ed.). Boston: Allyn and Bacon, 1995.

Freud, S. (1910). The future prospects of psychoanalytic therapy. In *Standard edition of the complete psychological works of Sigmund Freud*, Vol. 11, 139–151. London: Hogarth Press.

Freud, S. (1912). The dynamics of transference. In J. Strachey (Ed. and Trans.), *The standard edition of the complete psychological works of Sigmund Freud: Vol. 12*. London: Hogarth.

Freud, S. (1914). Remembering, repeating and working through. *The standard edition of the complete psychological works of Sigmund Freud: Vol. 12* (pp. 145–156). London: Hogarth Press.

Freud, S. (1917). Resistance and repression. *The standard edition of the complete psychological works of Sigmund Freud: Vol. 12* (pp. 286–301). London: Hogarth Press.

Freud, S. (1949). *An outline of psychoanalysis*. New York: Norton.

Fromm, E. (1941). *Escape from freedom*. New York: Holt, Rinehart & Winston.

Fromm, E. (1956). *The art of loving*. New York: Bantam Books.

Garner, B. (Ed.). (2001). *Black's law dictionary*. New York: West Group Publishing.

Gelfer, M. (1996). *Survey of communication disorders, a social and behavioral perspective*. New York: McGraw-Hill.

George, R. & Cristiani, T. (1995). *Counseling: Theory and practice* (4th ed.). Boston: Allyn and Bacon.

Gill, M. M. (1982). *The analysis of transference*. New York: International University Press.

Gladding, S. (2000). *Counseling: A comprehensive profession*. Upper Saddle River, New Jersey: Prentice-Hall, Inc.

Goldenberg, I., & Goldenberg, H. (2000). *Family therapy: An overview* (4th ed.). Pacific Grove, CA: Brooks/Cole Publishing Co.

Goldfried, M. R. (1982). On the history of therapeutic integration. *Behavior Therapy, 13*, 572–593.

Goldfried, M. R., & Davison, G. L. (1976). *Clinical behavior therapy*. New York: Holt, Rinehart & Winston.

Goleman, D. (1995). *Emotional intelligence, why it can matter more than IQ*. New York: Bantam Books.

Gordon, T. (2000). *Parent effectiveness training.* New York: P. H. Wyden, Publisher.

Gravell, R., & France, J. (1992). *Speech and communication problems in psychiatry.* San Diego, CA: Singular Publishing Group.

Greenberg, J. (1999). *Sharing bad news: A module for the Hanen Program for Early Childhood Educators on sharing sensitive information with parents.* Toronto, Canada: The Hanen Center.

Greenson, R. (1967). *The technique and practice of psychoanalysis*: Vol. 1. Madison, CT: International University Press.

Guitar, B. (1998). *Stuttering: An integrated approach to its nature and treatment.* Baltimore: Williams & Wilkins.

Gurman, A. E., & Messer, S. B. (Eds.). (1995). *Essential psychotherapies: Theory and practice.* New York: Guilford Press.

Hackney, H., & Cormier, L. (1999). *Counseling strategies and interventions* (5th ed.). Boston: Allyn and Bacon.

Hagen, C. (1998). *Rancho levels of cognitive functioning* (Rev. ed.). Communication Disorders Department, Rancho Los Amigos Medical Center, Downey, California.

Hagen, C., Malkmus, D., & Stenderup-Bowman, K. (1973, March). *A clinical approach to treatment of cognitive-communicative problems resulting from traumatic head injury.* Paper presented at the California Speech-Language-Hearing Association State Convention, San Diego.

Haley, J., & Hoffman, L. (1968). *Techniques of family therapy.* New York: Badic Books.

Hartley, L. (1995). *Cognitive-communicative abilities following brain injury, a functional approach.* San Diego, CA: Singular Publishing Group.

Health Insurance Portability and Accountability Act of 1996 (HIPAA). Office of the Federal Register, National Archives and Records Administration, United States Government Printing Office.

Hegde, M. (1995). *Introduction to communicative disorders* (2nd ed.). Austin, TX: Pro-Ed.

Henry, W. P. (1997). Interpersonal case formulation: Describing and explaining interpersonal patterns using the structured analysis of social behaviors. In T. Eells (Ed.), *Handbook of psychotherapy case formulation.* New York: Guilford Press.

Hoffman, L. (1981). *Foundations of family therapy.* New York; Basic Books.

Hoffman, L. (2002). *Family therapy: An intimate journey.* New York: Norton.

Holcomb, R. (1996). *Deaf culture our way.* San Diego, CA: Dawn Sign Press.

Holmes, T., & Rahe, R. (1967). The social readjustment rating scale. *Journal of Psychosomatic Research, 11,* 213–218.

Hooyman, N. R., & Kiyak, H. A. (2001). *Social gerontology: A multidisciplinary perspective* (5th ed.). Boston: Allyn and Bacon.

Horowitz, M., Marmar, C., Krupnick, J., Wilner, N., Kaltreider, N., & Wallerstein, R. (1984). *Personality styles and brief psychotherapy.* New York: Basic Books.

Hull, R. (1987). *Aural rehabilitation: Serving children and adults.* San Diego, CA: Singular Publishing Group.

Hull, R. (1997). *Aural rehabilitation: Serving children and adults* (3rd ed.). San Diego, CA: Singular Publishing Group.

Hummell, D., Talbutt, L., & Alexander, M. (1985). *Law and ethics in counseling.* New York: Van Nostrand Reinhold.

Iskowitz, M. (1999). Assessing and managing CAPD. *Advance for Speech-Language Pathologists and Audiologists*, July, pp. 6–8.

Ivey, A. (1994). *Intentional interviewing and counseling: Facilitating client development in a multicultural society* (3rd ed.). Pacific Grove, CA: Brooks-Cole Publishing Co.

Ivey, A. (1998). *Intentional interviewing and counseling: Facilitating client development in a multicultural society* (4th ed.). Pacific Grove, CA: Brooks-Cole Publishing Co.

Izard, C. (1977). *Human emotions*. New York: Plenum Press.

Johnson, A., & Jacobson, B. (1998). *Medical speech-language pathology: A practitioner's guide*. New York: Thieme.

Kahn, M. (1999). *Between therapist and client: The new relationship*. New York: W. H. Freeman and Company.

Kelly, D. (2001). *Central auditory processing disorder: Identification and intervention*. Gaylord, MI: Northern Speech-National Rehab.

Kelly, K. (1991). Theoretical integration is the future for mental health counseling. *Journal of Mental Health Counseling, 13*(1), 106–111.

Keltner, N., Schwecke, L., & Bostrom, C. (1999). *Psychiatric nursing* (3rd ed.). St. Louis: Mosby.

Kernberg, O. (1965). Notes on countertransference. *Journal of the American Psychoanalytic Association, 13*, 38–56.

Kiesler, D. J. (1982). Confronting the client-therapist in psychotherapy. In J. Anchin & D. Kiesler (Eds.), *Handbook of interpersonal psychotherapy*. New York: Pergamon Press.

Kiesler, D. J. (1988). *Therapeutic metacommunication: Therapist impact disclosure as feedback in psychotherapy*. Palo Alto, CA: Consulting Psychologist Press.

Klerman, G. L., & Weissman, M. M. (Eds.). (1993). *New application of interpersonal therapy*. Washington, DC: American Psychiatric Press.

Kolvin, I., & Fundudis, T. (1981). Elective mute children: Psychological development and background factors. *Journal of Child Psychology and Psychiatry, 22*, 219–232.

Komaroff, A. (1999). *Harvard medical school family health guide*. Cambridge, MA: Harvard Publications.

Kottler, J. (1993). *On being a therapist* (Rev. ed.). San Francisco, CA: Joessey-Bass Publishers.

Kottler, J., & Blau, D. (1989). *The imperfect therapist: Learning form failure in therapeutic practice*. San Francisco: Joessey-Bass Publishers.

Kriege, M. (1993, October). *Managing the behavioral challenges of the patients with traumatic brain injury and/or CVA, a workshop for rehabilitation specialists*. Paper presented at a workshop on Managing the Unmanageable, Long Beach, California.

Kubler-Ross, E. (1969). *On death and dying*. New York: Macmillan Publishing Co.

Kuo, J., & Hu, X. (2002). Counseling Asian American adults with speech, language, and swallowing disorders. *Contemporary Issues in Communication Sciences and Disorders, 29*, 35–42.

La Greca, A., Silverman, W., Vernberg, E., & Roberts, M. (2002). *Helping children cope with disaster and terrorism*. Washington, DC: American Psychological Association.

Lang, P. (1985). The cognitive psychophysiology of emotion: Fear and anxiety. In A. Tuma & J. Maser (Eds.), *Anxiety and the anxiety disorders*. Hillsdale, NJ: Laurence Erlbaum.

Langdon, H. (2002). Communicating effectively with clients during a speech-language pathologists/interpreter conference: Results of a survey. *Contemporary Issues in Communication Science and Disorders, 29*, 17–34.

Lavorato, A.S., & McFarlane, S.C. (1988). Counseling clients with voice disorders. *Seminars in Speech and Language Pathology, 9*, 237–255.

Lazarus, A. (1996). The utility and futility of combining treatments in psychotherapy. *Clinical Psychology: Science and Practice, 3*(1), 59–68.

Lazarus, A. & Beutler, L. (1993). On technical eclecticism. *Journal of Counseling and Development, 71*, 381–385.

Lineham, M. M., & Kehrer, C. A. (1993). Borderline personality disorder. In D. H. Barlow (Ed.), *Clinical handbook of psychological disorders* (2nd ed.). New York: Guilford Press.

Lubinski, R. & Frattali, C. (2001). *Professional issues in speech-language pathology and audiology* (2nd ed.). Clifton Park, NY: Singular/Thomson Learning.

Luterman, D. (1984, 1991, 1996, 2001). *Counseling persons with communication disorders and their families* (4th ed.). Austin, TX: Pro-Ed.

Macinick, C., & Macinick, J. (1990). Strategies for burnout prevention in the mental health setting. *International Nursing Review, 37*, 247–250.

Mahoney, M. J. (1974). *Cognitive and behavior modification*. Cambridge, MA: Ballinger.

Manning, W. (2001). *Clinical decision making in fluency disorders* (2nd ed.). Vancouver, Canada: Singular Publishing.

Marschark, M. (1993). *Psychological development of deaf children.*New York: Oxford University Press.

Martin, D. (1999). *Counseling and therapy skills*. Prospect Heights, IL: Therapy Press.

Martin, T. & Doka, K. (1996). Masculine grief. In K. Doka (Ed.), *Living with grief: After sudden loss*. Washington, DC: Hospice Foundation of America.

Maslach, C. (1982). *Burnout: The cost of caring*. Englewood Cliffs, NJ: Prentice-Hall.

Maurer, J., & Martin, D. (1997). Counseling the older adult who is hearing impaired. In R. Hull (Ed.), *Aural rehabilitation: Serving children and adults* (3rd ed., pp. 337–345). San Diego, CA: Singular Publishing Group.

Maxmen, J., & Ward, N. (1995). *Essential psychopathology and its treatment* (2nd ed.). New York: W. W. Norton and Company.

May, R. (1953). *Man's search for himself*. New York: Norton.

May, R. (Ed.). (1961). *Existential psychology*. New York: Random House.

May, R. (1975). *The courage to create*. New York: Norton Press.

May, R., Remen, N., Young, D., & Berland, W. (1985). The wounded healer. *Saybrook Review, 5*, 84–93.

McCay, V. & Andrews, J. (1990). *The psychology of deafness: Understanding deaf and hard of hearing people*. New York: Longman.

McGonigel, M., Kaufman, J., & Johnson, B. (Eds.). (1991). *Guidelines and recommended practices for the individualized family service plan* (2nd ed.). Bethesda, MD: Association for the Care of Children's Health.

MedicAlert. (2001). Turlock, CA.

Meichenbaum, D. (1977). *Cognitive-behavior modification: An integrative approach*. New York: Plenum

Meichenbaum, D. (1999). *Cognitive-behavior modification*. New York: Plenum.

Meir, S., & Davis, S. (2000). *The elements of counseling* (2nd ed.). Pacific Grove, CA: Brooks/Cole Publishing Co.

Minuchin, S. (1974). *Families and family therapy*. Cambridge, MA: Harvard University Press.

Minuchin, S. (1978). *Psychosomatic families*. Cambridge, MA: Harvard University Press.

Moeller, D. (1975). *Speech pathology & audiology: Iowa origins of a disciple*. Iowa City: The University of Iowa Press.

Moore, M. (2001). Amid chaos, Air Force Major finds her role. *The ASHA Leader, 6*(20), 6.

Morrison, J. (1995). *The first interview, revised for DSM-IV*. New York: Guilford Press.

Morrison, J. (1997). *Psychological symptoms that mask medical disorders*. New York: Guilford Press.

Morrison, J., & Anders, T. (1999). *Interviewing children and adolescents: Skills and strategies for effective DSM-IV diagnosis*. New York: The Guilford Press.

Mosak, H., & Maniacci, M. (1998). *Tactics in counseling and psychotherapy*. Itasca, IL: F.E. Peacock Publishers, Inc.

Norcross, J., & Newman, C. (1992). Psychotherapy integration: Setting the context. In J. Norcross & M. Goldfried (Eds.), *Handbook of psychotherapy integration* (pp. 3–45). New York: Basic Books.

Norcross, J. & Prochaska, J. (1988). A study of eclectic (and integrative) views revisited. *Professional Psychology: Research and Practice, 19*(2), 170–174.

Novaco, R. W. (1976). Treatment of chronic anger through cognitive and relaxation controls. *Journal of Consulting and Clinical Psychology, 45*, 600–608.

Novaco, R. W. (1983). *Stress inoculation therapy for anger control: A manual for therapists*. (Available from Raymond W. Novaco, University of California, Irvine.)

Novak, J. (2002). Counseling: an approach for speech-language pathologists. *Contemporary Issues in Communication Science and Disorders, 29*, 79–90.

Nystul, M. (1999) *Introduction to counseling: An art and science perspective*. Boston: Allyn and Bacon.

Padden, C., & Humphries, T. (1990). *Deaf in America: Voices from a culture*. Cambridge, MA: Harvard University Press.

Papalia, D. & Olds, S. (1997). *Human development* (7th ed.). New York: McGraw-Hill.

Parker, R. (1990). *Traumatic brain injury and neuropsychological impairment: Sensorimotor, cognitive, emotional, and adaptive problems of children and adults*. New York: Springer-Verlag.

Patterson, C. (1986). *Theories of counseling and psychology*. New York: Harper & Row.

Paul, P., & Jackson, D. (1993). *Toward a psychology of deafness*. Boston: Allyn and Bacon.

Pedersen, P., Draguns, J., Lonner, W., & Trimble, J. (Eds.). (2002). *Counseling across cultures* (5th ed.). Thousand Oaks, CA: SAGE Publications.

Pipes, R. & Davenport, D. (1998). *Introduction to psychotherapy: Common clinical wisdom*. Englewood Cliffs, NJ: Prentice Hall.

Pipp-Siegel, S. & Biringen, Z. (2000). Assessing the quality of relationships between parents and chilren: The Emotional Availability Scales. *Volta Review, 100*(5) (monograph), 237–249.

Preston, P. (1995). *Mother-father deaf: Living between sound and silence*. Cambridge, MA: Harvard University Press.

Prochaska, J., & Norcross, J. (2003). *Systems of psychotherapy, a transtheoretical analysis*. Pacific Grove, CA: Thomson-Brooks/Cole Publishing Co.

Pruitt, D. (1981). *Negotiation behavior*. New York: Academic Press.

Pynoos, R., Frederick, C., Nader, K., Arroyo, W., Steinberg, A., Eth, S., Nunez, F., & Fairbanks, L. (1987). Life threat and posttraumatic stress in school-age children. *Archives of General Psychiatry, 44*, 1057–1063.

Pyszczynski, T., Solomon, S., & Greenberg, J. (2003). *In the wake of 9/11: The psychology of terror*. Washington, DC: American Psychological Association.

Renwick, M. (2002, August 19). [Interview with the author].

Ridley, C. R., & Lingle, D. W. (1996). Cultural empathy in multicultural counseling. In P. B. Pedersen, J. G. Draguns, W. J. Lonner, & J.E. Trimble (Eds.), *Counseling across cultures* (4th ed.). Thousand Oaks, CA: Sage.

Riley, J. (2002). Counseling: an approach for speech-language pathologists. *Contemporary Issues in Communication Science and Disorders, 29*, 6–16.

Roeser, R. J. & Downs, M. P. (1995). *Auditory disorders in school children: The law, identification, remediation*. New York: Thieme Medical Publishers.

Rogers, C. (1951). *Client-centered therapy*. Boston: Houghton Miffin.

Rogers, C. (1957). The necessary and sufficient conditions of therapeutic personality change. *Journal of Consulting Psychology, 21*, 95–103.

Rogers, C. (1961). *On becoming a person*. Boston: Houghton Miffin.

Rogers, C. (1980). *A way of being*. Boston: Houghton Miffin.

Rolland, J. (1994). *Families, illness, & disability: An integrative treatment model*. New York: Harper-Collins.

Rollin, W. (1987). *Counseling individuals with communication disorders: Psychodynamic and family aspects*. Boston: Butterworth-Heinemann.

Rollin, W. (2000). *Counseling individuals with communication disorders: Psychodynamic and family aspects* (2nd ed.). Boston: Butterworth-Heinemann.

Roseberry-McKibbin, C. (2002). *Multicultural students with special language needs, practical strategies for assessment and intervention*. Oceanside, CA: Academic Communication Associates, Inc.

Roy, A. (1991). Suicide. In H. Kaplan and B. Sadock (Eds.), *Comprehensive textbook of psychiatry* (5th ed.). Baltimore: Williams & Wilkins.

Rubalcaba, M. (May 21, 2000). *Department of Speech-Language Pathology Commencement Address*. University of the Pacific, Stockton, California.

Ryan, E. (1995). Normal aging and language. In R. Lubinski (Ed.), *Dementia and communication*. San Diego, CA: Singular Publishing Group.

Ryan, E., Bourhis, R., & Knops, U. (1991). Evaluating perceptions of patronizing speech addressed to elders. *Psychology and Aging, 6*, 442–450.

Ryan, E., Hummert, M., & Boisch, L. (1995). Communication predicaments of aging: Patronizing behavior toward older adults. *Journal of Language and Social Psychology, 14*, 144–166.

Saba, G., Karrer, B. & Hardy, K. (1995). *Minorities and family therapy*. New York: Haworth Press.

Safran, J. D., & Segal, Z. V. (1990). *Interpersonal process in cognitive therapy*. New York: Basic Books.

Salas-Provance, M., Erickson, J., & Reed, J. (2002). Disability as viewed by four generations of one Hispanic family. *American Journal of Speech-Language Pathology, 11*, 151–162.

Sanders, C. (1995). The grief of children and parents. In K. Doka (Ed.), *Children mourning, mourning children*. Washington, DC: Hospice Foundation of America.

Sanders, C. (1998). Gender differences in bereavement expression across the life span. In R. Doka & J. Davidson (Eds.), *Living with grief: Who we are, how we grieve*. Washington, DC: Hospice Foundation of America.

Satir, V. (1964). *Conjoint family therapy*. Palo Alto, CA: Science and Behavior Books, Inc.

Satir, V. (1976). *Making contact*. Berkeley, CA: Celestial Arts.

Satir, V. (1983). *Conjoint family therapy* (3rd ed., Rev. ed.). Palo Alto, CA: Science and Behavior Books, Inc.

Schaefer, E. (1965). Children's report of parental behavior, an inventory. *Child Development, 36*, 413–424.

Schafer, R. (1983). *The analytic attitude*. New York: Basic Books.

Scheller, M. (1990). *Building partnerships in hospital care*. Palo Alto, CA: Bull Publishing.

Scheuerle, J. (1992). *Counseling in speech-language pathology and audiology*. New York: Macmillan Publishing.

Schow, R., & Nerbonne, M. (2002). *Introduction to audiologic rehabilitation* (4th ed.). Boston: Allyn and Bacon.

Schultz, D., & Carnevale, F. (1996). Engagement and suffering in responsible caregiving: On overcoming maleficience in health care. *Theoretical Medicine, 17*, 189–207.

Shadden, B., & Toner, M. (Eds.). (1997). *Aging and communication*. Austin, TX: Pro-Ed.

Shames, G. (2000). *Counseling the communicatively disabled and their families: A manual for clinicians*. Boston: Allyn and Bacon.

Sheehan (1970). *Stuttering: Research and therapy*. New York: Harper & Row.

Shipley, K. (1992). *Interviewing and counseling in communicative disorders: Principles and procedures*. Boston: Allyn and Bacon.

Shipley, K. (1997). *Interviewing and counseling in communicative disorders: Principles and procedures*. Boston: Allyn and Bacon.

Shipley, K., & McAfee, J. (1998). *Assessment in speech-language pathology, a resource manual* (2nd ed.). San Diego, CA: Singular Publishing Group.

Shneidman, E. (1984). Aphorisms of suicide and some implications for psychotherapy. *American Journal of Psychotherapy, 38*, 319–328.

Skinner, B. (1953). *Science and human behavior*. New York: Free Press.

Skinner, B. (1974). *About behaviorism*. New York: Vintage Books.

Smith, P. (1981). Empirically based models for viewing the dynamics of violence. In Keltner, N., Schwecke, L., & Bostrom, C. (Eds.), *Psychiatric nursing* (3rd ed.). St. Louis: Mosby.

Sohlberg, M., & Mateer, C. (1989). *Introduction to cognitive rehabilitation, theory and practice*. New York: Guilford Press.

Sommers-Flanagan, J., & Sommers-Flanagan, R. (1993). *Foundations of therapeutic interviewing*. Boston: Allyn and Bacon.

Springhouse Corporation. (1997). *Mastering geriatric care*. Springhouse, PA: Springhouse Corporation.

Sroufe, L., & Cooper, R. (1996). *Child development: Its nature and course*. New York: McGraw-Hill.

Staab, A., & Hodges, L. (1996). *Essential of gerontological nursing, adaptation to the aging process.* Philadelphia: J.B. Lippincott Company.

Stewart, W. (1997). *An A–Z of counseling theory and practice.* London: Chapman & Hall.

St. Louis, K. (2001). *Living with stuttering.* Morgantown, WV: Populore Publishing Company.

Stolorow, R. D., Brandcraft, B., & Atwood, G. E. (1987). *Psychoanalytic treatment: An intersubjective approach.* Hillsdale, NJ: Analytic Press.

Stone, J. & Olswang, L. (1989). The hidden challenge in counseling. *ASHA, 31,* 27–31.

Stone, J., Shapiro, J., & Pasino, J. (1990). *The boundaries of counseling: Strategies for habilitation/rehabilitation professionals.* Conference, Reno, NV.

Stromstra, C. (1986). *Elements of stuttering.* Oshtemo, MI: Atsmorts Publishing.

Strupp, H. H., & Binder, J. L. (1984). *Psychotherapy in a new key.* New York: Basic Books.

Sullivan, H. (1953). *The interpersonal theory of psychiatry.* New York: Norton.

Sullivan, H. (1972). *Personal psychopathology.* New York: Norton.

Sweet, A. A. (1984). The therapeutic relationship in behavior therapy. *Clinical Psychology Review, 4,* 253–272.

Tannen, D. (2001). *You just don't understand: Women and men in conversation.* New York: Ballantine Books.

Tanner, D. (1980). Loss and grief: Implications for the speech-language pathologist and audiologist. *Asha, A Journal of the American Speech-Language-Hearing Association, 22(*11), 915–928.

Tanner, D. (1999). *The family guide to surviving stroke and communication disorders.* Boston: Allyn and Bacon.

Tarasoff v. Board of Regents of the University of California, 13 Cal. 3d 177,529 P.2d 553 (1974), vacated, 17 Cal. 3d 425, 551 P2d 334 (1976).

Taylor, J. (2001). *Helping your ADD child* (3rd ed.). Roseville, CA: Prima Publishing.

Teyber, E. (2000). *Interpersonal process in psychotherapy* (4th ed.). Belmont, CA: Brooks/Cole, Thomson Learning.

Tompkins, C. (1995). *Right hemisphere communication disorders, theory and management.* San Diego, CA: Singular Publishing Group.

Toner, M., & Shadden, B. (2002). Counseling challenges: Working with older clients and caregivers. *Contemporary Issues in Communication Sciences and Disorders, 29,* 68–78.

Tschudin, V. (1990). Support yourself. *Nursing Times, 86,* 40–42.

Tye-Murray, N. (1998). *Foundations of aural rehabilitation, children, adults, and their family members.* San Diego, CA: Singular Publishing Group.

Ulmer, S. (2002, July 26). [Interview with the author].

Van Hoose, W. H., & Kottler, J. (1985). *Ethical and legal issues in counseling and psychotherapy.* Cranston, RI: Carrol.

Van Riper, C. (1953). *Speech therapy, a book of readings.* New York: Prentice-Hall, Inc.

Visher, E., & Visher, J. (1996). *Therapy with stepfamilies.* New York: Brunner/Mazel, Publishing.

Wachtel, P. L. (1977). *Psychoanalysis and behavior therapy.* New York: Basic Books.

Wachtel, P. (1993). *Therapeutic communication: Principles and effective practice.* New York: Guilford Press.

Watzlawick, P. (1978). *The language of change.* New York: Basic Books.

Watzlawick, P., Weakland, J., & Fisch, R. (1974). *Change: The principles of problem formation and problem resolution.* New York: Norton.

Weakland, J. (1976). Communication theory and clinical change. In P. J. Guerin, Jr. (Ed.), *Family therapy: Theory and practice*. New York: Gardner Press.

Weinrich, D. (2002). Elder abuse: A hidden tragedy. American Speech-Language-Hearing Association Special Interest Division, *Gerontology, 7*(1), 5–10.

Weissman, M. M., & Klerman, G. L. (1991). Interpersonal psychotherapy for depression. In B. D. Beitman & G. L. Klerman (Eds.), *Integrating pharmacotherapy and psychotherapy*. Washington, DC: American Psychological Assocation.

Wepman, J. (1951). *Recovery from aphasia*. New York: Ronald Press.

Williams-Quinlan, S. (2002, June 26). Private interview.

Wilson, G. T., & Franks, C. M. (Eds.). (1982). *Cognitive behavior therapy: Conceptual and empirical foundations*. New York: Guilford Press.

Wolpe, J. (1958). *Psychotherapy by reciprocal inhibition*. Stanford, CA: Stanford University Press.

Wolpe, J. (1987). *Essential principles and practices of behavior therapy*. Phoenix, AZ: Milton H. Erickson Foundation.

Worrall, L., & Frattali, C. (2000). *Neurogenic communication disorders, a functional approach*. New York: Thieme.

Yairi, E. (1970). *Perceptions of parental attitudes by stuttering and by nonstuttering children*. Unpublished doctoral dissertation, University of Iowa, Iowa City.

Yairi, E., & Williams, D. (1971). Reports of parental attitudes by stuttering and by nonstuttering children. *Journal of Speech and Hearing Research, 14*, 596–603.

Yalom, I. (1980). *Existential psychotherapy*. New York: Basic Books.

Zaner, R. (1993). *Troubled voices*. Cleveland, OH: The Pilgrim Press.

Zaro, J., Barach, R., Nedelman, D., & Dreiblatt, I. (1995). *A guide for beginning psychotherapists*. Cambridge, England: Cambridge University Press.

Zebrowski, P. (2000). *Counseling parents of children who stutter*. Memphis, TN: Stuttering Foundation of America.

Zebrowski, P. (2002). Counseling: An approach for speech-language pathologists. *Contemporary Issues in Communication Science and Disorders, 29*, 91–100.

INDEX

failures, 278-80
  benefits of, 279-80
  interventions, value of, 7
  relationship, variables contributing to the, 88-90
"Therapist Noises", 125
Therapy, humanistic, 42-48
Threat of harm to others, 265-67
  role of SLP and audiologist, 266-67
Three-stage crisis intervention model, 249-54
Tolerance for ambiguity, 17
Tone of voice, 96
Top-down model, 10
Touch, 107-8
  hypersensitivity to, 108
Training
  cue, 244
  relaxation, 186
Transference, 90-92, 303
  client romantic, 92
Traumatic
  brain injury, 5, 30-31, 162, 248
  events, experiencing, 272-73
Triangulation, 63-64, 303
Trigger, 163
Triggering phase, 231. (*See also* Assault cycle)

Uncertainty, existential, 67-68, 301
Unconditional positive regard, 12, 14, 42, 44-45, 236 303
Understanding
  checking for, 136
  empathic, 12-13
Unhealthy personality development, 42-43

Verbal
  encouragers, 124-25
  people, overly, 215-16
Visual imagery (Visualizations), 252
Voice
  disorders, 11
  tone of, 96

Warning signs of
  child abuse/neglect, 267
  elder maltreatment/abuse, 269-70
Western cultures, 127
Within boundaries, 20, 32
World view, 77, 303
Written Expression, Disorders of, 11

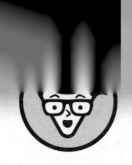

Agile Project Management

2nd Edition

by Mark C. Layton and Steven J Ostermiller

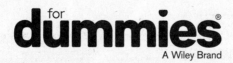

A Wiley Brand

Agile Project Management For Dummies®, 2nd Edition

Published by: **John Wiley & Sons, Inc.,** 111 River Street, Hoboken, NJ 07030-5774, www.wiley.com

Copyright © 2017 by John Wiley & Sons, Inc., Hoboken, New Jersey

Published simultaneously in Canada

For general information on our other products and services, please contact our Customer Care Department within the U.S. at 877-762-2974, outside the U.S. at 317-572-3993, or fax 317-572-4002. For technical support, please visit https://hub.wiley.com/community/support/dummies.

Wiley publishes in a variety of print and electronic formats and by print-on-demand. Some material included with standard print versions of this book may not be included in e-books or in print-on-demand. If this book refers to media such as a CD or DVD that is not included in the version you purchased, you may download this material at http://booksupport.wiley.com. For more information about Wiley products, visit www.wiley.com.

Library of Congress Control Number: 2017948508

ISBN 978-1-119-40569-6 (pbk); ISBN 978-1-119-40574-0 (ebk); ISBN 978-1-119-40573-3 (ebk)

Manufactured in the United States of America

10 9 8 7 6 5 4 3 2 1

Contents at a Glance

Table of Contents

Introduction

Welcome to *Agile Project Management For Dummies*. Agile project management has grown to be as common as any management technique in business today. Over the past decade and a half, we have trained and coached companies big and small, all over the world, about how to successfully run agile projects. Through this work, we found that there was a need to write a digestible guide that the average person could understand and use.

In this book, we will clear up some of the myths about what agile project management is and what it is not. The information in this book will give you the confidence to know you can be successful using agile techniques.

About This Book

Agile Project Management For Dummies, 2nd Edition is more than just an introduction to agile practices and methodologies; you also discover the steps to execute agile techniques on a project. The material here goes beyond theory and is meant to be a field manual, accessible to the everyday person, giving you the tools and information you need to be successful with agile processes in the trenches of project management.

Foolish Assumptions

Because you're reading this book, you might have a passing familiarity with project management. Perhaps you are a project manager, a member of a project team, or a stakeholder on a project. Or perhaps you don't have experience with formal project management approaches but are looking for a solution now. You may even have heard the term *agile* and want to know more. Or you might already be part of a project team that's trying to be more agile.

Regardless of your experience or level of familiarity, this book provides insights you may find interesting. If nothing else, we hope it brings clarity to any confusion or myths regarding agile project management you may have encountered.

Icons Used in This Book

Throughout this book, you'll find the following icons.

Tips are points to help you along your agile project management journey. Tips can save you time and help you quickly understand a particular topic, so when you see them, take a look!

The Remember icon is a reminder of something you may have seen in past chapters. It also may be a reminder of a commonsense principle that is easily forgotten. These icons can help jog your memory when an important term or concept appears.

The Warning icon indicates that you want to watch out for a certain action or behavior. Be sure to read these to steer clear of big problems!

The Technical Stuff icon indicates information that is interesting but not essential to the text. If you see a Technical Stuff icon, you don't need to read it to understand agile project management, but the information there might just pique your interest.

On the Web means that you can find more information on the book's website at www.dummies.com/go/agileprojectmanagementfd2e.

Beyond the Book

Although this book broadly covers the agile project management spectrum, we can cover only so much in a set number of pages! If you find yourself at the end of this book thinking, "This was an amazing book! Where can I learn more about how to advance my projects under an agile approach?" check out Chapter 22 or head over to www.dummies.com for more resources.

We've provided a cheat sheet for tips on assessing your current projects in relation to agile principles and free tools for managing projects using agile techniques. To get to the cheat sheet, go to www.dummies.com, and then type *Agile Project Management For Dummies Cheat Sheet* in the Search box. This is also where you'll find any significant updates or changes that occur between editions of this book.

Where to Go from Here

We wrote this book so that you could read it in just about any order. Depending on your role, you may want to pay extra attention to the appropriate sections of the book. For example:

>> If you're just starting to learn about project management and agile approaches, start with Chapter 1 and read the book straight through to the end.

>> If you are a member of a project team and want to know the basics of how to work on an agile project, check out the information in Part 3 (Chapters 7 through 11).

>> If you are a project manager and are wondering how agile approaches affect your job, review Part 4 (Chapters 12 through 15).

>> If you know the basics of agile project management and are looking at bringing agile practices to your company or scaling agile practices across your organization, Part 5 (Chapters 16 through 18) provides you with helpful information.

1

Understanding Agile

Understand why project management needs to modernize due to the flaws and weaknesses in historical approaches to project management.

Find out why agile methods are growing as an alternative to traditional project management, and become acquainted with the foundation of agile project management: the Agile Manifesto and the 12 Agile Principles.

Discover the advantages that your products, projects, teams, customers, and organization can gain from adopting agile project management processes and techniques.

Chapter **1**

Modernizing Project Management

Agile project management is a style of project management that focuses on early delivery of business value, continuous improvement of the project's product and processes, scope flexibility, team input, and delivering well-tested products that reflect customer needs.

In this chapter, you find out why agile processes emerged as an approach to software development project management in the mid-1990s and why agile methodologies have caught the attention of project managers, customers who invest in the development of new software, and executives whose companies fund software development departments. This chapter also explains the advantages of agile methodologies over long-standing approaches to project management.

Project Management Needed a Makeover

A *project* is a planned program of work that requires a definitive amount of time, effort, and planning to complete. Projects have goals and objectives and often must be completed in some fixed period of time and within a certain budget.

Because you are reading this book, it's likely that you are either a project manager or someone who initiates projects, works on projects, or is affected by projects in some way.

Agile approaches are a response to the need to modernize project management. To understand how agile approaches are revolutionizing projects, it helps to know a little about the history and purpose of project management and the issues that projects face today.

The origins of modern project management

Projects have been around since ancient times. From the Great Wall of China to the Mayan pyramids at Tikal, from the invention of the printing press to the invention of the Internet, people have accomplished endeavors big and small in projects.

As a formal discipline, project management as we know it has only been around since the middle of the twentieth century. Around the time of World War II, researchers around the world were making major advances in building and programming computers, mostly for the United States military. To complete those projects, they started creating formal project management processes. The first processes were based on step-by-step manufacturing models the United States military used during World War II.

People in the computing field adopted these step-based manufacturing processes because early computer-related projects relied heavily on hardware, with computers that filled up entire rooms. Software, by contrast, was a smaller part of computer projects. In the 1940s and 1950s, computers might have thousands of physical vacuum tubes but fewer than 30 lines of programming code. The 1940s manufacturing process used on these initial computers is the foundation of the project management methodology known as waterfall.

In 1970, a computer scientist named Winston Royce wrote "Managing the Development of Large Software Systems," an article for the IEEE that described the phases in the waterfall methodology. The term *waterfall* was coined later, but the phases, even if they are sometimes titled differently, are essentially the same as originally defined by Royce:

1. Requirements

2. Design

3. Development

4. Integration

5. Testing

6. Deployment

On waterfall projects, you move to the next phase only when the prior one is complete — hence, the name waterfall.

TECHNICAL STUFF

Pure waterfall project management — completing each step in full before moving to the next step — is actually a misinterpretation of Royce's suggestions. Royce identified that this approach was inherently risky and recommended developing and testing within iterations to create products — suggestions that were overlooked by many organizations that adopted the waterfall methodology.

SOFTWARE PROJECT SUCCESS AND FAILURE

Unfortunately, the stagnation in traditional project management approaches is catching up with the software industry. In 2015, a software statistical company called the Standish Group did a study on the success and failure rates of 10,000 projects in the US. The results of the study showed that

- *29 percent of traditional projects failed outright.* The projects were cancelled before they finished and did not result in any product releases. These projects delivered no value whatsoever.

- *60 percent of traditional projects were challenged.* The projects were completed, but they had gaps between expected and actual cost, time, quality, or a combination of these elements. The average difference between the expected and actual project results — looking at time, cost, and features not delivered — was well over 100 percent.

- *11 percent of projects succeeded.* The projects were completed and delivered the expected product in the originally expected time and budget.

Of the hundreds of billions of dollars spent on application development projects in the US alone, billions of dollars were wasted on projects that never deployed a single piece of functionality.

The waterfall methodology was the most common project management approach in software development until it was surpassed by improved approaches based on agile techniques around 2008.

The problem with the status quo

Computer technology has, of course, changed a great deal since the last century. Many people have a computer on their wrist with more power, memory, and capabilities than the largest, most expensive machine that existed when people first started using waterfall methodologies.

At the same time, the people using computers have changed as well. Instead of creating behemoth machines with minimal programs for a few researchers and the military, people create hardware and software for the general public. In many countries, almost everyone uses a computer, directly or indirectly, every day. Software runs our cars, our appliances, our homes; it provides our daily information and daily entertainment. Even young children use computers — a 2-year-old is almost more adept with the iPhone than her parents. The demand for newer, better software products is constant.

Somehow, during all this growth of technology, processes were not left behind. Software developers are still using project management methodologies from the 1950s, and all these approaches were derived from manufacturing processes meant for the hardware-heavy computers of the mid-twentieth century.

Today, traditional projects that do succeed often suffer from one problem: *scope bloat*, the introduction of unnecessary product features in a project.

Think about the software products you use every day. For example, the word-processing program we're typing on right now has many features and tools. Even though we write with this program every day, we use only some of the features all the time. We use other elements less frequently. And we have never used quite a few tools — and come to think of it, we don't know anyone else who has used them, either. The features that few people use are the result of scope bloat.

Scope bloat appears in all kinds of software, from complex enterprise applications to websites that everyone uses. Figure 1-1 shows data from a Standish Group study that illustrates just how common scope bloat is. In the figure, you can see that 64 percent of requested features are rarely or never used.

The numbers in Figure 1-1 illustrate an enormous waste of time and money. That waste is a direct result of traditional project management processes that are unable to accommodate change. Project managers and stakeholders know that change is not welcome mid-project, so their best chance of getting a potentially desirable feature is at the start of a project. Therefore, they ask for

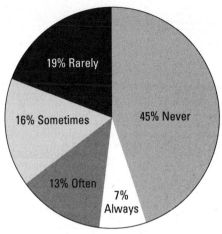

FIGURE 1-1: Actual use of requested software features.

>> Everything they need

>> Everything they think they may need

>> Everything they want

>> Everything they think they may want

The result is the bloat in features that results in the statistics in Figure 1-1.

The problems associated with using outdated management and development approaches are not trivial. These problems waste billions of dollars a year. The billions of dollars lost in project failure in 2015 (see the sidebar, "Software project success and failure") could equate to millions of jobs around the world.

Over the past two decades, people working on projects have recognized the growing problems with traditional project management and have been working to create a better model: agile project management.

Introducing Agile Project Management

The seeds for agile techniques have been around for a long time. In fact, agile values, principles, and practices are simply a codification of common sense. Figure 1-2 shows a quick history of agile project management, dating to the 1930s with Walter Sherwart's Plan-Do-Study-Act (PDSA) approach to project quality.

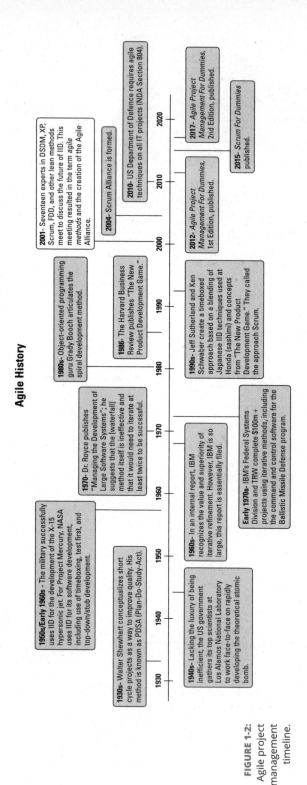

Agile History

1930s- Walter Shewhart conceptualizes short cycle projects as a way to improve quality. His method is known as PDSA (Plan-Do-Study-Act).

1940s- Lacking the luxury of being inefficient, the US government gathers its top scientists at Los Alamos National Laboratory to work face-to-face on rapidly developing the theoretical atomic bomb.

1950s/Early 1960s - The military successfully uses IID for the development of the X-15 hypersonic jet. For Project Mercury, NASA uses IID for its software development, including use of timeboxing, test first, and top-down/stub development.

1960s- In an internal report, IBM recognizes the value and superiority of iterative refinement. However, IBM is so large, this report is essentially filed.

1970- Dr. Royce publishes "Managing the Development of Large Software Systems"; he suggests that the [waterfall] method itself is ineffective and that it would need to iterate at least twice to be successful.

Early 1970s- IBM's Federal Systems Division and TRW complete $100m + projects using iterative methods, including the command and control software for the Ballistic Missile Defense program.

1980s- Object-oriented programming guru Grady Booch articulates the spiral development method.

1986- The Harvard Business Review publishes "The New Product Development Game."

1990s- Jeff Sutherland and Ken Schwaber create a timeboxed approach based on a blending of Japanese IID techniques used at Honda (sashimi) and concepts from "The New Product Development Game." They called the approach Scrum.

2001- Seventeen experts in DSDM, XP, Scrum, FDD, and other lean methods meet to discuss the future of IID. This meeting resulted in the term *agile methods* and the creation of the Agile Alliance.

2004- Scrum Alliance is formed.

2010- US Department of Defence requires agile techniques on all IT projects (NDA Section 804).

2012- *Agile Project Management For Dummies,* 1st Edition, published.

2015- *Scrum For Dummies* published.

2017- *Agile Project Management For Dummies,* 2nd Edition, published.

FIGURE 1-2: Agile project management timeline.

In 1986, Hirotaka Takeuchi and Ikujiro Nonaka published an article called "New New Product Development Game" in the *Harvard Business Review*. Takeuchi and Nonaka's article described a rapid, flexible development strategy to meet fast-paced product demands. This article first paired the term *scrum* with product development. (*Scrum* originally referred to a player formation in rugby.) Scrum eventually became one of the most popular agile project management frameworks.

In 2001, a group of software and project experts got together to talk about what their successful projects had in common. This group created the *Agile Manifesto*, a statement of values for successful software development:

> ### Manifesto for Agile Software Development*
>
> We are uncovering better ways of developing
> software by doing it and helping others do it.
> Through this work we have come to value:
>
> **Individuals and interactions** over processes and tools
> **Working software** over comprehensive documentation
> **Customer collaboration** over contract negotiation
> **Responding to change** over following a plan
>
> That is, while there is value in the items on
> the right, we value the items on the left more.
>
> ** Agile Manifesto Copyright © 2001: Kent Beck, Mike Beedle, Arie van Bennekum, Alistair Cockburn, Ward Cunningham, Martin Fowler, James Grenning, Jim Highsmith, Andrew Hunt, Ron Jeffries, Jon Kern, Brian Marick, Robert C. Martin, Steve Mellor, Ken Schwaber, Jeff Sutherland, Dave Thomas.*
>
> *This declaration may be freely copied in any form, but only in its entirety through this notice.*

These experts also created the *Principles behind the Agile Manifesto*, 12 practices that help support the values in the Agile Manifesto. We list the Agile Principles and describe the Agile Manifesto in more detail in Chapter 2.

Agile, in product development terms, is a descriptor for project management approaches that focus on people, communications, the product, and flexibility. If you're looking for *the* agile methodology, you won't find it. However, all agile methodologies (for example, crystal), frameworks (for example, scrum), techniques (for example, user story requirements), and tools (for example, relative estimating) have one thing in common: adherence to the Agile Manifesto and the 12 Agile Principles.

How agile projects work

Agile approaches are based on an *empirical control method* — a process of making decisions based on the realities observed in the project. In the context of software development methodologies, an empirical approach can be effective in both new product development and enhancement and upgrade projects. By using frequent and firsthand inspection of the work to date, you can make immediate adjustments, if necessary. Empirical control requires

>> **Unfettered transparency:** Everyone involved in an agile project knows what is going on and how the project is progressing.

>> **Frequent inspection:** The people who are invested in the product and process the most regularly evaluate the product and process.

>> **Immediate adaptation:** Adjustments are made quickly to minimize problems; if an inspection shows that something should change, it is changed immediately.

To accommodate frequent inspection and immediate adaptation, agile projects work in *iterations* (smaller segments of the overall project). An agile project involves the same type of work as in a traditional waterfall project: You create requirements and designs, develop the product, document it, and if necessary, integrate the product with other products. You test the product, fix any problems, and deploy it for use. However, instead of completing these steps for all product features at once, as in a waterfall project, you break the project into iterations, also called *sprints*.

Figure 1-3 shows the difference between a linear waterfall project and an agile project.

WARNING

Mixing traditional project management methods with agile approaches is like saying, "I have a Porsche 911 Turbo. However, I'm using a wagon wheel on the front left side. How can I make my car as fast as the other Porsches?" The answer, of course, is you can't. If you fully commit to an agile approach, you will have a better chance of project success.

Why agile projects work better

Throughout this book, you see how agile projects work better than traditional projects. Agile project management approaches can produce more successful projects. The Standish Group study, mentioned in the sidebar "Software project success and failure," found that while 29 percent of traditional projects failed outright, that number dropped to only 9 percent on agile projects. The decrease in failure for agile projects is a result of agile project teams making immediate adaptations based on frequent inspections of progress and customer satisfaction.

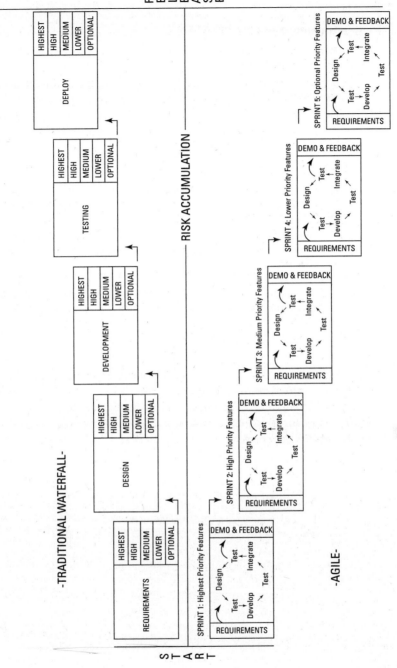

FIGURE 1-3:
Waterfall versus
agile project.

Here are some key areas where agile approaches are superior to traditional project management methods:

>> **Project success rates:** In Chapter 15, you find out how the risk of catastrophic project failure falls to almost nothing on agile projects. Agile approaches of prioritizing by business value and risk ensure early success or failure. Agile approaches to testing throughout the project help ensure that you find problems early, not after spending a large amount of time and money.

>> **Scope creep:** In Chapters 7, 8, and 12, you see how agile approaches accommodate changes throughout a project, minimizing scope creep. On agile projects, you can add new requirements at the beginning of each sprint without disrupting development flow. By fully developing prioritized features first, you prevent scope creep from threatening critical functionality.

>> **Inspecting and adaptation:** In Chapters 10 and 14, you find details of how regular inspections and adaptation work on agile projects. Agile project teams — armed with frequent feedback from complete development cycles and working, shippable functionality — can improve their processes and their products with each sprint.

Throughout many chapters in this book, you discover how you gain control of the outcome of agile projects. Testing early and often, adjusting priorities as needed, using better communication techniques, and regularly demonstrating and releasing product functionality allow you to fine-tune your control over a wide variety of factors on agile projects.

Chapter **2**

Applying the Agile Manifesto and Principles

This chapter describes the basics of what it means to be agile: the Agile Manifesto, with its four values, and the 12 agile principles behind the Agile Manifesto. We also expand on these basics with three additional Platinum Principles, which Platinum Edge (owned by Mark) crafted after years of experience supporting organizations' agile transitions.

This foundation provides product development teams with the information needed to evaluate whether the project team is following agile principles, as well as whether their actions and behaviors are consistent with agile values. When you understand these values and principles, you'll be able to ask, "Is this agile?" and be confident in your answer.

Understanding the Agile Manifesto

In the mid-1990s, the Internet was changing the world right before our eyes. The people working in the booming dot-com industry were under constant pressure to be the first to market with fast-changing technologies. Development teams worked day and night, struggling to deliver new software releases before competitors made their companies obsolete. The information technology (IT) industry was completely reinvented in a few short years.

Given the pace of change at that time, cracks inevitably appeared in conventional project management practices. Using traditional methodologies such as waterfall, which is discussed in Chapter 1, didn't allow developers to be responsive enough to the market's dynamic nature and to emerging new approaches to business. Development teams started exploring alternatives to these outdated approaches to project management. In doing so, they noticed some common themes that produced better results.

In February 2001, 17 of these new methodology pioneers met in Snowbird, Utah, to share their experiences, ideas, and practices; to discuss how best to express them; and to suggest ways to improve the world of software development. They couldn't have imagined the effect their meeting would have on the future of project management. The simplicity and clarity of the manifesto they produced and the subsequent principles they developed transformed the world of information technology and continue to revolutionize project management in every industry, not just software development.

Over the next several months, these leaders constructed the following:

>> **The Agile Manifesto:** An intentionally streamlined expression of core development values

>> **The Agile Principles:** A set of 12 guiding concepts that support agile project teams in implementing agile techniques and staying on track

>> **The Agile Alliance:** A community development organization focused on supporting individuals and organizations that are applying agile principles and practices

The group's work was destined to make the software industry more productive, more humane, and more sustainable.

The Agile Manifesto is a powerful statement, carefully crafted using fewer than 75 words:

Manifesto for Agile Software Development

We are uncovering better ways of developing software by doing it and helping others do it. Through this work we have come to value:

Individuals and interactions over processes and tools
Working software over comprehensive documentation
Customer collaboration over contract negotiation
Responding to change over following a plan

That is, while there is value in the items on
the right, we value the items on the left more.

No one can deny that the Agile Manifesto is both a concise and an authoritative statement. Whereas traditional approaches emphasize a rigid plan, avoid change, document everything, and encourage hierarchal-based control, the manifesto focuses on

>> People

>> Communications

>> The product

>> Flexibility

The Agile Manifesto represents a big shift in focus in how projects are conceived, conducted, and managed. If we read only the items on the left, we understand the new paradigm that the manifesto signers envisioned. They found that by focusing more attention on individuals and interactions, teams would more effectively produce working software through valuable customer collaboration and by responding well to change. In contrast, the traditional primary focus on processes and tools often produces comprehensive or excess documentation to comply with contract negotiations and to follow an unchanging plan.

Research and experience illustrate why agile values are so important:

>> **Individuals and interactions over processes and tools:** Why? Because research shows a 50 times increase in performance when we get individuals and interactions right. One of the ways we get this right is by collocating a development team with an empowered product owner.

>> **Working software over comprehensive documentation:** Why? Because failure to test for and correct defects during the sprint can take up to 24 times more effort and cost in the next sprint. And after the functionality is deployed to the market, if a production support team that wasn't involved in product development performs the testing and fixing, the cost is up to 100 times more.

>> **Customer collaboration over contract negotiation:** Why? Because a dedicated and accessible product owner can generate a fourfold increase in productivity by providing in-the-moment clarification to the development team, aligning customer priorities with the work being performed.

>> **Responding to change over following a plan:** Why? Because 64 percent of features developed under a waterfall model are rarely or never used (as discussed in Chapter 1). Starting with a plan is vital, but that is when we know the least. Agile teams don't plan less than waterfall teams — they plan as much or more. However, agile teams take a just-in-time approach, planning just enough when needed. Adaptation of the plan to the realities along the way is how agile teams deliver products that delight customers.

The creators of the Agile Manifesto originally focused on software development because they worked in the IT industry. However, agile project management techniques have spread beyond software development and even outside computer-related products. Today, people use agile approaches to create products in a variety of industries, including biotech, manufacturing, aerospace, engineering, market-ing, nonprofit work, and even building construction. If you want early empirical feedback on the product or service you're providing, you can benefit from agile methods.

REMEMBER

The Agile Manifesto and 12 Agile Principles directly refer to software; we leave these references intact when quoting the manifesto and principles throughout the book. If you create non-software products, try substituting your product as you read on.

Outlining the Four Values of the Agile Manifesto

The Agile Manifesto was generated from experience, not from theory. As you review the values described in the following sections, consider what they would mean if you put them into practice. How do these values support meeting time-to-market goals, dealing with change, and valuing human innovation?

Value 1: Individuals and interactions over processes and tools

When you allow each person to contribute his or her unique value to a project, the result can be powerful. When these human interactions focus on solving problems, a unified purpose can emerge. Moreover, the agreements come about through processes and tools that are much simpler than conventional ones.

A simple conversation in which you talk through a project issue can solve many problems in a relatively short time. Trying to emulate the power of a direct conversation with email, spreadsheets, and documents results in significant overhead costs and delays. Instead of adding clarity, these types of managed, controlled communications are often ambiguous and time-consuming and distract the development team from the work of creating a product.

Consider what it means if you value individuals and interactions highly. Table 2-1 shows some differences between valuing individuals and valuing interactions and valuing processes and tools.

TABLE 2-1   **Individuals and Interactions versus Processes and Tools**

	Individuals and Interactions Have High Value	Processes and Tools Have High Value
Pros	Communication is clear and effective.	Processes are clear and can be easy to follow.
	Communication is quick and efficient.	Written records of communication exist.
	Teamwork becomes strong as people work together.	
	Development teams can self-organize.	
	Development teams have more chances to innovate.	
	Development teams can customize processes as necessary.	
	Development team members can take personal ownership of the project.	
	Development team members can have deeper job satisfaction.	
Cons	Development team members must have the *capacity* to be involved, responsible, and innovative.	People may over-rely on processes instead of finding the best ways to create good products.
	People may need to let go of ego to work well as members of a team.	One process doesn't fit all teams — different people have different work styles.
		One process doesn't fit all projects.
		Communication can be ambiguous and time-consuming.

You can find a blank template of Table 2-1 on the book's companion website at www.dummies.com/go/agileprojectmanagementfd2e — jot down the pros and cons of each approach that apply to you and your projects.

If processes and tools are seen as the way to manage product development and everything associated with it, people and the way they approach the work must conform to the processes and tools. Conformity makes it hard to accommodate new ideas, new requirements, and new thinking. Agile approaches, however, value people over process. This emphasis on individuals and teams puts the focus on their energy, innovation, and ability to solve problems. You use processes and tools in agile project management, but they're intentionally streamlined and directly support product creation. The more robust a process or tool, the more you spend on its care and feeding and the more you defer to it. With people front and center, however, the result is a leap in productivity. An agile environment is human-centric and participatory and can be readily adapted to new ideas and innovations.

Value 2: Working software over comprehensive documentation

A development team's focus should be on producing working functionality. On agile projects, the only way to measure whether you are truly finished with a product requirement is to produce the working functionality associated with that requirement. For software products, working software means the software meets what we call the *definition of done:* at the very least, developed, tested, integrated, and documented. After all, the working product is the reason for the project.

Have you ever been in a status meeting where you reported that you were, say, 75 percent done with your project? What would happen if your customer told you, "We ran out of money. Can we have our 75 percent now?" On a traditional project, you would not have any working software to give the customer — "75 percent done" traditionally means you are 75 percent in progress and 0 percent done. On an agile project, however, by using the definition of done, you would have working, potentially shippable functionality for 75 percent of your project requirements — the highest-priority 75 percent of requirements.

Although agile approaches have roots in software development, you can use them for other types of products. This second agile value can easily read, "Working functionality over comprehensive documentation."

Tasks that distract from producing valuable functionality must be evaluated to see whether they support or undermine the job of creating a working product. Table 2-2 shows a few examples of traditional project documents and their use-fulness. Think about the documents produced on a recent project you were involved in.

TABLE 2-2   # Identifying Useful Documentation

Document	Does the Document Support Product Development?	Is the Document Barely Sufficient or Gold-Plated?
Project schedule created with expensive project management software, complete with Gantt Chart.	No. Start-to-finish schedules with detailed tasks and dates tend to provide more than what is necessary for product development. Also, many of these details change before you develop future features.	Gold-plated. Although project managers might spend a lot of time creating and updating project schedules, project team members tend to want to know only key deliverable dates. Management often wants to know only whether the project is on time, ahead of schedule, or behind.
Requirements documentation.	Yes. All projects have requirements — details about product features and needs. Development teams need to know those needs to create a product.	Possibly gold-plated; should be barely sufficient. Requirements documents can easily grow to include unnecessary details. Agile approaches provide simple ways to describe product requirements.
Product technical specifications.	Yes. Documenting how you created a product can make future changes easier.	Possibly gold-plated; should be barely sufficient. Agile documentation includes just what it needs — development teams often don't have time for extra flourishes and are keen to minimize documentation.
Weekly status report.	No. Weekly status reports are for management purposes but do not assist product creation.	Gold-plated. Knowing project status is helpful, but traditional status reports contain outdated information and are much more burdensome than necessary.
Detailed project communication plan.	No. Although a contact list can be helpful, the details in many communication plans are useless to product development teams.	Gold-plated. Communication plans often end up being documents about documentation — an egregious example of busywork.

REMEMBER

With agile project management, the term *barely sufficient* is a positive description, meaning that a task, document, meeting, or almost anything on a project includes only what it needs to achieve the goal. Being barely sufficient is practical and efficient — it's sufficient, just enough. The opposite of barely sufficient is *gold-plating*, adding unnecessary frivolity — and effort — to a feature, task, document, meeting, or anything else.

All projects require some documentation. On agile projects, documents are useful only if they support product development and are barely sufficient to serve the design, delivery, and deployment of a working product in the most direct, unceremonious way. Agile approaches dramatically simplify the administrative paperwork relating to time, cost control, scope control, or reporting.

You can find a blank template of Table 2-2 at www.dummies.com/go/agile projectmanagementfd2e. Use that form to assess how well your documentation directly contributed to the product and whether it was barely sufficient.

We often stop producing a document and see who complains. After we know the requestor of the document, we strive to better understand why the document is necessary. The *five whys* work great in this situation — ask "why" after each successive answer to get to the root reason for the document. After you know the core reason for the document, see how you can satisfy that need with an agile artifact or streamlined process.

Agile project teams produce fewer, more streamlined documents that take less time to maintain and provide better visibility into potential issues. In the coming chapters, you find out how to create and use simple tools (such as a product backlog, a sprint backlog, and a task board) that allow project teams to understand requirements and assess status daily. With agile approaches, project teams spend more time on development and less time on documentation, resulting in a more efficient delivery of a working product.

Value 3: Customer collaboration over contract negotiation

The customer is not the enemy. Really.

Historical project management approaches usually involve customers at three key points:

>> **Start of a project:** When the customer and the project manager — or another project team representative — negotiate contract details.

>> **Any time the scope changes during the project:** When the customer and the project manager negotiate changes to the contract.

>> **End of a project:** When the project team delivers a completed product to the customer. If the product doesn't meet the customer's expectations, the project manager and the customer negotiate additional changes to the contract.

This historical focus on negotiation discourages potentially valuable customer input and can even create an adversarial relationship between customers and project teams.

WARNING

You will never know less about a product than at the project's start. Locking product details into a contract at the beginning of your project means you have to make decisions based on incomplete knowledge. If you have flexibility for change as you learn more about a product, you'll ultimately create better products.

The agile pioneers understood that collaboration, rather than confrontation, produced better, leaner, more useful products. As a result of this understanding, agile methods make the customer part of the project on an ongoing basis.

Using an agile approach in practice, you'll experience a partnership between the customer and the development team in which discovery, questioning, learning, and adjusting during the course of the project are routine, acceptable, and systematic.

Value 4: Responding to change over following a plan

Change is a valuable tool for creating great products. Project teams that can respond quickly to customers, product users, and the market are able to develop relevant, helpful products that people want to use.

Unfortunately, traditional project management approaches attempt to wrestle the change monster and pin it to the ground so it goes out for the count. Rigorous change management procedures and budget structures that can't accommodate new product requirements make changes difficult. Traditional project teams often find themselves blindly following a plan, missing opportunities to create more valuable products.

Figure 2-1 shows the relationship between time, opportunity for change, and the cost of change on a traditional project. As time — and knowledge about your product — increases, the ability to make changes decreases and costs more.

By contrast, agile projects accommodate change systematically. The flexibility of agile approaches increases project stability because change in an agile project is predictable and manageable. In later chapters, you discover how the agile approaches to planning, working, and prioritization allow project teams to respond quickly to change.

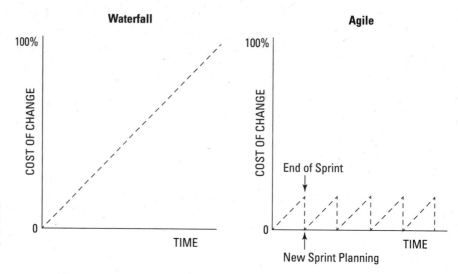

Waterfall

Agile

FIGURE 2-1:
Traditional
project
opportunity
for change.

As new events unfold, the project team incorporates those realities into the ongoing work. Any new item becomes an opportunity to provide additional value instead of an obstacle to avoid, giving development teams a greater opportunity for success.

Defining the 12 Agile Principles

In the months following the publication of the Agile Manifesto, the original signatories continued to communicate. To support teams making agile transitions, they augmented the four values of the manifesto with 12 principles behind the Agile Manifesto.

REMEMBER

These principles, along with the Platinum Principles (explained later in the "Adding the Platinum Principles" section) can be used as a litmus test to see whether the specific practices of your project team are true to the intent of the agile movement.

Following is the text of the original 12 principles, published in 2001 by the Agile Alliance:

1. Our highest priority is to satisfy the customer through early and continuous delivery of valuable software.

2. Welcome changing requirements, even late in development. Agile processes harness change for the customer's competitive advantage.

3. Deliver working software frequently, from a couple of weeks to a couple of months, with a preference to the shorter timescale.

4. Business people and developers must work together daily throughout the project.

5. Build projects around motivated individuals. Give them the environment and support they need, and trust them to get the job done.

6. The most efficient and effective method of conveying information to and within a development team is face-to-face conversation.

7. Working software is the primary measure of progress.

8. Agile processes promote sustainable development. The sponsors, developers, and users should be able to maintain a constant pace indefinitely.

9. Continuous attention to technical excellence and good design enhances agility.

10. Simplicity — the art of maximizing the amount of work not done — is essential.

11. The best architectures, requirements, and designs emerge from self-organizing teams.

12. At regular intervals, the team reflects on how to become more effective, then tunes and adjusts its behavior accordingly.

These agile principles provide practical guidance for development teams.

Another way of organizing the 12 principles is to consider them in the following four distinct groups:

>> Customer satisfaction

>> Quality

>> Teamwork

>> Project management

The following sections discuss the principles according to these groups.

Agile principles of customer satisfaction

Agile approaches focus on customer satisfaction, which makes sense. After all, the customer is the reason for developing the product in the first place.

While all 12 principles support the goal of satisfying customers, principles 1, 2, 3, and 4 stand out for us:

1. Our highest priority is to satisfy the customer through early and continuous delivery of valuable software.

2. Welcome changing requirements, even late in development. Agile processes harness change for the customer's competitive advantage.

3. Deliver working software frequently, from a couple of weeks to a couple of months, with a preference to the shorter timescale.

4. Business people and developers must work together daily throughout the project.

You may define the customer on a project in a number of ways:

» In project management terms, the customer is the person or group paying for the project.

» In some organizations, the customer may be a client, external to the organization.

» In other organizations, the customer may be a project stakeholder or stakeholders in the organization.

» The person who ends up using the product is also a customer. For clarity and to be consistent with the original 12 agile principles, in this book, we call that person *the user*.

How do you enact these principles? Simply do the following:

» Agile project teams include a *product owner*, a person who is responsible for ensuring translation of what the customer wants into product requirements.

» The product owner prioritizes product features in order of business value or risk and communicates priorities to the development team. The development team delivers the most valuable features on the list in short cycles of development, known as *iterations* or *sprints*.

» The product owner has deep and ongoing involvement throughout each day to clarify priorities and requirements, make decisions, provide feedback, and quickly answer the many questions that pop up during a project.

» Frequent delivery of working functionality allows the product owner and the customer to have a full sense of how the product is developing.

>> As the development team continues to deliver complete, working, potentially shippable functionality every four to eight weeks or less, the value of the total product grows incrementally, as do its functional capabilities.

>> The customer accumulates value for his or her investment regularly by receiving new, ready-to-use functionality throughout the project, rather than waiting until the end of what might be a long project for the first, and maybe only, delivery of releasable product features.

In Table 2-3, we list some customer satisfaction issues that commonly arise on projects. Use Table 2-3 and gather some examples of customer dissatisfaction that you've encountered. Do you think agile project management would make a difference? Why or why not?

TABLE 2-3 **Customer Dissatisfaction and How Agile Might Help**

Examples of Customer Dissatisfaction with Projects	How Agile Approaches Can Increase Customer Satisfaction
The product requirements were misunderstood by the development team.	Product owners work closely with the customer to define and refine product requirements and provide clarity to the development team.
	Agile project teams demonstrate and deliver working functionality at regular intervals. If a product doesn't work the way the customer thinks it should work, the customer is able to provide feedback at the end of the sprint, not before it's too late at the end of the project.
The product wasn't delivered when the customer needed it.	Working in sprints allows agile project teams to deliver high-priority functionality early and often.
The customer can't request changes without additional cost and time.	Agile processes are built for change. Development teams can accommodate new requirements, requirement updates, and shifting priorities with each sprint, offsetting the cost of these changes by removing the lowest-priority requirements — functionality that likely will never or rarely get used.

You can find a blank template of the form at www.dummies.com/go/agile projectmanagementfd2e.

Agile strategies for customer satisfaction include the following:

>> Producing, in each iteration, the highest-priority features first

>> Ideally, locating the product owner and the other members of the project team in the same place to eliminate communication barriers

>> Breaking requirements into groups of features that can be delivered in four to eight weeks or less

>> Keeping written requirements sparse, forcing more robust and effective face-to-face communication

>> Getting the product owner's approval as functionality is completed

>> Revisiting the feature list regularly to ensure that the most valuable requirements continue to have the highest priority

Agile principles of quality

An agile project team commits to producing quality in every product it creates — from development through documentation to integration and test results — every day. Each project team member contributes his or her best work all the time. Although all 12 principles support the goal of quality delivery, principles 1, 3, 4, 6–9, and 12 stand out for us:

1. Our highest priority is to satisfy the customer through early and continuous delivery of valuable software.

3. Deliver working software frequently, from a couple of weeks to a couple of months, with a preference to the shorter timescale.

4. Business people and developers must work together daily throughout the project.

6. The most efficient and effective method of conveying information to and within a development team is face-to-face conversation.

7. Working software is the primary measure of progress.

8. Agile processes promote sustainable development. The sponsors, developers, and users should be able to maintain a constant pace indefinitely.

9. Continuous attention to technical excellence and good design enhances agility.

12. At regular intervals, the team reflects on how to become more effective, then tunes and adjusts its behavior accordingly.

These principles, in practice on a day-to-day basis, can be described as follows:

>> The development team members must have full ownership and be empowered to solve problems. They carry the responsibility for determining how to create the product, assigning tasks, and organizing product development. People not doing the work don't tell them how to do it.

>> With software development projects, an agile approach requires architectures that make coding and the product modular, flexible, and extensible. The design should address today's problems and make inevitable changes as simple as possible.

- A set of designs on paper can never tell you that something will work. When the product quality is such that it can be demonstrated and ultimately shipped in short intervals, everyone knows that the product works — at the end of every sprint.

- As the development team completes features, the team shows the product owner the product functionality to get validation that it meets the acceptance criteria. The product owner's reviews should happen throughout the iteration, ideally the same day that development of the requirement was completed.

- At the end of every iteration (lasting one to four weeks or less), working code is demonstrated to the customer. Progress is clear and easy to measure.

- Testing is an integral, ongoing part of development and happens throughout the day, not at the end of the iteration.

- On software projects, checking that new code is tested and integrates with previous versions occurs in small increments and may even occur several times a day (or thousands of times a day in some organizations, such as Google, Amazon, and Facebook). This process, called *continuous integration (CI),* helps ensure that the entire solution continues to work when new code is added to the existing code base.

- On software projects, examples of technical excellence include establishing coding standards, using service-oriented architecture, implementing automated testing, and building for future change.

TIP

Agile approaches provide the following strategies for quality management:

- Defining what *done* means at the beginning of the project and then using that definition as a benchmark for quality

- Testing aggressively and daily through automated means

- Building only the functionality that is needed when it's needed

- Reviewing the software code and streamlining (refactoring)

- Showcasing to stakeholders and customers only the functionality that has been accepted by the product owner

- Having multiple feedback points throughout the day, iteration, and project

Agile principles of teamwork

Teamwork is critical to agile projects. Creating good products requires cooperation among all the members of the project team, including customers and stakeholders. Agile approaches support team-building and teamwork, and they emphasize trust in self-managing development teams. A skilled, motivated, unified, and empowered project team is a successful team.

Although all 12 principles support the goal of teamwork, principles 4–6, 8, 11, and 12 stand out for us as supporting team empowerment, efficiency, and excellence:

4. Business people and developers must work together daily throughout the project.

5. Build projects around motivated individuals. Give them the environment and support they need, and trust them to get the job done.

6. The most efficient and effective method of conveying information to and within a development team is face-to-face conversation.

8. Agile processes promote sustainable development. The sponsors, developers, and users should be able to maintain a constant pace indefinitely.

11. The best architectures, requirements, and designs emerge from self-organizing teams.

12. At regular intervals, the team reflects on how to become more effective, then tunes and adjusts its behavior accordingly.

TIP

Agile approaches focus on sustainable development; as knowledge workers, our brains are the value we bring to a project. If only for selfish reasons, organizations should want fresh, well-rested brains working for them. Maintaining a regular work pace, rather than having periods of intense overwork, helps keep team members' minds sharp and quality high.

Here are some practices you can adopt to make this vision of teamwork a reality:

>> Ensure that your development team members have the proper skills and motivation.

>> Provide training sufficient to the task.

>> Support the self-organizing development team's decisions about what to do and how to do it; don't have managers tell the team what to do.

>> Hold project team members responsible as a single team, not individuals.

>> Use face-to-face communication to quickly and efficiently convey information.

WARNING

Suppose that you usually communicate by email to Sharon. You take time to craft your message and then send it. The message sits in Sharon's inbox, and she eventually reads it. If Sharon has any questions, she writes an email in response and sends it. That message sits in your inbox until you eventually read it. And so forth. This type of table tennis communication is too inefficient to use in the middle of a rapid iteration.

>> Have spontaneous conversations throughout the day to build knowledge, understanding, and efficiency.

>> Collocate teammates in close proximity to increase clear and efficient communication. If collocation isn't possible, use video chat rather than email.

>> Make sure that *lessons learned* is an ongoing feedback loop. Retrospectives should be held at the end of each iteration, when reflection and adaptation can improve development team productivity going forward, creating ever higher levels of efficiency. A lessons learned meeting at the end of a project is of minimal value.

The first retrospective is often the most valuable because, at that point, the project team has the opportunity to make changes to benefit the rest of the project moving forward.

TIP

The following strategies promote effective teamwork:

>> Place the development team in the same location — this is called *collocation*.

>> Put together a physical environment that's conducive for collaboration: a team room with whiteboards, colored pens, and other tactile tools for developing and conveying ideas to ensure shared understanding.

>> Create an environment where project team members are encouraged to speak their minds.

>> Meet face-to-face whenever possible. Don't send an email if a conversation can handle the issue.

>> Get clarifications throughout the day as they're needed.

>> Encourage the development team to solve problems rather than having managers solve problems for the development team.

Agile principles of project management

Agility in project management encompasses three key areas:

>> Making sure the development team can be productive and can sustainably increase productivity over long periods of time

>> Ensuring that information about the project's progress is available to stakeholders without interrupting the flow of development activities by asking the development team for updates

>> Handling requests for new features as they occur and integrating them into the product development cycle

An agile approach focuses on planning and executing the work to produce the best product that can be released. The approach is supported by communicating openly, avoiding distractions and wasteful activities, and ensuring that the progress of the project is clear to everyone.

All 12 principles support project management, but principles 2, 8, and 10 stand out for us:

2. Welcome changing requirements, even late in development. Agile processes harness change for the customer's competitive advantage.

8. Agile processes promote sustainable development. The sponsors, developers, and users should be able to maintain a constant pace indefinitely.

10. Simplicity — the art of maximizing the amount of work not done — is essential.

Following are some advantages of adopting agile project management:

>> Agile project teams achieve faster time-to-market, and consequentially cost savings. They start development earlier than in traditional approaches because agile approaches minimize the exhaustive upfront planning and documentation that is conventionally part of the early stages of a water-fall project.

>> Agile development teams are self-organizing and self-managing. The managerial effort normally put into telling developers how to do their work can be applied to removing impediments and organizational distractions that slow down the development team.

>> Agile development teams determine how much work they can accomplish in an iteration and commit to achieving those goals. Ownership is fundamentally different because the development team is establishing the commitment, not complying with an externally developed commitment.

>> An agile approach asks, "What is the minimum we can do to achieve the goal?" instead of focusing on including all the features and extra refinements that could possibly be needed. An agile approach usually means streamlining: barely sufficient documentation, removal of unnecessary meetings, avoidance of inefficient communication (such as email), and less coding (just enough to make it work).

WARNING

Creating complicated documents that aren't useful for product development is a waste of effort. It's okay to document a decision, but you don't need multiple pages on the history and nuances of how the decision was made. Keep the documentation barely sufficient, and you will have more time to focus on supporting the development team.

>> By encapsulating development into short sprints that last one to four weeks or less, you can adhere to the goals of the current iteration while accommodating change in subsequent iterations. The length of each sprint remains the same throughout the project to provide a predictable rhythm of development for the team long-term.

>> Planning, elaborating on requirements, developing, testing, and demonstrating functionality occur within an iteration, lowering the risk of heading in the wrong direction for extended periods of time or developing something that the customer doesn't want.

>> Agile practices encourage a steady pace of development that is productive and healthy. For example, in the popular agile development set of practices called extreme programming (XP), the maximum workweek is 40 hours, and the preferred workweek is 35 hours. Agile projects are sustainable and more productive, especially long term.

WARNING

Traditional approaches routinely feature a *death march,* in which the project team puts in extremely long hours for days and even weeks at the end of a project to meet a previously unidentified and unrealistic deadline. As the death march goes on, productivity tends to drop dramatically. More defects are introduced, and because defects need to be corrected in a way that doesn't break a different piece of functionality, correcting defects is the most expensive work that can be performed. Defects are often the result of overloading a system — specifically demanding an unsustainable pace of work. Check out our presentation on the negative effects of "Racing in Reverse" (https://platinumedge.com/overtime).

>> Priorities, experience on the existing project, and, eventually, the speed at which development will likely occur within each sprint are clear, making for good decisions about how much can or should be accomplished in a given amount of time.

If you've worked on a project before, you might have a basic understanding of project management activities. In Table 2-4, we list a few traditional project management tasks, along with how you would meet those needs with agile approaches. Use Table 2-4 to capture your thoughts about your experiences and how agile approaches looks different from traditional project management.

ON THE WEB

A blank template of Table 2-4 is available at www.dummies.com/go/agile projectmanagementfd2e.

TABLE 2-4 **Contrasting Historical Project Management with Agile Project Management**

Traditional Project Management Tasks	Agile Approach to the Project Management Task
Create a fully detailed project requirement document at the beginning of the project. Try to control requirement changes throughout the project.	Create a product backlog — a simple list of requirements by priority. Quickly update the product backlog as requirements and priorities change throughout the project.
Conduct weekly status meetings with all project stakeholders and developers. Send out detailed meeting notes and status reports after each meeting.	The development team meets quickly, for no longer than 15 minutes, at the start of each day to coordinate and synchronize that day's work and any roadblocks. They can update the centrally visible burndown chart in under a minute at the end of each day.
Create a detailed project schedule with all tasks at the beginning of the project. Try to keep the project tasks on schedule. Update the schedule on a regular basis.	Work within sprints and identify only specific tasks for the active sprint.
Assign tasks to the development team.	Support the development team by helping remove impediments and distractions. On agile projects, development teams define and pull (as opposed to push) their own tasks.

TIP

Project management is facilitated by the following agile approaches:

>> Supporting the development team

>> Producing barely sufficient documents

>> Streamlining status reporting so that information is pushed out by the development team in seconds rather than pulled out by a project manager over a longer period of time

>> Minimizing nondevelopment tasks

>> Setting expectations that change is normal and beneficial, not something to be feared or evaded

>> Adopting a just-in-time requirements refinement to minimize change disruption and wasted effort

>> Collaborating with the development team to create realistic schedules, targets, and goals

>> Protecting the development team from organizational disruptions that could undermine project goals by introducing work not relevant to the project objectives

>> Understanding that an appropriate balance between work and life is a component of efficient development

Adding the Platinum Principles

Through in-the-trenches experience working with teams transitioning to agile project management — and field testing in large, medium, and small organizations worldwide — we developed three additional principles of agile software development that we call the Platinum Principles. They are

>> Resist formality.

>> Think and act as a team.

>> Visualize rather than write.

You can explore each principle in more detail in the following sections.

Resisting formality

Even the most agile project teams can drift toward excessive formalization. For example, it isn't uncommon for us to find project team members waiting until a scheduled meeting to discuss simple issues that could be solved in seconds. These meetings often have an agenda and meeting minutes and require a certain level of mobilization and demobilization just to attend. In an agile approach, this level of formalization isn't required.

WARNING

You should always question formalization and unnecessary, showy displays. For example, is there an easier way to get what you need? How does the current activity support the development of a quality product as quickly as possible? Answering these questions helps you focus on productive work and avoid unnecessary tasks.

In an agile system, discussions and the physical work environment are open and free-flowing; documentation is kept to the lowest level of quantity and complexity such that it contributes value to the project, not hampers it; flashy displays, such as well-decorated presentations, are avoided. Professional, frank communications are best for the project team, and the entire environment has to make that openness available and comfortable.

TIP

Strategies for success with resisting formality include the following:

>> Reducing organizational hierarchy wherever possible by eliminating titles in the project team

>> Avoiding aesthetic investments such as elaborate PowerPoint presentations or extensive meeting minute forms, especially when demonstrating shippable functionality at the end of a sprint

>> Identifying and educating stakeholders who may request complicated displays of work on the costs of such displays

Thinking and acting as a team

Project team members should focus on how the team as a whole can be most productive. This focus can mean letting go of individual niches and performance metrics. In an agile environment, the entire project team should be aligned in its commitment to the goal, its ownership of the scope of work, and its acknowledgment of the time available to achieve that commitment.

Following are some strategies for thinking and acting as a team:

>> Develop in pairs and switch partners often. Both pair programming (both partners are knowledgeable in the area) and shadowing (only one partner is knowledgeable in the area) raise product quality. You can learn more about pair programming in Chapter 15.

>> Replace individual work titles with a uniform product developer title. Development activities include all tasks required to take requirements through to functionality, including design, implementation (coding), testing, and documentation, not just writing code or turning a screwdriver.

>> Report at the project team level only, as opposed to creating special management reports that subdivide the team.

>> Replace individual performance metrics with project team performance metrics.

Visualizing rather than writing

An agile project team should use visualization as much as possible, whether through simple diagrams or computerized modeling tools. Images are much more powerful than words. When you use a diagram or mockup instead of a document, your customer can relate better to the concept and the content.

Our ability to define the features of a system increases exponentially when we step up our interaction with the proposed solution: A graphical representation is almost always better than a textual one, and experiencing functionality hands-on is best.

TIP

Even a sketch on a piece of paper can be a more effective communication tool than a formal text-based document. A picture is worth a thousand words. A textual description is the weakest form of communication if you're trying to ensure common understanding — especially when it's delivered by email with the request to "let me know if you have any questions."

CHANGES TO COME

Enterprises are leveraging agile techniques on a large-scale basis to solve business problems. Although the methodologies of agile IT groups, as well as non-IT groups, have undergone radical transformation, the organizations around these groups have often continued to use historical methodologies and concepts. For example, corporate funding and spending cycles are still geared toward the following:

- Long development efforts that deliver working software at the end of the project
- Annual budgeting
- An assumption that certainty is possible at the beginning of a project
- Corporate incentive packages focused on individual rather than team performance

The resulting tension keeps organizations from taking full advantage of the efficiency and significant savings that agile techniques promise.

A truly integrated agile approach encourages organizations to move away from yesterday's traditions and develop a structure at all levels that continually asks what's best for the customer, the product, and the project team.

An agile project team can be only as agile as the organization it serves. As the movement continues to evolve, the values articulated in the Agile Manifesto and its principles provide a strong foundation for the changes necessary to make individual projects and entire organizations more productive and profitable. This evolution will be driven by passionate practitioners who continue to explore and apply agile principles and practices.

Examples of strategies for visualization include the following:

- ❯❯ Stocking the work environment with plenty of whiteboards, poster paper, pens, and paper so that drawing tools are readily available
- ❯❯ Using models instead of text to communicate concepts
- ❯❯ Reporting project status through charts, graphs, and dashboards, such as those in Figure 2-2.

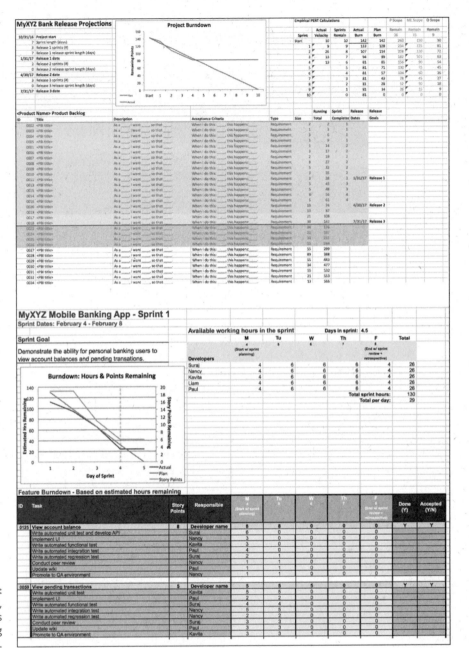

FIGURE 2-2: Charts, graphs, and dashboards for reporting project status.

Changes as a Result of Agile Values

The publication of the Agile Manifesto and the 12 Agile Principles legitimized and focused the agile movement in the following ways:

>> **Agile approaches changed attitudes toward project management processes.** In trying to improve processes, methodologists in the past worked to develop a universal process that could be used under all conditions, assuming that more process and greater formality would yield improved results. This approach, however, required more time, overhead, and cost and often diminished quality. The manifesto and the 12 principles acknowledged that too much process is a problem, not a solution, and that the right process in the right amount differs in each situation.

>> **Agile approaches changed attitudes toward knowledge workers.** IT groups began to remember that development team members aren't disposable resources but individuals whose skills, talents, and innovation make a difference to every project. The same product created by different team members will be a different product.

>> **Agile approaches changed the relationship between business and IT groups.** Agile project management addressed the problems associated with the historical separation between business and IT by bringing these contributors together on the same project team, at equal levels of involvement and with shared goals.

>> **Agile approaches corrected attitudes toward change.** Historical approaches viewed change as a problem to be avoided or minimized. The Agile Manifesto and its principles helped identify change as an opportunity to ensure that the most informed ideas were implemented.

The Agile Litmus Test

To be agile, you need to be able to ask, "Is this agile?" If you're ever in doubt about whether a particular process, practice, tool, or approach adheres to the Agile Manifesto or the 12 principles, refer to the following list of questions:

1. Does what we're doing at this moment support the early and continuous delivery of valuable software?

2. Does our process welcome and take advantage of change?

3. Does our process lead to and support the delivery of working functionality?

4. Are the developers and the product owner working together daily? Are customers and business stakeholders working closely with the project team?

5. Does our environment give the development team the support it needs to get the job done?

6. Are we communicating face to face more than through phone and email?

7. Are we measuring progress by the amount of working functionality produced?

8. Can we maintain this pace indefinitely?

9. Do we support technical excellence and good design that allows for future changes?

10. Are we maximizing the amount of work not done — namely, doing as little as necessary to fulfill the goal of the project?

11. Is this development team self-organizing and self-managing? Does it have the freedom to succeed?

12. Are we reflecting at regular intervals and adjusting our behavior accordingly?

If you answered "yes" to all these questions, congratulations; you're truly working on an agile project. If you answered "no" to any of these questions, what can you do to change that answer to "yes"? You can come back to this exercise at any time and use the agile litmus test with your project team and the wider organization.

Chapter **3**

Why Being Agile Works Better

A gile approaches work well in the real world. Why is this? In this chapter, you examine the mechanics of how agile processes improve the way people work and how they prevent burdensome overhead. Comparisons with historical methods highlight the improvements agile techniques bring.

When talking about agile project management advantages, the bottom line is two-fold: project success and stakeholder satisfaction.

Evaluating Agile Benefits

The agile concept of project management is different from previous methodologies. As mentioned in Chapter 1, agile approaches address key challenges of historical project management methods such as waterfall, but they also go much deeper. Agile processes provide a framework for how we *want* to work — how we naturally function when we solve problems and complete tasks.

Historical methods of project management were developed not for contemporary development lifecycles, such as software development, but for less complex systems. They also were adapted from other spheres, such as construction, manufacturing, and the military. It's no wonder that these project management methods don't fit when attempting to build more complex, modern products, such as mobile applications or web-centric, object-oriented applications, which require constant innovation to stay competitive. Even with older technologies, the track record of traditional methodologies is abysmal, especially when applied to software projects. For more details on the high failure rates of projects that are run traditionally, check out the studies from the Standish Group shown in Chapter 1.

REMEMBER

You can use agile project management techniques in many industries besides software development. If you're creating a product and want early feedback throughout the process, you can benefit from agile processes.

When you have a critical looming deadline, your instinct is to *go agile.* Formality goes out of the window as you roll up your sleeves and focus on what has to get done. You solve problems quickly, practically, and in descending order of necessity, making sure you complete the most critical tasks.

More than going agile — it's about *being agile.* When you become agile, you don't institute unreasonable deadlines to force greater focus. Instead, you realize that people function well as practical problem solvers, even under stress. For example, a popular team-building exercise titled the *marshmallow challenge* involves groups of four people building the tallest free-standing structure possible out of 20 sticks of spaghetti, a yard of tape, and a yard of string, and then placing a marshmallow on the top — in 18 minutes. See www.marshmallowchallenge.com for background information about the concept. On that site, you can also view the associated TED Talk by Tom Wujec.

Wujec points out that young children usually build taller and more interesting structures than most adults because children build incrementally on a series of successful structures in the time allotted. Adults spend a lot of time planning, produce one final version, and then run out of time to correct any mistakes. The youngsters provide a valuable lesson that *big bang development* — namely, excessive planning and then one shot at product creation — doesn't work. Formality, excessive time detailing uninformed future steps, and a single plan are often detriments to success.

The marshmallow challenge sets opening conditions that mimic those in real life. You build a structure (which equates to a software product in the IT industry) using fixed resources (four people, spaghetti, and so on) and a fixed time (18 minutes). What you end up with is anyone's guess, but an underlying assumption in historical project management approaches is that you can determine the precise destination (the features or requirements) in the beginning and then estimate the people, resources, and time required.

This assumption is upside down from how life really is. As you can see in Figure 3-1, the theories of historical methods are the reverse of agile approaches.

We pretend that we live in the world on the left, but we actually live in the world on the right.

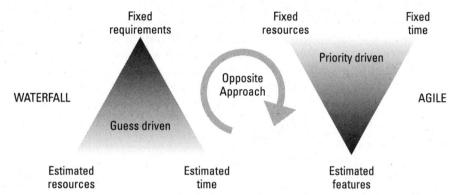

FIGURE 3-1:
A comparison of historical project management and agile concepts.

In the historical approach, which locks the requirements and delivers the product all in one go, the result is all or nothing. We either succeed completely or fail absolutely. The stakes are high because everything hinges on work that happens at the end (that is, putting the marshmallow on the top) of the final phase of the cycle, which includes integration and customer testing.

In Figure 3-2, you can see how each phase of a waterfall project is dependent on the previous one. Teams design and develop all features together, meaning you don't get the highest-priority feature until you've finished developing the lowest-priority feature. The customer has to wait until the end of the project to get final delivery of any element of the product.

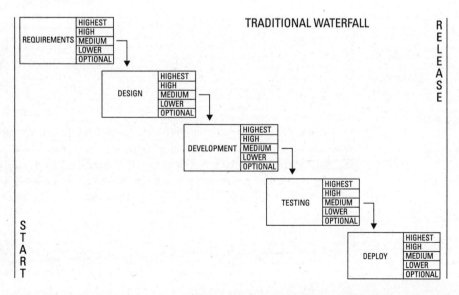

FIGURE 3-2:
The waterfall project cycle is a linear methodology.

In the testing phase of a waterfall project, the customers get to see their long-awaited product. By that time, the investment and effort have been huge, and the risk of failure is high. Finding defects among all completed product requirements is like looking for a weed in a cornfield.

Agile project management turns the concept of how software development should be done upside down. Using agile methods, you develop, test, and launch small groups of product requirements in short iterative cycles, known as *iterations,* or *sprints,* as illustrated in Figure 3-3. Testing occurs during each iteration. To find defects, the development team looks for a weed in a flowerpot, rather than in a cornfield.

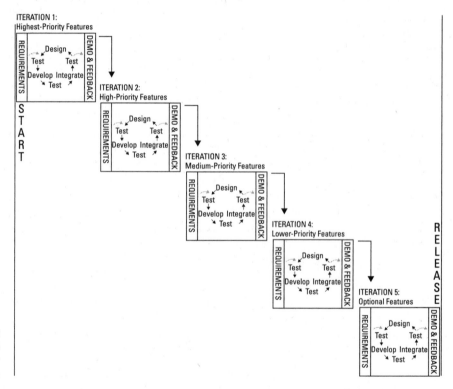

FIGURE 3-3:
Agile approaches
have an iterative
project cycle.

Product owner, scrum master, and *sprint* are terms from *scrum,* a popular agile framework for organizing work and exposing project progress. *Scrum* refers to a rugby huddle, in which a rugby team locks together over the ball. Scrum as an approach, like rugby, encourages the project team to work together closely and take responsibility for the result. (You find out more about scrum and other agile techniques in Chapter 4.)

WHERE THE WATERFALL FALLS SHORT

As we mention in Chapter 1, before 2008, waterfall was the most widely used traditional project management methodology. The following list summarizes the major aspects of the waterfall approach to project management:

- The team must know all requirements up front to estimate time, budgets, team members, and resources. Knowing all the requirements at the project start means you have a high investment in detailed requirements gathering before any development begins.

- Estimation is complex and requires a high degree of competence and experience and a lot of effort to complete.

- The customer and stakeholders may not be available to answer questions during the development period, because they may assume that they provided all the information needed during the requirements-gathering and design phases.

- The team needs to resist the addition of new requirements or document them as change orders, which adds more work to the project and extends the schedule and budget.

- The team must create and maintain volumes of process documentation to manage and control the project.

- Although some testing can be done as you go, final testing can't be completed until the end of the project, when all functionality has been developed and integrated.

- Full and complete customer feedback is not possible until the end of the project, when all functionality is complete.

- Funding is ongoing, but the value appears only at the end of the project, creating a high level of risk.

- The project has to be fully complete for value to be achieved. If funding runs out prior to the end of the project, the project delivers zero value.

Moreover, on an agile project, the customers get to see their product at the end of every short cycle. You can create the highest-priority features first, which gives you the opportunity to ensure maximum value early on, when less of the customer's money has been invested.

This agile concept is attractive, especially to risk-averse organizations. In addition, if your product has market value, revenue can be coming in even during development. Now you have a self-funding project!

How Agile Approaches Beat Historical Approaches

Agile frameworks promise significant advantages over historical methods, including greater flexibility and stability, less nonproductive work, faster delivery with higher quality, improved development team performance, tighter project control, and faster failure detection. We describe all these results in this section.

However, these results can't be achieved without a highly competent and functional development team. The development team is pivotal to the success of the project. Agile methods emphasize the importance of the support provided to the development team as well as the importance of project team members' actions and interactions.

REMEMBER

The first core value in the Agile Manifesto is "Individuals and interactions over processes and tools." Nurturing the development team is central to agile project management and the reason why you can have such success with agile approaches.

Agile project teams are centered on development teams (which include developers, testers, designers, and anyone else who does the actual work of creating the product), and also include project stakeholders, as well as the following two important team members, without which the development team couldn't function:

>> **Product owner:** The *product owner* is a project team member who is an expert on the product and the customer's business needs. The product owner works with the business community and prioritizes product requirements, and supports the development team by being available to provide daily clarifications and final acceptance to the development team. (Chapter 2 has more on the product owner.)

>> **Scrum master or agile coach:** The *scrum master or agile coach* acts as a buffer between the development team and distractions that might slow down the development effort. The scrum master also provides expertise on agile processes and helps remove obstacles that hinder the development team from making progress. The scrum master or agile coach facilitates consensus building and stakeholder communication.

You can find complete descriptions of the product owner, the development team, and the scrum master in Chapter 6. Later in this chapter, you see how the product owner and scrum master's highest priority is supporting and optimizing the development team's performance.

Greater flexibility and stability

By way of comparison, agile projects offer both greater flexibility and greater stability than traditional projects. First, you find out how agile projects offer flexibility, and then we discuss stability.

A project team, regardless of its project management approach, faces two significant challenges at the beginning of a project:

>> The project team has limited knowledge of the product end state.

>> The project team cannot predict the future.

This limited knowledge of the product and of future business needs almost guarantees project changes.

The fourth core value in the Agile Manifesto is "Responding to change over following a plan." The agile framework was created with flexibility in mind.

With agile approaches, project teams can adapt to new knowledge and new requirements that emerge as the project progresses. We provide many details about the agile processes that enable flexibility throughout this book. Here's a simple description of some processes that help agile project teams manage change:

>> At the start of an agile project, the product owner gathers high-level product requirements from project stakeholders and prioritizes them. The product owner doesn't need all the requirements — just enough to have a good understanding of what the product must accomplish.

>> The development team and the product owner work together to break down the initial highest-priority requirements into more detailed requirements. The result is small chunks of work that the development team can start developing immediately.

>> You focus on the top priorities in each sprint regardless of how soon before the sprint those priorities were set.

Iterations, or sprints, on agile projects are short — they last up to four weeks, and are often one or two weeks. You can find details about sprints in Chapters 8–10.

>> The development team works on groups of requirements within sprints and learns more about the product with each successive sprint.

>> The development team plans one sprint at a time and drills further into requirements at the beginning of each sprint. The development team generally works only on the highest-priority requirements.

>> Concentrating on one sprint at a time and on the highest-priority require-ments allows the project team to accommodate new high-priority require-ments at the beginning of each sprint.

>> When changes arise, the product owner updates a list of requirements that remains to be dealt with in future sprints. The product owner reprioritizes the list regularly.

>> The product owner can financially invest in high-priority features first and can choose which features to fund throughout the project.

>> The product owner and development team collect client feedback at the end of each sprint and act on that feedback. Client feedback often leads to changes to existing functionality or to new, valuable requirements. Feedback can also lead to removing or reprioritizing requirements that are not really necessary.

>> The product owner can stop the project once he or she deems that the product has sufficient functionality to fulfill project goals.

Figure 3-4 illustrates how making changes on agile projects can be more stable than making changes in waterfall. Think of the two images in the figure as steel bars. In the top image, the bar represents a two-year project. The bar's length makes it much easier to distort, bend, and break. Project changes can be thought of in the same way — long projects are structurally vulnerable to instability because the planning stage of a project is different than the execution, when real-ity sets in, and there is no natural point of give in a long project.

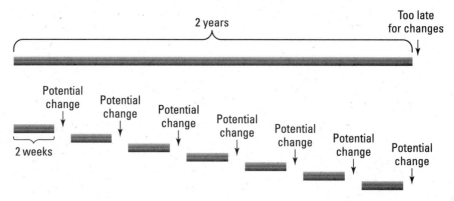

FIGURE 3-4:
Stability in
flexibility on
agile projects.

Now look at the bottom image in Figure 3-4. The small steel bars represent two-week iterations within a project. It is much easier for those small bars to be stable and unchanging than it is for the larger bar. In the same manner, it is easier to have project stability in smaller increments with known flexibility points.

Telling a business there can be no changes for two weeks is much easier and more realistic than saying there can be no changes for two years.

Agile projects are tactically flexible because they are strategically stable. They're great at accommodating change because the means for regular change are built into everyday processes. At the same time, iterations on agile projects offer distinct areas for project stability. Agile project teams accommodate changes to the product backlog anytime but do not generally accommodate external changes to scope during the sprint. The product backlog may be constantly changing, but, except in emergencies, the sprint is generally stable.

At the beginning of the iteration, the development team plans the work it will complete for that sprint. After the sprint begins, the development team works only on the planned requirements. A couple of exceptions to this plan can occur — if the development team finishes early, it can request more work; if an emergency arises, the product owner can cancel the sprint. In general, however, the sprint is a time of great stability for the development team.

This stability can lead to innovation. When development team members have stability — that is, they know what they will be working on in a set period of time — they will think about their tasks consciously at work. They may also think about tasks unconsciously away from work and tend to come up with solutions at any given time.

Agile projects provide a constant cycle of development, feedback, and change, allowing project teams the flexibility to create products with only the right features and the stability to be creative.

Reduced nonproductive tasks

When you're creating a product, at any point in your working day, you can work either on developing the product or on the peripheral processes that are supposed to manage and control the creation of the product. Clearly, there's more value in the first, which you should try to maximize, than in the second, which you want to minimize.

To finish a project, you have to work on the solution. As obvious as this statement sounds, it's routinely neglected on waterfall projects. Programmers on some software projects spend only 20 percent of their time generating functionality, with the rest of the time in meetings, writing emails, or creating unnecessary presentations and documentation.

Product development can be an intense activity that requires sustained periods of focus. Many developers can't get enough development time during their normal workday to keep up with the schedule of a project because they're doing other types of tasks. The following causal chain is the result:

Long workday = tired developers = unnecessary defects = more defect fixing = delayed release = longer time to value

To maximize productive work, the goal is to eliminate overtime and have developers creating functionality during the working day. To increase productive work, you have to reduce unproductive tasks, period.

Meetings

Meetings can be a large waste of valuable time. On traditional projects, development team members may find themselves in long meetings that provide little or no benefit to the developers. The following agile approaches can help ensure that development teams spend time only in productive, meaningful meetings:

» Agile processes include only a few formal meetings. These meetings are focused, with specific topics and limited time. On agile projects, you generally don't need to attend non-agile meetings.

» Part of the scrum master's job is to prevent disruptions to the development team's working time, including requests for non-agile meetings. When there's a demand to pull developers away from development work, the scrum master asks "why" to understand the true need. The scrum master then may figure out how to satisfy that need without disrupting the development team.

» On agile projects, the current project status is often visually available to the entire organization, removing the need for status meetings. You can find ways to streamline status reporting in Chapter 14.

Email

Email is not an efficient mode of communication; agile project teams aim to use email only sparingly. The email process is asynchronous and slow: You send an email, you wait for an answer; you have another question, you send another email. This process eats up time that could be spent more productively.

Instead of sending emails, agile project teams use face-to-face discussions to resolve questions and issues on the spot.

Presentations

When preparing for a presentation of the functionality to the customer, agile project teams often use the following techniques:

>> **Demonstrate, don't present.** In other words, show the customer what you've created, rather than describing what you've created.

>> **Show how the functionality delivers on the requirement and fulfills the acceptance criteria.** In other words, say, "This was the requirement. These are the criteria needed to indicate that the feature was complete. Here is the resulting functionality meeting those criteria."

>> **Avoid formal slide presentations and all the preparation they involve.** When you demonstrate the working functionality, it will speak for itself. Keep demonstrations raw and real.

Process documentation

Documentation has been the burden of project managers and developers for a long time. Agile project teams can minimize documentation with the following approaches:

>> **Use iterative development.** A lot of documentation is created to reference decisions made months or years ago. Iterative development shortens the time between decision and developed product from months or years to days. The product and associated automated tests, rather than extensive paperwork, documents the decisions made.

>> **Remember that one size doesn't fit all.** You don't have to create the same documents for every project. Choose what you need to fit the particular project.

>> **Use informal, flexible documentation tools.** Whiteboards, sticky notes, charts, and other visual representations of the work plan are great tools.

>> **Include simple tools that provide adequate information for management about project progress.** Don't create special project progress reports, such as extensive status reports, for the sake of reporting. Agile teams use visual charts, such as burndown charts, to readily convey project status.

Higher quality, delivered faster

On traditional projects, the period from completion of requirements gathering to the beginning of customer testing can be painfully long. During this time, the customer is waiting to see some sort of result, and the development team is wrapped up in developing. The project manager is making sure that the project team is following the plan, keeping changes at bay, and updating everyone with an interest in the outcome by providing frequent and detailed reports.

When testing starts, near the end of the project, defects can cause budget increases, create schedule delays, and even kill a project. Testing is a project's largest unknown, and in traditional projects, it is an unknown carried until the end.

Agile project management is designed to deliver high-quality, shippable functionality quickly. Agile projects achieve better quality and quick delivery with the following:

>> The client reviews working functionality at the end of each sprint, and gives immediate feedback to the team for inspection and adaptation as soon as the next sprint.

>> Short development iterations (sprints) limit the number and complexity of features in development at any given time, making the finished work easier to test in each sprint. Only so much can be created in each sprint. Development teams break down features too complex for one sprint.

>> The development team builds and tests daily and maintains a working product throughout the project.

>> The product owner is involved throughout the day to answer questions and clarify misunderstandings quickly.

>> The development team is empowered and motivated and has a reasonable workday. Because the development team is not worn out, fewer defects occur.

>> Errors are detected quickly because developers test their work as it's completed. Extensive automated testing happens frequently, at least every night.

>> Modern software development tools allow many requirements to be written as test scripts, without the need for programming, which makes automated testing quicker.

Improved team performance

Central to agile project management is the experience of the project team members. Compared with traditional approaches such as waterfall, agile project teams get more environmental and organizational support, can spend more time focusing on their work, and can contribute to the continuous improvement of the process. To find out what these characteristics mean in practice, continue reading.

Support for the team

The development team's ability to deliver potentially shippable functionality is central to getting results with agile approaches and is achieved with the following support mechanisms:

» A common agile practice is *collocation* — keeping the development team and, ideally, the product owner together in one place and physically close to the customer. Collocation encourages collaboration and makes communication faster, clearer, and easier. You can get out of your seat, have a direct conversation, and eliminate any vagueness or uncertainty immediately.

» The product owner can respond to development team questions and requests for clarification without delay, eliminating confusion and allowing work to proceed smoothly.

» The scrum master removes impediments and ensures that the development team has everything it needs to focus and achieve maximum productivity.

Focus

Using agile processes, the development team can focus as much of its work time as possible on the development of the product. The following approaches help agile development teams focus:

» Development team members are allocated 100 percent to one project, eliminating the time and focus lost by switching context among different projects.

» Development team members know that their teammates will be fully available.

» Developers focus on small units of functionality that are as independent as possible from other functionality. Every morning, the development team knows what it means to be successful that day.

» The scrum master has an explicit responsibility to help protect the development team from organizational distractions.

» The time the development team spends on coding and related productive activities increases because nonproductive work decreases.

Continuous improvement

An agile process isn't a mindless check-the-box approach. Different types of projects and different project teams are able to adapt around their specific situation, as you see in the discussion of sprint retrospectives in Chapter 10. Here are some ways that agile project teams can continuously improve:

» Iterative development makes continuous improvement possible because each new iteration involves a fresh start.

» Because sprints happen over only a few weeks, project teams can incorporate process changes quickly.

>> A review process called the *retrospective* takes place at the end of each iteration and gives all agile team members a specific forum for identifying and planning actions for improvements.

>> The entire scrum team — product owner, development team members, and scrum master — reviews aspects of the work it feels might need improvement.

>> The scrum team applies the lessons it learns from the retrospective to the sprints that follow, which thus become more productive.

Tighter project control

The work goes more quickly under agile projects than under waterfall conditions. Elevated productivity helps increase project control with the following:

>> Agile processes provide a constant flow of information. Development teams plan their work together every morning in daily scrum meetings, and they update task status throughout each day.

>> For every sprint, the customer has the opportunity to reprioritize product requirements based on business needs.

>> After you deliver working functionality at the end of each sprint, you finalize the workload for the next sprint according to current priorities. It makes no difference whether the priorities were set weeks or minutes before the next sprint.

>> When the product owner sets priorities for the next sprint, this action has no effect on the current sprint. On an agile project, a change in requirements adds no administrative costs or time and doesn't disrupt the current work.

>> Agile techniques make project termination easier. At the end of each iteration, you can determine whether the features of the product are now adequate. Low-priority items may never be developed.

In waterfall, project metrics may be outdated by weeks, and demonstrable functionality may be months away. In an agile context, metrics are fresh and relevant every day, work completed is often compiled and integrated daily, and working software is demonstrated every few weeks. From the first sprint to the close of the project, every project team member knows whether the project team is delivering. Up-to-the-minute project knowledge and the ability to quickly prioritize make high levels of project control possible.

Faster and less costly failure

In a waterfall project, opportunities for failure detection are theoretical until close to the end of the project schedule, when all the completed work comes together and when most of the investment is gone. Waiting until the final weeks or days of the project to find out that the product has serious issues is risky for all concerned. Figure 3-5 compares the risk and investment profile for waterfall with that for agile approaches.

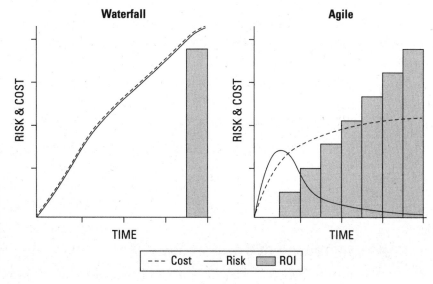

FIGURE 3-5: A risk and investment chart comparing waterfall and agile methodologies.

Along with opportunities for tighter project control, the agile framework offers you

>> Earlier and more frequent opportunities to detect failure

>> An assessment and action opportunity every few weeks

>> Reduction in failure costs

What sorts of failures have you seen on projects? Would agile approaches have helped? You can find out more about risk on agile projects in Chapter 15.

Why People Like Being Agile

You've seen how an organization can benefit from agile project management with faster product delivery and lower costs. In the following sections, you find out how the people involved in a project can benefit as well, whether directly or indirectly.

Executives

Agile project management provides two benefits that are especially attractive to executives: efficiency and a higher and quicker return on investment.

Efficiency

Agile practices allow for vastly increased efficiency in the development process in the following ways:

>> Agile development teams are very productive. They organize the work themselves, focus on development activities, and are protected from distractions by the scrum master.

>> Nonproductive efforts are minimized. The agile approach eliminates unfruitful work; the focus is on development.

>> By using simple, timely, on-demand visual aids — such as graphs and diagrams — to display what's been done, what's in progress, and what's to come, the progress of the project is easier to understand at a glance.

>> Through continuous testing, defects are detected and corrected early.

>> An agile project can be halted when it has enough functionality.

Increased ROI opportunity

ROI is significantly enhanced using agile approaches for the following reasons:

>> **Functionality is delivered to the marketplace earlier.** Features are fully completed and then released in groups, rather than waiting until the end of all development and releasing 100 percent of the features at once.

>> **Product quality is higher.** The scope of development is broken down into manageable chunks that are tested and verified on an ongoing basis.

>> **Revenue opportunity can be accelerated.** Increments of the product are released to the market earlier than with traditional approaches to project management.

>> **Projects can self-fund.** A release of functionality might generate revenue while development of further features is ongoing.

Product development and customers

Customers like agile projects because they can accommodate changing requirements and generate higher-value products.

Improved adaptation to change

Changes to product requirements, priorities, timelines, and budgets can greatly disrupt traditional projects. In contrast, agile processes handle project and product changes in beneficial ways. For example:

>> Agile projects create an opportunity for increased customer satisfaction and return on investment by handling change effectively.

>> Changes can be incorporated into subsequent iterations routinely and smoothly.

>> Because the team members and the sprint length remain constant, project changes pose fewer problems than with traditional approaches. Necessary changes are slotted into the features list based on priority, pushing lower-priority items down the list. Ultimately, the product owner chooses when the project will end, at the point where future investment won't provide enough value.

>> Because the development team develops the highest-value items first and the product owner controls the prioritization, the product owner can be confident that business priorities are aligned with developer activity.

Greater value

With iterative development, product features can be released as the development team completes them. Iterative development and releases provide greater value in the following ways:

>> Project teams deliver highest-priority product features earlier.

>> Project teams can deliver valuable products earlier.

>> Project teams can adjust requirements based on market changes and customer feedback.

Management

People in management tend to like agile projects for the higher quality of the product, the decreased waste of time and effort, and the emphasis on the value of the product over checking off lists of features of dubious usefulness.

Higher quality

With software development, through such techniques as test-driven development, continuous integration, and frequent customer feedback on working software, you can build higher quality into the product upfront.

With non-software development projects, what are ways you can think of to build in quality upfront?

Less product and process waste

In agile projects, wasted time and features are reduced through a number of strategies, including the following:

» **Just-in-time (JIT) elaboration:** Amplification of only the currently highest-priority requirements means that time isn't spent working on details for features that might never be developed.

» **Customer and stakeholder participation:** Customers and other stakeholders can provide feedback in each sprint, and the development team incorporates that feedback into the project. As the project and feedback continue, value to the customer increases.

» **A bias for face-to-face conversation:** Faster, clearer communication saves time and confusion.

» **Built-in exploitation of change:** Only high-priority features and functions are developed.

» **Emphasis on the evidence of working functionality:** If a feature doesn't work or doesn't work in a valuable way, it's discovered early at a lower cost.

Emphasis on value

The agile principle of simplicity supports the elimination of processes and tools that don't support development directly and efficiently, and the exclusion of features that add little tangible value. This principle applies to administration and documentation as well as development in the following ways:

- » Fewer, shorter, more focused meetings
- » Reduction in pageantry
- » Barely sufficient documentation
- » Joint responsibility between customer and project team for the quality and value of the product

Development teams

Agile approaches empower development teams to produce their best work under reasonable conditions. Agile methods give development teams

- » A clear definition of success through joint sprint goal creation and identification of the acceptance criteria during requirements development
- » The power and respect to organize development as they see fit
- » The customer feedback they need to provide value
- » The protection of a dedicated scrum master to remove impediments and prevent disruptions
- » A humane, sustainable pace of work
- » A culture of learning that supports both personal development and project improvement
- » A structure that minimizes non-development time

Under the preceding conditions, the development team thrives and delivers results faster and with higher quality.

REMEMBER

On Broadway and in Hollywood, performers who are on stage and onscreen to connect with the audience are often referred to as "the talent." They are the reason many entertainment customers come to a show, and the supporting writers, directors, and producers ensure that they shine. In an agile environment, the development team is "the talent." When the talent is successful, everyone succeeds.

2

Being Agile

Understand what it means to be agile and how to put agile practices into action.

Get an overview of the three most popular agile approaches, and discover how to create the right environment of physical space, communication, and tools to facilitate agile interactions.

Examine the behavior shift in values, philosophy, roles, and skills needed to operate in an agile team.

Chapter **4**

Agile Approaches

I n previous chapters, you read about the history of agile project management. You may have even heard of common agile frameworks and techniques. Are you wondering what agile frameworks, methods, and techniques actually look like? In this chapter, you get an overview of three of the most common approaches used today to implement an agile project.

Diving under the Umbrella of Agile Approaches

The Agile Manifesto and the agile principles on their own wouldn't be enough to launch you into an agile project, eager as you might be to do so. The reason is that principles and practices are different. The approaches described in this book, however, provide you with the necessary practices to be successful on an agile project.

Agile is a descriptive term for a number of techniques and methods that have the following similarities:

» Development within multiple iterations, called *iterative development*

» Emphasis on simplicity, transparency, and situation-specific strategies

>> Cross-functional, self-organizing teams

>> Working functionality as the measure of progress

Agile project management is an empirical project management approach. In other words, you do something in practice and adjust your approach based on experience rather than theory.

With regards to product development, the empirical approach is braced by the following pillars:

>> **Unfettered transparency:** Everyone involved in the process understands and can contribute to the development of the process.

>> **Frequent inspection:** The inspector must inspect the product regularly and possess the skills to identify variances from acceptance criteria.

>> **Immediate adaptation:** The development team must be able to adjust quickly to minimize further product deviations.

A host of approaches have agile characteristics. Three, however, are common to many agile projects: lean product development, scrum, and extreme programming (XP). These three approaches work perfectly together and share many common elements, although they use different terminology or have a slightly different focus. Broadly, lean and scrum focus on structure. Extreme programming does that, too, but is more prescriptive about development practices, focusing more on technical design, coding, testing, and integration. (From an approach called *extreme programming*, this type of focus is to be expected.)

When organizations we work with state that they're using an agile approach for managing projects, they're usually working in an environment that is lean, with constant attention to limiting work in progress, wasteful practices, and process steps; using scrum to organize their work and expose project progress; and using extreme programming practices to build in quality upfront. Each of these approaches is explained in more detail later in this chapter.

Like any systematic approach, agile techniques didn't arise out of nothing. The concepts have historical precedents, some of which have origins outside software development, which isn't surprising, given that software development hasn't been around that long in the history of human events.

The basis for agile approaches is not the same as that of traditional project management methodologies such as waterfall, which was rooted in a defined control method used for World War II materials procurement. Early computer hardware pioneers used the waterfall process to manage the complexity of the first computer systems, which were mostly hardware: 1,600 vacuum tubes but only 30 or so lines of hand-coded software. (See Figure 4-1.) An inflexible process is effective when the problems are simple and the marketplace is static, but today's product development environment is too complex for such an outdated model.

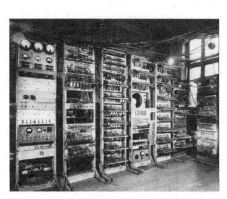

SSEM — "Baby"

FIGURE 4-1:
Early hardware
and software.

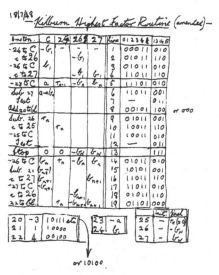

Tom Kilburn's program for "Baby"

Enter Dr. Winston Royce. In his article, "Managing the Development of Large Systems," published in 1970, Dr. Royce codified the step-by-step software development process known as waterfall. When you look at his original diagram in Figure 4-2, you can see where that name came from.

Over time, however, the computer development situation reversed. Hardware became repeatable through mass production, and software became the more complex and diverse aspect of a complete solution.

The irony here is that, even though the diagram implies that you complete tasks step by step, Dr. Royce himself added the cautionary note that you need iteration. Here's how he stated it:

> "If the computer program in question is being developed for the first time, arrange matters so that the version being delivered to the customer for operational deployment is actually the second version insofar as critical design/operations areas are concerned."

Royce even included the diagram shown in Figure 4-3 to illustrate that iteration.

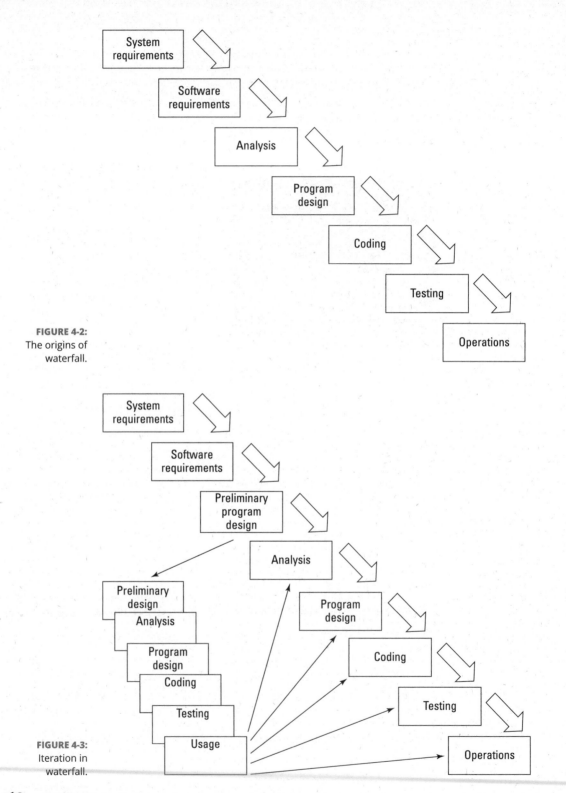

FIGURE 4-2:
The origins of waterfall.

FIGURE 4-3:
Iteration in waterfall.

Now, we're not sure if the diagram was stuck with chewing gum to other pages, but the software development community by and large lost this part of the story. After you allow the idea that you might not know everything when you first start developing a software component and might have to revisit the code to ensure that it's appropriate, you have the ray of light that lets in agile concepts. Agile might have come to prominence 40 years earlier if people had taken Dr. Royce's advice to heart!

Reviewing the Big Three: Lean, Scrum, and Extreme Programming

Now that you have a brief history of the waterfall approach to project management, you're ready to find out more about three popular agile approaches: lean, scrum, and extreme programming.

An overview of lean

Lean has its origins in manufacturing. Mass production methods, which have been around for more than 100 years, were designed to simplify assembly processes (for example, putting together a Model-T Ford). These processes use complex, expensive machinery and low-skilled workers to inexpensively churn out an item of value. The idea is that if you keep the machines and people working and stockpile inventory, you generate a lot of efficiency.

The simplicity is deceptive. Traditionally, mass production requires wasteful supporting systems and large amounts of indirect labor to ensure that manufacturing continues without pause. It generates a huge inventory of parts, extra workers, extra space, and complex processes that don't add direct value to the product. Sound familiar?

Cutting the fat as lean emerges in manufacturing

In the 1940s in Japan, a small company called Toyota wanted to produce cars for the Japanese market but couldn't afford the huge investment that mass production requires. The company studied supermarkets, noting how consumers buy just what they need because they know there will always be a supply and how the stores restock shelves only as they empty. From this observation, Toyota created a just-in-time process that it could translate to the factory floor.

The result was a significant reduction in inventory of parts and finished goods and a lower investment in machines, people, and space.

One big cost of the mass production processes at the time was that humans on the production line were treated like machines: People had no autonomy and could not solve problems, make choices, or improve processes. The work was boring and set aside human potential. By contrast, the just-in-time process gives workers the ability to make decisions about what is most important to do next, in real time, on the factory floor. The workers take responsibility for the results. Toyota's success with just-in-time processes has helped change mass manufacturing approaches globally.

Understanding lean and software development

The term *lean* was coined in the 1990s in *The Machine That Changed the World: The Story of Lean Production* (Free Press) by James P. Womack, Daniel T. Jones, and Daniel Roos. eBay was an early adopter of lean principles for software development. The company led the way with an approach that responded daily to customers' requests for changes to the website, developing high-value features in a short time.

The focus of lean is business value and minimizing activities outside product development. Mary and Tom Poppendieck discuss a group of lean principles on their blog and in their books on lean software development. Following are the lean principles from their 2003 book, *Lean Software Development* (Addison-Wesley Professional):

>> **Eliminate waste.** Doing anything that is beyond barely sufficient (process steps, artifacts, meetings) slows down the flow of progress. Waste includes failing to learn from work, building the wrong thing, and thrashing (context switching between tasks or projects) — which results in only partially creating lots of product features but not completely creating any.

>> **Amplify learning.** Learning drives predictability. Enable improvement through a mindset of regular and disciplined transparency, inspection, and adaptation. Encourage an organization-wide culture that allows failure for the sake of learning from it.

>> **Deliver as late as possible.** Allow for late adaptation. Don't deliver late, but leave your options open long enough to make decisions at the last responsible moment based on facts rather than uncertainty — when you know the most. Learn from failure. Challenge standards. Use the scientific method — experiment with hypotheses to find solutions.

>> **Deliver as fast as possible.** Speed, cost, and quality are compatible. The sooner you deliver, the sooner you receive feedback. Work on fewer things at once, limiting work in progress and optimizing flow. Manage workflow, rather than schedules. Use just-in-time planning to shorten development and release cycles.

>> **Empower the team.** Working autonomously, mastering skills, and believing in the purpose of work can motivate development teams. Managers do not tell developers how to do their jobs but instead support them to self-organize around the work to be done and remove their impediments. Make sure teams and individuals have the environment and tools they need to do their job well.

>> **Build quality in.** Establish mechanisms to catch and correct defects when they happen and before final verification. Quality is built in from the beginning, not at the end. Break dependencies, so you can develop and integrate functionality at any time without regressions.

>> **See the whole.** An entire system is only as strong as its weakest link. Solve problems, not just symptoms. Continually pay attention to bottlenecks throughout the flow of work and remove them. Think long-term when creating solutions.

Beyond the lean principles, one of the most common lean approaches used by agile teams is kanban, sometimes referred to as *lean-kanban*. Adapted from the Toyota Production System approach, *kanban* is essentially a method for removing waste to improve flow and throughput in a system.

Kanban practices can be applied in almost any situation because they're designed to start with where you are — you don't have to change anything about your existing workflow to get started. Kanban practices include the following:

>> Visualize.

>> Limit work in progress (WIP).

>> Manage flow.

>> Make process policies explicit.

>> Implement feedback loops.

>> Improve collaboratively, evolve experimentally.

The last three practices are commonly found in other agile frameworks, such as scrum and XP (both discussed later in this chapter). The first three enhance effectiveness for agile teams:

>> **Visualize:** Visualizing a team's workflow is the first step in identifying potential waste. Traditional bloated processes exist in many organizations but do not reflect reality, even if visualized. As agile teams visualize the flow of their work (on a whiteboard, on a wall, or in a drawing) and identify where productivity breaks down, they can easily analyze the root cause and see how to remove the constraint. And then do it again, and again, and again.

Kanban is Japanese for *visual signal*. Hanging on the factory wall or the development workspace wall, where everyone can see it, the kanban board shows the items that teams need to produce next. Slotted into the board are cards representing units of production. As production progresses, the workers remove, add, and move cards. As the cards move, they act as a signal to workers when work or inventory replenishment is needed. Agile teams use kanban boards or task boards to expose their progress and manage their flow of work (described in more detail in Chapters 5 and 9).

>> **Limit work in progress (WIP):** When teams keep starting work but don't finish it, their work in progress continues to grow. Being agile is all about getting to done, so the goal is to start things only when other things are completed. Working on multiple things at once does not mean you complete them all faster — you actually complete them more slowly than if you had worked on them one at a time. When agile teams limit their work in progress, items get completed faster, speeding the pace of completing each item in their queue.

>> **Manage flow:** We've all experienced what happens on a busy street during rush hour. When there are more cars than the lanes of traffic can handle, all cars move more slowly. Everyone wants to get somewhere at the same time, and so everyone has to wait longer to get there. To manage flow better, we need to regulate the entry of vehicles into the flow of traffic or increase the number of lanes of traffic where congestion is highest. Like cars in traffic, development work items move more slowly if developers try to take them all on at once. Working on one thing at a time and identifying and removing constraints increases the flow of all items through the system.

Measuring lead and cycle times helps agile teams monitor their management of flow. A team determines the lead time by tracking the amount of time it takes a request for functionality to go from arrival in the queue to completed. They know the cycle time by tracking the time from when work begins to when it is completed. And the agile team optimizes flow by identifying and removing bottlenecks that keep its lead and cycle times from decreasing.

To support good product development practices, remember the following:

>> Don't develop features that you're unlikely to use.

>> Make the development team central to the project because it adds the biggest value.

>> Have the customers prioritize features — they know what's most important to them. Tackle high-priority items first to deliver value.

>> Use tools that support great communication across all parties.

Today, lean principles continue to influence the development of agile techniques — and to be influenced by them. Any approach should be agile and adapt over time.

An overview of scrum

Scrum, the most popular agile framework in software development, is an iterative approach that has at its core the *sprint* (the scrum term for iteration). To support this process, scrum teams use specific roles, artifacts, and events. To make sure that they meet the goals of each part of the process, scrum teams use inspection and adaptation throughout the project. The scrum approach is shown in Figure 4-4.

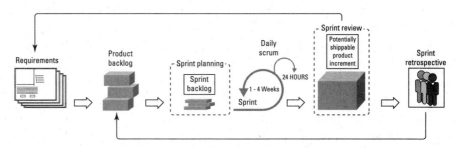

FIGURE 4-4: The scrum approach.

Going the distance with the sprint

Within each sprint, the development team develops and tests a functional part of the product until the product owner accepts it, often daily, and the functionality becomes a potentially shippable increment of the overall product. When one sprint finishes, another sprint starts. Releasing functionality to the market often occurs at the end of multiple sprints, when the product owner determines that enough value exists. However, the product owner may decide to release functionality after every sprint, or even as many times as needed during a sprint.

REMEMBER

A core principle of the sprint is its cyclical nature: The sprint, as well as the processes within it, repeats over and over, as shown in Figure 4-5.

You use the tenets of inspection and adaptation on a daily basis as part of a scrum project:

» During a sprint, you conduct *constant inspections* to assess progress toward the sprint goal, and consequentially, toward the release goal.

» You hold a *daily scrum* meeting to organize the day by reviewing what the team completed yesterday and coordinating what it will work on today. Essentially, the scrum team inspects its progress toward the sprint goal.

» At the end of the sprint, you use a *sprint retrospective* meeting to assess performance and plan necessary adaptations.

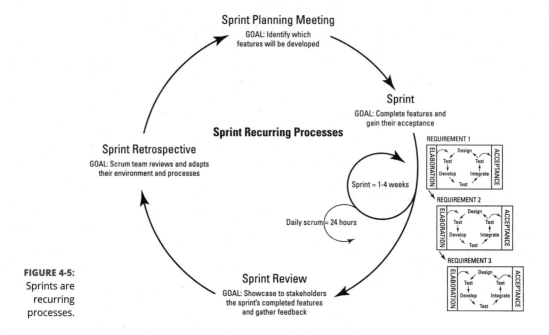

FIGURE 4-5:
Sprints are
recurring
processes.

These inspections and adaptations may sound formal and process–laden, but they aren't. Use inspection and adaptation to solve issues and don't overthink this process. The problem you're trying to solve today will often change in the future anyway.

Understanding scrum roles, artifacts, and events

The scrum framework defines specific roles, artifacts, and events for projects.

Scrum's three *roles* — people on the project — are as follows:

>> **Product owner:** Represents and speaks for the business needs of the project.

>> **Development team:** Performs the day-to-day work. The development team is dedicated to the project and each team member is *multi-skilled* — that is, although team members may have certain strengths, each member is capable of doing multiple jobs on the project.

>> **Scrum master:** Protects the team from organizational distractions, clears roadblocks, ensures that scrum is played properly, and continuously improves the team's environment.

Additionally, scrum teams find that they're more effective and efficient when they work closely with two non-scrum–specific roles:

>> **Stakeholders:** Anyone who is affected by or has input on the project. Although stakeholders are not official scrum roles, it is essential for scrum teams and stakeholders to work closely together throughout a project.

>> **Agile mentor:** An experienced authority on agile techniques and the scrum framework. Often this person is external to the project's department or organization, so he or she can support the scrum team objectively with an outsider's point of view.

In the same way that scrum has specific roles, scrum also has three tangible deliverables, called *artifacts:*

>> **Product backlog:** The full list of requirements that defines the product, often documented in terms of business value from the perspective of the end user. The product backlog can be fluid throughout the project. All scope items, regardless of level of detail, are in the product backlog. The product owner owns the product backlog, determining what goes in it and in what priority.

>> **Sprint backlog:** The list of requirements and tasks in a given sprint. The product owner and the development team select the requirements for the sprint in sprint planning, with the development team breaking down these requirements into tasks. Unlike the product backlog, the sprint backlog can be changed only by the development team.

>> **Product increment:** The usable, potentially shippable functionality. Whether the product is a website or a new house, the product increment should be complete enough to demonstrate its working functionality. A scrum project is complete after a product contains enough shippable functionality to meet the customer's business goals for the project.

Finally, scrum also has five events:

>> **Sprint:** Scrum's term for iteration. The *sprint* is the container for each of the other scrum events, in which the scrum team creates potentially shippable functionality. Sprints are short cycles, no longer than a month, typically between one and two weeks, and in some cases as short as one day. Consistent sprint length reduces variance; a scrum team can confidently extrapolate what it can do in each sprint based on what it has accomplished in previous sprints. Sprints give scrum teams the opportunity to make adjustments for continuous improvement immediately, rather than at the end of the project.

>> **Sprint planning:** Takes place at the start of each sprint. In sprint planning meetings, scrum teams decide which goal, scope, and supporting tasks will be part of the sprint backlog.

>> **Daily scrum:** Takes place daily for no more than 15 minutes. During the daily scrum, development team members make three statements:

- What the team member completed yesterday

- What the team member will work on today

- A list of items impeding the team member

The scrum master also participates in the context of impediments he or she is working to remove for the developers.

>> **Sprint review:** Takes place at the end of each sprint. In this meeting, the development team demonstrates to the stakeholders and the entire organization the accepted parts of the product the team completed during the sprint. The key to the sprint review is collecting feedback from the stakeholders, which informs the product owner how to update the product backlog and consider the next sprint goal.

>> **Sprint retrospective:** Takes place at the end of each sprint. The sprint retrospective is an internal team meeting in which the scrum team members (product owner, development team, and scrum master) discuss what went well during the sprint, what didn't work well, and how they can make improvements for the next sprint. This meeting is action-oriented (frustrations should be vented elsewhere) and ends with tangible improvement plans for the next sprint.

Scrum is simple: three roles, three artifacts, and five events. Each plays a part to ensure that the scrum team has continuous transparency, inspection, and adaptation throughout the project. As a framework, scrum accommodates many other agile techniques, methods, and tools for executing the technical aspects of building functionality.

An overview of extreme programming

One popular approach to product development, specific to software, is extreme programming (XP). Extreme programming takes the best practices of software development to an extreme level. Created in 1996 by Kent Beck, with the help of Ward Cunningham and Ron Jeffries, the principles of XP were originally described in Beck's 1999 book, *Extreme Programming Explained* (Addison-Wesley Professional), which has since been updated.

ESSENTIAL CREDENTIALS

If you are — or want to be — an agile practitioner, you may consider getting one or more agile certifications. The certification training alone can provide valuable information and the chance to practice agile processes — lessons you can use in your everyday work. Many organizations want to hire people with proven agile knowledge, so certification can also boost your career.

You can choose from a number of well-recognized, entry-level certifications, including the following:

- **Certified ScrumMaster (CSM):** The Scrum Alliance, a professional organization that promotes the understanding and use of scrum, offers a certification for scrum masters. The CSM requires a two-day training class, provided by a Certified Scrum Trainer (CST) and completing a CSM evaluation. CSM training provides an overall view of scrum and is a good starting point for people starting their agile journey. See http://scrumalliance.org.

- **Certified Scrum Product Owner (CSPO):** The Scrum Alliance also provides a certification for product owners. Like the CSM, the CSPO requires two days of training from a CST. CSPO training provides a deep dive into the product owner role. See http://scrumalliance.org.

- **Certified Scrum Developer (CSD):** For development team members, the Scrum Alliance offers the CSD. The CSD is a technical-track certification, requiring five days of training from a CST and passing an exam on agile engineering techniques. CSM or CSPO training can count toward a CSD; the remaining three days are a technical skills course. See http://scrumalliance.org.

- **PMI Agile Certified Practitioner (PMI-ACP):** The Project Management Institute (PMI) is the largest professional organization for project managers in the world. In 2012, PMI introduced the PMI-ACP certification. The PMI-ACP requires training, general project management experience, experience working on agile projects, and passing an exam on your knowledge of agile fundamentals. See http://pmi.org.

The focus of extreme programming is customer satisfaction. XP teams achieve high customer satisfaction by developing features when the customer needs them. New requests are part of the development team's daily routine, and the team is empowered to deal with these requests whenever they crop up. The team organizes itself around any problem that arises and solves it as efficiently as possible.

As XP has grown as a practice, XP roles have blurred. A typical project now consists of people in customer, management, technical, and project support groups. Each person may play a different role at different times.

Discovering extreme programming principles

Basic approaches in extreme programming are based on Agile principles. These approaches are as follows:

>> **Coding is the core activity.** Software code not only delivers the solution but can also be used to explore problems. For example, a programmer can explain a problem using code.

>> **XP teams do lots of testing.** If doing just a little testing helps you identify some defects, a lot of testing will help you find more. In fact, developers don't start coding until they've worked out the success criteria for the requirement and designed the unit tests. A defect is not a failure of code; it's a failure to define the right test.

>> **Communication between customer and programmer is direct.** The programmer must understand the business requirement to design a technical solution.

>> **For complex systems, some level of overall design, beyond any specific function, is necessary.** In XP projects, the overall design is considered during regular *refactoring* — namely, using the process of systematically improving the code to enhance readability, reduce complexity, improve maintainability, and ensure extensibility across the entire code base.

You may find extreme programming combined with lean or scrum because the process elements are so similar that they marry well.

Getting to know some extreme programming practices

In XP, some practices are similar to other agile approaches, but others aren't. Table 4-1 lists a few key XP practices, most of which are commonsense practices and many of which are reflected in agile principles.

Extreme programming intentionally pushes the limits of development customs by dramatically increasing the intensity of best practice rituals, which has resulted in a strong track record of XP improving development efficiency and success.

TABLE 4-1   ## Key Practices of Extreme Programming

XP Practice	Underpinning Assumption
Planning game	All members of the team should participate in planning. No disconnect exists between business and technical people.
Whole team	The customer needs to be collocated (physically located together) with the development team and be available. This accessibility enables the team to ask more minor questions, quickly get answers, and ultimately deliver a product more aligned with customer expectations.
Coding standards	Use coding standards to empower developers to make decisions and to maintain consistency throughout the product; don't constantly reinvent the basics of how to develop products in your organization. Standard code identifiers and naming conventions are two examples of coding standards.
System metaphor	When describing how the system works, use an implied comparison, a simple story that is easily understood (for instance, "the system is like cooking a meal"). This provides additional context that the team can fall back on in all product discovery activities and discussions.
Collective code ownership	The entire team is responsible for the quality of code. Shared ownership and accountability bring about the best designs and highest quality. Any engineer can modify another engineer's code to enable progress to continue.
Sustainable pace	Overworked people are not effective. Too much work leads to mistakes, which leads to more work, which leads to more mistakes. Avoid working more than 40 hours per week for an extended period of time.
Pair programming	Two people work together on a programming task. One person is strategic (the driver), and one person is tactical (the navigator). They explain their approach to each other. No piece of code is understood by only one person. Defects can more easily be found and fixed before merging and integrating code with the system.
Design improvement	Continuously improve design by refactoring code — removing duplications and inefficiencies within the code. A lean code base is simpler to maintain and operates more efficiently.
Simple design	The simpler the design, the lower the cost to change the software code.
Test-driven development (TDD)	Write automated customer acceptance and unit tests before you code anything. Write a test, run it, and watch it fail. Then write just enough code to make the test pass, refactoring until it does (red-green-clean). Test your success before you claim progress.
Continuous integration	Team members should be working from the latest code. Integrate code components across the development team as often as possible to identify issues and take corrective action before problems build on each other.
Small releases	Release value to the customer as often as possible. Some organizations release daily. Avoid building up large stores of unreleased code requiring extensive risky regression and integration efforts. Get feedback from your customer as early as possible, as often as possible.

Putting It All Together

All three agile approaches — lean, scrum, and extreme programming (XP) — have common threads. The biggest thing these approaches have in common is adherence to the Agile Manifesto and the 12 Agile Principles. Table 4-2 shows a few more of the similarities among the three approaches.

TABLE 4-2 **Similarities between Lean, Scrum, and Extreme Programming**

Lean	Scrum	Extreme Programming
Engaging everyone	Cross-functional development team	Entire team
		Collective ownership
Optimizing the whole	Product increment	Test-driven development
		Continuous integration
Delivering fast	Sprints of four weeks or less	Small release

In addition to more extensive agile frameworks and practices, scrum also accommodates a variety of accouterments that consistently increase success with agile projects. Just like a physical home is framed to support the plumbing, electrical, ventilation, and internal convenience features, scrum provides the framework for many other agile tools and techniques to do the job well. Here is a sampling, most of which you learn more about in the following chapters:

>> Product vision statement (elevator pitch, clear statement of direction for reaching the outer boundary of the project)

>> Product roadmap (a representation of the features required to achieve the product vision)

>> Velocity (a tool for scrum teams to plan the workload for each sprint and empirically predict the delivery of functionality long-term)

>> Release planning (establishing a specific mid-range goal, the trigger for releasing functionality to the market)

>> User stories (structuring requirements from an end-user's point of view to clarify business value)

>> Relative estimation (using self-correcting relative complexity and effort rather than inaccurate absolute measures, which give a false sense of precision)

>> Swarming (cross-functional teams working together on one requirement at a time until completion to get the job done faster)

» Rediscovering low-tech
communication and using the right
high-tech communication

» Finding and using the tools you need

Chapter **5**

Agile Environments in Action

C onjure up a mental picture of your current working environment. Perhaps it looks like the following setup. The IT team sits in cube city in one departmental area with the project manager somewhere within walking distance. You work with an offshore development team eight time zones away. The business customer is on the other side of the building. Your manager has a small office tucked away somewhere. Conference rooms are usually fully booked, and even if you were to get into one, someone would chase you out within the hour.

Your project documents are stored in folders on a shared drive. The development team gets at least 100 emails a day. The project manager holds a team meeting every week and, referring to the project plan, tells the developers what to work on. The project manager also creates a weekly status report and posts it on the shared drive. The product manager is usually too busy to talk to the project manager to review progress but periodically sends emails with some new thoughts about the application.

Although the description in the preceding paragraphs may not describe your particular situation, you can see something like it in any given corporate setting. Agile teams, however, execute projects in short, focused iterative cycles, relying on timely feedback from project team members. To operate and become more agile, your working environment is going to have to change.

This chapter shows you how to create a working space that facilitates communication, one that will help you best become agile.

Creating the Physical Environment

Agile project teams flourish when scrum team members work closely together in an environment that supports the process. As noted in other chapters, the development team members are central to the success of agile projects. Creating the right environment for them to operate in goes a long way toward supporting their success. You can even hire people who specialize in designing optimal agile work environments.

Collocating the team

If at all possible, the scrum team needs to be *collocated* — that is, physically located together. When a scrum team is collocated, the following practices are possible and significantly increase efficiency and effectiveness:

>> Communicating face to face

>> Physically standing up — rather than sitting — as a group for the daily scrum meeting (this keeps meetings brief and on topic)

>> Using simple, low-tech tools for communication

>> Getting real-time clarifications from scrum team members

>> Being aware of what others are working on

>> Asking for help with a task

>> Supporting others with their tasks

All these practices uphold agile processes. When everyone resides in the same area, it's much easier for one person to lean over, ask a question, and get an immediate answer. If the question is complex, a face-to-face conversation, with all the synergy it creates, is much more productive than an email exchange.

TECHNICAL
STUFF

This improved communication effectiveness is due to *communication fidelity* — the degree of accuracy between the meaning intended and the meaning interpreted. Albert Mehrabian, Ph.D., a professor at UCLA, has shown that for complex, incongruent communication, 55 percent of meaning is conveyed by physical body language, 38 percent is conveyed through cultural-specific voice tonality interpretation, and only 7 percent is conveyed by words. That's something to keep in mind during your next voice-over IP or smartphone conference call to discuss the design nuances of a system that doesn't exist.

Alistair Cockburn, one of the Agile Manifesto signatories, created the graph in Figure 5-1. This graph shows the effectiveness of different forms of communication. Notice the difference in effectiveness between paper communication and two people at a whiteboard — with collocation, you get the benefit of better communication.

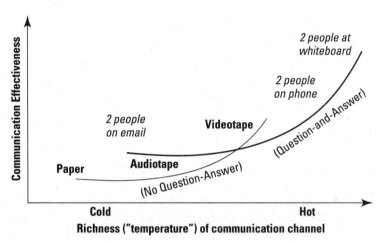

FIGURE 5-1:
Better
communication
through
collocation.

Setting up a dedicated area

If the scrum team members are in the same physical place, you want to create as ideal a working environment for them as you can. The first step is to create a dedicated area.

Set up an environment where the scrum team can work in close physical proximity. If possible, the scrum team should have its own room, sometimes called a *project room* or a *scrum room*. The scrum team members create the setup they need in this project room, putting whiteboards and bulletin boards on the walls and moving the furniture. By arranging the space for productivity, it becomes part of how they work. If a separate room isn't possible, a *pod* — with workspaces around the edges and a table or collaboration center in the middle — works well.

If you're stuck in cube city and can't tear down walls, ask for some empty cubes in a group and remove the dividing panels. Create a space that you can treat as your project room.

REMEMBER

The right space allows the scrum team to be fully immersed in solving problems and crafting solutions.

The situation you have may be far from perfect, but it's worth the effort to see how close you can get to the ideal. Before you start an agile transition in your organization, ask management for the resources necessary to create an optimal condition. Resources will vary from project to project, but at a minimum, they can include whiteboards, bulletin boards, markers, pushpins, and sticky notes. You'll be surprised at how quickly the efficiency gains pay for the investment and more.

For example, with one client company, dedicating a project room and making a $6,000 investment in multiple monitors for developers increased productivity, which saved the company almost two months and $60,000 over the life of the project. That's a pretty good return on a simple investment. We show you how to quantify these savings early on in the project in Chapter 13.

Removing distractions

The development team needs to focus, focus, focus. Agile methods are designed to create structure for highly productive work carried out in a specific way. The biggest threat to this productivity is distraction, such as . . . hold on a minute, I need to take a call.

Okay, I'm back. The good news is that an agile team has someone dedicated to deflecting or eliminating distractions: the scrum master. Whether you're going to be taking on a scrum master role or some other role, you need to understand what sorts of distractions can throw the development team off course and how to handle them. Table 5-1 is a list of common distractions and do's and don'ts for dealing with distractions.

REMEMBER

Distractions sap the development team's focus, energy, and performance. The scrum master needs strength and courage to manage and deflect interruptions. Every distraction averted is a step toward success.

TABLE 5-1   **Common Distractions**

Distraction	Do	Don't
Multiple projects	Do make sure that the development team is dedicated 100 percent to a single project at a time.	Don't fragment the development team between multiple projects, operations support, and special duties.
Multitasking	Do keep the development team focused on a single task, ideally developing one piece of functionality at a time. A task board can help keep track of the tasks in progress and quickly identify whether someone is working on multiple tasks at once.	Don't let the development team switch between requirements. Switching tasks creates a huge overhead (a minimum of 30 percent) in lost productivity.
Over-supervising	Do leave development team members alone after you collaborate on iteration goals; they can organize themselves. Watch their productivity skyrocket.	Don't interfere with the development team or allow others to do so. The daily scrum meeting provides ample opportunity to assess progress.
Outside influences	Do redirect any distracters. If a new task outside the sprint goal surfaces, ask the product owner to decide whether the task's priority is worth sacrificing sprint functionality.	Don't mess with the development team members and their work. They're pursuing the sprint goal, which is the top priority during an active sprint. Even a seemingly quick task can throw off work for an entire day.
Management	Do shield the development team from direct requests from management (unless management wants to give team members a bonus for their excellent performance).	Don't allow management to negatively affect the productivity of the development team. Make interrupting the development team the path of greatest resistance.

Going mobile

Judging by the "Going mobile" heading, you might have thought this section was about smartphone teleconferencing, but it isn't. Agile project teams take a responsive approach, and scrum team members require an environment that helps them respond to the project needs of the day. An agile team environment should be mobile — literally:

>> Use movable desks and chairs so that people can move about and reconfigure the space.

>> Get wirelessly connected laptops so that scrum team members can pick them up and move them about easily.

>> Have a large mobile whiteboard. Also see the next section on low-tech communication.

With this movable environment, scrum team members can configure and reconfigure their arrangement as needed. Given that scrum team members will be working with different members from day to day, mobility is important. Fixed furniture tends to dictate the communications that take place. Being mobile allows for freer collaboration and more freedom overall.

Low-Tech Communicating

When a scrum team is collocated, the members can communicate in person with ease and fluidity. Particularly when you begin your agile transition, you want to keep the communication tools low-tech. Rely on face-to-face conversations and good old-fashioned pen and paper. Low-tech promotes informality, allowing scrum team members to feel that they can change work processes and be innovative as they learn about the product.

The primary tool for communication should be face-to-face conversation. Tackling problems in person is the best way to accelerate production:

>> **Have short daily scrum meetings in person.** Some scrum teams stand throughout a meeting to discourage it from running longer than 15 minutes.

>> **Ask the product owner questions.** Also, make sure he or she is involved in discussions about product features to provide clarity when necessary. The conversation shouldn't end when planning ends.

>> **Communicate with your co-workers.** If you have questions about features, the project's progress, or integrating, communicate with co-workers. The entire development team is responsible for creating the product, and team members need to talk throughout the day.

As long as the scrum team is in close proximity, you can use physical and visual approaches to keep everyone on the same page. The tools should enable everyone to see

>> The goal of the sprint

>> The functionality necessary to achieve the sprint goal

>> What has been accomplished in the sprint

>> What's coming next in the sprint

>> Who is working on which task

>> What remains to be done

Only a few tools are needed to support this low-tech communication:

>> A whiteboard or two (ideally, mobile — on wheels or lightweight). Nothing beats a whiteboard for collaboration. The scrum team can use one for brainstorming solutions or sharing ideas.

>> A huge supply of sticky notes in different colors (including poster-sized ones for communicating critical information you want readily visible — such as architecture, coding standards, and the project's definition of done).

TIP

A personal favorite is giving each developer at least one tabletop dry erase/ sticky note easel pad combination, with a lightweight easel. These low-cost tools facilitate communication fantastically.

>> Lots of colorful pens.

>> A sprint-specific task or kanban board (described in Chapters 4 and 9) for tracking progress tactility.

If you decide to have a sprint-specific kanban board, use sticky notes to represent *units of work* (features broken down into tasks). For your work plan, you can place sticky notes on a large surface (a wall or your second whiteboard), or you can use a kanban board with cards. You can customize a kanban board in many ways, such as using different-colored sticky notes for different types of tasks, red flag stickers for features that have an impediment, and team member stickers to easily see who is working on which task.

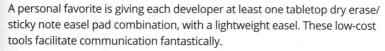
TECHNICAL STUFF

An *information radiator* is a tool that physically displays information to the scrum team and anyone else in the scrum team's work area. Information radiators include kanban boards, whiteboards, bulletin boards, *burndown charts,* which show the iteration's status, and any other sign with details about the project, the product, or the scrum team.

Basically, you move sticky notes or cards around the board to show the status (see Figure 5-2). Everyone knows how to read the board and how to act on what it shows. In Chapter 9, you find out the details of what to put on the boards.

TIP

Whatever tools you use, avoid spending time making things look perfectly neat and pretty. Formality in layout and presentation (what you might call *pageantry*) can give an impression that the work is tidy and elegant. However, the work is what matters, so focus your energy on activities that support the work.

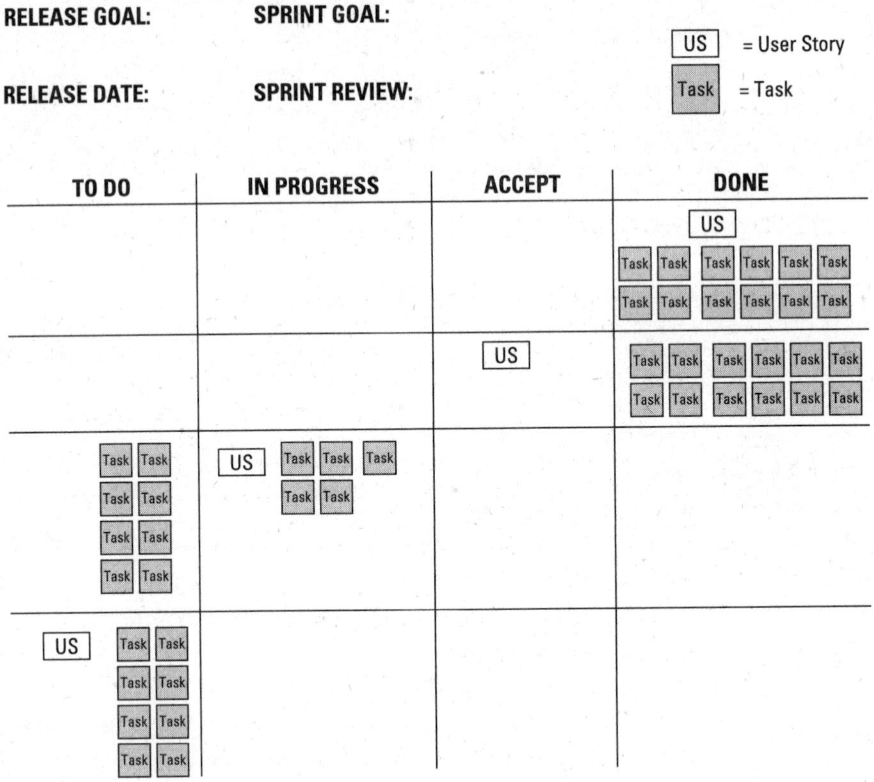

RELEASE GOAL: **SPRINT GOAL:**

RELEASE DATE: **SPRINT REVIEW:**

| US | = User Story |
| Task | = Task |

TO DO	IN PROGRESS	ACCEPT	DONE
			US Task Task Task Task Task Task Task Task Task Task Task Task
		US	Task Task Task Task Task Task Task Task Task Task Task Task
Task Task Task Task Task Task Task Task	US Task Task Task Task Task		
US Task Task Task Task Task Task Task Task			

FIGURE 5-2:
A scrum task board on a wall or whiteboard.

High-Tech Communicating

Although collocation almost universally improves effectiveness, many scrum teams can't be collocated. Some projects have teammates scattered across multiple offices; others have off-shore development teams around the world. If you have multiple, geographically scattered scrum teams, try first to reallocate existing talent to form scrum teams collocated within each geographic location. If this move isn't possible, don't give up on an agile transition. Instead, simulate collocation as much as possible.

When scrum team members work in different places, you have to make a greater effort to set up an environment that creates a sense of connectedness. To span distance and time zones, you need more sophisticated communication mechanisms.

DON'T REINVENT THE WHEEL!

In the past, manufacturing processes often involved partially completed items being shipped to another location for completion. In these situations, the kanban board on a factory wall in the first location needed to be seen by shop floor management at the second location. Electronic kanban board software was developed to resolve this problem, but interestingly, the software looked like a literal kanban board on the wall and was used in the same way. Don't fix what's already working.

When determining which types of high-tech communication tools to support, first consider the loss of face-to-face discussions. Some tools you can use follow:

>> **Videoconferencing and webcams:** These tools can create a sense of being together. If you have to communicate remotely, at the very least make sure you can see and hear each other clearly. Body language provides the majority of the message.

>> **Instant messaging:** Although instant messaging doesn't convey nonverbal communication, it is real time, accessible, and easy to use. Several people can also share a session and share files.

>> **Web-based desktop sharing:** Especially for the development team, sharing your desktop allows you to highlight issues and updates visually in real time. Seeing the problem is always better than just talking it out over the phone.

>> **Collaboration websites:** These sites allow you to do everything from sharing simple documentation so that everyone has the latest information to using a virtual whiteboard for brainstorming.

TIP

Using a collaboration site (such as SharePoint, Confluence, and Google Drive) allows you to post documents that show the status of the sprint. When managers request status updates, you can simply direct them to the collaboration site to pull the information they need, on demand. By updating these documents daily, you provide managers with better information than they would have with formalized status reporting procedures under a traditional project management cycle. Avoid creating separate status reports for management; these reports duplicate information in the sprint burndowns and don't support production.

WARNING

When you have a collaboration site with shared documentation, don't assume that everyone automatically understands everything in the documentation. Use a collaboration site to make sure everything is published, accessible, and transparent, but don't let it give your team a false sense of shared understanding.

Choosing Tools

As noted throughout the chapter, low-tech tools are best suited for agile projects, especially initially, while the scrum team becomes accustomed to the process. This section discusses a few points to consider when choosing agile tools: the purpose of the tool and organizational and compatibility constraints.

The purpose of the tool

When choosing tools, the primary question you need to ask is, "What is the purpose of the tool?" Tools should solve a specific problem and support agile processes, the focus of which is pushing forward with the work.

Above all, don't choose anything more complicated than you need. Some tools are sophisticated and take time to learn before you can use them to be productive. If you're working with a collocated scrum team, the training and adoption of agile practices can be enough of a challenge without adding a suite of complicated tools to the mix. If you're working with a dislocated scrum team, introducing new tools can be even more difficult.

WARNING

You can find a lot of agile-centric websites, software, and other tools on the market. Many are useful, but you shouldn't invest in expensive agile tools in your early days of implementing agile. This investment is unnecessary and adds another level of complexity to adoption. As you go through the first few iterations and modify your approach, the scrum team will start identifying procedures that can be improved or need to change. One of these improvements might be the need for additional tools or replacement tools. When a need emerges naturally, from the scrum team, finding organizational support for purchasing the necessary tools is often easier because the need can be tied to a project issue.

Organizational and compatibility constraints

Beyond the initial considerations noted in the preceding section, the tools you choose must operate in your organization. Unless you're using solely non-electronic tools, you'll likely have to take into account organizational policies with respect to hardware, software, and services as well as cloud computing, security, and telephony systems.

If you're part of a distributed organization, some scrum teams may not be able to support complex solutions, maintain the latest versions of desktop software, or have the robust Internet bandwidth you take for granted.

The key to creating an agile environment for agile teams is to do so at the strategic organizational level. Agile teams drive agile projects, so enlist your organization's leadership early to provide tools that will empower your teams to succeed.

Chapter **6**

Agile Behaviors in Action

I n this chapter, you look at the behavioral dynamics that need to shift for your organization to benefit from the performance advantages that agile techniques enable. You find out about the different roles on an agile project and see how you can change a project team's values and philosophy about project management. Finally, we discuss some ways for a project team to hone key skills for agile project success.

Establishing Agile Roles

In Chapter 4, we describe scrum, one of the most popular agile frameworks in use today. The scrum framework defines common agile roles in an especially succinct manner. We use scrum terms to describe agile roles throughout this book. These roles are

» Product owner

» Development team member

» Scrum master

The product owner, development team, and scrum master together make up the *scrum team.* Each role is a peer to the others — no one is the boss of anyone else on the team.

The following roles are not part of the scrum framework but are still critically important to agile projects:

>> Stakeholders

>> Agile mentor

The scrum team together with the stakeholders make up the agile *project team.* At the center of it all is the development team. The product owner and scrum master fulfill roles that ensure the development team's success. Figure 6-1 shows how these roles and teams fit together. This section discusses these roles in detail.

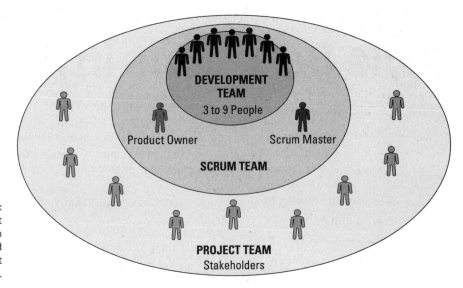

FIGURE 6-1: Agile project team, scrum team, and development team.

Product owner

The product owner, sometimes called the *customer representative* in non-scrum environments, is responsible for bridging the gaps between the customer, business stakeholders, and the development team. The product owner is an expert on the product and the customer's needs and priorities. The product owner, who is a peer member of the scrum team, shields the development team from business distractions, works with the development team daily to help clarify requirements, and accepts completed work throughout the sprint in preparation for the sprint review.

Product owners make the decisions about what the product does and does not include. Add to that the responsibility of deciding what to release to the market and when to do it, and you see that you need a smart and savvy person to fill this role.

On an agile project, the product owner will

>> Develop strategy and direction for the project and set long- and short-term goals.

>> Provide or have access to product expertise.

>> Understand and convey the customer's and other business stakeholders' needs to the development team.

>> Gather, prioritize, and manage product requirements.

>> Take responsibility for the product's budget and profitability.

>> Decide when to release completed functionality.

>> Work with the development team on a daily basis to answer questions and make decisions.

>> Accept or reject completed work — as it's completed — during the sprint.

>> Present the scrum team's accomplishments at the end of each sprint, before the development team demonstrates these accomplishments.

What makes a good product owner? Decisiveness. Good product owners understand the customer thoroughly and are empowered by the organization to make difficult business decisions every day. Although able to gather requirements from stakeholders, product owners are knowledgeable about the product in their own right. They can prioritize with confidence.

Good product owners interact well with the business stakeholder community, the development team, and the scrum master. They are pragmatic and able to make trade-offs based on reality. They are accessible to the development team and also ask for what they need. They are patient, especially with questions from the development team.

Table 6-1 outlines the responsibilities and matching characteristics of a product owner.

TABLE 6-1   **Characteristics of a Good Product Owner**

Responsibility	A Good Product Owner . . .
Supplies project strategy and direction	Envisions the completed product
	Firmly understands company strategy
Provides product expertise	Has worked with similar products in the past
	Understands the needs of the people who will use the product

(continued)

TABLE 6-1 *(continued)*

Responsibility	A Good Product Owner . . .
Understands customer and other stakeholder needs	Understands relevant business processes
	Creates a solid customer input and feedback channel
	Works well with business stakeholders
Manages and prioritizes product requirements	Is decisive
	Focuses on efficiency
	Remains flexible
	Turns stakeholder feedback into valuable, customer-focused functionality
	Is practical about prioritizing financially valuable features, high-risk features, and strategic system improvements
	Shields the development team from business distractions (competing stakeholder requests)
Is responsible for budget and profitability	Understands which product features can deliver the best return on investment
	Manages budgets effectively
Decides on release dates	Understands business needs regarding timelines
Works with development team	Is accessible for daily clarification of requirements
	Works with the development team to understand capabilities
	Works well with developers
	Adeptly describes product features
Accepts or rejects work	Understands requirements and ensures that completed features work correctly
Presents completed work at the end of each sprint	Clearly introduces the accomplishments of the sprint before the development team demonstrates the sprint's working functionality

The product owner takes on a great deal of business–related responsibility during the project. Although the project sponsor funds and owns the budget, the product owner manages how the budget is spent.

With a dedicated and decisive product owner, the development team has all the business support it needs to turn requirements into working functionality. The following section explains how the product owner helps ensure that the development team understands the product it will create.

Development team member

Development team members are the people who create the product. In software development, programmers, testers, designers, writers, data engineers, and anyone else with a hands-on role in product development are development team members. With other types of product, the development team members may have different skills.

On an agile project, the development team is

>> Directly accountable for creating project deliverables.

>> Self-organizing and self-managing. The development team members determine their own tasks and how they want to complete those tasks.

>> Cross-functional. Collectively, the development team possesses all skills required to elaborate, design, develop, test, integrate and document requirements into working functionality.

>> Multi-skilled. Development team members are versatile — they're not tied to a single skill set. They have existing skills to immediately contribute at the beginning of the project, but they are also willing to learn new skills and to teach what they know to other development team members.

>> Ideally dedicated to one project for the duration of the project.

>> Ideally collocated. The team should be working together in the same area of the same office.

What makes a good development team member? Take a look at the team responsibilities and matching characteristics in Table 6-2.

TABLE 6-2   **Characteristics of a Good Development Team Member**

Responsibility	A Good Development Team Member . . .
Creates the product	Enjoys creating products
	Is skilled in more than one of the jobs necessary to create the product
Is self-organizing and self-managing	Exudes initiative and independence
	Understands how to work through impediments to achieve goals
	Coordinates the work to be done with the rest of the team

(continued)

TABLE 6-2 *(continued)*

Responsibility	A Good Development Team Member . . .
Is cross-functional	Has curiosity
	Willingly contributes to areas outside his or her mastery
	Enjoys learning new skills
	Enthusiastically shares knowledge
Is dedicated and collocated	Is part of an organization that understands the gains in efficiency and effectiveness associated with focused, collocated teams

The two other members of the scrum team, the product owner and the scrum master, help support the development team's efforts in creating the product. Whereas the product owner ensures that the development team is effective (working on the right things), the scrum master helps clear the way for the development team to work as efficiently as possible.

Scrum master

A scrum master, sometimes called a *project facilitator* in non-scrum agile environments, is responsible for supporting the development team, clearing organizational roadblocks, and keeping processes true to agile principles.

A scrum master is different from a project manager. Teams using traditional project approaches work for a project manager. A scrum master, on the other hand, is a servant-leader peer who supports the team so that it is fully functional and productive. The scrum master role is an enabling role, rather than an accountability role. You can find more about servant leadership in Chapter 14.

On an agile project, the scrum master will

>> Act as a process coach, helping the project team and the organization follow scrum values and practices.

>> Help remove project impediments — both reactively and proactively — and shield the development team from external interferences.

>> Foster close cooperation between stakeholders and the scrum team.

>> Facilitate consensus building within the scrum team.

>> Protect the scrum team from organizational distractions.

We compare the scrum master to the aeronautical engineer whose job is to reduce drag on the aircraft. Drag is always there but can be reduced through innovative and proactive engineering. Likewise, all projects have organizational impediments creating drag on the team's efficiency, and there is always another constraint that can be identified and removed. One of the most significant parts of a scrum master's role is removing roadblocks and preventing distractions to the development team's work. A scrum master who is good at these tasks is priceless to the project and to the team. If a development team has seven people, the effect of a good scrum master is times seven.

The product owner may never have participated in an agile project, but the scrum master likely has. As such, a scrum master may coach new product owners and development teams and does everything possible to help them succeed.

What makes a good scrum master? A scrum master doesn't need project manager experience. A scrum master is an expert in agile processes and can coach others. The scrum master must also work collaboratively with the product owner and the stakeholder community.

Facilitation skills cut through the noise of group gatherings and ensure that everyone on the scrum team is focused on the right priority at the right time.

Scrum masters have strong communication skills, with enough organizational clout to secure the conditions for success by negotiating for the right environment, protecting the team from distractions, and removing impediments. Scrum masters are great facilitators and great listeners. They can negotiate their way through conflicting opinions and help the team help itself. Review the scrum master's responsibilities and matching characteristics in Table 6-3.

TABLE 6-3   **Characteristics of a Good Scrum Master**

Responsibility	A Good Scrum Master . . .
Upholds scrum values and practices	Is an expert on scrum processes
	Is passionate about agile techniques
Removes roadblocks and prevents disruptions	Has organizational clout and can resolve problems quickly
	Is articulate, diplomatic, and professional
	Is a good communicator and a good listener
	Is firm about the development team's need to focus only on the project and the current sprint

(continued)

TABLE 6-3 *(continued)*

Responsibility	A Good Scrum Master . . .
Fosters close cooperation between external stakeholders and the scrum team	Looks at the needs of the project as a whole
	Avoids cliques and helps break down group silos
Facilitates consensus building	Understands techniques to help groups reach agreements
Is a servant-leader	Does not need or want to be in charge or be the boss
	Ensures that all members of the development team have the information they need to do the job, use their tools, and track progress
	Truly desires to help the scrum team

TIP

Clout is not the same thing as authority. Organizations need to empower their scrum masters so they can influence change in the project team and organization, but clout involves earned respect, often through success and experience. Some types of clout that empower scrum masters come about through expertise (usually a niche knowledge), longevity ("I've been at the company a long time and know its history first hand"), charisma ("people generally like me"), or associations ("I know important people"). Don't underestimate the value of a scrum master with clout.

The members of the scrum team — the product owner, development team, and scrum master — work together on the project every day.

As we mention earlier in the chapter, the scrum team plus stakeholders make up the project team. Sometimes stakeholders have less active participation than scrum team members but still can have considerable effect and provide a great deal of value to a project.

Stakeholders

Stakeholders are anyone with an interest in the project. They are not ultimately responsible for executing the product, but they provide input and are affected by the project's outcome. The group of stakeholders is diverse and can include people from different departments or even different companies.

On an agile project, stakeholders

>> Include the customer

>> May include technical people, such as infrastructure architects or system administrators

GAINING CONSENSUS: THE FIST OF FIVE

Part of working as a team means agreeing on decisions as a team. An important part of being a scrum master is helping the team build consensus. We've all worked with groups where it was difficult to arrive at consensus, from how long a task would take to where to go for lunch. A quick, casual way to find out whether a group agrees with an idea is to use the *fist of five,* which appears similar to rock-paper-scissors.

On the count of three, each person holds up a number of fingers, reflecting the degree of comfort with the idea in question:

5: I love the idea.

4: I think it's a good idea.

3: I can support the idea.

2: I have reservations, so let's discuss.

1: I am opposed to the idea.

If some people have three, four, or five fingers up, and some have only one or two, discuss the idea. Find out why the people who support the idea think it will work, and what reservations the people who oppose the idea have. You want to get all group members showing at least three fingers — they don't need to love the idea, but they need to support it. The scrum master's consensus-building skills are essential for this task.

You can also quickly get an idea of consensus on a decision by asking for a simple thumb up (support), thumb down (don't support), or thumb to the side (undecided). It's quicker than a fist of five, and is great for answering yes-or-no questions.

>> May include the legal department, account managers, salespeople, marketing experts, and customer service representatives

>> May include product or subject matter experts besides the product owner

Stakeholders may help provide key insights about the product and its use. Stakeholders might work closely with the product owner during the sprint, and will give feedback about the product during the sprint review at the end of each sprint.

Stakeholders and the part they play vary among projects and organizations. Almost all agile projects have stakeholders outside the scrum team.

Some projects also have agile mentors, especially projects with project teams that are new to agile processes.

Agile mentor

A mentor is a great idea for any area in which you want to develop new expertise. The *agile mentor,* sometimes called an *agile coach,* is someone who has experience implementing agile projects and can share that experience with a project team. The agile mentor can provide valuable feedback and advice to new project teams and to project teams that want to perform at a higher level.

On an agile project, the agile mentor

>> Serves in a mentoring role only and is not part of the scrum team

>> Is often a person from outside the organization, and can provide objective guidance, without personal or political considerations

>> Is an agile expert with significant experience in implementing agile techniques and running agile projects of different sizes

You may want to think of an agile mentor the way you think of a golf coach. Most people use a golf coach not because they don't know how to play the game of golf but because a golf coach objectively observes things that a player engaged in the game never notices. Golf, like implementing agile techniques, is an exercise where small nuances make a world of difference in performance.

Establishing New Values

Lots of organizations post their core values on the wall. In this section, however, we are talking about values that represent a way of working together every day, supporting each other, and doing whatever it takes to achieve the scrum team's commitments.

In addition to the values from the Agile Manifesto, the five core values for scrum teams are

>> Commitment

>> Courage

>> Focus

>> Openness

>> Respect

The following sections provide details about each of these values.

Commitment

Commitment implies engagement and involvement. On agile projects, the scrum team pledges to achieve specific goals. Confident that the scrum team will deliver what it promises, the organization mobilizes around the pledge to meet each goal.

Agile processes, including the idea of self-organization, provide people with all the authority they need to meet commitments. However, commitment requires a conscious effort. Consider the following points:

>> Scrum teams must be realistic when making commitments, especially for short sprints. It is easier, both logistically and psychologically, to bring new features into a sprint than it is to take unachievable features out of a sprint.

>> Scrum teams must fully commit to goals. This includes having consensus among the team that the goal is achievable. After the scrum team agrees on a goal, the team does whatever it takes to reach that goal.

>> The scrum team is pragmatic but ensures that every sprint has a tangible value. Achieving a sprint goal and completing every item in the goal's scope are different. For example, a sprint goal of proving that a product can perform a specific action is much better than a goal stating that exactly seven requirements will be complete during the sprint. Effective scrum teams focus on the goal and remain flexible in the specifics of how to reach that goal.

>> Scrum teams are willing to be accountable for results. The scrum team has the power to be in charge of the project. As a scrum team member, you can be responsible for how you organize your day, the day-to-day work, and the outcome.

Consistently meeting commitments is central to using agile approaches for long-term planning. In Chapter 13, you read about how to use performance to accurately determine project schedules and budgets.

Courage

We all experience fear. We all have certain things we don't want to do, whether asking a team member to explain something we don't understand or confronting the boss. Embracing agile techniques is a change for many organizations. Successfully making changes requires courage in the face of resistance. Following are some tips that foster courage:

>> **Realize that the processes that worked in the past won't necessarily work now.** Sometimes you need to remind people of this fact. If you want to be successful with agile techniques, your everyday work processes need to change to improve.

>> **Be ready to buck the status quo.** The status quo will push back. Some people have vested interests and will not want to change how they work.

>> **Temper challenge with respect.** Senior members of the organization might be especially resistant to change; they often created the old rules for how things were done. Now you're challenging those rules. Respectfully remind these individuals that you can achieve the benefits of agile techniques only by following the 12 agile principles faithfully. Ask them to give change a try.

>> **Embrace the other values.** Have the courage to make commitments and stand behind those commitments. Have the courage to focus and tell distracters "no." Have the courage to be open and to acknowledge that there is always an opportunity to improve. And have the courage to be respectful and tolerant of other people's views, even when they challenge your views.

As you replace your organization's antiquated processes with more modern approaches, expect to be challenged. Take on that challenge; the rewards can be worth it in the end.

Focus

Working life is full of distractions. Plenty of people in your organization would love to use your time to make their day easier. Disruptions, however, are costly. Jonathan Spira, from the consulting firm Basex, published a report called "The Cost of Not Paying Attention: How Interruptions Impact Knowledge Worker Productivity." His report details how businesses in the United States lose close to $600 *billion* a year through workplace distractions.

Scrum team members can help change those dysfunctions by insisting on an environment that allows them to focus. To reduce distractions and increase productivity, scrum team members can

>> **Physically separate themselves from company distracters.** One of our favorite techniques for ensuring high productivity is to find an annex away from the company's core offices and have that be the scrum team's work area. Sometimes the best defense is distance.

>> **Ensure that you're not spending time on activities unrelated to the sprint goal.** If someone tries to distract you from the sprint goal with something that "has to be done," explain your priorities. Ask, "How will this request move the sprint goal forward?" This simple question can push a lot of activities off the to-do list.

>> **Figure out what needs to be done and do only that.** The development team determines the tasks necessary to achieve the sprint goal. If you're a development team member, use this ownership to drive your focus to the priority tasks at hand.

>> **Balance focused time with accessibility to the rest of the scrum team.** Francesco Cirillo's Pomodoro technique — splitting work into 25-minute time blocks, with breaks in between — helps achieve balance between focus and accessibility. We often recommend giving development team members noise-canceling headsets, the wearing of which is a "do not disturb" sign. However, we also suggest a team agreement that all scrum team members have a minimum set of office hours in which they are available for collaboration.

>> **Check that you're maintaining your focus.** If you're unsure of whether you are maintaining focus — it can be hard to tell — go back to the basic question, "Are my actions consistent with achieving the overall goal and the near-term goal (such as completing the current task)?"

As you can see, task focus is not a small priority. Extend the effort upfront to create a distraction-free environment that helps your team succeed.

Openness

Secrets have no place on an agile team. If the team is responsible for the result of the project, it only makes sense that they have all the facts at their disposal. Information is power, and ensuring that everyone has access to the information necessary to make the right decisions requires a willingness to be transparent. To leverage the power of openness, you can

>> **Ensure that everyone on the team has access to the same information.** Everything from the vision for the project down to the smallest detail about the status of tasks needs to be in the public domain as far as the team is concerned. Use a centralized repository as the single source for information, and then avoid the distraction of "status reporting" by putting all status (burndowns, impediment list, and so forth) and information in this one place. We often send a link to this repository to the project stakeholders and say, "All the information we have is a click away. There is no faster way to get updated."

- **Be open and encourage openness in others.** Team members must feel free to speak openly about problems and opportunities to improve, whether the issues are something that they're dealing with themselves or see elsewhere in the team. Openness requires trust within the team, and trust takes time to develop.

- **Defuse internal politics by discouraging gossip.** If someone starts talking to you about what another team member did or didn't do, ask him or her to take the issue to the person who can resolve it. Don't gossip yourself. Ever.

- **Always be respectful.** Openness is never an excuse to be destructive or mean. Respect is critical to an open team environment.

Small problems unaddressed often grow to become crises. Use an open environment to benefit from the input of the entire team and ensure that your development efforts are focused on the project's true priorities.

Respect

Each individual on the team has something important to contribute. Your background, education, and experiences have a distinctive influence on the team. Share your uniqueness and look for, and appreciate, the same in others. You encourage respect when you

- **Foster openness.** Respect and openness go hand in hand. Openness without respect causes resentment; openness with respect generates trust.

- **Encourage a positive work environment.** Happy people tend to treat one another better. Encourage positivity, and respect will follow.

- **Seek out differences.** Don't just tolerate differences; try to find them. The best solutions come from diverse opinions that have been considered and appropriately challenged.

- **Treat everyone on the team with the same degree of respect.** All team members should be accorded the same respect, regardless of their role, level of experience, or immediate contribution. Encourage everyone to give his or her best.

REMEMBER

Respect is the safety net that allows innovation to thrive. When people feel comfortable raising a wider range of ideas, the final solution can improve in ways that would never be considered without a respectful team environment. Use respect to your team's advantage.

Changing Team Philosophy

An agile development team operates differently from a team using a waterfall approach. Development team members must change their roles based on each day's priorities, organize themselves, and think about projects in a whole new way to achieve their commitments.

To be part of a successful agile project, development teams should embrace the following attributes:

>> **Dedicated team:** Each scrum team member works only on the project assigned to the scrum team, and not with outside teams or projects. Projects may finish and new projects may start, but the team stays the same.

>> **Cross-functionality:** The willingness and ability to work on different types of tasks to create the product.

>> **Self-organization:** The ability and responsibility to determine how to go about the work of product development.

>> **Self-management:** The ability and responsibility to keep work on track.

>> **Size-limited teams:** Right-size development teams to ensure effective communication. Smaller is better; the development team should never be larger than nine people.

>> **Ownership:** Take initiative for work and responsibility for results.

The following sections look at each of these ideas in more detail.

Dedicated team

A traditional approach to resource allocation (we prefer the term *talent allocation*) is to allocate portions of team members' time across multiple teams and projects to get to full 100 percent utilization to justify the expense of employing team members. For management, knowing that all hours of the week are accounted for and justified is gratifying. However, the result is lower productivity due to continual *context switching* — the cost associated with cognitive demobilization and remobilization to switch from one task to another.

Other common talent allocation practices include moving a team member from team to team to temporarily fill a skill gap or a manpower gap, and tasking a team with multiple projects at once. These tactics are often employed to try to do more with less, but all the input variances make it nearly impossible to predict outputs.

These approaches have similar results: a significant decrease in productivity and an inability to extrapolate performance. Studies clearly show a minimum of 30 percent increase in the time required to complete projects run in parallel instead of serially.

TECHNICAL STUFF

Thrashing is another term for context switching between tasks. Avoid thrashing by dedicating team members to a single project at a time.

The following results occur when you dedicate scrum teams to work on only one project at a time:

>> **More accurate release projections:** Because the same people are consistently doing the same tasks every sprint with the same amount of time allocated to the project from sprint to sprint, scrum teams can accurately and empirically extrapolate how long it will take to complete their remaining backlog items with more certainty than traditional splintered approaches.

>> **Effective, short iterations:** Sprints are short because the shorter the feedback loop, the more quickly scrum teams can respond to feedback and changing needs. There just isn't enough time for thrashing team members between projects.

>> **Fewer and less costly defects:** Context switching results in more defects because distracted developers produce lower quality functionality. It costs less to fix something while it is still fresh in your mind (during the sprint) than later, when you have to try to remember the context of what you were working on. Studies show that defects cost 6.5 times more to fix after the sprint ends and you've moved on to other requirements, 24 times more to fix when preparing for release, and 100 times more to fix after the product is in production.

TIP

If you want more predictability, higher productivity, and fewer defects, dedicate your scrum team members. We've found this to be one of the highest factors of agile transition success.

Cross-functionality

On traditional projects, experienced team members are often typecast as having a single skill. For example, a .NET programmer may always do .NET work, and a tester may always do quality control work. Team members with complementary skills are often considered to be part of separate groups, such as the programming group or the testing group.

Agile approaches bring the people who create products together into a cohesive group — the development team. People on agile development teams try to avoid titles and limited roles. Development team members may start a project with one skill, but learn to perform many different jobs throughout the project to help create the product.

Cross-functionality makes development teams more efficient. For example, suppose a daily scrum meeting uncovers testing as the highest priority task to complete the requirement. A programmer might help test to finish the task quickly. When the development team is cross-functional, it can *swarm* on product features, with as many people working on a single requirement as possible, to quickly complete the feature.

Cross-functionality also helps eliminate single points of failure. Consider traditional projects, where each person knows how to do one job. When a team member gets sick, goes on vacation, or leaves the company, no one else may be capable of doing his or her job. The tasks that person was doing are delayed. By contrast, cross-functional agile development team members are capable of doing many jobs. When one person is unavailable, another can step in.

Cross-functionality encourages each team member to

>> **Set aside the narrow label of what he or she can do.** Titles have no place on an agile team. Skills and an ability to contribute are what matter. Start thinking of yourself as a Special Forces commando — knowledgeable enough in different areas that you can take on any situation.

>> **Work to expand skills.** Don't work only in areas you already know. Try to learn something new each sprint. Techniques such as *pair programming* — where two developers work together to code one item — or shadowing other developers can help you learn new skills quickly and increase overall product quality.

>> **Step up to help someone who has run into a roadblock.** Helping someone with a real-world problem is a great way to learn a new skill.

>> **Be flexible.** A willingness to be flexible helps to balance workloads and makes the team more likely to reach its sprint goal.

With cross-functionality in place, you avoid waiting for key people to work on tasks. Instead, a motivated, even if somewhat less knowledgeable, development team member can work on a piece of functionality today. That development team member learns and improves, and the workflow continues to be balanced.

One big payback of cross-functionality is that the development team completes work quickly. Post-sprint review afternoons are often celebration time. Go to the movies together. Head to the beach or the bowling alley. Go home early.

Self-organization

Agile techniques emphasize self-organizing development teams to take advantage of development team members' varied knowledge and experience.

REMEMBER

If you've read Chapter 2, you may recall agile principle #11: The best architectures, requirements, and designs emerge from self-organizing teams.

Self-organization is an important part of being agile. Why? In a word: ownership. Self-organized teams are not complying with orders from others; they own the solution developed and that makes a huge difference in team member engagement and solution quality.

For development teams used to a traditional command-and-control project management model, self-organization may take some extra effort at first. Agile projects do not have a project manager to tell the development team what to do. Instead, self-organizing development teams

>> **Commit to their own sprint goals.** At the beginning of each sprint, the development team works with the product owner to identify an objective it can reach, based on project priorities.

>> **Identify their tasks.** Development team members determine the tasks necessary to meet each sprint goal. The development team works together to figure out who takes on which task, how to get the work done, and how to address risks and issues.

>> **Estimate the effort necessary for requirements and related tasks.** The development team knows the most about how much effort it will take to create specific product features.

>> **Focus on communication.** Successful agile development teams hone their communication skills by being transparent, communicating face-to-face, being aware of nonverbal communication, participating, and listening.

TIP

The key to communication is clarity. With complex topics, avoid one-way, potentially ambiguous modes of communication, such as email. Face-to-face communication prevents misunderstandings and frustration. You can always summarize the conversation in a quick email later if details need to be retained.

>> **Collaborate.** Getting the input of a diverse scrum team almost always improves the product but requires solid collaboration skills. Collaboration is the foundation of an effective agile team.

No successful project is an island. Collaboration skills help scrum team members take risks with ideas and bring innovative solutions to project problems. A safe and comfortable environment is a cornerstone of a successful agile project.

>> **Decide with consensus.** For maximum productivity, the entire development team must be on the same page and committed to the goal at hand. The scrum master often plays an active role in building consensus, but the development team ultimately takes responsibility for reaching agreement on decisions, and everyone owns the decisions.

>> **Actively participate.** Self-organization may be challenging for the shy. All development team members must actively participate. No one is going to tell the development team what to do to create the product. The development team members tell themselves what to do. And when. And how.

In our agile coaching experience, we've heard new agile development team members ask questions like, "So, what should I do now?" A good scrum master answers by asking the developer what he or she needs to do to achieve the sprint goal, or by asking the rest of the development team what they suggest. Answering questions with questions can be a helpful way to guide a development team toward being self-organizing.

Being part of a self-organizing development team takes responsibility, but it also has its rewards. Self-organization gives development teams the freedom to succeed. Self-organization increases ownership, which can result in better products, which can help development team members find more satisfaction in their work.

Self-management

Self-management is closely related to self-organization. Agile development teams have a lot of control over how they work; that control comes with the responsibility for ensuring the project is successful. To succeed with self-management, development teams

>> **Allow leadership to ebb and flow.** On agile projects, each person on the development team has the opportunity to lead. For different tasks, different leaders will naturally emerge; leadership will shift throughout the team based on skill expertise and previous experiences.

>> **Rely on agile processes and tools to manage the work.** Agile methods are tailored to make self-management easy. With an agile approach, meetings have clear purposes and time limits, and artifacts expose information but rely on minimal effort to create and maintain. Taking advantage of these processes allows development teams to spend most of their time creating the product.

>> **Report progress regularly and transparently.** Each development team member is responsible for accurately updating work status on a daily basis. Luckily, progress reporting is a quick task on agile projects. In Chapter 9, you find out about burndown charts, which provide status but only require a few minutes each day to update. Keeping status current and truthful makes planning and issue management easier.

>> **Manage issues within the development team.** Many obstacles can arise on a project: Development challenges and interpersonal problems are a couple of examples. The development team's first point of escalation for most issues is the development team itself.

>> **Create a team agreement.** Development teams sometimes make up a team agreement, a document that outlines the expectations each team member will commit to meet. Working agreements provide a shared understanding of behavioral expectations and empower the facilitator to keep the team on track according to what they've already agreed together.

>> **Inspect and adapt.** Figure out what works for your team. Best practices differ from team to team. Some teams work best by coming in early; others work best by coming in late. The development team is responsible for reviewing its own performance and identifying techniques to continue and techniques to change.

>> **Actively participate.** As with self-organization, self-management works only when development team members join in and commit to guiding the project's direction.

TIP

The development team is primarily responsible for self-organization and self-management. However, the scrum master can assist the development team in a number of ways. When development team members look for specific directions, the scrum master can remind them that they have the power to decide what to do and how to do it. If someone outside the development team tries to give orders, insist on tasks, or dictate how to create the product, the scrum master can intervene. The scrum master can be a powerful ally in the development team's self-organization and self-management.

Size-limited teams

Agile development teams are intentionally small. A small development team is a nimble team. As the development team size grows, so does the overhead associated with orchestrating task flow and communication flow.

Ideally, agile development teams have the least number of people necessary to be self-encapsulated (can do everything necessary to produce the product) and not have single points of failure. To have skill coverage, teams typically won't be any smaller than three people. Statistically, scrum teams are fastest with six developers, and cheapest with four to five developers. Keeping the development team size between three and nine people helps teams act as cohesive teams, and avoids creating subgroups, or *silos*.

Limiting development team size

>> Encourages diverse skills to be developed

>> Facilitates good team communication

>> Maintains the team in a single unit

>> Promotes joint code ownership, cross-functionality, and face-to-face communication

When you have a small development team, a similarly limited and focused project scope follows. Development team members are in close contact throughout the day as tasks, questions, and peer reviews flow back and forth among teammates. This cohesiveness ensures consistent engagement, increases communication, and reduces project risk.

When you have a large project and a correspondingly large development team, split the work between multiple scrum teams. For more on scaling agile projects across the enterprise, see Chapter 17.

Ownership

Being part of a cross-functional, self-organized, self-managing development team requires responsibility and ownership. The top-down management approaches on traditional projects do not always foster the maturity of ownership necessary for taking responsibility for projects and results. Even seasoned development team members may need to adjust their behavior to get used to making decisions on agile projects.

Development teams can adapt behavior and increase their level of ownership by doing the following:

>> **Take initiative.** Instead of waiting for someone else to tell you what to work on, take action. Do what is necessary to help meet commitments and goals.

>> **Succeed and fail as a team.** On agile projects, accomplishments and failures alike belong to the project team. If problems arise, be accountable as a group,

rather than finding blame. When you succeed, recognize the group effort necessary for that success.

>> **Trust the ability to make good decisions.** Development teams can make mature, responsible, and sound decisions about product development. This takes a degree of trust as team members become accustomed to having more control in a project.

Behavioral maturity and ownership doesn't mean that agile development teams are perfect. Rather, they take ownership for the scope they commit to, and they take responsibility for meeting those commitments. Mistakes happen. If they don't, you aren't pushing yourself outside your comfort zone. A mature development team identifies mistakes honestly, accepts responsibility for mistakes openly, and learns and improves from its mistakes consistently.

3

Agile Planning and Execution

Follow the Roadmap to Value, from vision to execution.

Define and estimate requirements.

Create working functionality and showcase it in iterations.

Inspect your work and adapt your processes for continuous improvement.

Chapter **7**

Defining the Product Vision and Product Roadmap

To start, let's dispel a common myth. If you've heard that agile projects don't include planning, dismiss that thought right now. You will plan not only the overall project but also every release, every sprint, and every day. Planning is fundamental to agile project success.

If you're a project manager, you probably do the bulk of your planning at the beginning of a project. You may have heard the phrase, "Plan the work, then work the plan," which sums up non-agile project management approaches.

Agile projects, in contrast, involve planning upfront and throughout the entire project. By planning at the last responsible moment, right before an activity starts, you know the most about that activity. This type of planning, called *just-in-time planning* or a *situationally informed strategy*, is a key to agile project success. Agile teams plan as much as, if not more than, traditional project teams. However, agile planning is more evenly distributed throughout the project and is done by the entire team that will be working on the project.

Helmuth von Moltke, a nineteenth-century German field marshal and military strategist, once said, "No plan survives contact with the enemy." That is, in the heat of a battle — much like in the thick of a project — plans always change. The agile focus on just-in-time planning allows you to accommodate real situations and to be well informed as you plan specific tasks.

This chapter describes how just-in-time planning works with agile projects. You also go through the first two steps of planning an agile project: creating the product vision and the product roadmap.

Agile Planning

Planning happens at a number of points in an agile project. A great way to look at the planning activities in agile projects is with the Roadmap to Value. Figure 7-1 shows the roadmap as a whole.

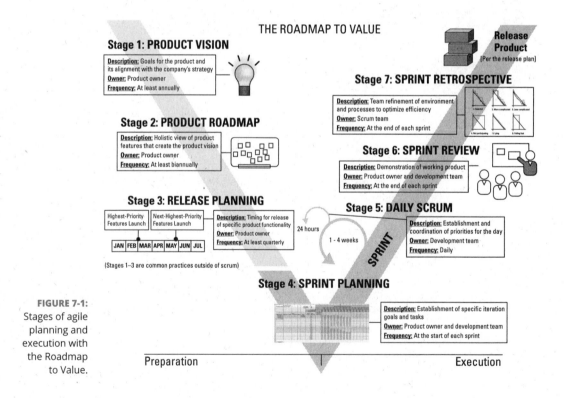

FIGURE 7-1:
Stages of agile planning and execution with the Roadmap to Value.

The Roadmap to Value has seven stages:

>> In stage 1, the product owner identifies the *product vision*. The product vision is your project's destination or end goal. The product vision includes the outer boundary of what your product will be, how the product is different from the competition, how the product will support your company or organization's strategy, who will use the product, and why people will use the product. On longer projects, revisit the product vision at least once a year.

>> In stage 2, the product owner creates a *product roadmap*. The product roadmap is a high-level view of the product requirements, with a general time frame for when you will develop those requirements. It also gives context to the vision by showing the tangible features that will be produced during the project. Identifying product requirements and then prioritizing and roughly estimating the effort for those requirements allow you to establish requirement themes and identify requirement gaps. The product owner, with support from the development team, should revise the product roadmap at least biannually.

>> In stage 3, the product owner creates a release plan. The *release plan* identifies a high-level timetable for the release of working functionality to the customer. The release serves as a mid-term boundary against which the scrum team can mobilize. An agile project will have many releases, with the highest-priority features appearing first. You create a release plan at the beginning of each release, which is usually at least quarterly. Find out more about release planning in Chapter 8.

>> In stage 4, the product owner, the development team, and the scrum master will plan iterations, also called sprints, and start creating the product function-ality in those sprints. *Sprint planning* sessions take place at the start of each sprint. During sprint planning, the scrum team determines a sprint goal, which establishes the immediate boundary of work that the team forecasts to accomplish during the sprint, with requirements that support the goal and can be completed in the sprint. The scrum team also outlines how to complete those requirements. Get more information about sprint planning in Chapter 8.

>> In stage 5, the development team has *daily scrum* meetings during each sprint to coordinate the day's priorities. In the daily scrum meeting, you discuss what you completed yesterday, what you will work on today, and any roadblocks you have, so that you can address issues immediately. Read about daily scrums in Chapter 9.

>> In stage 6, the scrum team holds a *sprint review* at the end of every sprint. In the sprint review, you demonstrate the working functionality to the product stakeholders. Find out how to conduct sprint reviews in Chapter 10.

>> In stage 7, the scrum team holds a *sprint retrospective*. The sprint retrospective is a meeting where the scrum team discusses the completed sprint with regard to their processes and environment, and makes plans for process improvements in the next sprint. Like the sprint review for inspecting and adapting the product, a sprint retrospective is held at the end of every sprint to inspect and adapt your processes and environment. Find out how to conduct sprint retrospectives in Chapter 10.

Each stage in the Roadmap to Value is repeatable, and each stage contains planning activities. Agile planning, like agile development, is iterative.

Progressive elaboration

During each stage in an agile project, you plan only as much as you need to plan. In the early stages of your project, you plan widely and holistically to create a broad outline of how the product will shape up over time. In later stages, you narrow your planning and add more details to ensure success in the immediate development effort. This process is called a *progressive elaboration of requirements*.

Planning broadly at first and in detail later, when necessary, prevents you from wasting time on planning lower-priority product requirements that may never be implemented. This model also lets you add high-value requirements during the project without disrupting the development flow.

The more just-in-time your detailed planning is, the more efficient your planning process becomes.

REMEMBER

Some studies show customers rarely or never use 64 percent of the features in an application. In the first few development cycles of an agile project, you complete features that have the highest priority and that people *will* use. Typically, you release those groups of features as early as possible to gain market share through first-mover advantage; receive customer feedback for viability; monetize functionality early to optimize return on investment (ROI); and avoid internal and external obsolescence.

Inspect and adapt

Just-in-time planning brings into play two fundamental tenets of agile techniques: inspect and adapt. At each stage of a project, you need to look at the product and the process (inspect) and make changes as necessary (adapt).

Agile planning is a rhythmic cycle of inspecting and adapting. Consider the following:

>> Each day during the sprint, the product owner provides feedback to help improve the product as the development team creates the product.

>> At the end of each sprint, in the sprint review, stakeholders provide feedback to further improve the product.

>> Also at the end of each sprint, in the sprint retrospective, the scrum team discusses the lessons it learned during the past sprint to improve the development process.

>> After a release, the customers can provide feedback for improvement. Feedback might be direct, when a customer contacts the company about the product, or indirect, when potential customers either do or don't purchase the product.

Inspect and adapt, together, are fantastic tools for delivering the right product in the most efficient manner.

REMEMBER

At the beginning of a project, you know the least about the product you're creating, so trying to plan fine details at that time just doesn't work. Being agile means you do the detailed planning when you need it, and immediately develop the specific requirements you defined with that planning.

Now that you know a little more about how agile planning works, it's time to complete the first step in an agile project: defining the product vision.

Defining the Product Vision

The first stage in an agile project is defining your product vision. The *product vision statement* is an elevator pitch, or a quick summary, to communicate how your product supports the company's or organization's strategies. The vision statement must articulate the end state for the product.

The product might be a commercial product for release to the marketplace or an internal solution that will support your organization's day-to-day functions. For example, say your company is XYZ Bank and your product is a mobile banking application. What company strategies does a mobile banking application support? How does the application support the company's strategies? Your vision statement clearly and concisely links the product to your business strategy.

Figure 7-2 shows how the vision statement — stage 1 of the Roadmap to Value — fits with the rest of the stages and activities in an agile project.

A common agile practice

FIGURE 7-2:
The product
vision statement
as part of the
Roadmap to
Value.

Stage 1: PRODUCT VISION

Description: Goals for the product and its alignment with the company's strategy
Owner: Product owner
Frequency: At least annually

The product owner is responsible for knowing about the product, its goals, and its requirements throughout the project. For those reasons, the product owner creates the vision statement, although other people may have input. After the vision statement is complete, it becomes a guiding light, the "what we are trying to achieve" statement that the development team, scrum master, and stakeholders refer to throughout the project.

When creating a product vision statement, follow these four steps:

1. **Develop the product objective.**

2. **Create a draft vision statement.**

3. **Validate the vision statement with product and project stakeholders and revise it based on feedback.**

4. **Finalize the vision statement.**

The look of a vision statement follows no hard-and-fast rules. However, anyone involved with the project, from the development team to the CEO, should be able to understand the statement. The vision statement should be internally focused, clear, nontechnical, and as brief as possible. The vision statement should also be explicit and avoid marketing fluff.

Step 1: Developing the product objective

To write your vision statement, you must understand and be able to communicate the product's objective. You need to identify the following:

>> **Customer:** Who will use the product? This question might have more than one answer.

>> **Key product goals:** How will the product benefit the company that is creating it? The goals may include benefits for a specific department in your company, such as customer service or the marketing department, as well as the company as a whole. What specific company strategies does the product support?

>> **Need:** Why does the customer need the product? What features are critical to the customer?

>> **Competition:** How does the product compare with similar products?

>> **Primary differentiation:** What makes this product different from the status quo or the competition or both?

Step 2: Creating a draft vision statement

After you have a good grasp of the product's objective, create a first draft of your vision statement.

You can find many templates for a product vision statement. For an excellent guide to defining the overall product vision, see *Crossing the Chasm*, by Geoffrey Moore (published by HarperCollins), which focuses on how to bridge the gap (chasm) between early adopters of new technologies and the majority who follow.

The adoption of any new product is a gamble. Will users like the product? Will the market take to the product? Will there be an adequate return on investment for developing the product? In *Crossing the Chasm*, Moore describes how early adopters are driven by vision, whereas the majority are skeptical of visionaries and interested in down-to-earth issues of quality, product maintenance, and longevity.

TECHNICAL STUFF

Return on investment, or ROI, is the benefit or value a company gets from paying for something. ROI can be quantitative, such as the additional money ABC Products makes from selling widgets online after investing in a new website. ROI can also be something intangible, such as better customer satisfaction for XYZ Bank customers who use the bank's new mobile banking application.

By creating your vision statement, you help convey your product's quality, maintenance needs, and longevity.

Moore's product vision approach is pragmatic. In Figure 7-3, we construct a template based on Moore's approach to more explicitly connect the product to the company's strategies. If you use this template for your product vision statement, it will stand the test of time as your product goes from early adoption to mainstream usage.

TIP

One way to make your product vision statement more compelling is to write it in the present tense, as if the product already exists. Using present tense helps readers imagine the product in use.

```
Vision Statement for Product

For _____ (target customer)
who _____ (needs)
the _____ (product name)
is a _____ (product category)
that _____ (product benefit, reason to buy)
Unlike _____ (competitors)
our product ____ (differentiation/value proposition)
```

Using our expansion of Moore's template, a vision statement for a mobile banking application might look like the following:

For XYZ Bank customers

who want access to banking capability while on the go,

the MyXYZ

is a mobile application

that allows secure, on-demand banking, 24 hours a day.

Unlike online banking from your home or office computer,

our product allows users immediate access,

which supports our strategy to provide quick, convenient banking services, anytime, anywhere. **(Platinum Edge addition)**

As you can see, a vision statement identifies a future state for the product when the product reaches completion. The vision focuses on the conditions that should exist when the product is complete.

WARNING

Avoid generalizations in your vision statement such as "make customers happy" or "sell more products." Also watch out for too much technological specificity, such as "using release 9.x of Java, create a program with four modules that . . ." At this early stage, defining specific technologies might limit you later.

Here are a few extracts from vision statements that should ring warning bells:

» Secure additional customers for the MyXYZ application.

» Satisfy our customers by December.

» Eliminate all defects and improve quality.

>> Create a new application in Java.

>> Beat the Widget Company to market by six months.

Step 3: Validating and revising the vision statement

After you draft your vision statement, review it against the following quality checklist:

>> Is this vision statement clear, focused, and written for an internal audience?

>> Does the statement provide a compelling description of how the product meets customer needs?

>> Does the vision describe the best possible outcome?

>> Is the business objective specific enough that the goal is achievable?

>> Does the statement deliver value that is consistent with corporate strategies and goals?

>> Is the product vision statement compelling?

>> Is the vision concise?

These yes-or-no questions will help you determine whether your vision statement is thorough and clear. If any answers are no, revise the vision statement.

When all answers are yes, move on to reviewing the statement with others, including the following:

>> **Project stakeholders:** The stakeholders will be able to identify that the vision statement includes everything the product should accomplish.

>> **Your development team:** The team, because it will create the product, must understand what the product needs to accomplish.

>> **Scrum master:** A strong understanding of the product will help the scrum master remove roadblocks and ensure that the development team is on the right path later in the project.

>> **Agile mentor:** Share the vision statement with your agile mentor, if you have one. The agile mentor is independent of the organization and can provide an external perspective, qualities that can make for a great objective voice.

See whether others think the vision statement is clear and delivers the message you want to convey. Review and revise the vision statement until the project stakeholders, the development team, and the scrum master fully understand the statement.

REMEMBER

At this stage of your project, you might not have a development team or scrum master. After you form a scrum team, be sure to review the vision statement with it.

Step 4: Finalizing the vision statement

After you finish revising the vision statement, make sure your development team, scrum master, and stakeholders have the final copy. You might even put a copy on the wall in the scrum team's work area, where you can see it every day. You will refer to the vision statement throughout the life of the project.

If your project is more than a year long, you may want to revisit the vision statement. We like to review the product vision statement at least once a year to make sure the product reflects the marketplace and supports any changes in the company's needs. Because the vision statement is the long-term boundary of the project, the project should end when the vision is no longer viable.

REMEMBER

The product owner owns the product vision statement and is responsible for its preparation and communication across the organization. The product vision sets expectations for stakeholders and helps the development team stay focused on the goal.

Congratulations. You've just completed the first stage in your agile project. Now it's time to create a product roadmap.

Creating a Product Roadmap

The product roadmap, stage 2 in the Roadmap to Value (see Figure 7-4), is an overall view of the product's requirements and a valuable tool for planning and organizing the journey of product development. Use the product roadmap to categorize requirements, prioritize them, identify gaps and dependencies, and determine a timetable for releasing to the customer.

As he or she does with the product vision statement, the product owner creates the product roadmap, with help from the development team and stakeholders. The development team participates to a greater degree than it did during the creation of the vision statement.

Stage 2: PRODUCT ROADMAP

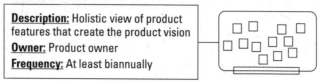

FIGURE 7-4:
The product
roadmap as part
of the Roadmap
to Value.

Description: Holistic view of product features that create the product vision
Owner: Product owner
Frequency: At least biannually

TIP

Keep in mind that you will refine requirements and effort estimates throughout the project. In the product roadmap phase, it's okay for your requirements, estimates, and time frames to be at a very high level.

To create your product roadmap, you do the following:

1. **Identify stakeholders.**

2. **Establish product requirements and add them to the roadmap.**

3. **Arrange the product requirements based on values, risks, and dependencies.**

4. **Estimate the development effort at a high level and prioritize the product's requirements.**

5. **Determine high-level time frames for releasing groups of functionality to the customer.**

Because priorities can change, expect to update your product roadmap throughout the project. We like to update the product roadmap at least twice a year.

TIP

Your product roadmap can be as simple as sticky notes arranged on a whiteboard, which makes updates as easy as moving a sticky note from one section of the whiteboard to another.

You use the product roadmap to plan releases — stage 3 in the Roadmap to Value. *Releases* are groups of usable product functionality that you release to customers to gather real-world feedback and to generate return on investment.

The following section details the steps to create a product roadmap.

Step 1: Identifying stakeholders

When initially establishing the product vision, it's likely you will have identified only a few key stakeholders who are available to provide high-level feedback. At the product roadmap stage, you put more context to the product vision and identify how you achieve the vision, which gives more insight into who will have a stake in your project.

This is the time to engage with existing and newly identified stakeholders to gather feedback on the functionality you want to implement to achieve the vision. The product roadmap is your first cut at a high-level product backlog, discussed later in this chapter. With this first round of detail identified, you'll want to engage more than just the scrum team, project sponsor, and obvious users. Consider including the following people:

>> **Marketing department:** Your customers need to know about your product, and that's what the marketing department provides. They need to understand your plans, and may have input into the order in which you release functionality to the market, based on their experience and research.

>> **Customer service department:** Once your product is in the market, how will it be supported? Specific roadmap items might identify the person you'll need to prepare for support. For instance, a product owner may not see much value in plugging in a live online chat feature, but a customer service manager may see it differently because his or her representatives can handle simultaneously only one phone call but as many as six chat sessions.

>> **Sales department:** Make sure that the sales team members see the product so that they start selling the same thing you are building. Like the marketing department, the sales department will have first-hand knowledge about what your customers are looking for.

>> **Legal department:** Especially if you're in a highly regulated industry, review your roadmap with legal counsel as early as possible to make sure you haven't missed anything that could put your project at risk if discovered later in the project.

>> **Additional customers:** While identifying features on your roadmap, you may discover additional people who will find value in what you will create. Give them a chance to review your roadmap to validate your assumptions.

Step 2: Establishing product requirements

The second step in creating a product roadmap is to identify, or define, the different requirements for your product.

When you first create your product roadmap, you typically start with large, high-level requirements. The requirements on your product roadmap will most likely be at two different levels: themes and features. *Themes* are logical groups of features and requirements at their highest levels. *Features* are parts of the product at a very high level and describe a new capability the customer will have once the feature is complete.

DECOMPOSING REQUIREMENTS

Throughout the project, you'll break down requirements into smaller, more manageable parts using a process called *decomposition,* or *progressive elaboration.* You can break down requirements into the following sizes, listed from largest to smallest:

Themes: A *theme* is a logical group of features and is also a requirement at its highest level. You may group features into themes in your product roadmap.

Features: *Features* are parts of products at a very high level. Features describe a new capability the customers will have once the feature is complete. You use features in your product roadmap.

Epic user stories: *Epics* are medium-sized requirements that are decomposed from a feature and often contain multiple actions or channels of value. You need to break down your epics before you can start creating functionality from them. You can find out how you use epics for release planning in Chapter 8.

User stories: *User stories* are requirements that contain a single action or integration and are small enough to start implementing into functionality. You see how you define user stories and use them at the release and sprint level in Chapter 8.

Tasks: *Tasks* are the execution steps required to develop a requirement into working functionality. You break down user stories into different tasks during sprint planning. You can find out about tasks and sprint planning in Chapter 8.

Keep in mind that each requirement may not go through all these sizes. For example, you may create a particular requirement at the user story level, and never think of it on the theme or epic scale. You may create a requirement at the epic user story level, but it may be a lower-priority requirement. Because of just-in-time planning, you may not take the time to decompose that lower-priority epic user story until you complete development of all the higher-priority requirements.

To identify product themes and features, the product owner can work with stakeholders and the development team. It may help to have a requirements session, where the stakeholders and the development team meet and write down as many requirements that they can think of.

TIP

When you start creating requirements at the theme and feature level, it can help to write those requirements on index cards or big sticky notes. Using a physical card that you can move from one category to another and back again can make organizing and prioritizing those requirements very easy.

While you create the product roadmap, the features you identify start to make up your *product backlog* — the full list of what is in scope for a product, regardless of level of detail. Once you have identified your first product features, you have your product backlog started.

Step 3: Arranging product features

After you identify your product features, you work with the stakeholders to group them into *themes* — common, logical groups of features. A stakeholder meeting works well for grouping features, just like it works for creating requirements. You can group features by usage flow, technical similarity, or business need.

Visualizing themes and features on your roadmap allows you to assign business value and risks associated with each feature relative to others. The product owner, along with the development team and stakeholders, can also identify dependencies between features, locate any gaps, and prioritize the order in which each feature should be developed based on each of these factors.

Here are questions to consider when grouping and ordering your requirements:

- >> How would customers use our product?
- >> If we offered this proposed feature, what else would customers need to do? What else might they want to do?
- >> Can the development team identify technical affinities or dependencies?

Use the answers to these questions to identify your themes. Then group the features by these themes. For example, in the mobile banking application, the themes might be

- >> Account information
- >> Transactions
- >> Customer service functions
- >> Mobile functions

Figure 7-5 shows features grouped by themes.

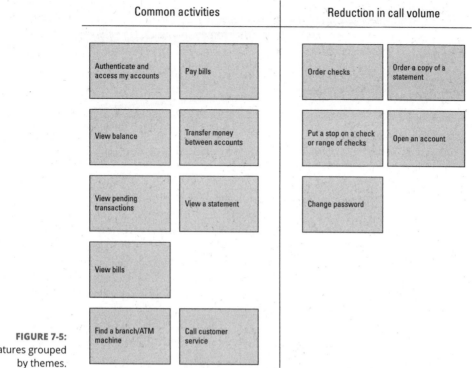

FIGURE 7-5: Features grouped by themes.

Step 4: Estimating efforts and ordering requirements

You've identified your product requirements and arranged those requirements into logical groups. Next, you estimate and prioritize the requirements. Here are a few terms you need to be familiar with:

» *Effort* is the ease or difficulty of creating functionality from a particular requirement.

» An *estimate,* as a noun, can be the number or description you use to express the estimated effort of a requirement.

» *Estimating* a requirement, as a verb, means to come up with an approximate idea of how easy or hard (how much effort) that requirement will be to create.

>> *Ordering*, or *prioritizing*, a requirement means to determine that requirement's value and risk in relation to other requirements, and in what order you will implement them.

>> *Value* means how beneficial a product requirement might be to the organization creating that product.

>> *Risk* refers to the negative effect a requirement can have on the project.

You can estimate and prioritize requirements at any level, from themes and features down to single user stories.

Prioritizing requirements is really about ordering them. You can find various methods — many of them complicated — for determining the priority of product backlog items. We keep things simple by creating an ordered to-do list of product backlog items, based on business value, risk, and effort, listed in the order in which you will implement them. Forcing an order requires making a priority decision for every requirement relative to every other requirement. A scrum team can work on one thing at a time, so it is important to format your product roadmap accordingly.

To score your requirements, you work with two different groups of people:

>> The development team determines the effort to implement the functionality for each requirement.

>> The product owner, with support from the stakeholders, determines the value and risk of the requirement to the customer and the business.

Estimating effort

To order requirements, the development team must first estimate the effort for each requirement relative to all other requirements.

In Chapter 8, we show you relative estimation techniques that agile teams use to accurately estimate effort. Traditional estimation methods aim for precision by using absolute time estimates at every level of the project schedule, whether the team is working on the work items today or two years from now. This practice gives non-agile teams a false sense of precision and isn't accurate in reality (as thousands of failed projects prove). How could you possibly know what each team member will be working on six months from now, and how long it will take to do that work, when you are just starting to learn about the project at the beginning?

Relative estimating is a self-correcting mechanism that allows agile teams to be more accurate because it's much easier to be right when comparing one requirement against another and determining whether one is bigger than another, and by roughly how much.

To order your requirements, you also want to know any dependencies. Dependencies mean that one requirement is a predecessor for another requirement. For example, if you were to have an application that needs someone to log in with a username and password, the requirement for creating the username would be a dependency for the requirement for creating the password, because you generally need a username to set up a password.

Assessing business value and risk

Together with stakeholders, the product owner identifies the highest business value items (either high potential ROI or other perceived value to the end customer), as well as those items with high negative impact on the project if unresolved.

Similar to effort estimates, values or risks can be assigned to each product roadmap item. For example, you might assign value using monetary ROI amounts or, for an internally used product, assign value or risk by using high, medium, or low.

Effort, business value, and risk estimates inform the product owner's prioritization decisions for each requirement. The highest value and risk items should be at the top of the product roadmap. High-risk items should be explored and implemented first to avoid rear-loading the project's risk. If a high-risk item will cause a project to fail (an issue that cannot be resolved), agile teams learn about it early. If a project is going to fail, you want to fail early, fail cheap, and move on to a new project that has value. In that sense, failure is a form of success for an agile team.

After you have your value, risk, and effort estimates, you can determine the relative priority, or order, of each requirement.

>> A requirement with high value or high risk (or both) and low effort will have a high relative priority. The product owner might order this item at the top of the roadmap.

>> A requirement with low value or low risk (or both) and high effort will have a lower relative priority. This item will likely end up toward the bottom of the roadmap.

WARNING

Relative priority is only a tool to help the product owner make decisions and prioritize requirements. It isn't a mathematical universal that you must follow. Make sure your tools help rather than hinder.

Prioritizing requirements

To determine the overall priority for your requirements, answer the following questions:

>> What is the relative priority of the requirement?

>> What are the prerequisites for any requirement?

>> What set of requirements belong together and will constitute a solid set of functionality you can release to the customer?

Using the answers to these questions, you can place the highest-priority requirements first in the product roadmap. When you've finished prioritizing your requirements, you'll have something that looks like Figure 7-6.

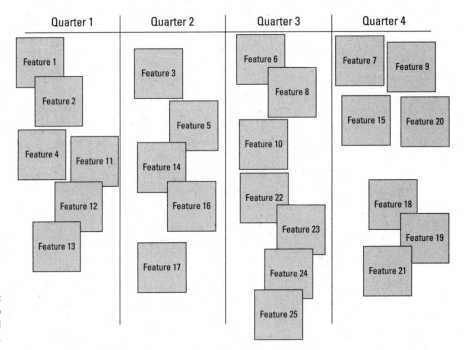

FIGURE 7-6:
Product roadmap with ordered requirements.

Your prioritized list of requirements is called a *product backlog.* Your product backlog is an important agile document, or *artifact.* You use this backlog throughout your entire project.

With a product backlog in hand, you can start adding target releases to your product roadmap.

Step 5: Determining high-level time frames

When you create your product roadmap, your time frames for releasing product requirements are at a very high level. For the initial roadmap, choose a logical time increment for your project, such as a certain number of days, weeks, months, quarters (three-month periods), or even larger increments. Using both the requirement and the priority, you can add requirements to each increment of time.

REMEMBER

Creating a product roadmap might seem like a lot of work, but after you get the hang of it, you can create one in a short time. Some scrum teams can create a product vision, a product roadmap, and a release plan and be ready to start their sprint in as little as one day! To begin developing the product, you need only enough requirements for your first sprint. You can determine the rest as the project progresses.

Saving your work

Up until now, you could do all your roadmap planning with whiteboards and sticky notes. After your first full draft is complete, however, save the product roadmap, especially if you need to share the roadmap with remote stakeholders or development team members. You could take a photo of your sticky notes and whiteboard, or you could type the information into a document and save it electronically.

You update the product roadmap throughout the project, as priorities change. For now, the contents of the first release should be clear — and that's all you need to worry about at this stage.

Completing the Product Backlog

The product roadmap contains high level features and some tentative release timelines. The requirements on your product roadmap are the first version of your *product backlog.*

The product backlog is the list of all requirements associated with the project. The product owner is responsible for creating and maintaining the product backlog by adding and prioritizing requirements. The scrum team uses the prioritized product backlog throughout the project to plan its work — like a streamlined project plan.

Figure 7-7 shows a sample product backlog. At a minimum, when creating your product backlog, be sure to do the following:

» Include a description of each requirement.

» Order the requirements based on priority.

» Add the effort estimate.

PRODUCT BACKLOG

Order	ID	Item	Type	Status	Estimate
1	121	As an Administrator, I want to link accounts to profiles, so that customers can access new accounts.	Requirement	Not Started	5
2	113	Update requirements traceability matrix.	Overhead	Not Started	2
3	403	Test automation training for Michael.	Improvement	Not Started	3
4	97	Refactor Login Class.	Maintenance	Not Started	8
5	68	As a Site Visitor, I want to find locations, so that I can use bank services.	Requirement	Not Started	8

FIGURE 7-7:
Product backlog
items sample.

We also like to include the type of backlog item as well as the status. Scrum teams will work mainly on developing features as described in the words of the user (user stories). But there may be need for other types of product backlog items, such as overhead items (things the scrum team determines are needed but don't contribute to the functionality), maintenance items (design improvements that need to be done to the product or system but don't directly increase value to the customer), or improvement items (action items for process improvements identified in the sprint retrospective). You can see examples of each of these in Figure 7-7.

REMEMBER

In Chapter 2, we explain how documents for agile projects should be barely sufficient, with only information that is absolutely necessary to create the product. If you keep your product backlog format simple and barely sufficient, you'll save time updating it throughout the project.

The scrum team refers to the product backlog as the main source for project requirements. If a requirement exists, it's in the product backlog. The requirements in your product backlog will change throughout the project in several ways. For example, as the team completes requirements, you mark those requirements as complete in the product backlog. You also record any new requirements gathered based on feedback from stakeholders and customers. Some requirements will be updated with new or clarified information, broken down into smaller user stories, or refined in other ways. Additionally, you update the priority and effort scores of existing requirements as needed.

The total number of story points in the product backlog — all user story points added together — is your current *product backlog estimate.* This estimate changes daily as user stories are completed and new user stories are added. Discover more about using the product backlog estimate to predict the project length and cost in Chapter 13.

REMEMBER

Keep your product backlog up to date so that you always have accurate cost and schedule estimates. A current product backlog also gives you the flexibility to prioritize newly identified product requirements — a key agile benefit — against existing features.

After you have a product backlog, you can begin planning releases and sprints, which we show you in the next chapter.

Chapter **8**

Planning Releases and Sprints

After you create a product roadmap for your agile project (see Chapter 7), it's time to start elaborating on your product details. In this chapter, you discover how to break down your requirements to a more granular level, refine your product backlog, create a release plan, and build a sprint backlog for execution. First, you see how to break down the larger requirements from your product roadmap into smaller, more manageable requirements called *user stories*.

REMEMBER

The concept of breaking down requirements into smaller pieces is called *decomposition*.

Refining Requirements and Estimates

You start agile projects with very large requirements. As the project progresses and you get closer to developing those requirements, you will break them down into smaller parts — small enough to begin developing.

One clear, effective format for defining product requirements is the user story. The user story and its larger cousin, the epic user story, are good-sized requirements for release planning and sprint planning. In this section, you find out how to create a user story, prioritize user stories, and estimate user story effort.

What is a user story?

The *user story* is a simple description of a product requirement in terms of what that requirement must accomplish for whom. Traditional requirements usually read something like this: "The system shall [insert technical description]." This requirement addresses only the technical nature of what will be done; the overall business objective is unclear. Because the development team has the context to engage more deeply, it clearly knows the benefit to the user (or the customer or the business) of each requirement and delivers what the customer wants faster and with higher quality.

Your user story will have, at a minimum, the following parts:

> Title (recognizable name for the user story)
>
> As a (type of user)
>
> I want to (take this action)
>
> so that (I get this benefit)

The user story also includes a list of validation steps *(acceptance criteria)* to take so you know that the working requirement for the user story is correct:

> When I (take this action), (this happens)

User stories may also include the following:

- **A user story ID:** A number to differentiate this user story from other user stories.

- **The user story value and effort estimate:** *Value* is how beneficial a user story might be to the organization creating that product. *Effort* is the ease or difficulty in creating that user story. We introduce how to score a user story's business value, risk, and effort in Chapter 7.

- **The name of the person who thought of the user story:** Anyone on the project team can create a user story.

TIP

Although agile project management approaches encourage low-tech tools, the scrum team should also find out what works best for it in each situation. A lot of electronic user story tools are available, some of which are free. Some are simple and are only for user stories. Others are complex and will integrate with other product documents. We love index cards, but that solution may not be for everyone. Use what works best for your scrum team and your project.

Figure 8-1 shows a typical user story card, front and back. The front has the main description of the user story. The back shows how you will confirm that the requirement works correctly, after the development team has created the functionality.

FIGURE 8-1:
Card-based user
story example.

Title Transfer money between accounts		When I do this:	This happens:
As Carol,		When I view my account balances,	I see an option to transfer funds.
I want to transfer funds between accounts		When I select the transfer option,	I choose between which accounts I want to transfer funds.
so that each account has the correct amount of funds		When I select the "transfer from" option,	I see a list of my available accounts and balances.
_____ Jennifer _____		When I select the "transfer to" option,	I see a list of my available accounts and balances.
Value Author Estimate			

The product owner gathers the user stories and manages them (that is, determines the priority and initiates the decomposition discussions). The development team and other stakeholders are also involved in creating and decomposing user stories.

TIP

Note that user stories aren't the only way to describe product requirements. You could simply make a list of requirements without any given structure. However, because user stories include a lot of useful information in a simple, compact format, we find that they are very effective in conveying exactly what a requirement needs to do for the customer.

The big benefit of the user story format is when the development team starts to create and test requirements. The development team members know exactly for whom they are creating the requirement, what the requirement should do, and how to double-check that the requirement satisfies the intention of the requirement.

We use user stories as examples of requirements throughout the chapter and the book. Keep in mind that anything we describe that you can do with user stories, you can do also with more generically expressed requirements.

Steps to create a user story

When creating a user story, follow these steps:

1. **Identify the project stakeholders.**

2. **Identify who will use the product.**

3. **Working with the stakeholders, write down the requirements that the product will need and use the format described earlier to create your user stories.**

Find out how to follow these three steps in the following sections.

REMEMBER

Being agile and adaptive requires iterating. Don't spend a ton of time trying to identify every single requirement your product might have. You can always add requirements later in the project. The best changes often come at the end of a project, when you know the most about the product and the customers.

Identifying project stakeholders

You probably have a good idea about who your project stakeholders are — anyone involved with, affected by, or who can affect the product and its creation.

REMEMBER

You will also work with stakeholders when you create your product vision and your product roadmap.

Make sure the stakeholders are available to help you create requirements. Stakeholders of the sample mobile banking application introduced in Chapter 7 might include the following:

>> People who interact with customers on a regular basis, such as customer service representatives or bank branch personnel.

>> Business experts for the different areas where your product's customers interact. For example, XYZ Bank might have one manager in charge of checking accounts, another manager in charge of savings accounts, and a third manager in charge of online bill payment services. If you're creating a mobile banking application, all these people would be project stakeholders.

>> Users of your product, if they're available.

>> Experts of the type of product you're creating. For example, a developer who has created mobile applications, a marketing manager who knows how to create mobile campaigns, and a user experience specialist who specializes in mobile interfaces all might be helpful on the sample XYZ Bank mobile banking project.

> » Technical stakeholders. These are people who work with the systems that might need to interact with your product.

Identifying users

Your customers and stakeholders provide requirements for the product owner to vet for placement on your product backlog. Your customers may or may not be the same people who will use your product. Knowing who your end users are and how they will interact with your product drive how you define and implement each requirement on your product roadmap.

With your product roadmap visualized, you can identify each type of user. For the mobile banking application, you would have individual and business bankers. The individual category would include youth, young adults, students, and single, married, retired, and wealthy users. Businesses of all sizes might be represented. Employee users would include tellers, branch managers, account managers, and fund managers. Each type of user will interact with your application in different ways and for different reasons. Knowing who these people are enables you to better define the purpose and desired benefits of each of their interactions.

We like to define users using *personas,* or a written description about a type of user represented by a fictitious person. For instance, "Robert is a 65-year-old retired engineer who is spending his retirement traveling the world. His net worth is $1,000,000, and he has residual income from several investment real estate properties."

"Robert" represents 30 percent of XYZ Bank's customers, and a good portion of the product roadmap includes features that someone like Robert will use. Instead of repeating all the details about Robert every time the scrum team discusses these features, they can simply refer to the type of user as "Robert." The product owner might identify several of these, as needed, and will even print the descriptions with a stock photo of what Robert might look like and post them on the wall in the team's work area to refer to throughout the project.

TIP

Know who your users are, so you can develop features they'll actually use.

Suppose that you're the product owner for the XYZ Bank's mobile banking project. You're responsible for the department that will bring the product to market, preferably in the next six months. You have the following ideas about the application's users:

> » The customers (the end users of the application) probably want quick access to up-to-date information about their balances and recent transactions.

> » Maybe the customers are about to buy a large-ticket item, and they want to make sure they can charge it.

>> Maybe the customers' ATM cards were just refused, but they have no idea why, and they want to check recent transactions for possible fraudulent activities.

>> Maybe the customers just realized that they forgot to pay their credit card bill and will have penalty charges if they don't pay the card today.

Who are your personas for this application? Here are a few examples:

>> **Persona #1:** Jason is a young, tech-savvy executive who travels a lot. When he has a spare moment, he wants to handle personal business quickly. He carefully invests his money in high-interest portfolios. He keeps his available cash low.

>> **Persona #2:** Carol is a small-business owner who stages properties when clients are trying to sell their home. She shops at consignment centers and often finds furnishings she wants to buy for her clients.

>> **Persona #3:** Nick is a student who lives on student loans and a part-time job. He knows he can be flaky with money because he's flaky with everything else. He just lost his checkbook.

TIP

Your product stakeholders can help you create personas. Find people who are experts on the day-to-day business for your product. Those stakeholders will know a lot about your potential customers.

Determining product requirements and creating user stories

After you have identified your different customers, you can start to determine product requirements and create user stories for the personas. A good way to create user stories is to bring your stakeholders together for a user story creation session.

Have the stakeholders write down as many requirements as they can think of, using the user story format. One user story for the project and personas from the preceding sections might be as follows:

>> Front side of card:

- **Title** See bank account balance

- **As** Jason,

- **I want to** see my checking account balance on my smartphone

- **so that** I can see how much money I have in my checking account

» Back side of card:

- **When I** sign into the XYZ Bank mobile application, my checking account balance appears at the top of the page.

- **When I** sign into the XYZ Bank mobile application after making a purchase or a deposit, my checking account balance reflects that purchase or deposit.

You can see sample user stories in card format in Figure 8-2.

Title Transfer money between accounts

As Carol,

I want to categorize expenses,

so that I can easily identify my purchases made for my clients.

	Jennifer	
Value	Author	Estimate

Title Put stop on a check

As Nick,

I want to stop payment on a lost or stolen check,

so that I can avoid any unauthorized activity on my account.

	Caroline	
Value	Author	Estimate

FIGURE 8-2: Sample user stories.

Be sure to continuously add and prioritize new user stories to your product backlog. Keeping your product backlog up-to-date will help you have the highest-priority user stories when it is time to plan your sprint.

Throughout an agile project, you will create new user stories. You'll also take existing large requirements and decompose them until they're manageable enough to work on during a sprint.

Breaking down requirements

You refine requirements many times throughout an agile project. For example:

>> When you create the product roadmap (see Chapter 7), you create features (capabilities your customers will have after you develop the features), as well as themes (logical groups of features). Although features are intentionally large, we require features at the product roadmap level to be no larger than 144 story points on the Fibonacci scale.

>> When you plan releases, you break down the features into more concise user stories. User stories at the release plan level can be either *epics,* very large user stories with multiple actions, or individual user stories, which contain a single action. For our clients, user stories at the release plan level should be no larger than 34 story points. You find out more about releases later in this chapter.

>> When you plan sprints, you can break down user stories even further. You also identify individual tasks associated with each user story in the sprint. For our clients, user stories at the sprint level should be no larger than eight story points. Tasks will be estimated in hours and should be no larger than what can be accomplished in a day.

To decompose requirements, you'll want to think about how to break down the requirement into individual actions. Table 8-1 shows a requirement from the XYZ Bank application introduced in Chapter 7 that is decomposed from the theme level down to the user story level.

TABLE 8-1   ## Decomposing a Requirement

Requirement Level	Requirement
Theme	See bank account data on a mobile device.
Features	See account balances.
	See a list of recent withdrawals or purchases.
	See a list of recent deposits.
	See my upcoming automatic bill payments.
	See my account alerts.
Epic user stories — decomposed from "see account balances"	See checking account balance.
	See savings account balance.
	See loan balance.
	See investment account balance.
	See retirement account balance.

Requirement Level	Requirement
User stories — decomposed from "see checking account balance"	See a list of my accounts once securely logged in.
	Select and view my checking account.
	See account balance changes after withdrawals.
	See account balance changes after purchases.
	See day's end account balance.
	See available account balance.
	See mobile application navigation items.
	Change account view.
	Log out of mobile application.

USER STORIES AND THE INVEST APPROACH

You may be asking, just how decomposed does a user story have to be? Bill Wake, in his blog at XP123.com, describes the INVEST approach to ensure quality in user stories. We like his method so much we include it here.

Using the INVEST approach, user stories should be

- **I**ndependent: To the extent possible, a story should need no other stories to implement the feature that the story describes.

- **N**egotiable: Not overly detailed. The user story has room for discussion and an expansion of details.

- **V**aluable: The story demonstrates product value to the customer. The story describes features, not technical tasks to implement it. The story is in the user's language and is easy to explain. The people using the product or system can understand the story.

- **E**stimable: The story is descriptive, accurate, and concise, so the developers can generally estimate the work necessary to create the functionality in the user story.

- **S**mall: It is easier to plan and accurately estimate small user stories. A good rule of thumb is that the development team can complete 6-10 user stories in a sprint.

- **T**estable: You can easily validate the user story, and the results are definitive.

Estimation poker

As you refine your requirements, you need to refine your estimates as well. It's time to have some fun!

One of the most popular ways of estimating user stories is by playing *estimation poker*, sometimes called *planning poker*, a game to determine user story size and to build consensus among the development team members.

The scrum master can help coordinate estimation, and the product owner can provide information about features, but the development team is responsible for estimating the level of effort required for the user stories. After all, the development team has to do the work to create the features that those stories describe.

To play estimation poker, you need a deck of cards like the one in Figure 8-3. You can get a digital version online at our website (`www.platinumedge.com/estimationpoker`), or you can make your own with index cards and markers. The numbers on the cards are from the Fibonacci sequence.

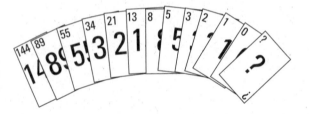

FIGURE 8-3:
A deck of estimation poker cards.

The Fibonacci sequence follows this progression:

1, 2, 3, 5, 8, 13, 21, 34, 55, 89, 144, and so on

Each number after the first two is the sum of the previous two numbers.

Each user story receives an estimate relative to other user stories. For instance, a user story that is a 5 requires more work than a 3, a 2, and a 1. It is about 5 times as much effort as a 1, more than double the effort of a 2, and roughly the amount of effort as a 3 and a 2 combined. It is not as much effort as an 8, but is just over half the effort of an 8.

As user stories and epic user stories increase in size, the difference between Fibonacci numbers gets bigger. Acknowledging these increasing gaps in precision for larger requirements is why the Fibonacci sequence works so well for relative estimation.

To play estimation poker, follow these steps:

1. **Provide each member of the development team with a deck of estimation poker cards.**

2. **From the list of user stories presented by the product owner, the team agrees on one user story that would be a 5.**

   The team follows two rules: (1) The development team should not allow any single user story larger than an 8 to be pulled into a sprint, and (2) scrum teams should be able to complete roughly 6-10 user stories in a sprint.

   The scrum master helps the development team reach consensus by using fist of five or thumbs up/thumbs down (as described in Chapter 6). This user story becomes the *anchor story*.

3. **The product owner reads a high-priority user story to the players.**

4. **Each player selects a card representing his or her estimate of the effort involved in the user story and lays the card facedown on the table.**

   The players should compare the user story to other user stories they have estimated. (The first time through, the players compare the user story to only the anchor story.) Make sure no other players can see your card.

5. **All players turn over their cards simultaneously.**

6. **If the players have different story points:**

   a. *It's time for discussion.*

      The players with the highest and lowest scores talk about their assumptions and why they think the estimate for the user story should be higher or lower, respectively. The players compare the effort for the user story against the anchor story. The product owner provides more clarification about the story, as necessary.

   b. *Once everyone agrees on assumptions and has any necessary clarifications, the players reevaluate their estimates and place their new selected cards on the table.*

   c. *If the story points are different, the players repeat the process, usually up to three times.*

   d. *If the players can't agree on the estimated effort, the scrum master helps the development team determine a score that all the players can support (he or she may use fist of five or thumbs up/thumbs down, as described in Chapter 6), or determine that the user story requires more detail or needs to be further broken down.*

7. **The players repeat Steps 3 through 6 for each user story.**

Consider each part of the definition of *done* — developed, integrated, tested, and documented — when you create estimates.

You can play estimation poker at any point — but definitely play during the product roadmap development and as you progressively break down user stories for inclusion in releases and sprints. With practice, the development team will get into a planning rhythm and become more adept at quickly estimating.

On average, development teams will spend about 10 percent of their time on a project decomposing requirements, including estimating and reestimating. Make your estimation poker games fun! Bring in snacks, take breaks as needed, use humor, and keep the mood light.

Affinity estimating

Estimation poker can be effective, but what if you have many user stories? Playing estimation poker for, say, 500 user stories could take a long time. You need a way to focus on only the user stories you must discuss to gain consensus.

When you have a large number of user stories, many of them are probably similar and would require a similar amount of effort to complete. One way to determine the right stories for discussion is to use affinity estimating. In *affinity estimating*, you quickly categorize your user stories and then apply estimates to these categories of stories.

When estimating by affinity, write your user stories on index cards or sticky notes. These types of user story cards work well when quickly categorizing stories.

Affinity estimating can be a fast and furious activity — the development team may choose to have the scrum master help facilitate affinity estimating sessions. To estimate by affinity, follow these steps:

1. **Taking no more than 60 seconds for each category, the development team agrees on a single user story in each of the following categories:**

   - Extra-small user story

   - Small user story

   - Medium user story

   - Large user story

   - Extra-large user story

   - Epic user story that is too large to come into the sprint

   - Needs clarification before estimating

2. **Taking no more than 60 seconds per user story, the development team puts all remaining stories into the categories listed in Step 1.**

   If you're using index cards or sticky notes for your user stories, you can physically place those cards into categories on a table or a whiteboard, respectively. If you split the user stories among the development team members, having each development team member categorize a group of stories, this step can go quickly!

3. **Taking another 30 minutes, maximum, for each 100 stories, the development team reviews and adjusts the placement of the user stories.**

   The entire development team must agree on the placement of the user stories into size categories.

4. **The product owner reviews the categorization.**

5. **When the product owner's expected estimate and the team's actual estimate differ by more than one story size, they discuss that user story.**

   The development team may or may not decide to adjust the story size.

6. **The development team plays estimation poker on the user stories in both the epic and the needs clarification categories.**

   The number of user stories in these categories should be minimal.

   Note that after the product owner and the development team discuss clarifications, the development team has the final say on the user story size.

REMEMBER

User stories in the same size category will have the same user story score. You can play a round of estimation poker to double-check a few, but you won't need to waste time in unnecessary discussion for every user story.

Story sizes are like T-shirt sizes and should correspond to Fibonacci scale numbers, as shown in Figure 8-4.

SIZE	POINTS
Extra small (XS)	1
Small (S)	2
Medium (M)	3
Large (L)	5
Extra large (XL)	8

FIGURE 8-4:
Story sizes as T-shirt sizes and their Fibonacci numbers.

TIP

You can use the estimating and prioritizing techniques in this chapter for requirements at any level, from themes and features down to single user stories.

That's it. In a few hours, your entire product backlog was estimated. In addition, your scrum team has a shared understanding of what the requirements mean, having discussed them face to face rather than relying on interpretations of extensive documentation.

Release Planning

A *release* is a group of usable product features that you deploy to the market. A release does not need to include all the functionality outlined in the product roadmap but should include at least the *minimal marketable features,* the smallest group of product features that you can effectively deploy and promote in the marketplace. Your early releases will exclude many of the medium- and low-priority requirements you identified during the product roadmap stage.

When planning a release, you establish the next set of minimal marketable features and identify an imminent product launch date around which the team can mobilize. As when creating the vision statement and the product roadmap, the product owner is responsible for creating the release goal and establishing the release date. However, the development team's estimates, with the scrum master's facilitation, contribute to the process.

Release planning is stage 3 in the Roadmap to Value (refer to Chapter 7 to see the roadmap as a whole). Figure 8-5 shows how release planning fits into an agile project.

Stage 3: RELEASE PLANNING

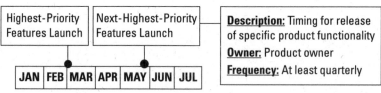

FIGURE 8-5:
Release planning
as part of the
Roadmap to
Value.

(Stages 1-3 are common practices outside of scrum)

Release planning involves completing two key activities:

>> **Revising the product backlog:** In Chapter 7, we tell you that the product backlog is a comprehensive list of all the user stories you currently know for

your project, whether or not they belong in the current release. Keep in mind that your list of user stories will probably change throughout the project.

» **Creating the release plan:** This activity consists of the release goal, release target date, and prioritization of product backlog items that support the release goal. The release plan provides a midrange goal that the team can accomplish.

WARNING

Don't create a new, separate backlog during release planning. The task is unnecessary and reduces the product owner's flexibility. Prioritizing the existing product backlog based on the release goal is sufficient and enables the product owner to have the latest information when he or she commits to the scope during sprint planning.

The product backlog and release plan are some of the most important communication channels between the product owner and the development team. In Chapter 7, you find out how to complete a product backlog. How to create a release plan is described next.

The release plan contains a release schedule for a specific set of features. The product owner creates a release plan at the start of each release. To create a release plan, follow these steps:

1. **Establish the release goal.**

The release goal is an overall business goal for the product features in your release. The product owner and development team collaborate to create a release goal based on business priorities and the development team's development speed and capabilities.

2. **Identify a target release date.**

Some scrum teams determine release dates based on the completion of functionality; others may have hard dates, such as March 31 or September 1.

3. **Review the product backlog and the product roadmap to determine the highest-priority user stories that support your release goal (the minimum marketable features).**

These user stories will make up your first release.

TIP

We like to achieve releases with about 80 percent of the user stories, using the final 20 percent to add robust features that will meet the release goal while adding to the product's "wow" factor.

4. **Refine the user stories in your release goal.**

During release planning, dependencies, gaps, or new details are often identified that affect estimates and prioritization. This is the time to make sure the portion of the product backlog supporting your release is sized appropriately. We like to make sure that requirements supporting the current release goal are sized no larger than 34. The development team helps the product owner by updating estimates for any added or revised user stories, and commits to the release goal and scope with the product owner.

5. **Estimate the number of sprints needed, based on the scrum team's velocity.**

Scrum teams use velocity to plan how much work they can take on in a release and sprint. *Velocity* is the sum of all user story points completed within a sprint. So, if a scrum team completed six user stories during its first sprint with sizes 8, 5, 5, 3, 2, 1, their velocity for the first sprint is 24. The scrum team would plan its second sprint keeping in mind that it completed 24 story points during the first sprint.

After multiple sprints, scrum teams can use their running average velocity as an input to determine how much work they can take on in a sprint, as well as to extrapolate their release schedule by dividing the total number of story points in the release by their average velocity. You learn more about velocity in Chapter 13.

6. **Identify work necessary to release that can't be completed within a sprint. Plan a release sprint, if necessary, and determine how long it should be.**

Some project teams add a *release sprint* to some releases to conduct activities that are unrelated to product development but necessary to release the product to customers. If you need a release sprint, be sure to factor that into the date you choose. You can find more about release sprints in Chapter 11.

Some tasks, such as security testing or load testing a software project, can't be completed within a sprint, because the security or load testing environments take time to set up and request. Although release sprints allow scrum teams to plan for these types of activities, doing so is an anti-pattern, or the opposite of being agile. Your goal should be to complete all work required for functionality to be shippable at the end of each sprint.

Not all agile projects use release planning. Some scrum teams release functionality for customer use with every sprint, or even every day. The development team, product, organization, customers, stakeholders, and the project's technological complexity can all help determine your approach to product releases.

The planned releases now go from a tentative plan to a more concrete goal. Figure 8-6 represents a typical release plan.

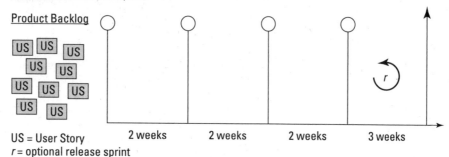

Release Goal: Enable customers to access, view, and transact against their active accounts
Release Date: March 31, 2021

Product Backlog

US = User Story
r = optional release sprint

2 weeks   2 weeks   2 weeks   3 weeks

FIGURE 8-6:
Sample release
plan.

TIP

Bear in mind the pen-pencil rule: You can commit to (write in pen) the plan for the first release, but anything beyond the first release is tentative (written in pencil). In other words, use just-in-time planning (see Chapter 7) for each release. After all, things change, so why bother getting microscopic too early?

Sprint Planning

In agile projects, a *sprint* is a consistent iteration of time in which the development team creates a specific group of product capabilities from start to finish. At the end of each sprint, the functionality that the development team has created should be working, ready to demonstrate, and potentially shippable to the customer.

Sprints should be the same length within a project. Keeping the sprint lengths consistent helps the development team measure its performance and plan better at each new sprint.

Sprints generally last one to four weeks. Four weeks is the longest amount of time any sprint should last; longer iterations make changes riskier, defeating the purpose of being agile. We rarely see sprints lasting longer than two weeks, and more often see sprints lasting a week. One-week sprints are a natural cycle with the Monday-to-Friday business week that structurally prevents weekend work. Some scrum teams work in one-day sprints where priorities change on a daily basis. Market and customer needs are changing more and more quickly, and the amount of time you can afford between opportunities to gather customer feedback only gets shorter. Our rule of thumb is that your sprint shouldn't be longer than your stakeholders can consistently go without changes in priority regarding what the scrum team should be working on in the sprint.

Each sprint includes the following:

>> Sprint planning at the beginning of the sprint

>> Daily scrum meetings

>> Development time — the bulk of the sprint

>> A sprint review and a sprint retrospective at the end of the sprint

Discover more about daily scrums, sprint development, the sprint review, and the sprint retrospective in Chapters 9 and 10. In this chapter, you find out how to plan sprints.

Sprint planning is stage 4 in the Roadmap to Value, as you can see in Figure 8-7. The entire scrum team — the Product owner, the scrum master, and the development team — works together to plan sprints.

Stage 4: SPRINT PLANNING

FIGURE 8-7:
Sprint planning as
part of the
Roadmap to
Value.

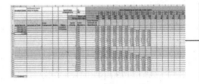

Description: Establishment of specific iteration goals and tasks

Owner: Product owner and development team

Frequency: At the start of each sprint

The sprint backlog

The *sprint backlog* is a list of user stories associated with the current sprint and related tasks. When planning your sprint, you do the following:

>> Establish goals for your sprint.

>> Choose the user stories that support those goals.

>> Break user stories into specific development tasks.

>> Create a *sprint backlog*. The sprint backlog consists of the following:

   • The list of user stories within the sprint in order of priority.

   • The relative effort estimate for each user story.

   • The tasks necessary to develop each user story.

   • The effort, in hours, to complete each task.

   At the task level, you estimate the number of hours each task will take to complete, instead of using story points. Because your sprint has a specific length, and thus a set number of available working hours, you can use the time each task takes to determine whether the tasks will fit into your sprint.

Each task should take one day or less for the development team to complete.

TIP

Some mature development teams may not need to estimate their tasks as they get more consistent at breaking down their user stories into executable tasks. Estimating tasks is helpful for newer development teams to ensure that they understand their capacity and plan each sprint appropriately.

- A *burndown chart,* which shows the status of the work the development team has completed.

TECHNICAL STUFF

Tasks in agile projects should take a day or less to complete for two reasons. The first reason involves basic psychology: People are motivated to get to the finish line. If you have a task that you know you can complete quickly, you are more likely to finish it on time, just to check it off your to-do list. The second reason is that one-day tasks provide good red flags that a project might be veering off course. If a development team member reports that he or she is working on the same task for more than one or two days, that team member probably has a roadblock. The scrum master should take the opportunity to investigate what might be keeping the team member from finishing work. (For more on managing roadblocks, see Chapter 9.)

The development team collaborates to create and maintain the sprint backlog, and only the development team can modify the sprint backlog. The sprint backlog should reflect an up-to-the-day snapshot of the sprint's progress. Figure 8-8 shows a sample sprint backlog at the end of the sprint planning meeting. You can use this example, find other samples, or even use a whiteboard.

The sprint planning meeting

On the first day of each sprint, often a Monday morning, the scrum team holds the sprint planning meeting.

TIP

For a successful sprint planning meeting, make sure everyone involved in the session (the product owner, the development team, the scrum master, and anyone else the scrum team requests) is dedicated to the effort for the entire meeting.

Base the length of your sprint planning meeting on the length of your sprints: Meet for no more than two hours for every week of your sprints. This timebox is one of the rules of scrum and helps ensure that the meeting stays focused and on track. Figure 8-9 illustrates this and is a good quick reference for your sprint planning meeting lengths.

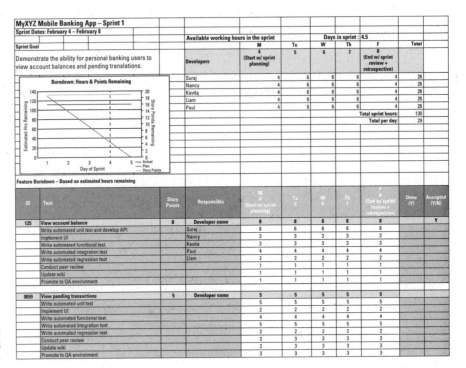

MyXYZ Mobile Banking App – Sprint 1

Sprint Dates: February 4 – February 8

Sprint Goal

Demonstrate the ability for personal banking users to view account balances and pending translations.

Burndown: Hours & Points Remaining

Developers	M (Start w/ sprint planning)	Tu 5	W 6	Th 7	F (End w/ sprint review + retrospective)	Total
	4	5	6	7	8	
Suraj	4	6	6	6	4	26
Nancy	4	6	6	6	4	26
Kavita	4	6	6	6	4	26
Liam	4	6	6	6	4	26
Paul	4	6	6	6	4	26
					Total sprint hours:	130
					Total per day:	29

Available working hours in the sprint — Days in sprint: 4.5

Feature Burndown – Based on estimated hours remaining

ID	Task	Story Points	Responsible	M 4 (Start w/ sprint planning)	Tu 5	W 6	Th 7	F 8 (End w/ sprint review + retrospective)	Done (Y)	Accepted (Y/N)
125	View account balance	8	Developer name	8	8	8	8	8		Y
	Write automated unit test and develop API		Suraj	6	6	6	6	6		
	Implement UI		Nancy	3	3	3	3	3		
	Write automated functional test		Kavita	3	3	3	3	3		
	Write automated integration test		Paul	4	4	4	4	4		
	Write automated regression test		Liam	2	2	2	2	2		
	Conduct peer review			1	1	1	1	1		
	Update wiki			1	1	1	1	1		
	Promote to QA environment			1	1	1	1	1		
0059	View pending transactions	5	Developer name	5	5	5	5	5		
	Write automated unit test			5	5	5	5	5		
	Implement UI			2	2	2	2	2		
	Write automated functional test			4	4	4	4	4		
	Write automated integration test			5	5	5	5	5		
	Write automated regression test			2	2	2	2	2		
	Conduct peer review			3	3	3	3	3		
	Update wiki			3	3	3	3	3		
	Promote to QA environment			3	3	3	3	3		

FIGURE 8-8:
Sprint backlog example.

If my sprint is this long...	My sprint planning meeting should last no longer than...
One week	Two hours
Two weeks	Four hours
Three weeks	Six hours
Four weeks	Eight hours

FIGURE 8-9:
Ratio of sprint planning meeting to sprint length.

TECHNICAL STUFF

On agile projects, the practice of limiting the time of your meetings is sometimes called *timeboxing*. Keeping your meetings timeboxed ensures that the development team has the time it needs to create the product.

You'll split your sprint planning meetings into two parts: one to set a sprint goal (the "why") and choose user stories for the sprint (the "what"), and another to break down your user stories into individual tasks (the "how" and "how much"). The details on each part are discussed next.

Part 1: Setting goals and choosing user stories

In the first part of your sprint planning meeting, the product owner and development team, with support from the scrum master, do the following:

1. Discuss and set a sprint goal.

2. Review the user stories from the product backlog that support the sprint goal and revisit their relative estimates.

3. If needed, create user stories to fill gaps to achieve the sprint goal.

4. Determine what the team can commit to in the current sprint.

At the beginning of your sprint planning meeting, the product owner should propose a sprint goal and then together with the development team discuss and agree on the sprint goal. The sprint goal should be an overall description of the working customer functionality that the team will demonstrate and possibly release at the end of the sprint. The goal is supported by the highest-priority user stories in the product backlog. A sample sprint goal for the mobile banking application (refer to Chapter 7) might be as follows:

> Demonstrate the ability of a mobile banking customer to log in and view account balances and pending and prior transactions.

Using the sprint goal, you determine the user stories that belong in the sprint. You also take another look at the estimates for those stories and make changes to the estimates if necessary. For the mobile banking application sample, the group of user stories for the sprint might include the following:

>> Log in and access my accounts.

>> View account balances.

>> View pending transactions.

>> View prior transactions.

All these would be high-priority user stories in the product backlog that support the sprint goal.

The second part of reviewing user stories is confirming that the effort estimates for each user story have been reviewed and adjusted if needed, and reflect the development team's current knowledge of the user story. Adjust the estimate if necessary. With the product owner in the meeting, resolve any outstanding questions. At the beginning of the sprint, the scrum team has the most up-to-date knowledge about the system and the customer's needs up to this point in the project, so make sure the development team and product owner have one more chance to clarify and size the user stories going into the sprint.

Finally, after you know which user stories support the sprint goal, the development team should agree and confirm that it can complete the goal planned for the sprint. If any of the user stories you discussed earlier don't fit in the current sprint, remove them from the sprint and add them back into the product backlog.

WARNING Always plan and work one sprint at a time. An easy trap to fall into is to place user stories into specific future sprints. For example, when you're still planning sprint 1, don't decide that user story X should go into sprint 2 or 3. Instead, keep the ordered list of user stories up to date in the product backlog and focus on always developing the next highest-priority stories. Commit to planning only for the current sprint.

After you have a sprint goal, user stories for the sprint, and a commitment to the goal, move on to the second part of sprint planning.

TIP Because a sprint planning meeting for sprints longer than one week might last a few hours, you might want to take a break between the two parts of the meeting.

Part 2: Breaking down user stories into tasks for the sprint backlog

In the second part of the sprint planning meeting, the scrum team does the following:

1. The development team creates the sprint backlog tasks associated with each user story. Make sure that tasks encompass each part of the definition of done: developed, integrated, tested, and documented.

2. The development team double-checks that it can complete the tasks in the time available in the sprint.

3. Each development team member should choose his or her first task to accomplish before leaving the meeting.

TIP Development team members should each work on only one task on one user story at a time to enable *swarming* — the practice of the entire development team working on one user story until completion. Swarming can be an efficient way to complete work in a short amount of time. In this way, scrum teams avoid getting to the end of the sprint with all user stories started but few finished.

At the beginning of part two of the meeting, break the user stories into individual tasks and allocate a number of hours to each task. The development team's target should be completing a task in a day or less. For example, a user story for the XYZ Bank mobile application might be as follows:

Log in and access my accounts.

The team decomposes this user story into tasks, such as the following:

- ▶▶ Write the unit test.
- ▶▶ Create an authentication screen for a username and password, with a Submit button.
- ▶▶ Create an error screen for the user to reenter credentials.
- ▶▶ Create a screen (once logged in) displaying a list of accounts.
- ▶▶ Using authentication code from the online banking application, rewrite code for an iPhone/iPad application.
- ▶▶ Create calls to the database to verify the username and password.
- ▶▶ Refactor code for mobile devices.
- ▶▶ Write the integration test.
- ▶▶ Update the wiki documentation.

After you know the number of hours that each task will take, do a final check to make sure that the number of hours available to the development team reasonably matches the total of the tasks' estimates. If the tasks exceed the hours available, one or more user stories will have to come out of the sprint. Discuss with the product owner what tasks or user stories are the best to remove.

If extra time is available within the sprint, the development team might be able to include another user story. Just be careful about over-committing at the beginning of a sprint, especially in the project's first few sprints.

After you know which tasks will be part of the sprint, choose what you will work on first. Each development team member should select his or her initial task to accomplish for the sprint. Team members should focus on one task at a time.

TIP

As the development team members think about what they can complete in a sprint, use the following guidelines to ensure that they don't take on more work than they can handle while they're learning new roles and techniques:

- ▶▶ **Sprint 1:** 25 percent of what the development team thinks it can accomplish. Include overhead for learning the new process and starting a new project.

>> **Sprint 2:** 50 percent of what the development team thinks it can accomplish.

>> **Sprint 3:** 75 percent of what the development team thinks it can accomplish.

>> **Sprint 4 and forward:** 100 percent. The development team will have developed a rhythm and velocity, gained insight into agile principles and the project, and will be working at close to full pace.

The scrum team should constantly evaluate the sprint backlog against the development team's progress on the tasks. At the end of the sprint, the scrum team can also assess estimation skills and capacity for work during the sprint retrospective (see Chapter 10). This evaluation is especially important for the first sprint.

TIP

For the sprint, how many total working hours are available? In a 40-hour week, you could wisely assume, for a two-week sprint, that nine working days are available to develop user stories. If you assume each full-time team member has 35 hours per week (7 productive hours per day) to focus on the project, the number of working hours available is

$$\text{Number of team members} \times 7 \text{ hours} \times 9 \text{ days}$$

Why nine days? Half of day one is taken up with planning, and half of day ten is taken up with the sprint review (when the stakeholders review the completed work) and the sprint retrospective (when the scrum team identifies improvements for future sprints). That leaves nine days of development.

After the sprint planning is finished, the development team can immediately start working on the tasks to create the product!

The scrum master should make sure the product roadmap, product backlog, and sprint backlog are in a prominent place and accessible to everyone. This allows managers and other interested parties to view the artifacts and get the status of progress without interrupting the development team.

Chapter **9**

Working throughout the Day

t's Tuesday, 9 a.m. Yesterday, you completed sprint planning, and the development team started work. For the rest of the sprint, you'll be working *cyclically*, where each day follows the same pattern.

In this chapter, you find out how to use agile principles daily throughout each sprint. You see the work that you will do every day as part of a scrum team: planning and coordinating your day, tracking progress, creating and verifying usable functionality, and identifying and dealing with impediments to your work. You see how the different scrum team members work together each day during the sprint to help create the product.

Planning Your Day: The Daily Scrum

On agile projects, you make plans throughout the entire project — and on a daily basis. Agile development teams start each workday with a *daily scrum* meeting to note completed items, to identify impediments, or roadblocks, requiring scrum master involvement, and to synchronize and plan what each team member will do during the day to achieve the sprint goal.

The daily scrum is Stage 5 on the Roadmap to Value. You can see how the sprint and the daily scrum fit into an agile project in Figure 9-1. Note how they both repeat.

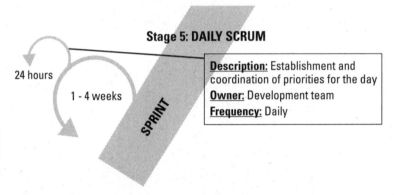

Stage 5: DAILY SCRUM

24 hours

1 - 4 weeks

SPRINT

Description: Establishment and coordination of priorities for the day
Owner: Development team
Frequency: Daily

FIGURE 9-1:
The sprint and the daily scrum in the Roadmap to Value.

In the daily scrum meeting, each development team member makes the following three statements, which enable team coordination:

>> **Yesterday, I completed** (state items completed).

>> **Today, I'm going to take on** (state task).

>> **My impediments are** (state impediments, if any).

TECHNICAL STUFF

Other names you might hear for the daily scrum meeting are the *daily huddle* or the *daily standup* meeting. Daily scrum, daily huddle, and daily standup all refer to the same thing.

We also have the scrum master address these three statements regarding the team's impediments:

>> **Yesterday, I resolved to** (state impediments completed).

>> **Today, I'm going to work on removing** (state impediment).

>> **The impediments I'm going to escalate are** (state impediments you need assistance with, if any).

One of the rules of scrum is that the daily scrum meeting lasts 15 minutes or less; longer meetings eat into the development team's day. The meeting is also referred to as the daily standup because standing encourages shorter meetings. You can also use props to keep daily scrum meetings quick.

TIP

We start meetings by tossing a squeaky burger–shaped dog toy — don't worry; it's clean — to a random development team member. Each person makes his or her three statements and then passes the squeaky toy to someone else. If people are long-winded, we change the prop to a 500–page ream of copy paper, which weighs about five pounds. Each person can talk for as long as he or she can hold the ream out to one side. Either meetings will quickly become shorter, or development team members will quickly build up their arm strength — in our experience, it's the former.

To keep daily scrums brief and effective, the scrum team can follow several guidelines:

>> **Anyone may attend a daily scrum, but only the development team, the scrum master, and the product owner may talk.** The daily scrum is the scrum team's opportunity to coordinate daily activities, not take on additional requirements or changes from stakeholders. Stakeholders can discuss questions with the scrum master or product owner afterward, but stakeholders should not approach the development team.

>> **The focus is on immediate priorities.** The scrum team should review only completed tasks, tasks to be done, and roadblocks.

>> **Daily scrum meetings are for coordination, not problem-solving.** The development team and the scrum master are responsible for removing roadblocks during the day.

>> **To keep meetings from drifting into problem-solving sessions, scrum teams can**

- Create a list on a whiteboard to keep track of issues that need immediate attention, and then address those issues directly after the meeting with only those team members who need to be involved.

- Hold a meeting, called an *after-party,* to solve problems after the daily scrum is finished. Some scrum teams schedule time for an after-party every day; others meet only as needed.

>> **The daily scrum is for peer-to-peer coordination.** It is not used for an individual to report status to one person, such as the scrum master or product owner. Status is reported at the end of each day in the sprint backlog.

>> **Such a short meeting must start on time.** It is not unusual for the scrum team to have creative punishments for tardiness (such as doing pushups or adding penalty money into a team celebration fund or another inconvenience). Whatever method is used, the scrum team agrees on it together; the method is not dictated to them by someone outside the team, such as a manager.

>> **The scrum team may request that daily scrum attendees stand up — rather than sit down — during the meeting.** Standing up makes people eager to finish the meeting and get on with the day's work.

When you have only 15 minutes to meet, every minute counts. Scrum teams should not be afraid to make being late to the daily scrum appropriately unpleasant. If members of the team love to sing, for example, performing a karaoke song probably won't have much of an effect. We've helped cure perpetual tardiness problems overnight by suggesting that the scrum team change its punishment from a $1 to a $20 contribution to the team celebration fund.

Daily scrum meetings are effective for keeping the development team focused on the right tasks for any given day. Because the development team members are accountable for their work in front of their peers, they are less likely to stray from their daily commitments. Daily scrum meetings also help ensure that the scrum master and development team can deal with roadblocks immediately. These meetings are so useful that even organizations that are not using any other agile techniques sometimes adopt daily scrums.

We like to hold daily scrum meetings one hour after the development team's normal start time to allow for traffic jams, emails, coffee, and other rituals when starting the day. Having a later scrum meeting also allows the development team time to review defect reports from automated testing tools that were run the night before.

The daily scrum is for discussing progress and planning each upcoming day. As you see next, you also track progress — not just discuss it — every day.

Tracking Progress

You also need to track the progress of your sprint daily. This section discusses ways to keep track of the tasks in your sprint.

Two tools for tracking progress are the sprint backlog and a task board. Both the sprint backlog and the task board enable the scrum team to show the sprint's progress to anyone at any given time.

The Agile Manifesto values individuals and interactions over processes and tools. Make sure your tools support, rather than hinder, your scrum team. Modify or even replace tools if you have to. Read more about the Agile Manifesto in Chapter 2.

The sprint backlog

During sprint planning, you concentrate on adding user stories and tasks to the spring backlog. During the sprint itself, you update the sprint backlog daily, tracking progress of the development team's tasks for each working day. Figure 9-2 shows the sprint backlog for this book's sample application, the XYZ Bank's mobile banking application, as it would appear after day 4 of the first sprint. (Chapter 8 discusses details of the sprint backlog.)

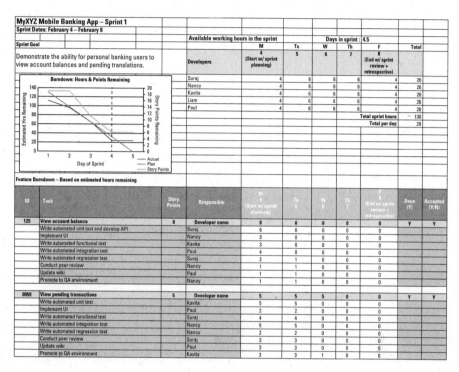

FIGURE 9-2: Sample sprint backlog.

Make the sprint backlog available to the entire project team every day. That way, anyone who needs to know the sprint status can find it instantly.

Near the top left of Figure 9-2, note the *sprint burndown chart*, which shows the progress that the development team is making. You can see that the development team members have completed tasks close to the even burn rate of their available hours, and the product owner has accepted several user stories as complete.

You can include burndown charts on your sprint backlog and on your product backlog. (This chapter concentrates on the sprint backlog.) Figure 9-3 shows the burndown chart in detail.

A burndown chart is a powerful tool for visualizing progress and the work remaining. The chart shows the following:

» The outstanding work (in hours) on the first vertical axis

» Time, in days along the horizontal axis

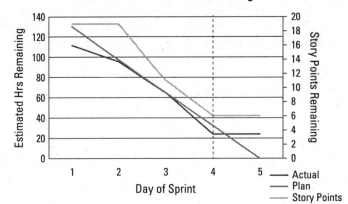

Burndown: Hours & Points Remaining

FIGURE 9-3:
A burndown
chart.

Some sprint burndown charts, like the one in Figure 9-3, also show the outstanding story points on a second vertical axis that is plotted against the same horizontal time axis as hours of work remaining.

A burndown chart enables anyone, at a glance, to see the status of the sprint. Progress is clear. By comparing the realistic number of hours available to the work remaining, you can find out daily whether the effort is going as planned, is in better shape than expected, or is in trouble. This information helps you determine whether the development team is likely to accomplish the targeted number of user stories and helps you make informed decisions early in the sprint.

ON THE WEB

You can create a sprint backlog using a spreadsheet and charting program such as Microsoft Excel. You can also download our sprint backlog template, which includes a burndown chart, from the book's website at www.dummies.com/go/ agileprojectmanagementfd2e.

Figure 9-4 shows samples of burndown charts for sprints in different situations. Looking at these charts, you can tell how the work is progressing:

» **1. Expected:** This chart shows a normal sprint pattern. The remaining work hours rise and fall as the development team completes tasks, ferrets out details, and identifies tactical work it may not have initially considered. Although work occasionally increases, it is manageable, and the team mobilizes to complete all user stories by the end of the sprint.

» **2. More complicated:** In this sprint, the work increased beyond the point at which the development team felt it could accomplish everything. The team identified this issue early, worked with the product owner to remove some user stories, and still achieved the sprint goal. The key to scope changes within a sprint is that they are always initiated by the development team — no one else.

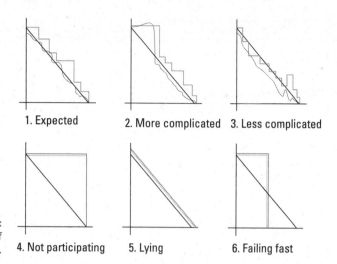

1. Expected   2. More complicated   3. Less complicated

4. Not participating   5. Lying   6. Failing fast

FIGURE 9-4:
Profiles of
burndown charts.

>> **3. Less complicated:** In this sprint, the development team completed some critical user stories faster than anticipated and worked with the product owner to identify additional user stories it could add to the sprint.

>> **4. Not participating:** A straight line in a burndown means that the team didn't update the burndown or made zero progress that day. Either case is a red flag for future problems.

Just like on a heartbeat graph, a horizontal straight line on a sprint burndown chart is never a good thing.

WARNING

>> **5. Lying (or conforming):** This burndown pattern is common for a new agile development team that might be accustomed to reporting the hours that management expects, instead of the time the work really takes, and consequently tends to adjust the team's work estimates to the exact number of remaining hours. This pattern often reflects a fear-based environment, where the managers lead by intimidation.

>> **6. Failing fast:** One of the strongest benefits of this simple visualization of progress is the immediate proof of progress or lack thereof. This pattern shows an example of a team that wasn't participating or progressing. Halfway through the sprint, the product owner decided to cut losses by killing the sprint and starting a new sprint with a new sprint goal. Only product owners can end a sprint early.

The sprint backlog helps you track progress throughout each sprint. You can also refer to earlier sprint backlogs to compare progress from sprint to sprint. You make changes to your process in each sprint (read more about the concept of inspect and adapt in Chapter 10). Constantly inspect your work and adapt to make it better. Hold on to those old sprint backlogs.

Another way to keep track of your sprint is by using a task board. Read on to find out how to create and use one.

The task board

Although the sprint backlog is a great way to track and show project progress, it's probably in an electronic format, so it might not be immediately accessible to anyone who wants to see it. Some scrum development teams use a task board along with their sprint backlog. A *task board* provides a quick, easy view of the items in the sprint that the development team is working on and has completed.

We like task boards because you can't deny the status they show. Like the product roadmap, the task board can be made up of sticky notes on a whiteboard. The task board will have at least the following four columns, from left to right:

>> **To Do:** The user stories and tasks that remain to be accomplished are in the far left column.

>> **In Progress:** User stories and tasks that the development team is currently working on are in the In Progress column. Only one user story should be in this column. Having more user stories in progress is an alert that development team members are not working cross-functionally and, instead, are hoarding desired tasks. You risk having multiple user stories partially done instead of more user stories completely done by the end of the sprint.

>> **Accept:** After the development team completes a user story, it moves it to the Accept column. User stories in the Accept column are ready for the product owner to review and either provide feedback or accept.

>> **Done:** When the product owner has reviewed a user story and verifies that the user story is complete, the product owner can move that user story to the Done column.

TIP

Limit your work in progress! Only select one task at a time. Leave other tasks available in the To Do column. Ideally, a development team will work on only one user story at a time and swarm on the tasks of that user story to complete it quickly.

Because the task board is tactile — people physically move a user story card through its completion — it can engage the development team more than an electronic document ever could. The task board encourages thought and action just by existing in the scrum team's work area, where everyone can see the board.

TIP

Allowing only the product owner to move user stories to the Done column prevents misunderstandings about user story status.

Figure 9-5 shows a typical task board. As you can see, the task board is a strong visual representation of the work in progress.

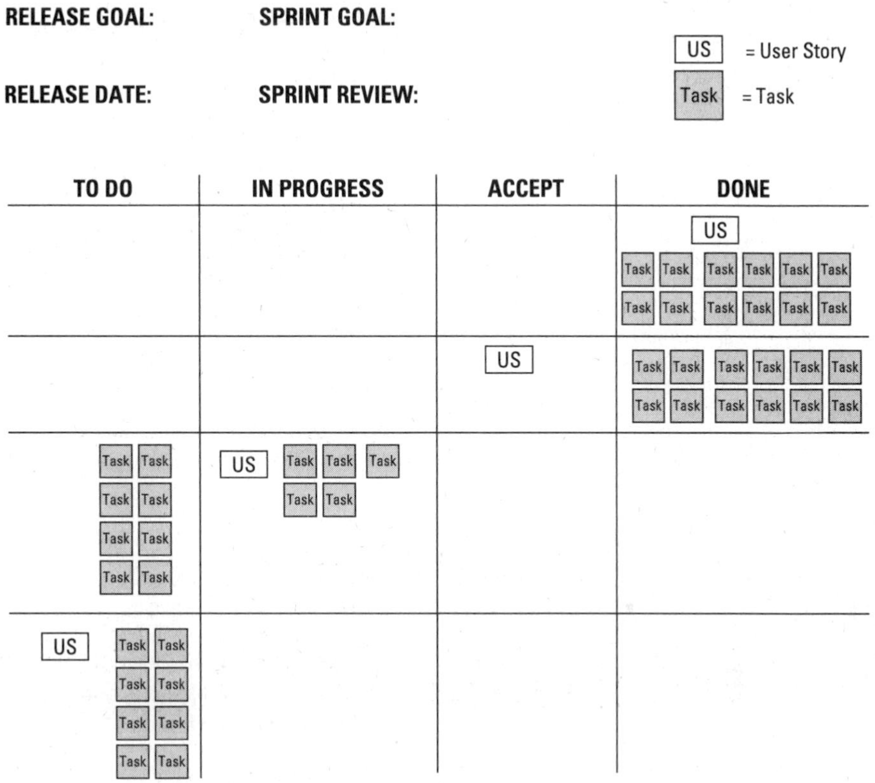

RELEASE GOAL: **SPRINT GOAL:**

RELEASE DATE: **SPRINT REVIEW:**

| US | = User Story |
| Task | = Task |

TO DO	IN PROGRESS	ACCEPT	DONE
			US Task Task Task Task Task Task Task Task Task Task Task Task
		US	Task Task Task Task Task Task Task Task Task Task Task Task
Task Task Task Task Task Task Task Task	US Task Task Task Task Task		
US Task Task Task Task Task Task Task Task			

FIGURE 9-5:
Sample task board.

The task board is a lot like a kanban board. *Kanban* is a Japanese term that means *visual signal.* (For more on kanban boards, see Chapter 4.) Toyota created these boards as part of its lean manufacturing process.

TECHNICAL STUFF

In Figure 9-5, the task board shows four user stories, each separated by a horizontal line called *swim lanes.* The first user story is done. All tasks are completed, and the product owner has accepted the work done. For the second user story, the development work is completed but is waiting for acceptance by the product owner. The third user story is in progress, and the fourth user story has not yet been started. At a glance, the status of each user story is clear not only to the scrum team, making tactical coordination faster and easier, but also to interested stakeholders.

Day-to-day work on an agile project involves more than just planning and tracking progress. In the next section, you see what most of your day's work will include, whether you're a member of the development team, a product owner, or a scrum master.

Some development teams report status only with a task board and ask the scrum master to convert the status into the sprint backlog. This process helps the scrum master see trends and potential issues.

Agile Roles in the Sprint

Each member of a scrum team has specific daily roles and responsibilities during the sprint. The day's focus for the development team is producing shippable functionality. For the product owner, the focus is on preparing the product backlog for future sprints while supporting the development team's execution of the sprint backlog with real-time clarifications. The scrum master is the agile coach and maximizes the development team's productivity by removing roadblocks and protecting the development team from external distractions.

Following are descriptions of the tasks each member of the scrum team performs during the sprint. If you're a member of the development team, you

>> Select the tasks of highest need and complete them as quickly as possible.

>> Request clarification from the product owner when you are unclear about a user story.

>> Collaborate with other development team members to design the approach to a specific user story, seek help when you need it, and provide help when another development team member needs it.

>> Conduct peer reviews on one another's work.

>> Take on tasks beyond your normal role as the sprint demands.

>> Fully develop functionality as agreed to in the definition of done (described in the next section, "Creating Shippable Functionality").

>> Report daily on your progress completing tasks in the sprint backlog.

>> Alert the scrum master to any roadblocks you can't effectively remove on your own.

>> Achieve the sprint goal you committed to during sprint planning.

The product owner has the following tasks during the sprint:

>> Make investments required to keep development speed high.

>> Prioritize product functionality.

>> Represent the product stakeholders to the development team.

>> Report on cost and schedule status to project stakeholders.

>> Elaborate user stories with the development team so that the team clearly understands what it is creating.

>> Provide immediate clarification and decisions about requirements to keep the development team developing.

>> Remove business impediments brought to you by other members of the scrum team.

>> Review completed functionality for user stories and provide feedback to the development team.

>> Add new user stories to the product backlog as necessary and ensure that new user stories support the product vision, the release goal, and the sprint goal.

>> Look forward to the next sprint and elaborate user stories in readiness for the next sprint planning meeting.

REMEMBER

Nonverbal communication says a lot. Scrum masters can benefit from understanding body language to identify unspoken tensions in the scrum team.

If you're a scrum master, you do the following during the sprint:

>> Uphold agile values and practices by coaching the product owner, the development team, and the organization when necessary.

>> Shield the development team from external distractions.

>> Remove roadblocks, both tactically for immediate problems and strategically for potential long-term issues. In Chapter 6, we compare the scrum master to an aeronautical engineer, continually removing and preventing organizational drag on the development team.

>> Facilitate consensus building in the scrum team.

>> Build relationships to foster close cooperation with people working with the scrum team.

TIP

We often tell scrum masters, "Never lunch alone. Always be building relationships." You never know when you will need to call in a favor on a project.

As you can see, each scrum team member has a specific job in the sprint. In the next section, you see how the product owner and the development team work together to create the product.

Creating Shippable Functionality

The objective of the day-to-day work of a sprint is to create shippable functionality for the product in a form that can be delivered to a customer or user.

Within the context of a single sprint, a *product increment* or *shippable functionality* means that a work product has been developed, integrated, tested, and documented according to the project definition of done and is deemed ready to release. The development team may or may not release that product at the end of the sprint — release timing depends on the release plan. The project may require multiple sprints before the product contains the set of minimum marketable features necessary to justify a market release.

TIP

It helps to think about shippable functionality in terms of user stories. A user story starts out as a written requirement on a card. As the development team creates functionality, each user story becomes an action a user can take. Shippable functionality equals completed user stories.

To create shippable functionality, the development team and the product owner are involved in three major activities:

>> Elaborating

>> Developing

>> Verifying

During the sprint, any or all of these activities can be happening at any given time. As you review them in detail, remember that they don't always occur in a linear way.

Elaborating

In an agile project, *elaboration* is the process of determining the details of a product feature. Whenever the development team tackles a new user story, elaboration ensures that any unanswered questions about a user story are answered so that the process of development can proceed.

The product owner works with the development team to elaborate user stories, but the development team should have the final say on design decisions. The product owner should be available for consultation if the development team needs further clarification on requirements throughout the day.

Collaborative design is a major factor for successful projects. Remember these agile principles: "The best architectures, requirements, and designs emerge from self-organizing teams," and "Business people and developers must work together daily throughout a project." Watch out for development team members who have a tendency to try to work alone on elaborating user stories. If a member of the development team separates himself or herself from the team, perhaps part of the scrum master's job should be coaching that person on upholding agile values and practices.

Developing

During product development, most of the activity, naturally, falls to the development team. The product owner continues to work with the development team on an as-needed basis to provide clarification and to approve developed functionality.

The development team should have immediate access to the product owner. Ideally, the product owner sits with the development team when he or she is not interacting with customers and stakeholders.

The scrum master should focus on protecting the development team from outside disruptions and removing impediments that the development team encounters.

To sustain agile practices during development, be sure to implement the type of development practices from extreme programming we show you in Chapter 4, including the following:

>> **Pair up development team members to complete tasks.** Doing so enhances the quality of the work and encourages the sharing of skills.

>> **Follow the development team's agreed-upon design standards.** If you can't follow them for whatever reason, revisit these standards and improve them.

>> **Start development by setting up automated tests.** You can find more about automated testing in the following section and in Chapter 15.

>> **If new, nice-to-have features become apparent during development, add them to the product backlog.** Avoid coding new features that are outside the sprint goal.

>> **Integrate changes that were coded during the day, one set at a time.** Test for 100 percent correctness. Integrate changes at least once a day; some teams integrate many times a day.

>> **Undertake code reviews to ensure that the code follows development standards.** Identify areas that need revising. Add the revisions as tasks in the sprint backlog.

>> **Create technical documentation as you work.** Don't wait until the end of the sprint or, worse, the end of the sprint prior to a release.

Continuous integration is the term used in software development for integrating and comprehensively testing with every code build. Continuous integration helps identify problems before they become crises.

Verifying

Verifying the work done in a sprint has three parts: automated testing, peer review, and product owner review.

It is exponentially cheaper to prevent a defect than it is to rip it out of a deployed system.

Automated testing

Automated testing means using a computer program to do the majority of your code testing for you. With automated testing, the development team can quickly develop and test code, which is a big benefit for agile projects.

Often, agile project teams code during the day and let the tests run overnight. In the morning, the project team can review the defect report that the testing program generated, report on any problems during the daily scrum, and correct those issues immediately during the day.

Automated testing can include the following:

>> **Unit testing:** Testing source code in its smallest parts — the component level

>> **System testing:** Testing the code with the rest of the system

>> **Static testing:** Verifying that the product's code meets standards based on rules and best practices that the development team has agreed upon

Peer review

Peer review simply means that development team members review one another's code. If Sam writes program A and Joan writes program B, Sam could review Joan's code, and vice versa. Objective peer review helps ensure code quality.

Pair programming is another form of peer review, but the review takes place during development. While one developer (the pilot) sits at the keyboard and writes the code, another developer (the navigator) is thinking strategically, looking ahead, and actively listening and responding to decisions made tactically by the pilot. Not only is the review happening in the moment — catching defects and making more informed decisions — but there are two developers, instead of only one, who are intimately familiar with the part of the system being developed.

TIP

Pair programming is a great way to develop cross-functional individuals to reduce single points of failure.

The development team can conduct peer reviews during development. Collocation helps make this easy — you can turn to the person next to you and ask him or her to take a quick look at what you just completed. The development team can also set aside time during the day specifically for reviewing code. Self-managing teams should decide what works best for them.

Product owner review

When a user story has been developed and tested, the development team moves the stories to the Accept column on the task board. The product owner then reviews the functionality and verifies that it meets the goals of the user story, per the user story's acceptance criteria. The product owner verifies user stories throughout each day.

As discussed in Chapter 8, the back side of each user story card has verification steps. These steps allow the product owner to review and confirm that the code works and supports the user story. Figure 9-6 shows a sample user story card's verification steps.

FIGURE 9-6: User story verification.

When I do this:	This happens:
When I go to the accounts page :	I am able to see my active account balance.
When I select transfer funds :	I am able to select "Transfer to Account" and amount.
When I submit transfer requests :	I get an account confirmation funds were transferred.

Finally, the product owner should run through some checks to verify that the user story in question meets the definition of done. When a user story meets the definition of done, the product owner updates the task board by moving the user story from the Accept column to the Done column.

While the product owner and the development team are working together to create shippable functionality for the product, the scrum master helps the scrum team to identify and clear roadblocks that appear along the way.

Identifying roadblocks

It's a major part of the scrum master's role to manage and help resolve roadblocks that the scrum team identifies. Roadblocks are anything that thwarts a team member from working to full capacity.

Although the daily scrum is a good place for the development team to identify roadblocks, the development team may come to the scrum master with issues anytime throughout the day.

Examples of roadblocks follow:

>> **Local, tactical issues,** such as

- A manager trying to pull away a team member to work on a "priority" sales report.

- The development team needing additional hardware or software to facilitate progress.

- A development team member who doesn't understand a user story and says the product owner isn't available to help.

>> **Organizational impediments,** such as

- An overall resistance to agile techniques, especially when the company established and maintained prior processes at significant cost.

- Managers who might not be in touch with the work on the ground. Technologies, development practices, and project management practices are always progressing.

- External departments that may not be familiar with scrum needs and the pace of development when using agile techniques.

- An organization that enforces policies that don't make sense for agile project teams. Centralized tools, budget restrictions, and standardized processes that don't align with agile processes can all cause issues for agile teams.

REMEMBER

The most important trait a scrum master can have is organizational clout or influence. Organizational clout gives the scrum master the ability to have difficult conversations and make the small and large changes necessary for the scrum team to be successful. We provide examples of different types of clout in Chapter 4.

Beyond the primary focus of creating shippable functionality, other things happen during the day on an agile project. Many of these tasks fall to the scrum master. Table 9-1 shows potential roadblocks and the action that the scrum master can take to remove the impediments.

TABLE 9-1   **Common Roadblocks and Solutions**

Roadblock	Action
The development team needs simulation software for a range of mobile devices so that it can test the user interface and code.	Do some research to estimate the cost of the software, prepare a summary of that for the product owner, and have a discussion about funding. Process the purchase through procurement, and deliver the software to the development team.
Management wants to borrow a development team member to write a couple of reports. All your development team members are fully occupied.	Tell the requesting manager that the person is not available and probably will not be for the duration of the project. Recommend that the requester discuss the need with the product owner so he or she can prioritize it against the rest of the product backlog. As you're likely a problem solver, you may want to suggest alternative ways in which the manager could get what he or she needs.
A development team member can't move forward on a user story because he or she does not fully understand the story. The product owner is out of the office for the day on a personal emergency.	Work with the development team member to determine if any work can happen around this user story while waiting for an answer. Help locate another person who could answer the question. Failing that, ask the development team to review upcoming tasks (not related to this stopped one) and move things around to keep productivity up.
A user story has grown in complexity and now appears to be too large for the sprint length.	Have the development team work with the product owner to break the user story down so that some demonstrable value can be completed in the current sprint and the rest can be put back into the product backlog. The goal is to ensure that the sprint ends with completed user stories, even smaller ones, rather than incomplete user stories.

So far in this chapter, you have seen how the scrum team starts its day and works throughout the day. The scrum team wraps up each day with a few tasks as well. The next section shows you how to end a day within a sprint.

The End of the Day

At the end of each day, the development team reports on task progress by updating the sprint backlog with which tasks were completed and how much work, in hours, remains to be done on new tasks started. Depending on the software that the scrum team uses, the sprint backlog data may automatically update the sprint burndown chart as well.

WARNING

Update the sprint backlog with the amount of work remaining — not the amount of time already spent — on open tasks. The important point is how much time is left, which informs the project team as to whether the scrum team is on track to meet its sprint goal. If possible, avoid spending time tracking how many hours were spent working on tasks, which is less necessary with self-correcting agile models.

The product owner should also update the task board, at least at the end of the day, and move any user stories that have passed review to the Done column.

The scrum master can review the sprint backlog or task board for any risks before the next day's daily scrum.

The scrum team follows this daily cycle until the end of the sprint, when it will be time to step back, inspect, and adapt at the sprint review and the sprint retrospective meetings.

Chapter **10**

Showcasing Work, Inspecting, and Adapting

A t the end of each sprint, the scrum team gets a chance to put the results of its hard work on display in the sprint review. The sprint review is where the product owner and the development team demonstrate the sprint's completed, potentially shippable functionality to the stakeholders. In the sprint retrospective, the scrum team (the product owner, development team, and scrum master) review how the sprint went and determine whether they need any adjustments for the next sprint.

Underpinning both of these events is the agile concept of inspect and adapt, which Chapter 7 explains.

In this chapter, you find out how to conduct a sprint review and a sprint retrospective.

The Sprint Review

The *sprint review* is a meeting to review and demonstrate the functionality created from the user stories that the development team completed during the sprint, and for the product owner to collect feedback and update the product backlog accordingly. The sprint review is open to anyone interested in reviewing the sprint's accomplishments. This means that all stakeholders get a chance to see product progress and accuracy, and provide feedback.

The sprint review is stage 6 in the Roadmap to Value. Figure 10-1 shows how the sprint review fits into an agile project.

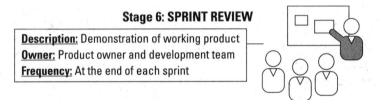

Stage 6: SPRINT REVIEW

Description: Demonstration of working product
Owner: Product owner and development team
Frequency: At the end of each sprint

FIGURE 10-1:
The sprint review
in the Roadmap
to Value.

The following sections show you what you need to do to prepare for a sprint review, how to run a sprint review meeting, and the importance of collecting feedback.

Preparing to demonstrate

Preparation for the sprint review meeting should not take more than a few minutes at most. Even though the sprint review might sound formal, the essence of showcasing for agile teams is informality. The meeting needs to be prepared and organized, but it doesn't require a lot of flashy materials. Instead, the sprint review focuses on demonstrating what the development team has done.

WARNING

If your sprint review is overly showy, ask yourself if you're covering up for not spending enough time developing. Get back to working on value — creating a working product. Pageantry is the enemy of agility.

The preparation for the sprint review meeting involves the product owner and the development team, facilitated by the scrum master as needed. The product owner needs to know which user stories the development team completed during the sprint. The development team needs to be ready to demonstrate completed, shippable functionality.

The time needed to prepare for a sprint review should not be more than 20 minutes — just enough time to make sure everyone knows who is doing what and when so the demonstration goes smoothly.

REMEMBER

Work not delivered has no business value. Within the context of a single sprint, *shippable functionality* means that the development team has satisfied its definition of done for each requirement, and the product owner has verified that the work product meets all acceptance criteria and could be released to the market, or *shipped*, if the value and timing are right for the marketplace. The actual release may be at a later time, per the communicated release plan. Find out more about shippable functionality in Chapter 9.

For the development team to demonstrate the code in the sprint review, it must be complete according to the definition of done. This means that the code is fully

>> Developed

>> Tested

>> Integrated

>> Documented

As user stories are moved to a status of done throughout the sprint, the product owner and development team should check that the functionality meets these standards. This continuous validation throughout the sprint reduces end-of-sprint risks and helps the scrum team spend as little time as possible preparing for the sprint review.

Knowing the completed user stories and being ready to demonstrate those stories' functionality prepares you to confidently start the sprint review meeting.

The sprint review meeting

Sprint review meetings have two activities: demonstrate and showcase the scrum team's finished work, and allow stakeholders to provide feedback on that work. Figure 10-2 shows the different loops of feedback a scrum team receives about a product.

This cycle of feedback repeats throughout the project as follows:

>> Each day, development team members work together in a collaborative environment that encourages feedback through peer reviews and informal communication.

>> Throughout each sprint, as soon as the development team completes each requirement, the product owner provides feedback by reviewing the working functionality for acceptance. The development team then immediately incorporates that feedback, if any, to satisfy the user story's acceptance

criteria. When the user story is complete, the product owner gives final acceptance of the functionality created for the user story, according to the user story's acceptance criteria.

» At the end of each sprint, project stakeholders provide feedback about completed functionality in the sprint review meeting.

» With each release, customers who use the product provide feedback about new working functionality.

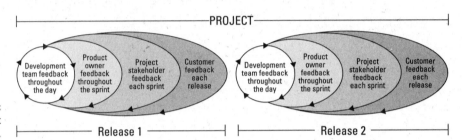

FIGURE 10-2:
Agile project
feedback loops.

The sprint review usually takes place later in the day on the last day of the sprint, often a Friday. One of the rules of scrum is to spend no more than one hour in a sprint review meeting for every week of the sprint — Figure 10-3 shows a quick reference.

If my sprint is this long...	My sprint review meeting should last no more than...
One week	One hour
Two weeks	Two hours
Three weeks	Three hours
Four weeks	Four hours

FIGURE 10-3:
Ratio of sprint
review meeting to
sprint length.

Here are some guidelines for your sprint review meeting:

» No PowerPoint slides! Show actual working functionality. Refer to the sprint backlog if you need to display a list of completed user stories.

» The entire scrum team should participate in the meeting.

>> Anyone who is interested in the meeting may attend. The project stakeholders, the summer interns, and the CEO could all theoretically be in a sprint review. Customers may also be invited whenever available.

>> The product owner introduces the release goal, the sprint goal, and the new capabilities included.

>> The development team demonstrates what it *completed* during the sprint. Typically, the development team showcases new features or architecture.

>> The demonstration should be on equipment as close as possible to the planned production environment. For example, if you're creating a mobile application, present the features on a smartphone — perhaps hooked up to a monitor — rather than on a laptop.

>> The stakeholders can ask questions and provide feedback on the demonstrated product.

>> No non-disclosed rigged functionality, such as hard-coded values and other programming shortcuts that make the application look more mature than it currently is. Rigged functionality creates more overhead work for the scrum team in future sprints to catch up to what the stakeholders think already exists.

>> The product owner can lead a discussion about what is coming next based on the features just presented and new items that have been added to the product backlog during the current sprint.

By the time you get to the sprint review, the product owner has already seen the functionality for each of the user stories that are going to be presented and has agreed that they are complete.

The sprint review meeting is valuable to the development team. The sprint review provides an opportunity for the development team to show its work directly. The meeting allows the stakeholders to recognize the development team for its efforts. The meeting contributes to development team morale, keeping the team motivated to try and produce ever-increasing volumes of quality work. The sprint review even establishes a certain level of friendly comparative competition between scrum teams that keeps everyone focused.

Sometimes, healthy competition can result in developers trying to create the coolest features or exceed the requirements of a user story — an issue known as *gold plating.* A tenet of agility is to produce only what a user story needs to pass the acceptance test. There is a risk that development team members will go beyond requirement needs in their enthusiasm, essentially wasting time that should be spent on useful product functionality. The product owner should be watchful for this. Gold-plating can be identified and avoided on a daily basis at the daily scrum or as the development team seeks clarification from the product owner.

Next, you see how to note and use the stakeholders' feedback during the sprint review meeting.

Collecting feedback in the sprint review meeting

Gather sprint review feedback informally. The product owner or scrum master can take notes on behalf of the development team, as team members often will be engaged in the presentation and resulting conversation.

Keep in mind the example project we use throughout the book: a mobile application for XYZ Bank. Stakeholders responding to functionality they saw for the XYZ Bank mobile application might have comments such as the following:

» From a person in sales or marketing: "You might want to consider letting the customers save their preferences, based on the results you showed. It will make for a more personalized experience going forward."

» From a functional director or manager: "Given what I've seen, you might be able to leverage some of the code modules that were developed for the ABC project last year. They needed to do similar data manipulation."

» From someone who works with the quality or user experience professionals in the company: "I noticed your logins were pretty straightforward; will the application be able to handle special characters?"

New user stories may come out of the sprint review. These new user stories might be new features or changes to the existing functionality.

TIP

In the first few sprint reviews, the scrum master may need to remind stakeholders about agile practices. Some people hear the word "demonstration" and immediately expect fancy slides and printouts. The scrum master has a responsibility to manage these expectations and uphold agile values and practices.

The product owner needs to add any new user stories to the product backlog and order those stories by priority. The product owner also adds back into the product backlog any stories that were scheduled for the current sprint but not completed, and reorders those stories based on the most recent priorities.

The product owner needs to complete updates to the product backlog in time for the next sprint planning meeting.

When the sprint review is over, it is time for the sprint retrospective.

TIP

You may want to take a brief break between the sprint review and the sprint retrospective so that scrum team members can come to the retrospective discussion fresh and relaxed.

Having just completed the sprint review, the scrum team will come into the retrospective ready to inspect its processes and will have ideas for adaptation.

The Sprint Retrospective

The *sprint retrospective* is a meeting in which the product owner, development team, and scrum master discuss how the sprint went and what they can do to improve the next sprint. The scrum team should conduct this meeting in a self-directed way. If managers or supervisors attend sprint retrospectives, scrum team members will avoid being open with each other, which limits the effectiveness of the team inspecting and adapting in a self-organizing way.

If the scrum team likes, members can invite other stakeholders to attend as well. If the scrum team regularly interacts with outside stakeholders, those stakeholders' insights can be valuable.

The sprint retrospective is stage 7 in the Roadmap to Value. Figure 10-4 shows how the sprint retrospective fits into an agile project.

Stage 7: SPRINT RETROSPECTIVE

FIGURE 10-4:
The sprint retrospective in the Roadmap to Value.

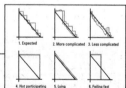

Description: Team refinement of environment and processes to optimize efficiency
Owner: Scrum team
Frequency: At the end of each sprint

The goal of the sprint retrospective is to continuously improve your processes. Improving and customizing processes according to the needs of each individual scrum team increases scrum team morale, improves efficiency, and increases *velocity* — work output. (Find details on velocity in Chapter 13.) However, what works for one team won't necessarily work for another team. Managers outside the scrum team should not dictate how all scrum teams should overcome their challenges and should instead allow them to find the best solutions for themselves.

Your sprint retrospective results may be unique for your scrum team. For example, members of one scrum team we worked with decided that they would like to come into work early and leave early, and spend summer afternoons with their families. Another team at the same organization felt that they did better work late at night, and decided to come to the office in the afternoon and work into the evenings. The result for both teams was increased morale and increased velocity.

Use the information you learn in the retrospective to review and revise your work processes and make your next sprint better.

REMEMBER

Agile approaches — particularly scrum — quickly reveal problems in projects. Scrum doesn't fix problems; it simply exposes them and provides a framework for inspecting and adapting exposed issues. Data from the sprint backlog shows exactly where the development team has been slowed down. The development team talks and collaborates. All these tools and practices help reveal inefficiencies and allow the scrum team to refine practices to improve sprint after sprint. Pay attention to what gets exposed. Don't ignore it, and don't work around it.

In the following sections, you find out how to plan for a retrospective, how to run a sprint retrospective meeting, and how to use the results of each sprint retrospective to improve future sprints.

STOPPING THE LINE

Taiichi Ohno, who built the Toyota Production System in the 1950s and 1960s — the beginning of lean manufacturing — decentralized assembly-line management to empower line workers to make decisions. Line workers actually had a responsibility to stop the line by pushing a red button when they found a defect or a problem on the assembly line. Traditionally, plant managers viewed stopping the line as a failure and focused on running the assembly line at capacity as many hours of the day as possible to maximize throughput. Ohno's philosophy was that by removing constraints as they occur, you proactively create a better system rather than trying to optimize your existing process.

When first introduced, the productivity of managers who implemented this practice took an initial drop because they spent more time fixing defects in the system than the managers' teams who did not adopt the practice. The old teams declared this a victory at first. However, it didn't take long until the new teams not only caught up but also began producing more quickly, more cheaply, and with fewer defects and variance than the teams who weren't making continuous improvements in their system. This process of regular and continuous improvement is what made Toyota so successful.

Planning for sprint retrospectives

For the first sprint retrospective, everyone on the scrum team should think about a few key questions and be ready to discuss them. What went well during the sprint? What would you change, and how?

Everyone on the scrum team may want to make a few notes beforehand, or even take notes throughout the sprint. The scrum team could keep the roadblocks from the sprint's daily scrum meetings in mind. For the second sprint retrospective forward, you can also start to compare the current sprint with prior sprints, and track progress on the improvement efforts from sprint to sprint. In Chapter 9, we mention saving sprint backlogs from prior sprints; this is where they might come in handy.

If the scrum team has honestly and thoroughly thought about what went right and what could be better, it can go into the sprint retrospective ready to have a useful conversation.

The sprint retrospective meeting

The sprint retrospective meeting is an action-oriented meeting. The scrum team immediately applies what it learned in the retrospective to the next sprint.

The sprint retrospective meeting is an action-oriented meeting, not a justification meeting. If you are hearing words like "because," the conversation is moving away from action and toward rationale.

One of the rules of scrum is to spend no more than 45 minutes in a sprint retrospective meeting for every week of the sprint. Figure 10-5 shows a quick reference.

If my sprint is this long…	My sprint retrospective meeting should last no more than…
One week	45 minutes
Two weeks	1.5 hours
Three weeks	2.25 hours
Four weeks	3 hours

FIGURE 10-5: Ratio of sprint retrospective meeting to sprint length.

The sprint retrospective should cover three primary questions:

>> What went well during the sprint?

>> What would we like to change?

>> How can we implement that change?

The following areas are also open for discussion:

>> **Results:** Compare the amount of work planned with what the development team completed. Review the sprint burndown chart (see Chapter 9) and what it tells the development team about how it's working.

>> **People:** Discuss team composition and alignment.

>> **Relationships:** Talk about communication, collaboration, and working in pairs.

>> **Processes:** Go over support, development, and peer review processes.

>> **Tools:** How are the different tools working for the scrum team? Think about the artifacts, electronic tools, communication tools, and technical tools.

>> **Productivity:** How can the team improve productivity and get the most work done in the next sprint?

It helps to have these discussions in a structured format. Esther Derby and Diana Larsen, authors of *Agile Retrospectives: Making Good Teams Great* (Pragmatic Book-shelf, 2006), have a great agenda for sprint retrospectives that keeps the team focused on discussions that will lead to real improvement:

1. **Set the stage.**

   Establishing the goals for the retrospective upfront will help keep your scrum team focused on providing the right kind of feedback later in the meeting. As you progress into later sprints, you may want to have retrospectives that focus on one or two specific areas for improvement.

2. **Gather data.**

   Discuss the facts about what went well in the last sprint and what needed improvement. Create an overall picture of the sprint; consider using a whiteboard to write down the input from meeting attendees.

3. **Generate insights.**

   Take a look at the information you just gathered and come up with ideas about how to make improvements for the next sprint.

4. **Decide what to do.**

   Determine — as a team — which ideas you'll put into place. Decide on specific actions you can take to make the ideas a reality.

5. **Close the retrospective.**

   Reiterate your plan of action for the next sprint. Thank people for contributing. Also find ways to make the next retrospective better!

For some scrum teams, it might be difficult to open up at first. The scrum master may need to ask specific questions to start discussions. Participating in retrospectives takes practice. What matters is to encourage the scrum team to take responsibility for the sprint — to truly embrace being self-managing.

In other scrum teams, a lot of debate and discussion ensues during the retrospective. The scrum master can find it challenging to manage these discussions and keep the meeting within its allotted time, but that is what needs to be done.

Be sure to use the results from your sprint retrospectives to inspect and adapt throughout your project.

Inspecting and adapting

The sprint retrospective is one of the best opportunities you have to put the ideas of inspect and adapt into action. You came up with challenges and solutions during the retrospective. Don't leave those solutions behind after the meeting; make the improvements part of your work every day.

You could record your recommendations for improvement informally. Some scrum teams post the actions identified during the retrospective meeting in the team area to ensure visibility and action on the items listed. Many teams also add action items to the product backlog to ensure that they implement them during an upcoming sprint.

TIP

To become more agile, scrum teams focus on small changes with big value. We like teams to take at least one improvement into each sprint, a process sometimes referred to as *scrumming the scrum*.

In subsequent sprint retrospective meetings, it's important to review the evaluations of the prior sprint and make sure you put the suggested improvements into place.

Chapter **11**

Preparing for Release

Releasing new product features to customers has a special set of challenges. The development team has specific tasks for a product release that differ from the tasks involved with creating functionality during normal sprints. The organization sponsoring the product may need to prepare to support the product. You want customers to be able to correctly use the released product.

This chapter covers how to manage the final sprint, if needed — the release sprint — before product release. You also discover how to prepare your organization and the marketplace for the product release.

Preparing the Product for Deployment: The Release Sprint

The work that takes place during regular development sprints should be whole and complete, including testing and technical documentation, before you demonstrate your product. The product of a development sprint is working functionality.

However, there may be activities, not related to creating product features, that the development team can't realistically complete within development sprints and that might even introduce unacceptable overhead. To accommodate prerelease activities and help ensure that the release goes well, scrum teams may schedule a release sprint as the final sprint prior to releasing functionality to customers.

If a scrum team requires a release sprint, it probably means that the broader organization can't support it, which is an anti-pattern to becoming agile. Every type of work or activity required to release functionality to the market should be part of the sprint-level definition of done. That is the goal for agile teams.

The release sprint contains only those things needed to move working functionality to the marketplace. The following are examples of release sprint backlog items. See if you can think of possible ways to shift any of these into the development sprint:

>> Creating user documentation for the most recent version of the product

>> Performance testing, load testing, security testing, and any other checks to ensure that the working software will perform acceptably in production

>> Integrating the product with enterprise-wide systems, where testing might take days or weeks

>> Completing organizational or regulatory procedures that are mandatory prior to release

>> Preparing release notes — final notes about changes to the product

>> Preparing the deployment package, enabling all the code for the product features to move to production at one time

>> Deploying your code to the production environment

Some aspects of a release sprint are different from a development sprint:

>> You do not develop any new functionality requirements from the product backlog. Although you have functionality freeze, you do not have code freeze because the development team will need to make adjustments to respond to feedback from release sprint activities, such as performance testing or focus groups.

>> Based on the work you need to do, your release sprint may be a different length than your regular development sprints. In addition, you won't have the concept of velocity because you won't be doing the same type of work that you do in development sprints.

>> The definition of done is different for work completed during a release sprint. In a development sprint, *done* means the completion of working functionality for a user story. In a release sprint, the definition is the completion of all tasks required for release.

UNDERSTANDING THE ROLE OF DOCUMENTATION

What's the difference between the technical documentation that you create during a sprint and the user documentation that you may create in your release sprint?

Your *technical documentation* should be barely sufficient, with no frills and just enough information to tell the development team — and perhaps future development teams — how to create and update the product. If, on the last day of the sprint, the development team won the lottery and retired to Costa Rica, a new development team should be able to review the technical documentation and easily pick up where the former team left off.

Your *user documentation* tells your customers how to use your product. You may want user documentation crafted specifically for each of your customers. For example, a mobile banking application might need a frequently asked questions (FAQs) section for banking customers. The same application might have a feature that enables marketing managers to upload ad messages to the application; you'd want to make sure those managers have instructions for the upload feature as well. Because your product will have changes throughout each sprint of the release, it might be more efficient to wait until the last responsible minute to create your user documentation, after the stakeholders agree that the functionality is ready for release.

>> A release sprint includes tests and approvals that may not be practical to do in a development sprint, such as performance testing, load testing, security testing, focus groups, and legal review.

REMEMBER

Agile development teams may create two definitions of done: one for sprints and one for releases.

Table 11-1 shows a comparison between the activities of a development sprint and a release sprint. For detailed descriptions of the key elements in a sprint, see Chapters 8 through 10.

TABLE 11-1 ## Development Sprint Elements versus Release Sprint Elements

Element	Used in Development Sprint	Used in Release Sprint
Sprint planning	Yes	Yes
Product backlog	Yes	No

(continued)

TABLE 11-1 *(continued)*

Element	Used in Development Sprint	Used in Release Sprint
Sprint backlog	Yes For a development sprint, your sprint backlog contains user stories and the tasks needed to create each user story. You estimate user stories relatively, with story points. (See Chapters 7 and 8.)	Yes In a release sprint, you no longer need to put your requirements in the user story format. Instead, you create only a list of tasks needed for the release. You also do not use story points. Instead, add the estimated hours each task will take when planning the release sprint, in the same way you break down and estimate tasks during the development sprint planning.
Burndown chart	Yes	Yes
Daily scrum	Yes	Yes Involve stakeholders from outside the scrum team who have tasks associated with releasing the product, such as enterprise build managers or other configuration managers.
Daily activities	In a development sprint, your daily activities focus on creating shippable functionality.	In a release sprint, your daily activities focus on preparing your working functionality for external release.
End-of-day reporting	Yes	Yes
Sprint review	Yes	Yes Some organizations use a release sprint review as a *go or no-go meeting* to authorize launching the functionality.
Sprint retrospective	Yes	Yes This can be an opportunity to inspect the entire sprint and plan for adapting in the next release.

WARNING

A release sprint should not be a parking lot for tasks that the development team didn't finish in the development sprints. You may not be surprised to hear that development teams are sometimes tempted to delay tasks until the release sprint. You can avoid this by ensuring that the scrum team has created a proper definition of done for requirements in development sprints, including testing, integration, and documentation.

While running a release sprint, you also need to prepare your organization for the product release. The next sections discuss how to prepare for supporting the new functionality in the marketplace and how to get stakeholders in your company or organization ready for product deployment.

Preparing for Operational Support

After your product is released to the customer, someone will have to support it. Supporting your product involves responding to customer inquiries, maintaining the system in a production environment, and enhancing existing functionality to fill minor gaps. Although new development work and operational support work are both important, they involve different approaches and cadences.

Separating new development and support work ensures that new development teams can focus on continuing to bring innovative solutions to customers at a faster rate than if the team frequently switches between the two types of work.

A scrum team doing new development can plan and develop new working functionality within a one- to two-week sprint, but it's difficult to plan when operational or maintenance issues will arise. Maintenance work usually requires shorter timeboxed iterations, typically no more than one day, which is usually the longest the organization can go without changing priorities with any issues in production.

We recommend a model that separates new development and maintenance work, as illustrated in Figure 11-1.

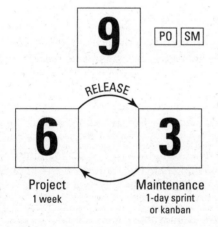

FIGURE 11-1: Operational support scrum team model.

For a scrum team of nine developers, for instance, we would divide the development team into two teams, one with six developers, and the other with three. (These numbers are flexible.) The team of six does new development project work from the product backlog in one-week to two-week sprints, as described in Chapters 7 through 10. The work that the team commits to during the sprint planning meeting will be the only work they do.

The team of three are our firefighters and do maintenance and support work in one-day sprints or by using kanban. (You learn about kanban in Chapter 4.) Single-day sprints allow the scrum team to triage all incoming requests from the previous day, plan the highest-priority items, implement those items as a team, and review the results at the end of the day (or even earlier) for go or no-go approval before pushing the changes to production. For continuity, the product owner and scrum master are the same for each team.

REMEMBER

Although the newly modified project development team is smaller than before, there are still enough developers to keep new development efforts moving forward, uninterrupted by maintenance work. By the time you begin releasing functionality to the market, your scrum team will be working well together and the developers will have increased their versatility by being able to complete more types of tasks than when the project first started.

The project development team will have periodic releases to production, such as once every 90 days. At each release, one developer will rotate to the maintenance team, armed with first-hand knowledge of the functionality being deployed to production. At the same time, one developer from the maintenance team will be rotated into the project development team, equipped with first-hand knowledge of what it's like to support the product in the real world. This rotation continues at each release.

TECHNICAL
STUFF

Development Operations (DevOps) is the collaboration and integration between software developers and IT operations (which includes functions such as systems administration and server maintenance). Taking a DevOps approach enables developers and operations to work together to tighten cycle times of deployment.

This DevOps model ensures that everyone gets to do new product development as well as maintenance work, and that product knowledge is continually shared effectively between the two development teams. This approach improves DevOps and facilitates cross-functional team members. It also minimizes any disruption the teams may experience from changing team members because the rotations happen only at each release rather than daily or weekly.

When preparing for release, establishing expectations upfront of how the functionality will be supported in production allows the scrum team to develop the product in a way that enables the team to effectively support the product after it is deployed. It increases ownership across the scrum team and heightens the team's awareness and dedication to long-term success.

ONE-DAY SPRINTS

We recommend running one-day sprints for maintenance teams. By framing each day in the sprint cycle, the scrum team operates in a solid feedback loop, ensuring continuous inspection and adaptation as well as regular stakeholder involvement.

By using the same formulas for timeboxing scrum events, you won't spend hours in planning or reviews as you would with one- to four-week sprints. Dividing one-week scrum event timeboxes by five days means you spend about 25 minutes triaging the maintenance product backlog and planning the day, about 12-15 minutes for the sprint review to determine go or no-go to production, and an additional 10 minutes to inspect and adapt the team's processes and identify any issues that should be continued or discontinued the next day.

The key to operating in one-day sprints is making sure maintenance items are broken down small enough so that developers can complete them in less than a day. This approach ensures that customers get something every day rather than wait for weeks.

Preparing the Organization for Product Deployment

A product release often affects a number of departments in a company or organization. To get the organization ready for the new product, the product owner and scrum master need to add items relevant to the organization to the *release sprint backlog*. (See how to create a sprint backlog in Chapter 8.)

The release sprint backlog should also cover activities for the development team. It also needs to address activities to be performed by groups in the organization but outside the scrum team to prepare for the product deployment. These departments might include the following:

>> **Marketing:** Do marketing campaigns related to the new product need to launch at the same time as the product?

>> **Sales:** Are there specific customers who need to know about the product? Will the new product cause an increase in sales?

>> **Logistics:** Is the product a physical item that includes packaging or shipping?

>> **Product support:** Does the customer service group have the information it needs to answer questions about the new product? Will this group have enough people on hand in case customer questions increase when the product launches?

>> **Legal:** Does the product meet legal standards, including pricing, licensing, and correct verbiage, for release to the public?

The departments that need to be ready for the product launch and the specific tasks these groups need to complete will, of course, vary from organization to organization. A key to release success, however, is that the product owner and scrum master involve the right people and ensure that those people clearly understand what they need to do to be ready for the functionality release.

As with development sprints, in your release sprint, you can effectively use daily scrums, sprint review meetings, and sprint retrospectives with department colleagues involved in preparing for product deployment. You can even use a task board, like the one we describe in Chapter 9.

During your release sprint, you also need to include one more group in your planning: the product customer. The next section discusses getting the marketplace ready for your product.

Preparing the Marketplace for Product Deployment

The product owner is responsible for working with other departments to ensure that the marketplace — existing customers and potential customers — is ready for what's coming. The marketing or sales teams may lead this effort; team members look to the product owner to keep them informed on the release date and the features that will be part of the release.

REMEMBER

Some software products are only for internal employee use. Certain things you're reading in this section might seem like overkill for an internal application — an application released only within your company. However, many of these steps are still good guidelines for promoting internal applications. Preparing customers, whether internal or external, for new products can be a key part of product success.

To help prepare customers for the product release, the product owner may want to work with different teams to ensure the following:

>> **Marketing support:** Whether you're dealing with a new product or new features for an existing product, the marketing department should leverage the excitement of the new product functionality to help promote the product and the organization.

>> **Customer testing:** If possible, work with your customers (some people use focus groups) to get real-world feedback about the product from a subset of end users. Your marketing team can also use this feedback translate into testimonials for promoting the product right away.

>> **Marketing materials:** An organization's marketing group also prepares the promotional and advertising plans, as well as packaging for physical media. Media materials, such as press releases and information for analysts, need to be ready, as do marketing and sales materials.

>> **Support channels:** Ensure that customers understand the available support channels in case they have questions about the product.

Review the tasks on your release sprint backlog from the customer's standpoint. Think of the personas you used when creating your user stories. Do those personas need to know something about the product? Update your launch checklist with items that would be valuable to customers represented by your personas. You can find more information about personas in Chapter 8.

Finally, you're there — release day. Whatever role you played along the way, this is the day you worked hard to achieve. It's time to celebrate!

4

Agile Management

» Managing scope and scope changes
with agile processes

» Seeing the different approach agile
processes bring to procurement

» Managing procurement on agile
projects

Chapter **12**

Managing Scope and Procurement

S cope management is part of every project. To create a product, you have to understand basic product requirements and the work it will take to fulfill those requirements. You need to be able to prioritize and manage scope changes as new requirements arise. You have to verify that finished product features fulfill customers' needs.

Procurement is also part of many projects. If you need to look outside your organization for help completing a project, you should know how to go about procuring goods and services. You will want to know how to collaborate with vendor teams during the project. You should also know something about creating contracts and different cost structures.

In this chapter, you find out how to manage scope in an agile project and take advantage of agile methods' welcoming approach to informed change. You also find out how to manage procurement of goods and services to deliver product scope on an agile project. First, we review traditional scope management.

What's Different about Agile Scope Management?

Historically, a large part of project management is scope management. *Product scope* is all the features and requirements that a product includes. *Project scope* is all the work involved in creating a product.

Traditional project management treats changing requirements as a sign of failure in upfront planning. Agile projects, however, have variable scope so that project teams can immediately and incrementally incorporate learning and feedback, and ultimately create better products. The signers of the Agile Manifesto recognized that scope change is natural and beneficial. Agile approaches specifically embrace change and use it to make better-informed decisions and more useful products.

TIP

If you run an agile project and your requirements don't change because you learned nothing along the way, that is a failure. Your product backlog should change often as you learn from stakeholder and customer feedback. It's unlikely that you knew everything at the beginning of the project.

REMEMBER

Chapter 2 details the Agile Manifesto and the 12 Agile Principles. (If you haven't yet checked out that chapter, flip back to it now. We'll wait.) The manifesto and the principles answer the question, "How agile are we?" The degree to which your project approach supports the manifesto and the principles helps determine how agile your methods are.

The agile principles that relate the most to scope management follow:

1. Our highest priority is to satisfy the customer through early and continuous delivery of valuable software.

2. Welcome changing requirements, even late in development. Agile processes harness change for the customer's competitive advantage.

3. Deliver working software frequently, from a couple of weeks to a couple of months, with a preference to the shorter timescale.

10. Simplicity — the art of maximizing the amount of work not done — is essential.

Agile approaches to scope management are fundamentally different than traditional methods for scope management. Consider the differences you see in Table 12-1.

TABLE 12-1 **Traditional versus Agile Scope Management**

Scope Management with Traditional Approaches	Scope Management with Agile Approaches
Project teams attempt to identify and document complete scope at the beginning of the project, when the teams are the least informed about the product.	The product owner gathers high-level requirements at the beginning of the project, breaking down and further detailing requirements that are going to be implemented in the immediate future. Requirements are gathered and refined throughout the project as the team's knowledge of customer needs and project realities grows.
Organizations view scope change after the requirements phase is complete as negative.	Organizations view change as a positive way to improve a product as the project progresses. Changes late in the project, when you know the most about the product, are often the most valuable changes.
Project managers rigidly control and discourage changes after stakeholders sign off on requirements.	Change management is an inherent part of agile processes. You assess scope and have an opportunity to include new requirements with every sprint. The product owner determines the value and priority of new requirements and adds those requirements to the product backlog.
The cost of change increases over time, while the ability to make changes decreases.	You fix resources and schedule initially. New features with high priority don't necessarily cause budget or schedule slip; they simply push out the lowest-priority features. Iterative development allows for changes with each new sprint.
Projects often include *scope bloat,* unnecessary product features included out of fear of mid-project change.	The scrum team determines scope by considering which features directly support the product vision, the release goal, and the sprint goal. The development team creates the most valuable features first to guarantee their inclusion and to ship those features as soon as possible. Less valuable features might never be created, which may be acceptable to the business and the customer after they have the highest-value features.

At any point in an agile project, anyone — the scrum team, stakeholders, or anyone else in the organization with a good idea — can identify new product requirements. The product owner determines the value and priority of new requirements and prioritizes those requirements against other requirements in the product backlog.

TECHNICAL STUFF

Traditional project management has a term to describe requirements that change after the project's initial definition phase: *scope creep.* Waterfall doesn't have a positive way to incorporate changes mid–project, so scope changes often cause large problems with a waterfall project's schedule and budget. (For more on the waterfall methodology, see Chapter 1.) Mention "scope creep" to a seasoned project manager, and you might even see him or her shudder.

During sprint planning at the beginning of each sprint, the scrum team can use the product backlog priority to help decide whether a new requirement should be part of the sprint. Lower-priority requirements stay in the product backlog for future consideration. You can read about planning sprints in Chapter 8.

The next section addresses how to manage scope on an agile project.

Managing Agile Scope

Welcoming scope change helps you create the best product possible. Embracing change, however, requires that you understand the current scope and know how to deal with updates as they arise. Luckily, agile approaches have straightforward ways to manage new and existing requirements:

>> The product owner ensures that the rest of the project team — the scrum team plus the project stakeholders — clearly understands the existing scope for the project, the product vision, the current release goal, and the current sprint goal.

>> The product owner determines the value and priority of new requirements in relation to the product vision, release goal, sprint goals, and existing requirements.

>> The development team creates product requirements in order of priority to release the most important parts of the product first.

In the following sections, you find out how to understand and convey scope in different parts of an agile project. You see how to evaluate priorities as new requirements arise. You also find out how to use the product backlog and other agile artifacts to manage scope.

Understanding scope throughout the project

At each stage in an agile project, the scrum team manages scope in different ways. A good way to look at scope management throughout a project is by using the Roadmap to Value, first presented in Chapter 7 and shown again in Figure 12-1.

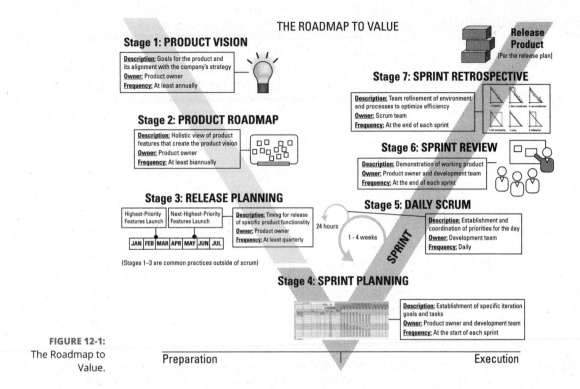

FIGURE 12-1:
The Roadmap to Value.

Consider each part of the Roadmap to Value:

>> **Stage 1, product vision:** The product vision statement establishes the outer boundary of the functionality that the product will include, and is the first step in establishing project scope. The product owner is responsible for ensuring that all members of the project team know the product vision statement and that everyone on the project team interprets the statement correctly.

>> **Stage 2, product roadmap:** During product roadmap creation, the product owner refers to the vision statement and ensures that features support the vision statement. As new features materialize, the product owner needs to understand them and be able to clearly communicate to the development team and stakeholders the scope of these features and how they support the product vision.

>> **Stage 3, release planning:** During release planning, the product owner needs to determine a release goal — the midterm boundary of functionality that is planned to go to market at the next release — and select only the scope that supports that release goal.

>> **Stage 4, sprint planning:** During sprint planning, the product owner needs to ensure that the scrum team understands the release goal and plans each

sprint goal — the immediate boundary of functionality to be potentially shippable at the end of the sprint — based on that release goal. The product owner and development team select only the scope that supports the sprint goal as part of the sprint. The product owner will also ensure that the development team understands the scope of the individual user stories selected for the sprint.

>> **Stage 5, daily scrum:** The daily scrum meeting can be a launching point for scope change for future sprints. The daily scrum meeting is a focused, 15-minute meeting for the development team to state three things: the preceding day's completed work, the scope of work for the coming day, and any roadblocks the development team may have. However, the three subjects of the daily scrum often reveal larger opportunities for scope changes.

When topics come up that warrant a bigger discussion than the time and format of the daily scrum meeting allows, a scrum team can decide to have an after-party meeting. In the after-party, scrum team members talk about issues affecting their progress toward the sprint goal. If opportunities for new functionality — new scope — are identified during the sprint, the product owner evaluates them and may add and prioritize them on the product backlog for a future sprint.

>> **Stage 6, sprint review:** The product owner sets the tone of each sprint review meeting by reiterating the scope of the sprint — the sprint goal that the scrum team pursued and what was completed. Especially during the first sprint review, it's important that the stakeholders in the meeting have the right expectations about scope.

Sprint reviews can be inspiring. When the entire project team is in one room, interacting with the working product, members may look at the product in new ways and come up with ideas to improve the product. The product owner updates the product backlog with new scope based on feedback received in the sprint review.

>> **Stage 7, sprint retrospective:** In the sprint retrospective, the scrum team members can discuss how well they met the scope commitments they made at the beginning of the sprint. If the development team was not able to achieve the sprint goal identified during sprint planning, its members will need to refine planning and work processes to make sure they can select the right amount of work for each sprint. If the development team met its goals, it can use the sprint retrospective to come up with ways to add more scope to future sprints. Scrum teams aim to improve productivity with every sprint.

Introducing scope changes

Many people, even people outside the organization, can suggest a new product feature on an agile project. You might see new ideas for features from the following:

>> User community feedback, including groups or people who are given an opportunity to preview the product

>> Business stakeholders who see a new market opportunity or threat

>> Executives and senior managers who have insight into long-term organizational strategies and changes

>> The development team, which is learning more about the product every day, and is closest to the working product

>> The scrum master, who may find an opportunity while working with external departments or clearing development team roadblocks

>> The product owner, who often knows the most about the product and the stakeholders' needs

Because you will receive suggestions for product changes throughout an agile project, you want to determine which changes are valid and manage the updates. Read on to see how.

Managing scope changes

When you get new requirements, use the following steps to evaluate and prioritize the requirements and update the product backlog.

WARNING

Do not add new requirements to sprints already in progress, unless the development team requests them, usually due to unexpected increased capacity.

1. **Assess whether the new requirement should be part of the product, the release, or the sprint by asking some key questions about the requirement:**

   a. *Does the new requirement support the product vision statement?*

   ● If yes, add the requirement to the product backlog and product roadmap.

   ● If no, the requirement shouldn't be part of the project. It may be a good candidate for a separate project.

b. *If the new requirement supports the product vision, does the new requirement support the current release goal?*

- If yes, the requirement is a candidate for the current release plan.

- If no, leave the requirement on the product backlog for a future release.

c. *If the new requirement supports the release goal, does the new requirement support the current sprint goal?*

- If yes and if the sprint has not started, the requirement is a candidate for the current sprint backlog.

- If no or the sprint has already started or both, leave the requirement on the product backlog for a future sprint.

2. **Estimate the effort for the new requirement.**

   The development team estimates the effort. Find out how to estimate requirements in Chapter 7.

3. **Prioritize the requirement against other requirements in the product backlog and add the new requirement to the product backlog, in order of priority.**

   Consider the following:

   - The product owner knows the most about the product's business needs and how important the new requirement may be in relation to other requirements. The product owner may also reach out to project stakeholders for additional insight to a requirement's priority.

   - The development team may also have technical insight about a new requirement's priority. For example, if Requirement A and Requirement B have equal business value, but you need to complete Requirement B for Requirement A to be feasible, the development team will need to alert the product owner. Requirement B may need to be completed first.

   - Although the development team and project stakeholders can provide information to help prioritize a requirement, determining priority is ultimately the product owner's decision.

   - Adding new requirements to the product backlog may mean other requirements move down the list in the product backlog. Figure 12-2 shows the addition of a new requirement in the product backlog.

The product backlog is a complete list of all known scope for the product and is your most important tool for managing scope change on an agile project.

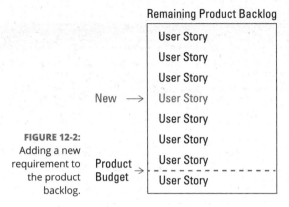

Remaining Product Backlog

	User Story
	User Story
	User Story
New →	User Story
	User Story
	User Story
Product	User Story
Budget →	User Story

FIGURE 12-2:
Adding a new requirement to the product backlog.

Keeping the product backlog up to date will allow you to quickly prioritize and add new requirements. With a current product backlog, you always understand the scope left in a project. Chapter 7 has more information about prioritizing requirements.

Using agile artifacts for scope management

From the vision statement through the sprint plan, all the artifacts in agile project management support you in your scope management efforts. Progressively decompose, or break down, requirements as features rise to the top of the priority list. We talk about decomposition and progressive elaboration of requirements in Chapter 7.

Table 12-2 reveals how each agile artifact, including the product backlog, contributes to ongoing scope refinement.

TABLE 12-2   **Agile Artifacts and Scope Management Roles**

Artifact	Role in Establishing Scope	Role in Scope Change
Vision statement: A definition of the product's end goal. Chapter 7 has more about the vision statement.	Use the vision statement as a benchmark to judge whether features belong in the scope for the current project.	When someone introduces new requirements, those requirements must support the product vision statement.
Product roadmap: A holistic view of product features that create the product vision. Chapter 7 has more about the product roadmap.	Product scope is part of the product roadmap. Requirements at a feature level are good for business conversations about what it means to realize the product vision.	Update the product roadmap as new requirements arise. The product roadmap provides visual communication of the new feature's inclusion in the project.

(continued)

TABLE 12-2 *(continued)*

Artifact	Role in Establishing Scope	Role in Scope Change
Release plan: A digestible mid-term target focused around a minimum set of marketable features. Chapter 8 has more about the release plan.	The release plan shows the scope of the current release. You may want to plan your releases by themes — logical groups of requirements.	Add new features that belong in the current release to the release plan. If the new user story doesn't belong in the current release, leave it on the product backlog for a future release.
Product backlog: A complete list of all known scope for the product. Chapters 7 and 8 offer more about the product backlog.	If a requirement is in the scope of the product vision, it is part of the product backlog.	The product backlog contains all scope changes. New, high-priority features push lower-priority features down on the product backlog.
Sprint backlog: The user stories and tasks in the scope of the current sprint. Chapter 8 has more about the sprint backlog.	The sprint backlog contains the user stories that are in scope for the current sprint.	The sprint backlog establishes what is allowed in the sprint. After the development team commits to the sprint goal in the sprint-planning meeting, only the development team can modify the sprint backlog.

What's Different about Agile Procurement?

Another part of project management is *procurement,* managing the purchase of services or goods needed to deliver the product's scope. Like scope, procurement is part of the investment side of a project.

Chapter 2 explains that the Agile Manifesto values *customer collaboration over contract negotiation.* This sets an important tone for procurement relationships on agile projects.

Valuing customer collaboration more than contract negotiation doesn't mean that agile projects have no contracts: Contracts and negotiation are critical to business relationships. However, the Agile Manifesto sets forth the idea that a buyer and seller should work together to create products, and that the relationship between the two is more important than quibbling over ill-informed details and checking off contract items that may or may not ultimately be valuable to customers.

All 12 Agile Principles apply to procurement on agile projects. However, the following seem to stand out the most when securing goods and services for an agile project:

2. Welcome changing requirements, even late in development. Agile processes harness change for the customer's competitive advantage.

3. Deliver working software frequently, from a couple of weeks to a couple of months, with a preference to the shorter timescale.

4. Business people and developers must work together daily throughout the project.

5. Build projects around motivated individuals. Give them the environment and support they need, and trust them to get the job done.

10. Simplicity — the art of maximizing the amount of work not done — is essential.

11. The best architectures, requirements, and designs emerge from self-organizing teams.

Table 12-3 highlights the differences between procurement on traditional projects and procurement on agile projects.

TABLE 12-3   **Traditional versus Agile Procurement Management**

Procurement Management with Traditional Approaches	Procurement Management with Agile Approaches
The project manager and the organization are responsible for procurement activities.	The self-managing development team plays a larger part in identifying items needing procurement. The scrum master facilitates the acquisition of needed items for the development team.
Contracts with service providers often include provisions for fixed requirements, extensive documentation, a comprehensive project plan, and other traditional deliverables based on a waterfall lifecycle.	Contracts for agile projects are based on the evaluation of working functionality at the end of each sprint, not on fixed deliverables and documentation that may or may not contribute to delivering quality products.
Contract negotiation between buyers and sellers can sometimes be challenging. Because negotiation is often a stressful activity, it can damage the relationship between the buyer and the seller before work even starts on a project.	Agile project teams focus on keeping a positive, cooperative relationship between buyers and sellers from the start of the procurement process.
Switching vendors after a project starts can be costly and time-consuming because a new vendor must try to understand the old vendor's massive amount of work in progress.	Vendors provide completed, working functionality at the end of each sprint. If vendors change mid-project, the new vendor can immediately start developing requirements for the next sprint, avoiding a long, costly transition.

TECHNICAL STUFF

Both waterfall and agile project teams are interested in vendor success. Traditional project approaches were firm in their accountability for compliance, defining success as checking off documents and deliverables in a list. Agile project approaches, by contrast, are firm in their accountability for end results, defining success with working functionality.

The next section shows how to manage procurement on agile projects.

Managing Agile Procurement

This section focuses on how agile project teams go through the procurement process: from determining need, selecting a vendor, and creating a contract through working with a vendor and closing out the contract at the end of a buyer–seller project.

Determining need and selecting a vendor

On agile projects, procurement starts when the development team decides it needs a tool or the services of a third-party to create the product.

REMEMBER

Agile project development teams are self-managing and self-organizing, and they get to make the decisions about what is best for maximizing development output. Self-management applies to all project management areas, including procurement. Find out more about self-managing teams in Chapters 6 and 14.

Development teams have a number of opportunities to consider outside goods and services:

>> **Product vision stage:** The development team may start thinking about the tools and skills necessary to help reach the product vision. At this stage, it may be prudent to research needs but not begin the purchase process.

>> **Product roadmap stage:** The development team starts to see specific features to create and may know some of the goods or services necessary to help create the product.

>> **Release planning:** The development team knows more about the product and can identify specific goods or services that will help meet the next release goal.

>> **Sprint planning:** The development team is in the trenches of development and may identify urgent needs for the sprint.

>> **Daily scrum:** Development team members state impediments. Procuring goods or services may help remove these impediments.

>> **Throughout the day:** Development team members communicate with one another and collaborate on tasks. Specific needs may arise from the development team's conversations.

>> **Sprint review meeting:** Project stakeholders may identify new requirements for future sprints that warrant procurement of goods or services.

>> **Sprint retrospective:** The development team may discuss how having a specific tool or service could have helped the past sprint and suggest a purchase for future sprints.

TIP

Sometimes you can find the goods or services you need for a project in your organization. Before looking at buying an item or working with vendors, the scrum master determines whether the tool or the person with the skills to fulfill the services the development team needs is available internally. If internal resources or people can meet the development team's needs, the scrum team saves money.

After the development team determines it needs a good or service, the development team and the scrum master work with the product owner to procure any necessary funds. The product owner is responsible for managing project scope against the project budget, so the product owner is ultimately responsible for any project purchases. The scrum master usually manages the vendor relationship on behalf of the scrum team after procurement is initiated with the vendor.

When procuring goods, the development team may need to compare tools and vendors before deciding on a purchase. When procuring goods, after you choose what to buy and where to get it, the process is usually straightforward: Make the purchase and take delivery.

Procuring services is usually a longer and more complex process than purchasing goods. Some agile-specific considerations for selecting a services vendor include the following:

>> Whether the vendor can work in an agile project environment and, if so, how much experience the vendor has with agile projects

>> Whether the vendor can work on-site with the development team

>> Whether the relationship between the vendor and the scrum team is likely to be positive and collaborative

WARNING

The organization or company you work for may be subject to laws and regulations for choosing vendors. Companies involved in government work, for example, often need to gather multiple proposals and bids from companies for work that will cost more than a certain amount of money. Although your cousin or your friend from college might be the most qualified person to complete the work, you may run into trouble if you don't follow applicable laws. Check with your company's legal department if you're in doubt about how to streamline bloated processes.

After you choose a service vendor, you need to create a contract so that the vendor can start work. The next section explains how contracts work on agile projects.

Understanding cost approaches and contracts for services

After the development team and the product owner have chosen a vendor, they need a contract to ensure agreement on the services and pricing. To start the contract process, you should know about different pricing structures and how they work with agile projects. After you understand these approaches, you see how to create a contract.

Cost structures

When you are procuring services for an agile project, it is important to know the difference between a *fixed-price* project, a *fixed-time* project, a *time-and-materials* project, and a *not-to-exceed* project. Each approach has its own strengths in an agile setting:

>> **Fixed-price project:** Starts out with a set budget. In a fixed-price project, a vendor works on the product and creates releases until that vendor has spent all the money in the budget or until you have delivered enough product features, whichever comes first.

 For example, if you have a $250,000 budget, and your vendor costs are $10,000 a week, the vendor's portion of the project will be able to last 25 weeks. Within those 25 weeks, the vendor creates and releases as much shippable functionality as possible.

>> **Fixed-time project:** Has specific deadlines. For example, you may need to launch a product in time for the next holiday season, for a specific event, or to coincide with the release of another product. With fixed-time projects, you determine costs based on the cost of the vendor's team for the duration of the project, along with any additional resource costs, such as hardware or software.

>> **Time-and-materials project:** Is more open-ended than fixed-priced or fixed-time projects. In a time-and-materials project, your work with the vendor lasts until enough product functionality is complete, without regard to total project cost. You know the total project cost at the end of the project, after your stakeholders have determined that the product has enough features to call the project complete.

 For example, suppose your project costs $10,000 a week. After 20 weeks, the stakeholders feel that they have enough valuable product features, so your project cost is $200,000. If the stakeholders instead deem that they have enough value by the end of 10 weeks, the project cost is half that amount, $100,000.

>> **Not-to-exceed project:** Is a project in which time and materials have a fixed-price cap.

THE FALLACY OF LOW-BALLING THE VENDOR

Trying to bully vendors into providing the lowest possible price is always a lose-lose situation. Contractors in industries where projects always go to the lowest bidder have a saying: *Bid it low, and watch it grow.* It is common for vendors to provide a low price during a project's proposal process and then add multiple change orders until the buyer ends up paying as much or more than he or she would have for higher-priced offers.

Waterfall project management supports this practice by locking in scope and price at the project start, when you know almost nothing about the project. Change orders — and their accompanying cost increases — are inevitable.

A better model is for the vendor and buyer to collaborate on defining the project scope, within fixed cost and schedule constraints, as the project unfolds. Both parties can reap the benefits of what they learn during the project, and you end up with a better product full of the highest-value functionality delivered and identified at the end of each sprint. Instead of trying to be a tough negotiator, be a good collaborator.

REMEMBER

Regardless of the cost approach, on agile projects, concentrate on completing the highest-value product features first.

Contract creation

After you know the project's cost approach, the scrum master might help create a contract. Contracts are legally binding agreements between buyers and sellers that set expectations about work and payment.

The person responsible for creating contracts differs by organization. In some cases, a person from the legal or procurement department drafts a contract and then asks the scrum master to review it. In other cases, the opposite occurs: The scrum master drafts the contract and has a legal or procurement expert review it.

Regardless of who creates the contract, the scrum master usually acts on behalf of the scrum team to do any of the following: Initiate the contract creation, negotiate the contract details, and route the contract through any necessary internal approvals.

The agile approach of placing value on collaboration over negotiation is a key to maintaining a positive relationship between a buyer and a seller while creating and negotiating a contract. The scrum master works closely with the vendor and communicates openly and often with the vendor throughout the contract creation process.

WARNING

The Agile Manifesto does *not* state that contracts are unnecessary. Regardless of the size of your company or organization, it is a very good idea to create a contract between your company and your vendor for services. Skipping the contract can leave buyers and sellers open to confusion about expectations, unfinished work, and even legal problems.

At the very least, most contracts have legal language describing the parties and the work, the budget, the cost approach, and payment terms. A contract for an agile project may also include the following:

>> **A description of the work that the vendor will complete:** The vendor may have its own product vision statement, which may be a good starting point to describe the vendor's work. You may want to refer to the product vision statement in Chapter 7.

>> **Agile approaches that the vendor may use:** They may include

- Meetings that the vendor will attend, such as the daily scrum, sprint planning, sprint review, and sprint retrospective meetings

- Delivery of working functionality at the end of each sprint

- The definition of done (discussed in Chapter 9): work that is developed, tested, integrated, and documented, per an agreement between the product owner, the development team, and the scrum master

- Artifacts that the vendor will provide, such as a sprint backlog with a burndown chart for status

- People whom the vendor will have on the project, such as the development team

- Where the vendor will work, such as on-site at your company

- Whether the vendor will work with its own scrum master and product owner, or if it will work with your scrum master and product owner

- A definition of what may constitute the end of the engagement: the end of a fixed budget or fixed time, or enough complete, working functionality

>> **For a vendor that doesn't use an agile approach, a description of how the vendor and the vendor's work will integrate with the buyer's development team and sprints.**

This is not a comprehensive list; contract items vary by project and organization.

The contract will likely go through a few rounds of reviews and changes before the final version is complete. One way to clearly communicate changes and maintain a good relationship with a vendor is to speak with the vendor each time you propose a change. If you email a revised contract, follow up with a call to explain what you changed and why, to answer any questions, and to discuss any ideas for further revision. Open discussion helps the contract process to be positive.

If anything substantial about the vendor's services changes during contract discussions, it is a good idea for the product owner or the scrum master to review those changes with the development team. The development team especially needs to know and provide input about changes to the service the vendor will provide, the vendor's approach, and the people on the vendor's team.

TIP

It is quite likely that your company and the vendor will require reviews and approvals by people outside their respective project teams. People who review contracts might include high-level managers or executives, procurement specialists, accounting people, and company attorneys. This differs by organization; the scrum master needs to ensure that anyone who needs to read the contract does so.

Now that you understand a little about how to select a vendor and create a contract, it's time to look at how procurement differs among companies and organizations.

Organizational considerations for procurement

The way your company approaches procurement will make a difference in how you go about selecting a vendor and creating and negotiating a contract. Because procurement involves money and legal contracts, purchase procedures and decisions are sometimes outside a project team's control. Considerations for procurement activities can include the following:

>> **Company or organization size and experience:** Smaller and newer companies may have less formality, allowing more autonomy over purchases. Larger and more established companies tend to have more overhead with purchasing. Some companies have entire departments with people working full-time on procurement.

>> **Company or organization type:** Some organizations, such as government agencies, have legally required procurement processes and documents to complete. Private companies may have fewer restrictions on procurement than publicly traded companies because of differences in laws for public companies.

>> **Company or organization culture:** Many organizations involve the project team in procurement decisions. However, this is not always the case, and project teams sometimes find themselves working with goods or service

providers they had no part in choosing. Some companies are rather informal and don't require much documentation or process for procurement. Other companies require documents to justify the need for a good or service, formal proposals from sellers, and multiple approvals at each step in procurement.

If you're working on an agile project in an organization with heavy procurement processes and a separate procurement department, you must balance those processes with agile processes. A good way to ensure agile processes during procurement is for the scrum master to work closely with the procurement department staffers.

In Chapter 6, we note that the scrum master makes sure that the organization follows agile practices and principles. In this role, the scrum master helps explain agile approaches to procurement specialists. The scrum master may find it worthwhile to help adjust organizational requirements to support agile processes.

REMEMBER

The scrum master makes sure procurement people understand why a contract may need to accommodate changing requirements and iterations. The scrum master sets the tone for the contract creation process to be collaborative.

If an agile project team has support from an organization's upper management, it will usually be easier to work agile approaches into an organization's procurement processes.

TIP

One good way to get support for moving agile approaches into your organization's procurement processes is to ensure that upper management understands how agile methods enable agile teams and organizations to deliver higher customer value more often. Benefits such as better product quality, reduced risk, and more control and visibility of project performance help make a strong argument for using agile processes when working with vendors. Chapter 19 provides a list of key benefits of agile project management.

Organizations with light or no procurement processes provide different challenges for an agile project — or for any project, for that matter. Scrum masters may find themselves starting procurement activities from scratch, with little precedent or support.

WARNING

People who sign contracts should have the authorization to make financial decisions for a company, and they often are people at the executive level. Scrum masters and product owners usually don't have this type of authorization. When in doubt, ask around. Find the right signatory.

After you choose a vendor and have a signed contract, the vendor can start work. In the next section, you see that, like the initial procurement processes, working with vendors has special considerations for agile projects.

Working with a vendor

How you work with a vendor on an agile project depends in part on the vendor team's structure. In an ideal situation, vendor teams are fully integrated with the buyer's organization. The vendor's team members are collocated with the buyer's scrum team. Vendor team members work as part of the buyer's development team for as long as necessary.

TIP

Some development teams include vendor team members in their daily scrum meetings. This can be a good way to get an idea of what the vendor team is doing every day and to help the development team work more closely with the vendor. You can also invite vendors to your sprint reviews to keep them informed on your progress.

Vendor teams also can be integrated but dislocated. If the vendor can't work on-site at the buyer's company, it can still be part of the buyer's scrum team. Chapter 14 has more information on team dynamics on agile projects.

If a vendor can't be collocated, or if the vendor is responsible for a discrete, separate part of the product, the vendor may have a separate scrum team. The vendor's scrum team works on the same sprint schedule as the buyer's scrum team. See Chapters 13 and 17 to find out how to work with more than one scrum team on a project.

If a vendor doesn't use agile project management processes, the vendor's team works separately from the buyer's scrum team, outside the sprints, and on its own schedule. The vendor's traditional project manager helps ensure that the vendor can deliver its services when the development team needs them. The buyer's scrum master may need to step in if the vendor's processes or timeline becomes a roadblock or a disruption for the development team. See the "Managing projects with dislocated teams" section in Chapter 14 for information about working with non-agile teams.

Vendors may provide services for a defined amount of time, or for the life of the project. After the vendor's work is complete, the contract is closed.

Closing a contract

After a vendor completes work on a contract, the buyer's scrum master usually has some final tasks to close the contract.

If the project finishes normally, according to the contract terms, the scrum master may want to acknowledge the end of the contract in writing. If the project is a time-and-materials project, the scrum master should definitely end it in writing to ensure that the vendor doesn't keep working on lower-priority requirements — and billing for them.

Depending on the organizational structure and the contract's cost structure, the scrum master may be responsible for notifying the buyer's company accounting department after work is complete to ensure that the vendor is paid properly.

If the project finishes before the contract dictates the end, the scrum master needs to notify the vendor in writing and follow any early termination instructions from the contract.

TIP

End the engagement on a positive note. If the vendor did a good job, the scrum team may want to acknowledge the people on the vendor's team at the sprint reviews. Everyone on the project could potentially work together again, and a simple, sincere "thank-you" can help maintain a good relationship for future projects.

Chapter **13**

Managing Time and Cost

M anaging project time and controlling project costs are key aspects of managing a project. In this chapter, you see agile approaches to time and cost management. You find out how to use a scrum team's development speed to determine time and cost on a given project and how to increase development speed to lower your project's time and cost.

What's Different about Agile Time Management?

In project management terms, *time* refers to the processes that ensure timely project completion. To understand agile time management, it helps to review some of the Agile Principles we discuss in Chapter 2:

1. Our highest priority is to satisfy the customer through early and continuous delivery of valuable software.

2. Welcome changing requirements, even late in development. Agile processes harness change for the customer's competitive advantage.

3. Deliver working software frequently, from a couple of weeks to a couple of months, with a preference to the shorter timescale.

8. Agile processes promote sustainable development. The sponsors, developers, and users should be able to maintain a constant pace indefinitely.

Table 13-1 shows some of the differences between time management on traditional projects and on agile projects.

TABLE 13-1   Traditional versus Agile Time Management

Time Management with Traditional Approaches	Time Management with Agile Approaches
Fixed scope directly drives the schedule.	Scope is not fixed on agile projects. Time can be fixed, and development teams can create the requirements that will fit into a specific time frame.
Project managers determine time based on the requirements gathered at the beginning of the project.	During the project, scrum teams assess and reassess how much work they can complete in a given time frame.
Teams work at one time in phases on all project requirements, such as requirements gathering, design, development, testing, and deployment. No schedule difference exists between critical requirements and optional requirements.	Scrum teams work in sprints and complete all the work on the highest-priority, highest-value requirements first.
Teams do not start actual product development until later in the project, after the requirements-gathering and design phases are complete.	Scrum teams start product development in the first sprint.
Time is more variable on traditional projects.	Timeboxed sprints on agile projects stay stable, enabling predictability.
Project managers try to predict schedules at the project start, when they know little about the product.	Scrum teams determine long-range schedules on actual development performance in sprints. Scrum teams adjust time estimates throughout the project as they learn more about the product and the development team's speed, or *velocity*. You find more about velocity later in this chapter.

REMEMBER

Fixed-schedule and fixed-price projects have lower risk with agile techniques because agile development teams always deliver the highest-priority functionality within the time or budget constraints.

A big benefit of agile time management techniques is that agile project teams can deliver products much earlier than traditional project teams. For example, starting development earlier and completing functionality in iterations often allow agile project teams that work with our company, Platinum Edge, to bring value to the market 30 percent to 40 percent faster.

TIP

The reason agile projects finish sooner isn't complicated; they simply start development sooner.

In the next section, find out how to manage time on an agile project.

Managing Agile Schedules

Agile practices support both strategic and tactical schedules and time management:

>> Your early planning is strategic in nature. The high-level requirements in the product roadmap and the product backlog can help you get an early idea of the overall schedule. Find out how to create a product roadmap and product backlog in Chapter 7.

>> Your detailed planning for each release and at each sprint is tactical. Read more about release planning and sprint planning in Chapter 8.

  • At release planning, you can plan your release to match a specific date, with minimal marketable features.

  • You also can plan your release with enough time to create a specific set of features.

  • During each sprint planning meeting, in addition to selecting the scope for the sprint, the development team estimates the time, in hours, to complete individual tasks for each of that sprint's requirements. Use the sprint backlog to manage detailed time allocations throughout the sprint.

>> After your project is underway, use the scrum team's velocity (development speed) to fine-tune your scheduling. We discuss velocity in the next section.

REMEMBER

In Chapter 8, we describe planning releases for *minimal marketable features*, the smallest group of product functionality providing enough value that you can effectively deploy and promote in the marketplace.

To determine how much functionality an agile development team can deliver within a set amount of time, you need to know your development team's velocity. In the next section, you take a look at how to measure velocity, how to use velocity for a project timeline, and how to increase velocity throughout the project.

DETERMINING AN AGILE PROJECT'S LENGTH

A few factors determine the length of agile projects:

Assigned deadline: For business reasons, agile project teams may want to set a specific end date. For example, you may want to get a product to market for a specific shopping season or to coincide with the timing of a competitor's product release. In that case, you set a specific end date, and create as much shippable functionality as possible from the project start until the end date.

Budget considerations: Agile project teams may also have budget considerations that affect the amount of time a project will last. For example, if you have a $1,600,000 budget, and your project costs $20,000 a week to run, your project will be able to last 80 weeks. You'll have 80 weeks to create and release as much shippable functionality as possible.

Functionality completed: Agile projects may also last only until enough functionality is complete. Project teams may run sprints until the requirements with the highest value are complete, and then determine that the lower-value requirements — the ones that few people will use or that will not generate much revenue — aren't necessary.

Introducing velocity

One of the most important things about time management on agile projects is the use of velocity, a powerful tool for forecasting long-term timelines. *Velocity,* in agile terms, is a development team's work speed. In Chapter 7, we describe measuring the effort for requirements, or user stories, in story points. You measure velocity by the number of user story points that the development team completes in each sprint.

REMEMBER

A *user story* is a simple description of a product requirement, identifying what a requirement must accomplish, and for whom. User story points are relative numbers that describe the amount of effort necessary to develop a user story. Chapter 8 delves into the details of creating user stories and estimating the effort using story points.

When you know the development team's velocity, you can use it as a long-range planning tool. Velocity can help you forecast how long the scrum team will take to complete a certain number of requirements and how much a project may cost.

In the next section, you dive into velocity as a tool for time management. You see how scope changes affect an agile project's timeline. You also find out how to work with multiple scrum teams and review agile artifacts for time management.

Monitoring and adjusting velocity

After a project starts, the scrum team starts to monitor its velocity. You measure velocity from sprint to sprint. You use velocity for long-term schedule and budget planning as well as for sprint planning.

In general, people are good at planning and estimating in the short term, so identifying hours for tasks in an upcoming sprint works well. At the same time, people are often terrible at estimating distant tasks in absolute terms such as hours. Tools such as relative estimating and velocity, which are based on performance, are more accurate measurements for longer-term planning.

Velocity is a good trending tool. You can use it to determine future timelines because the activities and development time within sprints is the same from sprint to sprint.

WARNING

Velocity is a post-sprint fact, not a goal. Avoid attempting to guess or commit to a certain velocity before a project starts or in the middle of a sprint. You'll only set unrealistic expectations about how much work the team can complete. If velocity turns into a target rather than a past measurement, scrum teams may be tempted to exaggerate estimated story points to meet that target, rendering velocity meaningless. Instead, use the scrum team's actual velocity to forecast how much longer the project may take and cost. Also focus on increasing velocity by removing constraints identified during the sprint and at the sprint retrospective.

In the next section, you see how to calculate velocity, how to use velocity to predict a project's schedule, and how to increase your scrum team's velocity.

Calculating velocity

At the end of each sprint, the scrum team looks at the requirements it has finished and adds up the number of story points associated with those requirements. The total number of completed story points is the scrum team's velocity for that sprint. After the first few sprints, you will start to see a trend and will be able to calculate the average velocity.

WARNING

Because velocity is a number, managers and executives may be tempted to use velocity as a performance metric for compensating and comparing teams. Velocity is not a performance metric, is team-specific, and should not be used outside the scrum team. It is no more than a planning tool scrum teams can use to forecast remaining work.

The *average velocity* is the total number of story points completed, divided by the total number of sprints completed. For example, if the development team's velocity was

Sprint 1 = 15 points

Sprint 2 = 13 points

Sprint 3 = 16 points

Sprint 4 = 20 points

your total number of story points completed will be 64. Your average velocity will be 16: 64 story points divided by 4 sprints.

After you have run a sprint and know the scrum team's velocity, you can start forecasting the remaining time on your project.

Using velocity to estimate the project timeline

When you know your velocity, you can determine how long your project will last. Follow these steps:

1. **Add up the number of story points for the remaining requirements in the product backlog.**

2. **Determine the number of sprints you'll need by dividing the number of story points remaining in the product backlog by the velocity:**

   - To get a pessimistic estimate, use the lowest velocity the development team has accomplished.

   - To get an optimistic estimate, use the highest velocity the development team has accomplished.

   - To get a most likely estimate, use the average velocity the development team has accomplished.

TIP

Using this empirical data — actual output speed — a product owner can give stakeholders a range of release outcomes, and they can work together to make business prioritization decisions early in the project. These decisions might include whether there is a need to spin up an additional scrum team to develop more scope items, adjust market release dates, or request project budget.

3. **Determine how much time it will take to complete the story points in the product backlog by multiplying sprint length by the number of remaining sprints.**

For example, assume that

- Your remaining product backlog contains 800 story points.

- Your development team velocity averages 20 story points per sprint.

How many more sprints will your product backlog need? Divide the number of story points by your velocity, and you get your remaining sprints. In this case, 800/20 = 40.

If you're using two-week sprints on your project, your project will last 80 weeks.

After the scrum team knows its velocity and the number of story points for the requirements, you can use the velocity to determine how long any given group of requirements will take to create. For example:

>> You can calculate the time an individual release may take if you have an idea of the number of story points that will go into that release. At the release level, your story point estimates will be more high level than at the sprint level. If you're basing your release timing on delivering specific functionality, your release date may change as you refine your user stories and estimates throughout the project.

>> You can calculate the time you need for a specific group of user stories — such as all high-priority stories or all stories relating to a particular theme — by using the number of story points in that group of user stories.

Velocity differs from sprint to sprint. In the first few sprints, when the project is new, the scrum team will typically have a low velocity. As the project progresses, velocity should increase because the scrum team will have learned more about the product and will have matured as a team working together. Setbacks within specific sprints can temporarily decrease velocity from time to time, but agile processes such as the sprint retrospective can help the scrum team ensure that those setbacks are temporary.

TIP

In the beginning of a project, velocity will vary considerably from sprint to sprint. Velocity will become more consistent over time, as long as the scrum team members remain consistent.

Scrum teams can also increase their velocity throughout agile projects, making projects shorter and less costly. In the next section, you find ways to increase velocity in each consecutive sprint.

Increasing velocity

If a scrum team has a product backlog with 800 story points and an average velocity of 20 story points, the project will last 40 sprints — 80 weeks, with 2-week sprints. But what if the scrum team could increase its velocity?

>> Increasing the average velocity to 23 story points per sprint would mean 34.78 sprints. If you round that up to 35 sprints, the same project would last 70 weeks.

>> An average velocity of 26 would take about 31 sprints, or 62 weeks.

>> An average velocity of 31 would take about 26 sprints, or 52 weeks.

As you can see, increasing velocity can save a good deal of time and, consequently, money.

Velocity can naturally increase with each sprint, as the scrum team finds its rhythm of working together on the project. However, opportunities exist to also raise velocity on agile projects, past the common increases that come with time. Everyone on a scrum team plays a part in helping get higher velocity with every successive sprint:

>> **Remove project roadblocks:** One way to increase velocity is to quickly remove project roadblocks, or impediments. Roadblocks are anything that keeps a development team member from working to full capacity. By definition, roadblocks can decrease velocity. Clearing roadblocks as soon as they arise increases velocity by helping the scrum team to be fully functional and productive. Find out more about removing project impediments in Chapter 9.

>> **Avoid project roadblocks:** The best way to increase velocity is to strategically create ways to avoid roadblocks in the first place. By knowing — or learning about — the processes and the specific needs of groups your team will work with, you can head off roadblocks before they arise.

>> **Eliminate distractions:** Another way to increase velocity is for the scrum master to protect the development team from distractions. By making sure people don't request work outside the sprint goal from the development team — even tasks that might take a small amount of time — the scrum master will be able to help keep the development team focused on the sprint.

REMEMBER

Having a dedicated scrum master who continually helps remove constraints for the scrum team will result in continually increasing velocity. The value of a dedicated scrum master is quantifiable.

PREVENTING ROADBLOCKS

One development team we worked with needed feedback from its company's legal department but had not been able to get a response via email or voicemail. In a daily scrum meeting, one of the development team members stated this lack of response as a roadblock. After the scrum meeting was over, the scrum master walked over to the legal department and found the right person to work with. After talking to that person, the scrum master found out that her email was constantly flooded with requests, and her voicemail was not much better.

The scrum master then suggested a process for future legal requests: Moving forward, the development team members could walk over to the legal department with requests and get feedback right there, in person, immediately. The new process took only a few minutes, but saved days on turnaround from the legal department, effectively preventing similar roadblocks in the future. Finding ways to prevent roadblocks helps increase the scrum team's velocity.

>> **Solicit input from the team:** Finally, everyone on the scrum team can provide ideas for increasing velocity in the sprint retrospective meeting. The development team knows its work the best, and may have ideas on how to improve output. The product owner may have insights into the requirements that can help the development team work faster. The scrum master will have seen any repetitive roadblocks and can discuss how to prevent the roadblocks in the first place.

TIP

Increasing velocity is valuable, but remember that you may not see changes overnight. Scrum team velocity often has a pattern of slow increases, some big velocity jumps, a flat period, and then slow increases again as the scrum team identifies, experiments, and corrects constraints that are holding it back.

Consistency for useful velocity

Because velocity is a measure of work completed in terms of story points, it's an accurate indicator and predictor of project performance only when you use the following practices:

>> **Consistent sprint lengths:** Each sprint should last the same amount of time throughout the life of the project. If sprint lengths are different, the amount of work the development team can complete in each sprint will be different, and velocity won't be relevant in predicting the remaining time on the project.

>> **Consistent work hours:** Individual development team members should work the same number of hours in each sprint. If Sandy works 45 hours in one sprint, 23 in another, and 68 in yet another, she will naturally complete a different amount of work from sprint to sprint. However, if Sandy always works the same number hours in one sprint, her velocity will be comparable between sprints.

>> **Consistent development team members:** Different people work at different rates. Tom might work faster than Bob, so if Tom works on one sprint and Bob works on the next sprint, the velocity of Tom's sprint will not be a good prediction for Bob's sprint.

When sprint lengths, work hours, and team members remain consistent throughout a project, you can use velocity to truly know whether development speed is increasing or decreasing and to accurately estimate the project timeline.

WARNING

Performance does not scale linearly with available time. For example, if you have two-week sprints with 20 story points per sprint, going to three-week sprints does not guarantee 30 story points. The new sprint length will generate an unknown change in velocity.

Although changing sprint lengths does introduce variance into a scrum team's velocity and projections, we rarely discourage scrum teams from decreasing their sprint lengths (from three weeks to two, or from two weeks to one) because shorter feedback loops allow scrum teams to react faster to customer feedback, enabling them to deliver more value to their customer. However, changing sprint lengths always comes with the same caution: Velocity does not scale linearly in the opposite direction either, and scrum teams will have to establish a new velocity for their shorter sprint before their projections will become reliable again.

When you know how to accurately measure and increase velocity, you have a powerful tool for managing time and cost on a project. In the next section, we talk about how to manage a timeline in an ever-changing agile environment.

Managing scope changes from a time perspective

Agile project teams welcome changing requirements at any time throughout a project, which means project scope reflects the real priorities of the business. It is "requirements Darwinism" at its purest — development teams complete requirements of highest priority first. Fixed sprint lengths force out requirements that sound like good ideas in theory but never win the "either this requirement or that requirement" contest.

New requirements may have no effect on a project's timeline; you just have to prioritize. Working with the project stakeholders, the product owner can determine to develop only the requirements that will fit in a certain window of time or budget. The priority ranking of items in the product backlog determines which requirements are important enough to develop. The scrum team can guarantee completing higher-priority requirements. The lower-priority requirements might be part of another project or may never be created.

In Chapter 12, we discuss how to manage scope changes with the product backlog. When you add a new requirement to an agile project, you prioritize that requirement against all other items in your product backlog and add the new item into the appropriate spot in the product backlog. This may move other product backlog items down in priority. If you keep your product backlog and its estimates up-to-date as new requirements arise, you'll always have a good idea of the project timeline, even with constantly changing scope.

On the other hand, the product owner and the project stakeholders may determine that all the requirements in the product backlog, including new requirements, are useful enough to include in the project. In this case, you extend the project end date to accommodate the additional scope, increase velocity, or divide the project scope among multiple scrum teams that will work simultaneously on different product features. Learn more about multi-team projects in Chapter 17.

Project teams often make schedule decisions about lower-priority requirements toward the end of a project. The reasons for these just-in-time decisions are because marketplace demands for specific scope items change, and also because velocity tends to increase as the development team gets into a rhythm. Changes in velocity increase your predictions about how many product backlog items the development team can complete in a given amount of time. On agile projects, you wait until the last responsible moment — when you know the most about the question at hand — to make decisions you'll be committed to for the rest of the project.

The next section shows you how to work with more than one scrum team on a project.

Managing time by using multiple teams

For larger projects, multiple scrum teams working in parallel may be able to complete a project in a shorter time frame.

You may want to create a project with multiple scrum teams if

>> Your project is very large and will require more than a single development team of nine or fewer development team members to complete.

>> Your project has a specific end date that you must meet, and the scrum team's velocity will not be sufficient to complete the most valuable requirements by that end date.

REMEMBER

The ideal size for a development team on an agile project is no less than three and no more than nine people. Groups of more than nine people start to build silos, and the number of communication channels makes self-management more difficult. (In some cases, we've seen these issues in teams smaller than nine.) When your product development requires more development team members than can effectively communicate, it may be time to consider using multiple scrum teams.

If you have multiple scrum teams on a project, break the work into themes, or logical groups of product features, for each team.

Before rushing into that, though, you need to consider the overall scope of the themes and the relationship between them. The work needs to be sufficiently separate to allow the teams to operate independently, with as few interdependencies as possible. In Chapter 17, we show you several techniques for scaling product development work across multiple teams.

Using agile artifacts for time management

The product roadmap, product backlog, release plan, and sprint backlog all play a part in time management. Table 13-2 shows how each artifact contributes to time management.

In the next sections, you dive into cost management for agile projects. Cost management is directly related to time management. You compare traditional approaches to cost management to those in agile projects. You find out how to estimate costs on an agile project and how to use velocity to forecast your long-term budget.

TABLE 13-2 **Agile Artifacts and Time Management**

Artifact	Role in Time Management
Product roadmap: The product roadmap is a prioritized, holistic view of the high-level requirements that support the product's vision. Find more about the product roadmap in Chapter 7.	The product roadmap is a strategic look at the overall project priorities. Although the product roadmap likely will not have specific dates, it will have general date ranges for groups of functionality and will allow an initial framing for bringing the product to market.
Product backlog: The product backlog is a complete list of all currently known product requirements. Find more about the product backlog in Chapters 7 and 8.	The requirements in your product backlog will have estimated story points. After you know your development team's velocity, you can use the total number of story points in the product backlog to determine a realistic project end date.
Release plan: The release plan contains a release schedule for a minimum set of requirements. Find more about the release plan in Chapter 8.	The release plan will have a target release date for a specific goal supported by a minimal set of marketable functionalities. Scrum teams plan and work on only one release at a time.
Sprint backlog: The sprint backlog contains the requirements and tasks for the current sprint. Find more about the sprint backlog in Chapter 8.	During your sprint-planning meeting, you estimate individual tasks in the backlog in hours. At the end of each sprint, you take the total completed story points from the sprint backlog to calculate your development team's velocity for that sprint.

What's Different about Agile Cost Management?

Cost is a project's financial budget. When you work on an agile project, you focus on value, exploit the power of change, and aim for simplicity. Agile Principles 1, 2, and 10 state the following:

1. Our highest priority is to satisfy the customer through early and continuous delivery of valuable software.

2. Welcome changing requirements, even late in development. Agile processes harness change for the customer's competitive advantage.

10. Simplicity — the art of maximizing the amount of work not done — is essential.

Because of this emphasis on value, change, and simplicity, agile projects have a different approach to budget and cost management than traditional projects. Table 13-3 highlights some of the differences.

TABLE 13-3 **Traditional versus Agile Cost Management**

Cost Management with Traditional Approaches	Cost Management with Agile Approaches
Cost, like time, is based on fixed scope.	Project schedule, not scope, has the biggest effect on cost. You can start with a fixed cost and a fixed amount of time, and then complete requirements as potentially shippable functionality that fit into your budget and schedule.
Organizations estimate project costs and fund projects before the project starts.	Product owners often secure project funding after the product roadmap stage is complete. Some organizations even fund agile projects one release at a time; product owners will secure funding after completing release planning for each release.
New requirements mean higher costs. Because project managers estimate costs based on what they know at the project start, which is very little, cost overruns are common.	Project teams can replace lower-priority requirements with new, equivalently sized high-priority requirements with no effect on time or cost.
Scope bloat (see Chapter 12) wastes large amounts of money on features that people simply do not use.	Because agile development teams complete requirements by priority, they concentrate on creating only the product features that users need, whether those features are added on day 1 or day 100 of the project.
Projects cannot generate revenue until the project is complete.	Project teams can release working, revenue-generating functionality early, creating a self-funding project.

TECHNICAL STUFF

When costs increase, project sponsors sometimes find themselves in a kind of hostage situation. A waterfall approach does not call for any complete product functionality until the end of a project. Because traditional approaches to development are all-or-nothing proposals, if costs increase and stakeholders don't pay more for the product, they will not get *any* finished requirements. The incomplete product becomes a kidnapped hostage; pay more, or get nothing.

In the following sections, you find out about cost approaches in agile projects, how to estimate costs for an agile project, how to control your budget, and how to lower costs.

Managing Agile Budgets

On agile projects, cost is mostly a direct expression of project time. Because scrum teams consist of full-time, dedicated team members, they have a set team cost — generally expressed as an hourly or fixed rate per person — that should be the same for each sprint. Consistent sprint lengths, work hours, and team members enable you to accurately use velocity to predict development speed. Once you use velocity to determine how many sprints your project will take — that is, how long your project will be — you can know how much your scrum team will cost for the whole project.

Project cost also includes the cost for resources like hardware, software, licenses, and any other supplies you might need to complete your project.

In this section, you find out how to create an initial budget and how to use the scrum team's velocity to determine long-range costs.

Creating an initial budget

To create your project budget, you need to know the cost for your scrum team, per sprint, and the cost for any additional resources you need to complete the project.

Typically, you calculate the cost for your scrum team by using an hourly rate for each team member. Multiply each team member's hourly rate by his or her available hours per week by the number of weeks in your sprints to calculate your scrum team's per-sprint cost. Table 13-4 shows a sample budget for a scrum team — the product owner, five development team members, and the scrum master — for a two-week sprint.

TABLE 13-4   **Sample Scrum Team Budget for a Two-Week Sprint**

Team Member	Hourly Rate	Weekly Hours	Weekly Cost	Sprint Cost (2 Weeks)
Don	$80	40	$3,200	$6,400
Peggy	$70	40	$2,800	$5,600
Bob	$70	40	$2,800	$5,600
Mike	$65	40	$2,600	$5,200
Joan	$85	40	$3,400	$6,800
Tommy	$75	40	$3,000	$6,000
Pete	$55	40	$2,200	$4,400
Total		280	$20,000	$40,000

The cost for additional resources will vary by project. In addition to scrum team member costs, take the following into account when determining your project costs:

>> Hardware costs

>> Software, including license costs

>> Hosting costs

>> Training costs

>> Miscellaneous team expenses, such as additional office supplies, team lunches, travel costs, and the price of any tools you may need

These costs may be one-time costs, rather than per-sprint costs. We suggest separating these costs in your budget; as you see in the next section, you need your cost for each sprint to determine the cost for the project. (To keep calculations simple throughout this chapter, we assume that the project cost of $40,000 includes scrum team member costs as well as any additional resources, such as those just listed.)

TIP

Resources typically refer to inanimate objects, not people. Resources need to be managed. When discussing resources on a project, refer to people as *team members, talent,* or just *people.* This issue may seem minor, but the more you focus on individuals and interactions over processes and tools, even in the details, the more your mindset will change to think and be more agile.

Creating a self-funding project

A big benefit of agile projects is the capability to have a self-funding project. Scrum teams deliver working functionality at the end of each sprint and make that functionality available to the marketplace at the end of each release cycle. If your product is an income-generating product, you could use revenue from early releases to help fund the rest of your project.

For example, an ecommerce website might generate $15,000 a month in sales after the first release, $40,000 a month after the second release, and so on. Tables 13-5 and 13-6 compare income on a sample traditional project to the income from a self-funding agile project.

TABLE 13-5

Income from a Traditional Project with a Final Release after Six Months

Month	Income Generated	Total Project Income
January	$0	$0
February	$0	$0
March	$0	$0
April	$0	$0
May	$0	$0
June	$0	$0
July	$100,000	$100,000

In Table 13-5, the project created $100,000 in income after six months of development. Now compare the income in Table 13-5 to the income generated in Table 13-6.

TABLE 13-6

Income from a Project with Monthly Releases and a Final Release after Six Months

Month/Release	Income Generated	Total Project Income
January	$0	$0
February	$15,000	$15,000
March	$25,000	$40,000
April	$40,000	$80,000
May	$70,000	$150,000
June	$80,000	$230,000
July	$100,000	$330,000

In Table 13-6, the project generated income with the first release. By the end of six months, the project had generated $330,000 — $230,000 more than the project in Table 13-5.

Using velocity to determine long-range costs

The "Using velocity to estimate the project timeline" section, earlier in this chapter, shows you how to determine how much time a project will take, using the scrum team's velocity and the remaining story points in the product backlog. You can use the same information to determine the cost for the project or for your current release.

After you know the scrum team's velocity, you can calculate the cost for the remainder of the project.

In the velocity example from earlier in this chapter, where your scrum team velocity averages 16 story points per sprint, your product backlog contains 800 story points, and your sprints are 2 weeks long, your project will take 50 sprints, or 100 weeks, to complete.

To determine the remaining cost for your project, multiply the cost per sprint by the number of sprints the scrum team needs to complete the product backlog.

If your scrum team cost is $40,000 per sprint and you have 50 sprints left, your remaining cost for your project will be $2,000,000.

In the next sections, you find out different ways to lower your project costs.

Lowering cost by increasing velocity

In the time management section of this chapter, we talk about increasing the scrum team's velocity. Using the examples from the earlier section, and the $40,000 per two-week sprint from Table 13-4, increasing velocity could reduce your costs, as follows:

>> If the scrum team increases its average velocity from 16 to 20 story points per sprint

- You will have 40 remaining sprints.

- Your project will cost $1.6 million, saving you more than $400,000.

>> If the scrum team increases its velocity to 23 story points

- You will have 35 remaining sprints.

- Your project will cost $1.4 million, saving you an additional $200,000.

>> If the scrum team increases its velocity to 26 story points

- You will have 31 remaining sprints.

- Your project will cost $1.24 million, an additional $160,000 savings.

As you can see, increasing the scrum team's velocity by removing impediments can provide real savings on project costs. See how to help the scrum team become more productive in the "Increasing velocity" section, earlier in this chapter.

Lowering cost by reducing time

You can also lower your project costs by not completing lower-priority requirements, thus lowering the number of sprints you need. Because completed functionality is delivered with each sprint in an agile project, the project stakeholders can make a business decision to end a project when the cost of future development is higher than the value of that future development.

Project stakeholders can then use the remaining budget from the old project to start a new, more valuable project. The practice of moving the budget from one project to another is called *capital redeployment.*

To determine a project's end based on cost, you need to know

>> The business value (V) of the remaining requirements in the product backlog

>> The actual cost (AC) of the work it will take to complete the requirements in the product backlog

>> The opportunity cost (OC), or the value of having the scrum team work on a new project

When $V < AC + OC$, the project can stop because the cost you'll sink into the project will be more than the value you will receive from the project.

Consider this example: A company is running an agile project and

>> The remaining features in the product backlog will generate $100,000 in income (V = $100,000).

>> It will take three sprints with a cost of $40,000 per sprint to create those features, a total of $120,000 (AC = $120,000).

>> The scrum team could be working on a new project that would generate $150,000 after three sprints, minus the scrum team's cost (OC = $150,000).

>> The project value, $100,000, is less than the actual costs plus opportunity costs, or $270,000. This would be a good time to end the project.

The opportunity for capital redeployment sometimes arises in emergencies, when an organization needs members of the scrum team to pause a project for critical unplanned work. Project sponsors sometimes evaluate a project's remaining value and cost before restarting a paused project.

WARNING

Pausing a project can be expensive. The costs associated with demobilization and remobilization — saving work in progress, documenting current state, debriefing paused project team members, retooling for the new project, briefing team members on the new project, learning new skills required on the new project — can be significant and should be evaluated before making the decision to pause a project that may need to be remobilized again in the future. V < AC + OC can help with this decision.

Project sponsors may also compare the product backlog value to remaining development costs throughout the project, so they know just the right time to end the project and receive the most value.

Determining other costs

Similar to time management, after you know the scrum team's velocity, you can determine the cost of anything in the project. For example:

>> You can calculate the cost for an individual release if you have an idea of the number of story points that will go into that release. Divide the number of story points in the release by the scrum team's velocity to determine how many sprints will be required. At the release, your story point estimates will be more high-level than at the sprint, so your costs may change, depending on how you determine your release date.

>> You can calculate the cost for a specific group of user stories, such as all high-priority stories or all stories relating to a particular theme, by using the number of story points in that group of user stories.

Using agile artifacts for cost management

You can use the product roadmap, release plan, and sprint backlog for cost management. Table 13-2 shows how each artifact helps you measure and evaluate project time and costs.

Time and cost forecasts based on actual development team performance are more accurate than forecasts based on hope.

Chapter **14**

Managing Team Dynamics and Communication

Team dynamics and communication are significant parts of project management. In this chapter, you find out about traditional and agile approaches to project teams and communication. You see how a high value on individuals and interactions makes agile project teams great teams to work on. You also find out how face-to-face communication helps make agile projects successful.

What's Different about Agile Team Dynamics?

What makes a project team on an agile project unique? The core reason agile teams are different from traditional teams is their team dynamics. The Agile Manifesto (refer to Chapter 2) sets the framework for how agile project team members work together: The very first item of value in the manifesto is *individuals and interactions over processes and tools.*

The following agile principles, also from Chapter 2, support valuing people on the project team and how they work together:

4. Business people and developers must work together daily throughout the project.

5. Build projects around motivated individuals. Give them the environment and support they need, and trust them to get the job done.

8. Agile processes promote sustainable development. The sponsors, developers, and users should be able to maintain a constant pace indefinitely.

11. The best architectures, requirements, and designs emerge from self-organizing teams.

12. At regular intervals, the team reflects on how to become more effective, then tunes and adjusts its behavior accordingly.

The agile principles apply to many different project management areas. You see some of these principles repeated in different chapters of this book.

REMEMBER

On agile projects, the development team contains the people who do the physical work of creating the product. The scrum team contains the development team, plus the product owner and the scrum master. The project team is the scrum team and your project stakeholder. Everyone on the scrum team has responsibilities related to self-management.

Table 14-1 shows some differences between team management on traditional projects and on agile projects.

TIP

We avoid the term *resources* when referring people. Referring to people and equipment with the same term is the beginning of thinking of team members as interchangeable objects that can be swapped in and out. Resources are things, utilitarian and expendable. The people on your project team are human beings, with emotions, ideas, and priorities inside and outside the project. People can learn and create and grow throughout the project. Respecting your fellow project team members by referring to them as *people* instead of *resources* is a subtle but powerful way to reinforce the fact that people are at the core of an agile mindset.

The following sections discuss how working with a dedicated, cross-functional, self-organizing, size-limited team benefits agile projects. You find out more about servant leadership and creating a good environment for a scrum team. In short, you find out how team dynamics help agile projects succeed.

TABLE 14-1   **Traditional versus Agile Team Dynamics**

Team Management with Traditional Approaches	Team Dynamics with Agile Approaches
Project teams rely on *command and control* — a top-down approach to project management, where the project manager is responsible for assigning tasks to team members and attempting to control what the team does.	Agile teams are self-managing, self-organizing, and benefit from *servant leadership.* Instead of top-down management, a servant-leader coaches, removes obstacles, and prevents distractions to enable the team to thrive.
Companies evaluate individual employee performance.	Agile organizations evaluate agile team performance. Agile teams, like any sports team, succeed or fail as a whole team. Whole-team performance encourages individual team members to increase the ways they can contribute to the team's success.
Team members often find themselves working on more than one project at a time, switching their attention back and forth.	Development teams are dedicated to one project at a time, and reap the benefits of focus.
Development team members have distinct roles, such as programmer or tester.	Agile organizations focus on skills instead of titles. Development teams work cross-functionally, doing different jobs within the team to ensure that they complete priority requirements quickly.
Development teams have no specific size limits.	Development teams are intentionally limited in size. Ideally, development teams have no fewer than three and no more than nine people.
Team members are commonly referred to as *resources,* a shortened term for *human resources.*	Team members are called *people, talent,* or simply *team members.* On an agile project, you probably will not hear the term *resource* used to refer to people.

Managing Agile Team Dynamics

Time and again, when we talk with product owners, developers, and scrum masters, we hear the same thing: People enjoy working on agile projects. Agile team dynamics enable people to do great work in the best way they know how. People on scrum teams have opportunities to learn, to teach, to lead, and to be part of a cohesive, self-managing team.

The following sections show you how to work as part of an agile team (using scrum as the context) and why agile approaches to teamwork make agile projects successful.

Becoming self-managing and self-organizing

On agile projects, scrum teams are directly accountable for creating deliverables. Scrum teams manage themselves, organizing their own work and tasks. No one person tells the scrum team what to do. This doesn't mean that agile projects have no leadership. Each member of the scrum team has the opportunity to lead informally, based on his or her skills, ideas, and initiative.

REMEMBER

On agile projects, the development team contains the people who are doing the physical work of creating the product. The scrum team contains the development team, plus the product owner and the scrum master. The project team is the scrum team and your project stakeholders. Both the development team and the overall scrum team have responsibilities related to self-management.

The idea of self-management and self-organization is a mature way of thinking about work. Self-management assumes that people are professional, motivated, and dedicated enough to commit to a job and see it through. At the core of self-management is the idea that the people who are doing a job from day to day know the most about that job and are best qualified to determine how to complete it. Working with a self-managing scrum team requires trust and respect within the team and within the team's organization as a whole.

Nonetheless, let's be clear: Accountability is at the core of agile projects. The difference is that in an agile project, teams are held accountable for tangible results that you can see and demonstrate. Traditionally, companies held teams accountable for compliance to the organization's step-by-step process — stripping them of the ability or incentive to be innovative. Self-management, however, returns innovation and creativity to development teams.

TIP

For a scrum team to be self-managing, you need an environment of trust. Everyone on the scrum team must trust one another to do his or her best for the scrum team and the project. The scrum team's company or organization must also trust the scrum team to be competent, to make decisions, and to manage itself. To create and maintain an environment of trust, each member of the scrum team must commit, individually and as a team, to the project and to one another.

Self-managing development teams create better product architectures, requirements, and design for a simple reason: ownership. When you give people the freedom and responsibility to solve problems, they are more mentally engaged in their work.

Scrum team members play roles in all areas of project management. Table 14-2 shows how scrum teams and development teams manage scope, procurement, time, cost, team dynamics, communication, stakeholders, quality, and risk.

TABLE 14-2   Project Management and Self-Managing Teams

Area of Project Management	How Product Owners Self-Manage	How Development Teams Self-Manage	How Scrum Masters Self-Manage
Scope	Use the product vision, the release goal, and each sprint goal to determine if and where scope items belong. Use product backlog prioritization to determine which requirements are developed.	May suggest features based on technical affinity. Work directly with the product owner to clarify requirements. Identify how much work they can take on in a sprint. Identify the tasks to complete scope in the sprint backlog. Determine the best way to create specific features.	Remove impediments that limit the amount of scope the development team can create. Through coaching, help development teams become more productive with each successive sprint.
Procurement	Secure necessary funding for tools and equipment for development teams.	Identify the tools they need to create the product. Work with the product owner to get those tools.	Help procure tools and equipment that accelerate development team velocity.
Time	Ensure that the development team correctly understands product features so that development teams can correctly estimate the effort to create those features. Use velocity — development speed — to forecast long-term timelines.	Provide effort estimates for product features. Identify what features they can create in a given time frame — the sprint. Often provide time estimates for tasks in each sprint. Choose their own daily schedules and manage their own time.	Facilitate estimation poker games. Help development teams increase velocity, which affects time. Shield the team from organizational time-wasters and distractions.
Cost	Ultimately responsible for the budget and return on investment on an agile project. Use velocity to forecast long-term costs, based on timelines.	Provide effort estimates for product features.	Facilitate estimation poker games. Help development teams increase velocity, which affects cost.

(continued)

TABLE 14-2 *(continued)*

Area of Project Management	How Product Owners Self-Manage	How Development Teams Self-Manage	How Scrum Masters Self-Manage
Team dynamics	Commit to their projects as an integrated peer member of the scrum team.	Prevent bottlenecks by working cross-functionally, and are willing to take on different types of tasks. Continuously learn and teach one another. Commit, both individually and as part of the scrum team, to their projects and to one another. Strive to build consensus when making important decisions.	Facilitate scrum team collocation. Help remove impediments to scrum team self-management. Commit to their projects and are integrated members of the scrum team. Strive to build consensus within the scrum team when making important decisions. Facilitate relationships between the scrum team and stakeholders.
Communication	Communicate information about the product and the business needs to development teams on an ongoing basis. Communicate information about the project progress to stakeholders. Help present working functionality to stakeholders at the sprint review meetings at the end of each sprint.	Report on progress, upcoming tasks, and identify roadblocks in their daily scrum meetings. Keep the sprint backlog up-to-date daily, providing accurate, immediate information about a project's status. Present working functionality to project stakeholders at the sprint review meetings at the end of each sprint.	Encourage face-to-face communication between all scrum team members. Foster close cooperation between the scrum team and other departments within the company or organization.
Stakeholders	Set vision, release, and sprint goal expectations. Shield development team from business noise. Collect feedback during sprint reviews. Gather requirements throughout project. Communicate release dates and how new feature requests affect release dates.	Demonstrate working functionality at sprint reviews. Work through product owner to decompose requirements. Report on project progress through release and sprint burndown charts. Update task status no less than at the end of each day.	Coach on scrum and agile principles as they relate to their interaction with the scrum team. Shield developers from non-business distractions. Facilitate sprint reviews for gathering feedback. Facilitate interactions outside sprint reviews.

Area of Project Management	How Product Owners Self-Manage	How Development Teams Self-Manage	How Scrum Masters Self-Manage
Quality	Add acceptance criteria to requirements. Ensure that the development team correctly understands and interprets requirements. Provide development teams with feedback about the product from the organization and from the marketplace. Accept functionality as done during each sprint.	Commit to providing technical excellence and good design. Test their work throughout the day and comprehensively test all development each day. Inspect their work and adapt for improvements at sprint retrospective meetings at the end of each sprint.	Help facilitate the sprint retrospective. Help ensure face-to-face communication between scrum team members, which in turn helps ensure quality work. Help create a sustainable development environment so that the development team can perform at its best.
Risk	Look at overall project risks as well as risks to their ROI commitment. Prioritize high-risk items on the product backlog near the top to address them sooner rather than later.	Identify and develop the risk mitigation approach for each sprint. Alert the scrum master to roadblocks and distractions. Use information from each sprint retrospective to reduce risk in future sprints. Embrace cross-functionality to reduce risk if one member unexpectedly leaves the team. Commit to delivering shippable functionality at the end of each sprint, reducing risk in the overall project.	Help prevent roadblocks and distractions. Help remove roadblocks and identified risks. Facilitate development team conversations about possible risks.

All in all, people on agile projects tend to find a great deal of job satisfaction. Self-management speaks to a deeply rooted human desire for autonomy — to control our own destiny — and allows people this control on a daily basis.

The next section discusses another reason that people on agile projects are happy: the servant-leader.

Supporting the team: The servant-leader

The scrum master serves as a servant-leader, someone who leads by removing obstacles, preventing distractions, and helping the rest of the scrum team do its job to the best of its ability. Leaders on agile projects help find solutions rather than assign tasks. Scrum masters coach, trust, and challenge the scrum team to manage itself.

Other members of the scrum team can also take on servant leadership roles. While the scrum master helps get rid of distractions and roadblocks, the product owner and members of the development team can also help where needed. The product owner can lead by proactively providing important details about the product needs and quickly providing answers to questions from the development team. Development team members can teach and mentor one another as they become more cross-functional. Each person on a scrum team may act as a servant-leader at some point in the project.

Larry Spears identified ten characteristics of a servant-leader in his paper, "The Understanding and Practice of Servant-Leadership" (Servant Leadership Round-table, School of Leadership Studies, Regent University, August 2005). Here are those characteristics, along with our additions for how each characteristic can benefit the team dynamics on an agile project.

>> **Listening:** Listening closely to other members of the scrum team will help the people on the scrum team identify areas to help one another. A servant-leader may need to listen to what people are saying, as well as what people are *not* saying, in order to remove obstacles.

>> **Empathy:** A servant-leader tries to understand and empathize with people on the scrum team, and to help them understand one another.

>> **Healing:** On an agile project, healing can mean undoing the damage of non-people-centric processes. These are processes that treat people like equipment and other replaceable parts. Many traditional project management approaches can be described as being non-people-centric.

>> **Awareness:** On an agile project, the people on the scrum team may need to be aware of activities on many levels to best serve the scrum team.

>> **Persuasion:** Servant-leaders rely on an ability to convince, rather than on top-down authority. Strong persuasion skills, along with organizational clout or influence, will help a scrum master advocate for the scrum team to the company or organization. A servant-leader can also pass along persuasion skills to the rest of the scrum team, helping maintain harmony and build consensus.

>> **Conceptualization:** Each member of a scrum team can use conceptualization skills on an agile project. The changing nature of agile projects encourages the scrum team to envision ideas beyond those at hand. A servant-leader will help nurture the scrum team's creativity, both for the development of the product and for team dynamics.

>> **Foresight:** Scrum teams gain foresight with each sprint retrospective. By inspecting its work, processes, and team dynamics on a regular basis, the scrum team can continuously adapt and understand how to make better decisions for future sprints.

>> **Stewardship:** A servant-leader is the steward of the scrum team's needs. Stewardship is about trust. Members of the scrum team trust one another to look out for the needs of the team and the project as a whole.

>> **Commitment to the growth of people:** Growth is essential to a scrum team's ability to be cross-functional. A servant-leader will encourage and enable a scrum team to learn and grow.

>> **Building community:** A scrum team is its own community. A servant-leader will help build and maintain positive team dynamics within that community.

Servant leadership works because it positively focuses on individuals and interactions, a key tenet of agile project management. Much like self-management, servant leadership requires trust and respect.

TECHNICAL STUFF

The concept of servant leadership is not specific to agile projects. If you have studied management techniques, you may recognize the works of Robert K. Greenleaf, who started the modern movement for servant-leadership — and coined the term *servant-leader* — in an essay in 1970. Greenleaf founded the Center for Applied Ethics, now known as the Greenleaf Center for Servant Leadership, which promotes the concept of servant leadership worldwide.

Another servant-leader expert, Kenneth Blanchard, co-wrote with Spencer Johnson the *One Minute Manager* (published by William Morrow), wherein he describes characteristics that make great managers of high-functioning people and teams. (The book has since been updated as *The New One-Minute Manager,* published by Harper Collins India.) The reason the managers Blanchard studied were so effective is because they focused on ensuring that the people doing the work had direction, resources, and protection from noise to do their job as quickly as possible.

The next two sections largely relate to team factors for agile project success: the dedicated team and the cross-functional team.

Working with a dedicated team

Having a dedicated scrum team provides the following important benefits to projects:

>> **Keeping people focused on one project at a time helps prevent distractions.** Dedication to one project increases productivity by reducing *task-switching* — moving back and forth between different tasks without really completing any of them.

>> **Dedicated scrum teams have fewer distractions — and fewer distractions mean fewer mistakes.** When a person doesn't have to meet the demands of more than one project, that person has the time and clarity to ensure his or her work is the best it can be. Chapter 15 discusses ways to increase product quality in detail.

>> **When people work on dedicated scrum teams, they know what they will be working on every day.** An interesting reality of behavioral science is that when people know what they will be working on in the immediate future, their minds engage those issues consciously at work and unconsciously outside the work environment. Stability of tasks engages your mind for much longer each day, enabling better solutions and higher quality products.

>> **Dedicated scrum team members are able to innovate more on projects.** When people immerse themselves in a product without distractions, they can come up with creative solutions for product functionality.

>> **People on dedicated scrum teams are more likely to be happy in their jobs.** By being able to concentrate on one project, a scrum team member's job is easier. Many, if not most, people enjoy producing quality work, being productive, and being creative. Dedicated scrum teams lead to higher satisfaction.

>> **When you have a dedicated scrum team working the same amount of time each week, you can accurately calculate *velocity* — the team's development speed.** In Chapter 13, we talk about determining a scrum team's velocity at the end of each sprint and using velocity to determine long-term timelines and costs. Because velocity relies on comparing output from one sprint to the next, using velocity to forecast time and cost works best if the scrum team's work hours are constant. If you are unable to have a dedicated scrum team, at least try to have team members allocated to your project for the same amount of time each week.

The idea of the productive multitasker is a myth. In the past 25 years, and especially in the last decade, a number of studies have concluded that task-switching reduces productivity, impairs decision-making skills, and results in more errors.

To have a dedicated scrum team, you need strong commitment from your organization. Many companies ask employees to work on multiple projects at one time, under the mistaken assumption that the company will save money by hiring fewer people. When companies start to embrace a more agile mindset, they learn that the least expensive approach is to reduce defects and raise development productivity through focus.

Each member of the scrum team can help ensure dedication:

>> If you're a product owner, make sure that the company knows that a dedicated scrum team is a good fiscal decision. You are responsible for project return on investment, so be willing to fight for your project's success.

>> If you're a member of the development team and anyone requests that you do work outside the project, you can push back and involve the product owner or scrum master, if necessary. A request for outside work, regardless of how benign, is a potential roadblock.

>> If you're a scrum master, as the expert on agile approaches, you can educate the company on why a dedicated scrum team means increased productivity, quality, and innovation. A good scrum master should also have the organizational clout to keep the company from poaching people from the scrum team for other projects.

Another characteristic of scrum teams is that they are cross-functional.

Working with a cross-functional team

Cross-functional development teams are also important on agile projects. The development team on an agile software project doesn't just include programmers; it could include all the people who will have a job on the project. For example, a development team on a software project might include programmers, database experts, quality assurance people, usability experts, and graphic designers. While each person has specialties, being cross-functional means that everyone on the team is willing to pitch in on different parts of the project, as much as possible.

On an agile development team, you continuously ask yourself two questions: "What can I contribute today?" and "How can I expand my contribution in the future?" Everyone on the development team will use his or her current skills and specialties in each sprint. Cross-functionality gives development team members the opportunity to learn new skills by working on areas outside of their expertise. Cross-functionality also allows people to share their knowledge with their fellow development team members. You don't need to be a jack-of-all-trades to work on an agile development team, but you should be willing to learn new skills and help with all kinds of tasks.

Although task-switching decreases productivity, cross-functionality works because you're not changing the context of what you are working on; you're looking at the same problem from a different perspective. Working on different aspects of the same problem increases knowledge depth and your ability to do a better job.

The biggest benefit of a cross-functional development team is the elimination of single points of failure. If you have worked on a project before, how many times have you experienced delays because a critical member of the team is on vacation, out sick, or, worse, has left the company? Vacations, illness, and turnover are facts of life, but with a cross-functional development team, other team members can jump in and continue work with minimal disruption. Even if an expert leaves the project team unexpectedly and abruptly, other development team members will know enough about the work to keep it progressing.

Development team members go on vacation or catch the flu. Don't sabotage your project by having only one person know a skill or functional area.

Cross-functionality takes strong commitment from the development team, both as individual members and as a group. The old phrase, "There is no *i* in *team*" is especially true on agile projects. Working on an agile development team is about skills, rather than titles.

Development teams without titles are more merit-based because team seniority and status is based on current knowledge, skills, and contribution.

Letting go of the idea that you're a "senior quality assurance tester" or a "junior developer" can require a new way of thinking about yourself. Embracing the concept of being part of a cross-functional development team may take some work, but it can be rewarding as you learn new skills and develop a rhythm of teamwork.

When developers also test, they create code that is test-friendly.

Having a cross-functional development team also requires commitment and support from your organization. Some companies eliminate titles or keep them intentionally vague (you might see something like "application development") to encourage teamwork. Other techniques for creating a strong cross-functional development team from an organizational standpoint include offering training, recognizing scrum teams as a whole, and being willing to make changes if a particular person does not fit in with a team environment. When hiring, your company can actively look for people who will work well in a highly collaborative environment, who want to learn new tasks, and who are willing to work on all areas of a project.

Both the physical environment and the cultural environment of an organization are important keys to success with agile projects. The next section shows you how.

Reinforcing openness

As we explain in other chapters, a collocated scrum team is ideal. The Internet has brought people together globally, but nothing — not the best combination of emails, instant messages, videoconferencing, phone calls, and online collaboration tools — can replace the simplicity and effectiveness of a face-to-face conversation. Figure 14-1 illustrates the difference between an email exchange and a conversation in person.

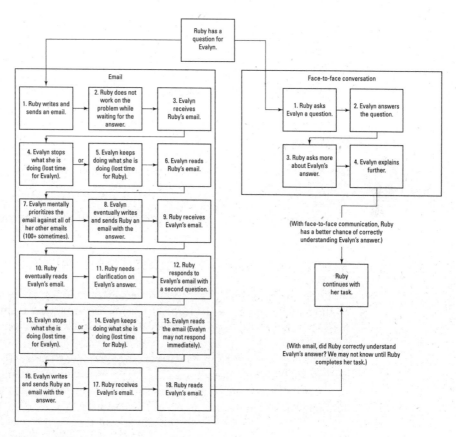

FIGURE 14-1: Email versus face-to-face conversation.

The idea of scrum team members working in the same physical location and being able to talk in person, instantly, is important to team dynamics. You find more details on communication later in this chapter. Also, Chapter 5 provides details on how to set up the physical environment for a scrum team.

Having a cultural environment of openness, which is conducive to scrum team growth, is another success factor for agile projects. Everyone on a scrum team should be able to

>> Feel safe.

>> Speak his or her mind in a positive way.

>> Challenge the status quo.

>> Be open about challenges without being penalized.

>> Request resources that will make a difference to the project.

>> Make mistakes and learn from them.

>> Suggest change and have other scrum team members seriously consider those changes.

>> Respect fellow scrum team members.

>> Be respected by other members of the scrum team.

Trust, openness, and respect are fundamental to team dynamics on an agile project.

TIP

Some of the best product and process improvements come from novices asking "silly" questions.

Another facet of agile team dynamics is the concept of the size-limited team.

Limiting development team size

An interesting psychological aspect of team dynamics on an agile project is the number of people on a development team. Development teams usually have between three and nine people. An ideal size is somewhere in the middle.

Limiting development team size to this range provides a team with enough diverse skills to take a requirement from paper to production while keeping communication and collaboration simple. Development team members can easily interact with one another and make decisions by consensus.

When you have development teams with more than nine people, the people on those teams tend to break into subgroups and build silos. This is normal social human behavior, but subgroups can be disruptive to a development team striving to be self-managing. It is also more difficult to communicate with larger development teams; there are more communication channels and opportunities to lose or misconstrue a message. With more than nine people on a development team, you often need an extra person just to help manage communication.

Development teams with fewer than nine people, on the other hand, tend to naturally gravitate to an agile approach. However, development teams that are too small may find working cross-functionally difficult because there may not be enough people with varying skills on the project.

TIP

If your product development requires more than nine development team members, consider breaking up the work between multiple scrum teams. Creating teams of people with similar personalities, skills, and work styles can improve productivity. Find details on how to work with multiple scrum teams in Chapters 13 and 17.

Managing projects with dislocated teams

As we say throughout the book, a collocated scrum team is ideal for agile projects. However, sometimes it isn't possible for a scrum team to work together in one place. *Dislocated teams*, teams with people who work in different locations, exist for many reasons and in different forms.

In some companies, the people with the right skills for a project may work in different offices, and the company may not want the cost of bringing those people together for the project's duration. Some organizations work jointly with other organizations on projects, but may not want or be able to share office space. Some people may telecommute, especially contractors, live long distances from the company they work with, and never visit that company's office. Some companies work with offshore groups and create projects with people from other countries.

The good news is that you can still have an agile project with a dislocated scrum team or teams. If you have to work with a dislocated team, we've found that an agile approach allows you to see working functionality much sooner and limits the risk of inevitable misunderstandings that a dislocated team will experience.

In *A Scrum Handbook* (Scrum Institute Training Press), Jeff Sutherland describes three models of distributed scrum teams:

>> **Isolated scrums:** With isolated scrums, individual scrum teams have collocated scrum team members, but each scrum team is in a separate geographic location and works separately. Product development with isolated scrums has only code-level integration; that is, the different teams don't communicate or work together but expect the code to work when it is time to integrate each module due to organizational coding standards. Isolated scrums tend to struggle because different people interpret coding standards differently.

>> **Distributed scrum of scrums:** With a distributed scrum of scrums model, scrum teams are in different locations, like in isolated scrums. To coordinate work, scrum teams hold a *scrum of scrums* — a meeting of multiple scrum masters — to integrate on a daily basis.

>> **Integrated scrums:** Integrated scrum teams are cross-functional, with scrum team members in different locations. A scrum of scrums still occurs but face-to-face communication is lost.

Table 14-3, from Ambysoft's "Agile Adoption Rate Survey Results" in 2008, shows a comparison of success rates for projects with collocated scrum teams against those with geographically dispersed scrum teams.

TABLE 14-3

Success of Collocated and Dislocated Scrum Teams

Team Location	Success Percentage
Collocated scrum team	83%
Dislocated but physically reachable	72%
Distributed across geographies	60%

"Agile Adoption Rate Survey Results" (Scott W. Ambler, Ambysoft, Copyright © 2008)

How do you have a successful agile project with a dislocated scrum team? We have three words: communicate, communicate, and communicate. Because daily in-person conversations are not possible, agile projects with dislocated scrum teams require unique efforts by everyone working on the project. Here are some tips for successful communication among non-collocated scrum team members:

>> **Use videoconferencing technology to simulate face-to-face conversations.** The majority of interpersonal communication is visual, involving facial cues, hand gestures, and even shoulder shrugs. Videoconferencing enables people to see one another and benefit from nonverbal communication as well as a discussion. Use videoconferencing, or even telepresence robots, liberally throughout the day, not just for sprint meetings. Make sure team members are ready for impromptu video chats, and that the technology makes it easy to initiate them.

>> **If possible, arrange for the scrum team members to meet in-person in a central location at least once at the beginning of the project, and preferably multiple times throughout the project.** The shared experience of meeting in-person, even once or twice, can help build teamwork among

dislocated team members. Working relationships built through face-to-face visits are stronger and carry on after the visit ends.

>> **Use an online collaboration tool.** Some tools simulate whiteboards and user story cards, track conversations, and enable multiple people to update artifacts at the same time.

>> **Include scrum team members' pictures on online collaboration tools, or even in email address signature lines.** Humans respond to faces more than written words alone. A simple picture can help humanize instant messages and emails.

>> **Be cognizant of time zone differences.** Put multiple clocks showing different time zones on the wall so you don't accidentally call someone's cellphone at 3 a.m. and wake up that person — or wonder why he or she isn't answering.

>> **Be flexible because of time zone differences as well.** You may need to take video calls or phone calls at odd hours from time to time to help keep project work moving. For drastic time zone differences, consider trading off on times you are available. One week, Team A can be available in the early morning. The next, Team B can be available later in the evening. That way, no one always has an inconvenience.

>> **If you have any doubt about a conversation or a written message, ask for clarification by phone or video.** It always helps to double-check when you're unsure of what someone meant. Follow up with a call to avoid mistakes from miscommunication.

>> **Be aware of language and cultural differences between scrum team members, especially when working with groups in multiple countries.** Understanding colloquialisms and pronunciation differences can increase the quality of your communication across borders. It helps to know about local holidays, too. We've been blindsided more than once by closed offices outside our region.

>> **Make an extra attempt to discuss non-work topics sometimes.** Discussing non-work topics helps you grow closer to scrum team members, regardless of location.

With dedication, awareness, and strong communication, distributed agile projects can succeed.

The unique approaches to team dynamics on agile projects are part of what make agile projects successful. Communication is closely related to team dynamics, and the communication methods on agile projects also have big differences from traditional projects, as you see in the following section.

What's Different about Agile Communication?

Communication, in project management terms, is the formal and informal ways the people on the project team convey information to each other. As with traditional projects, good communication is a necessity for agile projects.

However, the agile principles set a different tone for agile projects, emphasizing simplicity, directness, and face-to-face conversations. The following agile principles relate to communication:

4. Business people and developers must work together daily throughout the project.

6. The most efficient and effective method of conveying information to and within a development team is face-to-face conversation.

7. Working software is the primary measure of progress.

10. Simplicity — the art of maximizing the amount of work not done — is essential.

12. At regular intervals, the team reflects on how to become more effective, then tunes and adjusts its behavior accordingly.

The Agile Manifesto also addresses communication, valuing working software over comprehensive documentation. Although documentation has value, working functionality has more importance on an agile project.

Table 14-4 shows some differences between communication on traditional projects and on agile projects.

TIP

The question of how much documentation is required is not a volume question but an appropriateness question. Why do you need a specific document? How can you create it in the simplest way possible? You can use poster-sized sticky sheets to put on the wall and make information digestible. This can also work best for visually conveying artifacts such as the vision statement, the definition of done, the impediments log, and important architectural decisions. Pictures truly are worth a thousand words.

The following sections show how to take advantage of the agile framework's emphasis on in-person communication, focus on simplicity, and value of working functionality as a communication medium.

TABLE 14-4 **Traditional versus Agile Communication**

Communication Management with Traditional Approaches	Communication Management with Agile Approaches
Team members might make no special effort for in-person conversations.	Agile project management approaches value face-to-face communication as the best way to convey information.
Traditional approaches place high value on documentation. Teams may create a large number of complex documents and status reports based on process, rather than considering actual need.	Agile documents, or *artifacts*, are intentionally simple and provide information that is barely sufficient. Agile artifacts only contain essential information and can often convey project status at a glance. Project teams use the *show, don't tell* concept, showing working software to communicate progress on a regular basis in the sprint review.
Team members may be required to attend a large number of meetings, whether or not those meetings are useful or necessary.	Meetings on agile projects are, by design, as quick as possible and include only people who will add to the meeting and benefit from the meeting. Agile meetings provide all the benefits of face-to-face communication without wasting time. The structure of agile meetings is to enhance, not reduce, productivity.

Managing Agile Communication

To manage communication on agile projects, you need to understand how different agile communication methods work and how to use them together. You also need to know why status on an agile project is different and how to report project progress to stakeholders. The following sections show you how.

Understanding agile communication methods

You can communicate on an agile project through artifacts, meetings, and informally.

Face-to-face conversations are the heart and soul of agile projects. When scrum team members talk with one another about the project throughout every day, communication is easy. Over time, scrum team members understand each other's personality, communication style, and thought processes, and will be able to communicate quickly and effectively.

Figure 14-2, from Alistair Cockburn's presentation *Software Development as a Cooperative Game*, shows the effectiveness of face-to-face communication versus other types of communication.

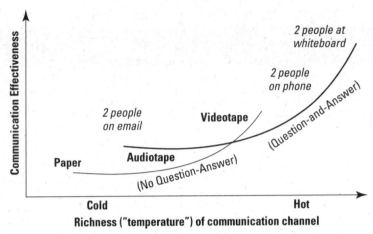

FIGURE 14-2:
Comparison of
communication
types.

Copyright © Humans and Technology, Inc.

In previous chapters, we describe a number of artifacts and meetings that fit with agile projects. All the agile artifacts and meetings play a role in communication. Agile meetings provide a format for communicating in a face-to-face environment. Meetings on agile projects have a specific purpose and a specific amount of time so that the development team can work, rather than sit in meetings. Agile artifacts provide a format for written communication that is structured but not cumbersome or unnecessary.

Table 14-5 provides a view of the different communication channels on an agile project.

TABLE 14-5 **Agile Project Communication Channels**

Channel	Type	Role in Communication
Project planning, release planning, and sprint planning	Meetings	Planning meetings have specific desired outcomes and concisely communicate the purpose and details of the project, the release, and the sprint to the scrum team. Learn more about planning meetings in Chapters 7 and 8.
Product vision statement	Artifact	The product vision statement communicates the end goal of the project to the project team and the organization. Find out more about the product vision in Chapter 7.
Product roadmap	Artifact	The product roadmap communicates a long-term view of the features that support the product vision and are likely to be part of the project. Find out more about the product roadmap in Chapter 7.
Product backlog	Artifact	The product backlog communicates the scope of the project as a whole to the project team. Find out more about the product backlog in Chapters 7 and 8.

Channel	Type	Role in Communication
Release plan	Artifact	The release plan communicates the goals and timing for a specific release. Find out more about the release plan in Chapter 8.
Sprint backlog	Artifact	When updated daily, the sprint backlog provides immediate sprint and project status to anyone who needs that information. The burndown chart on the sprint backlog provides a quick visual of the sprint progress. Find out more about the sprint backlog in Chapters 8 and 9.
Task board	Artifact	Using a task board visually radiates the status of the current sprint or release to anyone who walks by the scrum team's work area. Find out more about the task board in Chapter 9.
Daily scrum	Meeting	The daily scrum provides the scrum team with a verbal, face-to-face opportunity to coordinate the priorities of the day and identify any challenges. Find out more about daily scrum meetings in Chapter 9.
Face-to-face conversations	Informal	Face-to-face conversations are the most important mode of communication on an agile project.
Sprint review	Meeting	The sprint review is the embodiment of show, don't tell, philosophy. Displaying working functionality to the entire project team conveys project progress in a more meaningful way than a written report or a conceptual presentation ever could. Find out more about sprint reviews in Chapter 10.
Sprint retrospective	Meeting	The sprint retrospective allows the scrum team to communicate with one another specifically for improvement. Find out more about sprint retrospectives in Chapter 10.
Meeting notes	Informal	Meeting notes are an optional, informal communication method on an agile project. Meeting notes can capture action items from a meeting to ensure that people on the scrum team remember them for later. Notes from a sprint review include new features for the product backlog. Notes from a sprint retrospective can remind the scrum team of plans for improvement.
Collaborative solutions	Informal	Whiteboards, sticky notes, and electronic collaboration tools all help the scrum team communicate. Ensure that these tools augment, rather than replace, face-to-face conversations. Capturing and saving collaboration results is a low-fidelity way to remind the team of decisions made for immediate and future consideration.

Artifacts, meetings, and more informal communication channels are all tools. Keep in mind that even the best tools need people to use those tools correctly to be effective. Agile projects are about people and interactions; tools are secondary to success.

The next section addresses a specific area of agile project communication: status reporting.

Status and progress reporting

All projects have stakeholders, people outside the immediate scrum team who have a vested interest in the project. At least one of the stakeholders is the person responsible for paying for your project (the project sponsor). It is important for stakeholders, especially those responsible for budgets, to know how the project is progressing. This section shows how to communicate your project's status.

Status on an agile project is a measure of the features that the scrum team has completed. Using the definition of done from Chapters 2, 8, 10, and 15, a feature is complete if the scrum team has developed, tested, integrated, and documented that feature, per the agreement between the product owner and the development team.

If you've worked on a traditional software project, how many times have you been in a status meeting and reported that the project was, say, 64 percent complete? If your stakeholders had replied, "Great! We would like that 64 percent now; we ran out of funds," you and the stakeholders alike would be at a loss, because you didn't mean that 64 percent of your features were ready to use. You meant that each one of the product features was only 64 percent in progress, you had no working functionality, and you still had a lot of work to do before anyone could use the product.

On an agile project, working functionality that meets the definition of done is the primary measure of progress. You can confidently say that project features are complete. Because scope changes constantly on agile projects, you would not express status as a percentage. Instead, a list of potentially shippable features would be more interesting for stakeholders to see as it grows.

Track the progress of your sprint and the project daily. Your primary tools for communicating status and progress are the task board, sprint backlog, product backlog, release and sprint burndown charts, and the sprint review.

The sprint review is where you demonstrate working software to your project stakeholders. Resist creating slides or handouts; the key to the sprint review is showing your stakeholders progress as a demonstration, rather than only telling them what you completed. Show, don't tell.

Strongly encourage anyone who may have an interest in your project to come to your sprint reviews. When people see the working functionality in action, especially on a regular basis, they get a much better sense of the work you've completed.

Companies and organizations that are starting out using agile techniques may expect to see traditional status reports, in addition to agile artifacts. These organizations may also want members of the scrum team to attend regular status meetings, outside of the daily scrums and other agile meetings. This is called *double work agile*, because you are doing twice as much work as necessary. Double work agile is one of the top pitfalls for agile projects. Scrum teams will burn out quickly if they try to meet the demands of two drastically different project approaches. You can avoid double work agile by educating your company about why agile artifacts and events are a better replacement for old documents and meetings. Insist on experimenting with agile artifacts and events to conduct a successful agile project.

The sprint backlog is a report of the daily status of your current sprint. The sprint backlog contains the sprint's user stories and their related tasks and estimates. The sprint backlog also often has a burndown chart that visually shows the status of the work the development team has completed and the remaining work to complete the requirements in the sprint. The development team is in charge of updating the sprint backlog at least once a day by updating the number of hours of work remaining for each task.

If you're a project manager now, or if you study project management in the future, you may come across the concept of *earned value management* (EVM), as a way of measuring project progress and performance. Some agile practitioners try to use an agile-like version of EVM, but we avoid EVM for agile projects. EVM assumes that your project has a fixed scope, which is antithetical to an agile approach. Instead of trying to change agile approaches to fit into old models, use the tools here — they work.

The burndown chart quickly shows, rather than tells, status. When you look at a sprint burndown chart, you can instantly see whether the sprint is going well or might be in trouble. In Chapter 9, we show you an image of sample burndown charts for different sprint scenarios; here it is again in Figure 14-3.

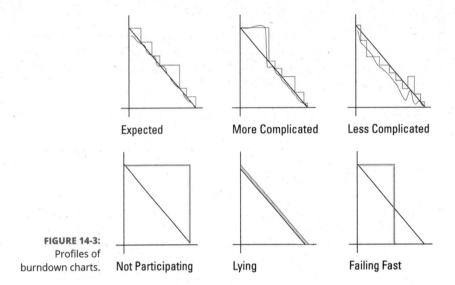

Expected   More Complicated   Less Complicated

FIGURE 14-3:
Profiles of
burndown charts.

Not Participating   Lying   Failing Fast

If you update your sprint backlog every day, you'll always have an up-to-date status for your project stakeholders. You can also show them the product backlog so that they know which features the scrum team has completed to date, which features will be part of future sprints, and the priority of the features.

REMEMBER

The product backlog will change as you add and reprioritize features. Make sure that people who review the product backlog, especially for status purposes, understand this concept.

TIP

A task board is a great way to quickly show your project team the status of a sprint, release, or even of the entire project. Task boards have sticky notes with user story titles in at least four columns: To Do, In Progress, Accept, and Done. If you display your task board in the scrum team's work area, anyone who walks by can see a high-level status of which product features are done and which features are in progress. The scrum team always knows where the project stands, because the scrum team sees the task board every day.

Always strive for simple, low-fidelity information radiators to communicate status and progress. The more you can make information accessible and on-demand, the less time you and your stakeholders will spend preparing and wondering about status.

Chapter 15

Managing Quality and Risk

Quality and risk are closely related parts of project management. In this chapter, you find out how to deliver quality products using agile project management methods. You understand how to take advantage of agile approaches to manage risk on your projects. You see how quality has historically affected project risk, and how quality management on agile projects fundamentally reduces project risk.

What's Different about Agile Quality?

Quality refers to whether a product works, and whether it fulfills the project stakeholders' needs. Quality is an inherent part of agile project management.

All 12 agile principles that we list in Chapter 2 promote quality either directly or indirectly. Those principles follow:

1. Our highest priority is to satisfy the customer through early and continuous delivery of valuable software.

2. Welcome changing requirements, even late in development. Agile processes harness change for the customer's competitive advantage.

3. Deliver working software frequently, from a couple of weeks to a couple of months, with a preference to the shorter timescale.

4. Business people and developers must work together daily throughout the project.

5. Build projects around motivated individuals. Give them the environment and support they need, and trust them to get the job done.

6. The most efficient and effective method of conveying information to and within a development team is face-to-face conversation.

7. Working software is the primary measure of progress.

8. Agile processes promote sustainable development. The sponsors, developers, and users should be able to maintain a constant pace indefinitely.

9. Continuous attention to technical excellence and good design enhances agility.

10. Simplicity — the art of maximizing the amount of work not done — is essential.

11. The best architectures, requirements, and designs emerge from self-organizing teams.

12. At regular intervals, the team reflects on how to become more effective, then tunes and adjusts its behavior accordingly.

These principles emphasize creating an environment where agile teams are able to produce valuable, working functionality. Agile approaches encourage quality both in the sense of products working correctly and meeting the needs of project stakeholders.

Table 15-1 shows some differences between quality management on traditional projects and on agile projects.

TABLE 15-1 **Traditional versus Agile Quality**

Quality Management with Traditional Approaches	Quality Dynamics with Agile Approaches
Testing is the last phase of a project before product deployment. Some features are tested months after they were created.	Testing is a daily part of each sprint and is included in each requirement's definition of done. You use automated testing, allowing quick and robust testing every day.
Quality is often a reactive practice, with the focus mostly on product testing and issue resolution.	You address quality both reactively, through testing, and proactively, encouraging practices to set the stage for quality work. Examples of proactive quality approaches include face-to-face communication, pair programming, and established coding standards.
Problems are riskier when found at the end of a project. Sunk costs are high by the time teams reach testing.	You can create and test riskier features in early sprints, when sunk costs are still low.
Problems or defects, sometimes called *bugs* in software development, are hard to find at the end of a project, and fixes for problems at the end of a project are costly.	Problems are easy to find when you test a smaller amount of work. Fixes are easier when you fix something you just created, rather than something you created months earlier.
Sometimes, to meet a deadline or save money, teams cut the testing phase short.	Testing is assured on agile projects because it is part of every sprint.

At the start of this chapter, we state that quality and risk are closely related. The agile approaches in Table 15-1 greatly reduce the risk and unnecessary cost that usually accompany quality management.

TECHNICAL STUFF

BUGS. BUGS? BUGS!

Why do we call computer problems *bugs?* The first computers were large, glass-encased machines that took up entire rooms. In 1945, one of these behemoth computers, the Mark II Aiken Relay Calculator at Harvard University, had problems with one of its circuits. Engineers traced the issue to a moth — a literal bug — in the machine. After that, the team's running joke was that any issue with the computer had to be a bug. The term stuck, and people still use *bug* today to describe hardware problems, software problems, and sometimes even problems outside of the computer science realm. The engineers at Harvard even taped the moth to a logbook. That first bug is now on display at the Smithsonian National Museum of American History.

Another difference about quality on agile projects is the multiple quality feedback loops throughout a project. In Figure 15-1, you see the different types of product feedback a scrum team receives in the course of a project. The development team can immediately incorporate this feedback into the product, increasing product quality on a regular basis.

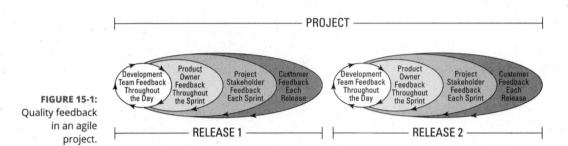

FIGURE 15-1:
Quality feedback in an agile project.

REMEMBER

In Chapter 14, we tell you that development teams on agile projects can include everyone who works on a product. Development teams on agile projects typically include people who are experts in creating and executing tests and ensuring quality. Development team members are cross-functional; that is, every team member may do different jobs at different times during the project. Cross-functionality extends to quality activities such as preventing issues, testing, and fixing bugs.

In the next section, you see how to use agile project management techniques to increase quality.

Managing Agile Quality

Agile development teams have the primary responsibility for quality on agile projects. The responsibility for quality is an extension of the responsibilities and free-doms that come with self-management. When the development team is free to determine its development methods, the development team is also responsible for ensuring that those methods result in quality work.

TECHNICAL STUFF

Organizations often refer to quality management as a whole as *quality assurance*, or *QA*. You may see QA departments, QA testers, QA managers, QA analysts, and all other flavors of QA-prefixed titles to refer to people who are responsible for quality activities. QA is also sometimes used as shorthand for testing, as in "we performed QA on the product" or "now we are in the QA phase." Quality control (QC) is also a common way to refer to quality management.

The other members of the scrum team — the scrum master and the product owner — also play parts in quality management. Product owners provide clarification on requirements and also accept those requirements as being done throughout each sprint. Scrum masters help ensure development teams have a work environment where the people on development teams can work to the best of their abilities.

Luckily, agile project management approaches have several ways to help scrum teams create quality products. In this section, you see how testing in sprints increases the likelihood of finding defects and reduces the cost of fixing them. You gain an understanding of the many ways agile project management proactively encourages quality product development. You see how inspecting and adapting on a regular basis addresses quality. Finally, you find out how automated testing is essential to delivering valuable products continuously throughout an agile project.

Quality and the sprint

Quality management is a daily part of agile projects. Scrum teams run agile projects in sprints, short development cycles that last one to four weeks. Each cycle includes activities from the different phases of a traditional project for each user story in the sprint: requirements, design, development, testing, and integration for deployment. Find out more about working in sprints in Chapters 8, 9, and 10.

TIP

Here's a quick riddle: Is it easier to find a quarter on a table or in a stadium? Obviously, the answer is a table. Just as obvious is that it is easier to find a defect in 100 lines of software code than in 100,000 lines. Iterative development makes quality product development easier.

Scrum teams test throughout each sprint. Figure 15-2 shows how testing fits into sprints on an agile project. Notice that testing begins in the first sprint, right after developers start creating the first requirement in the project.

When development teams test throughout each sprint, they can find and fix defects very quickly. With agile project management, development teams create product requirements, immediately test those requirements, and fix any problems immediately before considering the work done. Instead of trying to remember how to fix something they created weeks or months ago, development teams are, at the most, fixing the requirement they worked on one or two days earlier.

Testing every day on an agile project is a great way to ensure product quality. Another way to ensure product quality is to create a better product from the start. The next section shows you different ways that agile project management helps you avoid errors and create an excellent product.

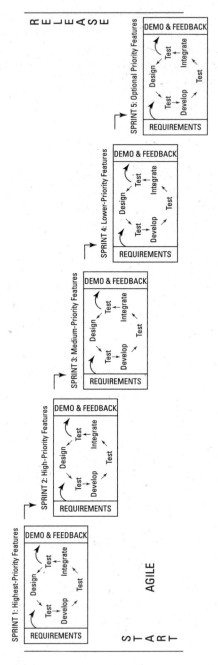

FIGURE 15-2:
Testing within sprints.

Proactive quality

An important and often-neglected aspect of quality is the idea of preventing problems. A number of agile approaches allow and encourage scrum teams to proactively create quality products. These practices include

>> An emphasis on technical excellence and good design

>> Incorporation of quality-specific development techniques into product creation

>> Daily communication between the development team and the product owner

>> Acceptance criteria built into user stories

>> Face-to-face communication and collocation

>> Sustainable development

>> Regular inspection and adaption of work and behavior

The following sections provide a detailed look at each of these proactive quality practices.

REMEMBER

Quality means both that a product works correctly and that the product does what the project stakeholders need it to do.

Continuous attention to technical excellence and good design

Agile teams focus on technical excellence and good design because these traits lead to valuable products. How do development teams provide great technical solutions and designs?

One way that development teams provide technical excellence is through self-management, which provides them with the freedom to innovate technically. Traditional organizations may have mandatory technical standards that may or may not make sense for a given project. Self-organizing development teams have the freedom to decide whether a standard will provide value in creating a product, or if a different approach will work better. Innovation can lead to good design, technical excellence, and product quality.

Self-management also provides development teams with a sense of product ownership. When people on development teams feel a deep responsibility for the product they're creating, they often strive to find the best solutions and execute those solutions in the best way possible.

Nothing is more sophisticated than a simple solution.

Organizational commitment also plays a role in technical excellence. Some companies and organizations, regardless of their project management approaches, have a commitment to excellence. Think about the products that you use every day and associate with quality; chances are those products come from companies that value good technical solutions. If you're working on an agile project for a company that believes in and rewards technical excellence, enacting this agile principle will be easy.

Other companies may undervalue technical excellence; agile project teams at these companies may struggle when trying to justify training or tools that will help create better products. Some companies do not make the connection between good technology, good products, and profitability. Scrum masters and product owners may need to educate their companies on why good technology and design are important and may need to lobby to get development teams what they need to create a great product.

Don't confuse technical excellence with using new technologies for the sake of using something new or trendy. Your technology solutions should efficiently support the product needs, not just add to a resume or a company skills profile.

By incorporating technical excellence and good design into your everyday work, you create a quality product that you are proud of.

Quality development techniques

During the past several decades of software development, the motivation to be more adaptive and agile has inspired a number of agile development techniques that focus on quality. This section provides a high-level view of a few extreme programming (XP) development approaches that help ensure quality proactively. For more information on XP practices, see Chapter 4.

Many agile quality management techniques were created with software development in mind. You can adapt some of these techniques when creating other types of products, such as hardware products or even building construction. If you're going to work on a non-software project, read about the development methods in this section with adaptability in mind:

>> **Test-driven development (TDD):** This development method begins with a developer creating a test for the requirement he or she wants to create. The developer then runs the test, which should fail at first because the

functionality does not yet exist. The developer develops until the test passes, and then refactors the code — takes out as much code as possible, while still having the test pass. With TDD, you know that the newly created functionality of a requirement works correctly because you test while you create the functionality and develop the functionality until the test passes.

>> **Pair programming:** With *pair programming,* developers work in groups of two. Both developers sit at the same computer and work as a team to create one product requirement. The developers take turns at the keyboard to collaborate. Usually, the one at the keyboard takes a direct tactical role, while the observing partner takes a more strategic or navigating role, looking ahead and providing in-the-moment feedback. Because the developers are literally looking over one another's shoulder, they can catch errors quickly. Pair programming increases quality by providing instant error checks and balances.

>> **Peer review:** Sometimes called *peer code review,* a *peer review* involves members of the development team reviewing one another's code. Like pair programming, peer reviews have a collaborative nature; when developers review each other's finished products, the developers work together to provide solutions for any issues they find. If development teams don't practice pair programming, they should at least practice peer reviews, which increase quality by allowing development experts to look for structural problems within product code.

>> **Collective code ownership:** In this approach, everyone on the development team can create, change, or fix any part of the code on the project. Collective code ownership can speed up development, encourage innovation, and with multiple pairs of eyes on the code, help development team members quickly find defects.

>> **Continuous integration:** This approach involves the creation of integrated code builds one or more times each day. Continuous integration allows members of the development team to check how the user story that the development team is creating works with the rest of the product. Continuous integration helps ensure quality by allowing the development team to check for conflicts regularly. Continuous integration is essential to automated testing on agile projects; you need to create a code build at the end of the day before running automated tests overnight. Find out more about automated testing later in this chapter.

On an agile project, the development team decides which tools and techniques will work best for the project, the product, and the individual development team.

Many agile software development techniques help ensure quality, and there is a lot of discussion and information about these techniques in the community of people who use agile project management approaches. We encourage you to learn more about these approaches if you're going to work on an agile project, especially if you're a developer. Entire books are dedicated to some of these techniques, such as test-driven development. The information we provide here is at the tip of the iceberg. See Chapter 22 for more recommendations.

The product owner and development team

Another aspect of agile project management that encourages quality is the close relationship between the development team and the product owner. The product owner is the voice of business needs for the product. In this role, the product owner works with the development team every day to ensure that the functionality meets those business needs.

During planning stages, the product owner's job is to help the development team understand each requirement correctly. During the sprint, the product owner answers questions that the development team has about requirements and is responsible for reviewing functionality and accepting them as done. When the product owner accepts requirements, he or she ensures that the development team correctly interpreted the business need for each requirement, and that the new functionality performs the task that it needs to perform.

In waterfall projects, feedback loops between developers and business owners are less frequent, so a development team's work typically strays from the original product goals set in the product vision statement.

A product owner who reviews requirements daily catches misinterpretations early. The product owner can then set the development team back on the right path, avoiding a lot of wasted time and effort.

The product vision statement communicates how your product supports the company's or organization's strategies. The vision statement articulates the product's goals. Chapter 7 explains how to create a product vision statement.

User stories and acceptance criteria

Another proactive quality measure on agile projects is the acceptance criteria you build into each user story. In Chapter 7, we explain that a user story is one format for describing product requirements. User stories increase quality by outlining the specific actions the user will take to correctly meet business needs. Figure 15-3 shows a user story and its acceptance criteria.

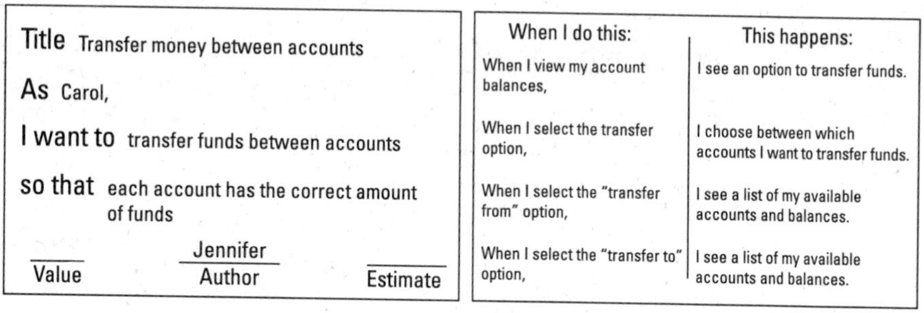

FIGURE 15-3:
A user story and
acceptance
criteria.

Title Transfer money between accounts		When I do this:	This happens:
As Carol,		When I view my account balances,	I see an option to transfer funds.
I want to transfer funds between accounts		When I select the transfer option,	I choose between which accounts I want to transfer funds.
so that each account has the correct amount of funds		When I select the "transfer from" option,	I see a list of my available accounts and balances.
_____ Jennifer _____ Value Author Estimate		When I select the "transfer to" option,	I see a list of my available accounts and balances.

Even if you don't describe your requirements in a user story format, consider adding validation steps to each of your requirements. Acceptance criteria don't just help the product owner review requirements; they help the development team understand how to create the product in the first place.

Face-to-face communication

Have you ever had a conversation with someone and known, just by looking at that person's face, that he or she didn't understand you? In Chapter 14, we explain that face-to-face conversations are the quickest, most effective form of communication. This is because humans convey information with more than just words; our facial expressions, gestures, body language, and even where we are looking contribute to communicating and understanding one another.

Face-to-face communication helps ensure quality on agile projects because it leads to better interpretation of requirements, roadblocks, and discussions between scrum team members. Regular face-to-face communication requires a collocated scrum team.

Sustainable development

Chances are, at some point in your life, you've found yourself working or studying long hours for an extended period of time. You may have even pulled an all-nighter or two, getting no sleep at all for a night. How did you feel during this time? Did you make good decisions? Did you make any silly mistakes?

Unfortunately, many teams on traditional projects find themselves working long, crazy hours, especially toward the end of a project, when a deadline is looming and it seems like the only way to finish is to spend weeks working extra-long days. Those long days often mean more problems later, as team members start making mistakes — some silly, some more serious — and eventually burn out.

On agile projects, scrum teams help ensure that they do quality work by creating an environment where members of the development team sustain a constant working pace throughout the project. Working in sprints helps sustain a constant working pace; when the development team chooses the work it can accomplish in each sprint, it shouldn't have to rush at the end.

The development team can determine what sustainable means for itself, whether that means working a regular 40-hour workweek, a schedule with more or fewer days or hours, or working outside a standard nine-to-five time frame.

TIP

If your fellow scrum team members start coming to work with their shirts on inside out, you might want to double-check that you're maintaining a sustainable development environment.

Keeping the development team happy, rested, and able to have a life outside of work can lead to fewer mistakes, more creativity and innovation, and better overall products.

Being proactive about quality saves you a lot of headaches in the long run. It is much easier and more enjoyable to work on a product with fewer defects to fix. The next section discusses an agile approach that addresses quality from both a proactive and a reactive standpoint: inspect and adapt.

Quality through regular inspecting and adapting

The agile tenet of inspect and adapt is a key to creating quality products. Throughout an agile project, you look at both your product and your process (inspect) and make changes as necessary (adapt). Chapters 7 and 10 have more information about this tenet.

In the sprint review and sprint retrospective meetings, agile project teams regularly step back and review their work and methods and determine how to make adjustments for a better project. We provide details on the sprint review and sprint retrospective in Chapter 10. Following is a quick overview of how these meetings help ensure quality on agile projects.

In a sprint review, agile project teams review requirements completed at the end of each sprint. Sprint reviews address quality by letting project stakeholders see working requirements and provide feedback on those requirements throughout the course of the project. If a requirement doesn't meet stakeholder expectations, the stakeholders tell the scrum team immediately. The scrum team can then adjust the product in a future sprint. The scrum team can also apply its revised understanding of how the product needs to work on other product requirements.

In a sprint retrospective, scrum teams meet to discuss what worked and what might need adjusting at the end of each sprint. Sprint retrospectives help ensure quality by allowing the scrum team to discuss and immediately fix problems. Sprint retrospectives also allow the team to come together and formally discuss changes to the product, project, or work environment that might increase quality.

The sprint review and sprint retrospective aren't the only opportunities for inspecting and adapting for quality on an agile project. Agile approaches encourage reviewing work and adjusting behavior and methods throughout each workday. Daily inspecting and adapting everything you do on the project help ensure quality.

Another way to manage and help assure quality on an agile project is to use automated testing tools. The next section explains why automated testing is important to agile projects and how to incorporate automated testing into your project.

Automated testing

Automated testing is the use of software to test your product. Automated testing is critical to agile projects. If you want to quickly create software functionality that meets the definition of done — coded, tested, integrated, and documented — you need a way to quickly test each piece of functionality as it's created. Automated testing means quick and robust testing on a daily basis. Agile teams continually increase the frequency with which they automatically test their system so they can continually decrease the time it takes them to complete and deploy new valuable functionality to their customers.

TIP

Project teams won't become agile without automated testing. Manual testing simply takes too long.

Throughout this book, we explain how agile project teams embrace low-tech solutions. Why, then, is there a section in this book about automated testing, a rather high-tech quality management technique? The answer to this question is efficiency. Automated testing is like the spell-check feature in word-processing programs. As a matter of fact, spell-checking is a form of automated testing. In the same way, automated testing is a much quicker and often more accurate — thus, more efficient — method of finding software defects than manual testing.

To develop a product using automated testing, development teams develop and test using the following steps:

1. **Develop code and automated tests in support of user stories during the day.**

2. **Create an integrated code build at the end of each day.**

3. **Schedule the automated testing software to test the newest build overnight.**

4. **Check the automated test results first thing each morning.**

5. **Fix any defects immediately.**

Comprehensive code testing while you're sleeping is cool.

Automated testing allows development teams to take advantage of non-working time for productivity and to have rapid create-test-fix cycles. Also, automated testing software can often test requirements quicker and with more accuracy and consistency than a person testing those requirements.

Today's market has a lot of automated testing tools. Some automated testing tools are open-source and free; others are available for purchase. The development team needs to review automated testing options and choose the tool that will work best.

Automated testing changes the work for people in quality roles on the development team. Traditionally, a large part of a quality management person's work involved manually testing products. The tester on a traditional project would use the product and look for problems. With automated testing, however, quality activities largely involve creating tests to run on automated testing software. Automated testing tools augment, rather than replace, people's skills, knowledge, and work.

It is still a good idea to have humans periodically check that the requirements you're developing work correctly, especially when you first start using an automated testing tool. Any automated tool can have hiccups from time to time. By manually double-checking (sometimes called smoke-testing) small parts of automated tests, you help avoid getting to the end of a sprint and finding out that your product doesn't work like it should.

You can automate almost any type of software test. If you're new to software development, you may not know that there are many different types of software testing. A small sample includes the following:

>> **Unit testing:** Tests individual units, or the smallest parts, of product code.

>> **Regression testing:** Tests an entire product from start to finish, including requirements you have tested previously.

>> **User acceptance testing:** Product stakeholders or even some of the product's end users review a product and accept it as complete.

>> **Functional testing:** Tests to make sure the product works according to acceptance criteria from the user story.

>> **Integration testing:** Tests to make sure the product works with other parts of the product.

>> **Enterprise testing:** Tests to make sure the product works with other products in the organization, as necessary.

>> **Performance testing:** Tests how fast a product runs on a given system under different scenarios.

>> **Load testing:** Tests how well a product handles different amounts of concurrent activity.

>> **Smoke testing:** Tests on small but critical parts of code or of a system to help determine if the system as a whole is likely to work.

>> **Static testing:** Focuses on checking code standards, rather than working software.

Automated testing works for these tests and the many other types of software tests out there.

As you may understand by now, quality is an integral part of agile projects. Quality is just one factor, however, that differentiates risk on agile projects from traditional projects. In the next sections, you see how risk on traditional projects compares to risk on agile projects.

What's Different about Agile Risk Management?

Risk refers to the factors that contribute to a project's success or failure. On agile projects, risk management doesn't have to involve formal risk documentation and meetings. Instead, risk management is built into scrum roles, artifacts, and events. In addition, consider the following agile principles that support risk management:

1. Our highest priority is to satisfy the customer through early and continuous delivery of valuable software.

2. Welcome changing requirements, even late in development. Agile processes harness change for the customer's competitive advantage.

3. Deliver working software frequently, from a couple of weeks to a couple of months, with a preference to the shorter timescale.

4. Business people and developers must work together daily throughout the project.

5. Working software is the primary measure of progress.

The preceding principles, and any practice that demonstrates those principles, significantly mitigate or eliminate many risks that frequently lead to project challenges and failure.

According to the Standish Group's "2015 Chaos Report," a study of 10,000 software projects, small agile projects are 30 percent more likely to succeed than traditional projects. See Figure 15-4. Medium-sized projects are four times (400 percent) more likely to succeed with an agile approach than a traditional approach, and large, complex projects are six times (600 percent) more likely to succeed with an agile approach.

CHAOS RESOLUTION BY AGILE VERSUS WATERFALL

SIZE	METHOD	SUCCESSFUL	CHALLENGED	FAILED
All Size Projects	Agile	39%	52%	9%
	Waterfall	11%	60%	29%
Large Size Projects	Agile	18%	59%	23%
	Waterfall	3%	55%	42%
Medium Size Projects	Agile	27%	62%	11%
	Waterfall	7%	68%	25%
Small Size Projects	Agile	58%	38%	4%
	Waterfall	44%	45%	11%

FIGURE 15-4: Standish Group's "2015 Chaos Report."

The resolution of all software projects from FY2011-2015 within the new CHAOS database, segmented by the agile process and waterfall method. The total number of software projects is over 10,000.

Table 15-2 shows some of the differences between risk on traditional projects and on agile projects.

TABLE 15-2 **Traditional versus Agile Risk**

Risk Management with Traditional Approaches	Risk Dynamics with Agile Approaches
Large numbers of projects fail or are challenged.	Risk of catastrophic failure — spending large amounts of money with nothing to show — is almost eliminated.
The bigger, longer, and more complex the project, the more risky it is. Risk is highest at the end of a project.	Product value is gained immediately, rather than sinking costs into a project for months or even years with the growing chance of failure.
Conducting all the testing at the end of a project means that finding serious problems can put the entire project at risk.	Testing occurs while you develop. If a technical approach, a requirement, or even an entire product is not feasible, the development team discovers this in a short time, and you have more time to course correct. If correction is not possible, stakeholders spend less money on a failed project.
Projects are unable to accommodate new requirements mid-project without increased time and cost because extensive sunk cost exists in even the lowest-priority requirements.	Change for the benefit of the product is welcomed. Agile projects accommodate new high-priority requirements without increasing time or cost by removing a low-priority requirement of equal time and cost.
Traditional projects require time and cost estimates at the project start, when teams know the least about the project. Estimates are often inaccurate, creating a gap between expected and actual project schedules and budgets.	Project time and cost is estimated using the scrum team's actual performance, or velocity. You refine estimates throughout the project, because the longer you work on a project, the more you learn about the project, the requirements, and the scrum team.
When stakeholders don't have a unified goal, they can end up confusing the project team with conflicting information about what the product should achieve.	A single product owner is responsible for creating a vision for the product and represents the stakeholders to the project team.
Unresponsive or absent stakeholders can cause project delays and result in products that do not achieve the right goals.	The product owner is responsible for providing information about the product immediately. In addition, the scrum master helps remove impediments on a daily basis.

Risk on agile projects declines as the project progresses. Figure 15-5 shows a comparison of risk and time between waterfall projects and agile projects.

All projects have some risk, regardless of your project approach. However, with agile project management, the days of catastrophic project failure — spending large amounts of time and money with no return on investment (ROI) — are over. The elimination of large-scale failure is the biggest difference between risk on traditional projects and on agile projects. In the next section, you see why.

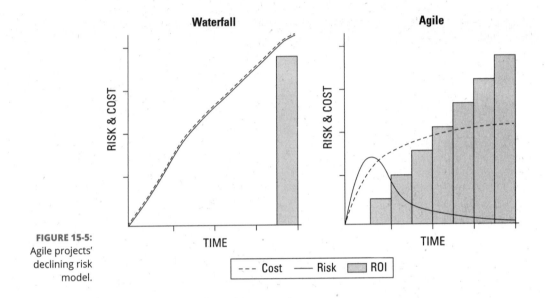

FIGURE 15-5:
Agile projects' declining risk model.

Managing Agile Risk

In this section, you examine key structures of agile projects that reduce risk over the life of the project. You find out how to use agile tools and events to find risks at the right time in a project and how to prioritize and mitigate those risks.

Reducing risk inherently

Agile approaches, when implemented correctly, inherently reduce risk in product development. Developing in sprints ensures a short time between project investment and proof that the product works. Sprints also provide the potential for a project to generate revenue early. The sprint review, the sprint retrospective, and the product owner's involvement during each sprint provide constant product feedback to the development team. Ongoing feedback helps prevent deviations between product expectations and the completed product.

Three especially important factors in risk reduction on agile projects are the definition of done, self-funding projects, and the idea of failing fast. You find out more about each of these factors in this section.

Risk and the definition of done

In Chapter 10, we discuss when a requirement is done. To consider a requirement complete and ready to demonstrate at the end of a sprint, that requirement must meet the scrum team's definition of done. The product owner and the development team agree upon the details of the definition; definitions of done usually include the following:

>> **Developed:** The development team must fully create the working product requirement.

>> **Tested:** The development team must have tested that the product works correctly and is defect-free.

>> **Integrated:** The development team must have ensured that the requirement works with the whole product and any related systems.

>> **Documented:** The development team must have created notes about how it created the product and the rationale behind key technical decisions made.

Figure 15-6 shows a sample definition of done, with details.

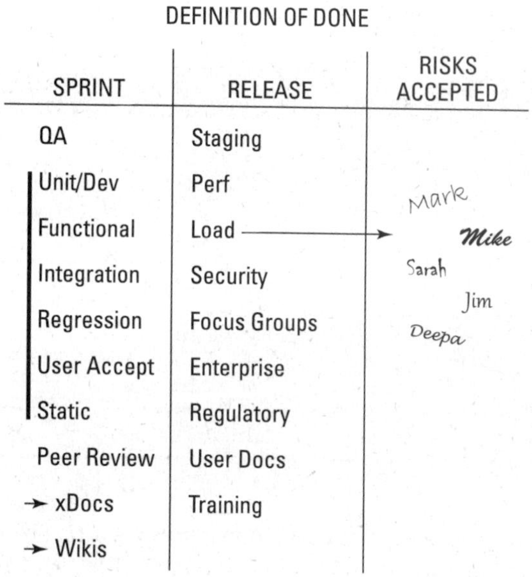

DEFINITION OF DONE

SPRINT	RELEASE	RISKS ACCEPTED
QA	Staging	
Unit/Dev	Perf	Mark
Functional	Load ⟶	Mike
Integration	Security	Sarah
Regression	Focus Groups	Jim
User Accept	Enterprise	Deepa
Static	Regulatory	
Peer Review	User Docs	
➔ xDocs	Training	
➔ Wikis		

FIGURE 15-6:
Sample definition of done.

The product owner and the development team may also create a list of acceptable risks. For example, they may agree that end-to-end regression testing or performance testing is overkill for the sprint definition of done. Or, with cloud computing, load testing may not be as crucial because additional capacity can be easily and quickly added on demand at nominal costs. Acceptable risks allow the development team to concentrate on the most important activities.

The definition of done drastically changes the risk factor for agile projects. By creating a product that meets the definition of done in every sprint, you end each sprint with a working build and usable functionality. Even if outside factors cause a project to end early, project stakeholders will always see some value and have working functionality to use now and build upon later.

Self-funding projects

Agile projects can mitigate financial risk in a unique way that traditional projects cannot: the self-funding project. Chapter 13 includes examples of self-funding projects. If your product is an income-generating product, you could use that income to help fund the rest of your project.

In Chapter 13, we show you two different project ROI models. Here they are again, in Tables 15-3 and 15-4. The projects in both tables create identical products.

TABLE 15-3   **Income from a Traditional Project with a Final Release after Six Months**

Month	Income Generated	Total Project Income
January	$0	$0
February	$0	$0
March	$0	$0
April	$0	$0
May	$0	$0
June	$0	$0
July	$100,000	$100,000

In Table 15-3, the project created $100,000 in income after six months of development. Now compare the ROI in Table 15-3 to the ROI in Table 15-4.

In Table 15-4, the project generated income with the very first release. By the end of six months, the project had generated $330,000 — $230,000 more than the project in Table 15-3.

TABLE 15-4   Income from an Agile Project with Monthly Releases and a Final Release after Six Months

Month/Release	Income Generated	Total Project Income
January	$0	$0
February	$15,000	$15,000
March	$25,000	$40,000
April	$40,000	$80,000
May	$70,000	$150,000
June	$80,000	$230,000
July	$100,000	$330,000

The capability to generate income in a short amount of time has a number of benefits for companies and project teams. Self-funding agile projects make good financial sense for almost any organization, but they can be especially useful to organizations that may not have the funds to create a product upfront. For groups short on cash, self-funding can enable projects that would otherwise not be feasible.

Self-funding projects also help mitigate the risk that a project will be cancelled due to lack of funds. A company emergency may dictate diverting a traditional project's budget elsewhere, delaying or cancelling the project. However, an agile project that generates additional revenue with every release has a good chance of continuing during a crisis.

Finally, self-funding projects help sell stakeholders on a project in the first place; it's hard to argue with a project that provides continuous value and pays for at least part of the project costs from the start.

Failing fast

All product development efforts carry some risk of failure. Testing within sprints introduces the idea of *failing fast:* Instead of sinking costs into a long effort for requirements, design, and development, and then finding problems that will prevent the project from moving forward during the testing phase, development teams on agile projects can identify critical problems within a few sprints. This quantitative risk mitigation can save organizations large amounts of money.

Tables 15-5 and 15-6 illustrate the difference in sunk costs for a failed waterfall project and a failed agile project. The projects in both tables are for identical products with identical costs.

TABLE 15-5   ## Cost of Failure on a Waterfall Project

Month	Phase and Issues	Sunk Project Cost	Total Sunk Project Cost
January	Requirements Phase	$80,000	$80,000
February	Requirements Phase	$80,000	$160,000
March	Design Phase	$80,000	$240,000
April	Design Phase	$80,000	$320,000
May	Design Phase	$80,000	$400,000
June	Development Phase	$80,000	$480,000
July	Development Phase	$80,000	$560,000
August	Development Phase	$80,000	$640,000
September	Development Phase	$80,000	$720,000
October	QA Phase: Large-scale problem uncovered during testing.	$80,000	$800,000
November	QA Phase: Development team attempted to resolve problem to continue development.	$80,000	$880,000
December	Project cancelled; product not viable.	0	$880,000

In Table 15-5, the project stakeholders spent 11 months and close to a million dollars to find out that a product idea would not work. Compare the sunk cost in Table 15-5 to that in Table 15-6.

TABLE 15-6   ## Cost of Failure on an Agile Project

Month	Sprint and Issues	Sunk Project Cost	Total Sunk Project Cost
January	Sprint 1: No issues. Sprint 2: No issues.	$80,000	$80,000
February	Sprint 3: Large-scale problem uncovered during testing resulted in failed sprint. Sprint 4: Development team attempted to resolve problem to continue development; sprint ultimately failed.	$80,000	$160,000
Final	Project cancelled; product not viable.	0	$160,000

By testing early, the development team from Table 15-6 determined that the product would not work by the end of February, spending less than one-sixth of the time and money spent in the project in Table 15-5.

REMEMBER

Because of the definition of done, even failed projects produce something tangible that an organization may leverage or improve. For example, the failed project in Table 15-5 would have provided working functionality in the first two sprints.

The concept of failing fast can apply beyond technical problems with a product. You can also use development within sprints and fast failure to see if a product will work in the marketplace, and to cancel the project early if it looks like customers won't buy or use the product. By releasing small parts of the product and testing the product with potential customers early in the project, you get a good idea of whether your product is commercially viable, and save large amounts of money if you find that people will not buy the product. You also discover important changes you might make to the product to better meet customer needs.

Finally, failing fast does not necessarily mean project cancellation. If you find catastrophic issues when sunk costs are low, you may have the time and budget to determine a completely different approach to create a product.

The definition of done, self-funding projects, and the idea of failing fast, along with the foundation of agile principles, all help lower risk on agile projects. In the next section, you see how to actively use agile project management tools to manage risk.

Identifying, prioritizing, and responding to risks early

Although the structure of agile projects inherently reduces many traditional risks, development teams still should be aware of the problems that can arise during a project. Scrum teams are self-managing; in the same way that they are responsible for quality, scrum teams are responsible for trying to identify risks and ways to prevent those risks from materializing.

TIP

On agile projects, you prioritize the highest-value and highest-risk requirements first.

Instead of spending hours or days documenting all of a project's potential risks, the likelihood of those risks happening, the severity of those risks, and ways to mitigate those risks, scrum teams use existing agile artifacts and meetings to manage risk. Scrum teams also wait until the last responsible minute to address risk, when they know the most about the project and problems that are more likely to arise. Table 15-7 shows how scrum teams can use the different agile project management tools to manage risk at the right time.

TABLE 15-7   **Agile Project Risk Management Tools**

Artifact or Meeting	Role in Risk Management
Product vision	The product vision statement helps unify the project team's definition of product goals, mitigating the risk of misunderstandings about what the product will need to accomplish.
	While creating the product vision, the project team might think of risks on a very high level, based on marketplace and customer feedback, and inline with organizational strategy. Find out more about the product vision in Chapter 7.
Product roadmap	The product roadmap provides a visual overview of the project's requirements and priorities. This overview allows the project team to quickly identify gaps in requirements and incorrectly prioritized requirements. Find out more about the product roadmap in Chapter 7.
Product backlog	The product backlog is a tool for accommodating change in the project. Being able to add changes to the product backlog and reprioritize requirements regularly helps turn the traditional risk associated with scope changes into a way to create a better product.
	Keeping the requirements and the priorities in the product backlog current helps ensure that the development team can work on the most important requirements at the right time. Find out more about the product backlog in Chapters 7 and 8.
Release planning	During release planning, the scrum team discusses risks to the release and how to mitigate those risks. Risk discussions in the release planning meeting should be high-level and relate to the release as a whole. Address risks with individual requirements in the sprint planning meetings. Find out more about release planning in Chapter 8.
Sprint planning	During each sprint-planning meeting, the scrum team discusses risks to the specific requirements and tasks in the sprint and how to mitigate those risks. Risk discussions during sprint planning can be done in depth, but should only relate to the current sprint. Find out more about sprint planning in Chapter 8.
Sprint backlog	The burndown chart on the sprint backlog provides a quick view of the sprint status. This quick view helps the scrum team manage risks to the sprint as they arise and minimize their effect by addressing problems immediately. Find out more about sprint backlogs and how burndown charts show project status in Chapter 9.
Daily scrum	During each daily scrum, development team members discuss roadblocks. Roadblocks, or impediments, are sometimes risks. Talking about roadblocks every day gives the development team and the scrum master the chance to mitigate those risks immediately. Find out more about the daily scrum in Chapter 9.

Artifact or Meeting	Role in Risk Management
Task board	The task board provides an unavoidable view of the sprint status, allowing the scrum team to catch risks to the sprint and manage them right away. Find out more about task boards in Chapter 9.
Sprint review	During the sprint review, the scrum team regularly ensures that the product meets stakeholders' expectations. The sprint review also provides opportunities for stakeholders to discuss changes to the product to accommodate changing business needs. Both aspects of the sprint review help manage the risk of getting to the end of a project with the wrong product. Find out more about sprint reviews in Chapter 10.
Sprint retrospective	During the sprint retrospective, the scrum team discusses issues with the past sprint and identifies which of those issues may be risks in future sprints. The development team needs to determine ways to prevent those risks from becoming problems again. Find out more about sprint retrospectives in Chapter 10.

The artifacts and meetings discussed in this section systematically help agile teams manage risk on an agile project by addressing risk by the responsible roles at appropriate times. The larger and more complex the project, the higher the likelihood that an agile approach can eliminate the risk of failure.

5

Ensuring Agile Success

Build a foundation through organizational and individual commitment to becoming more agile.

Choose a project and create an environment that will optimize agile transition success.

Scale agile techniques across multi-team projects appropriately.

Become a change agent in your organization and help avoid common pitfalls in agile transitions.

Chapter **16**

Building a Foundation

To successfully move from traditional project management processes to agile processes, you must start with a good foundation. You need commitment, both from your organization and from people as individuals, and you need to find a good project team for your first agile project, providing them an environment conducive to agile approaches. You want to find the right training for your project team, and sustainably support your organization's agile approach so that it can grow beyond your first project.

In this chapter, we show you how to build a strong agile foundation within your organization.

Organizational and Individual Commitment

Commitment to agile project management means making an active, conscious effort to work with new methods and to abandon old habits. Commitment at both an individual level and at an organizational level is critical to agile transition success.

Without organizational support, even the most enthusiastic agile project team members may find themselves forced back into old project management processes. Without the commitment of individual project team members, a company that embraces agile approaches may encounter too much resistance, or even sabotage, to be able to become an agile organization.

The following sections provide details on how organizations and people can support an agile transition.

Organizational commitment

Organizational commitment plays a large role in agile transition. When a company and the groups in that company embrace agile principles, the transition can be easier for the project team members.

Organizations can commit to an agile transition by doing the following:

» Engaging an experienced agile expert to create a realistic transition plan and to guide the company through that plan

» Investing in employee training, starting with the members of the company's first agile project team and the leadership at all levels who support them

» Allowing scrum teams to abandon waterfall processes, meetings, and documents in favor of streamlined agile approaches

» Ensuring all scrum team members necessary for each agile project are dedicated: an empowered product owner, a cross-functional development team of multi-skilled people, and an influential servant-leader scrum master

» Encouraging development teams to continuously increase their skill sets

» Providing automated testing tools and a continuous integration framework

» Logistically supporting scrum team collocation

» Allowing scrum teams to manage themselves

» Giving the agile project team the time and freedom to go through a healthy trial-and-error process

» Revising employee performance reviews to emphasize team performance

» Encouraging agile project teams and celebrating successes

Organizational support is also important beyond the agile transition. Companies can ensure that agile processes continue to work by hiring with agile project teams in mind and by providing agile training to new employees. Organizations can also engage the ongoing support of an agile mentor, who can guide project teams as they encounter new and challenging situations.

Organizations, of course, are made up of individuals. Organizational commitment and individual commitment go hand in hand.

Individual commitment

Individual commitment has an equal role to organizational commitment in agile transitions. When each person on a project team works at adopting agile practices, the changes become easier for everyone on the project team.

People can individually commit to an agile transition by using these methods:

>> Attending training and conferences and being willing to learn about agile methods

>> Being open to change, willing to try new processes, and making an effort to adapt new habits

>> Resisting the temptation to fall back on old processes

>> Acting as a peer coach for project team members who are less experienced in agile techniques

>> Allowing themselves to make mistakes and learn from those mistakes

>> Reflecting on each sprint honestly in the sprint retrospective and committing to improvement efforts

>> Actively becoming multi-skilled development team members

>> Letting go of ego and working as a part of a team

>> Taking responsibility for successes and failures as a team

>> Taking the initiative to be self-managing

>> Being active and present throughout each agile project

Like organizational commitment, individual commitment is important beyond the agile transition period. The people on the first agile project team will become change agents throughout the company, setting the stage and exemplifying for other project teams how to effectively work with agile methods.

Getting commitment

Commitment to agile methods may not be instant. You'll need to help people in your organization overcome the natural impulse to resist change.

A good early step in an agile transition is to find an *agile champion,* a senior-level manager or executive who can help ensure organizational change. The fundamental process changes that accompany agile transitions require support from the people who make and enforce business decisions. A good agile champion will be able to rally the organization and its people around process changes.

Another important way to get commitment is to identify challenges with the organization's current projects and provide potential solutions with agile approaches. Agile project management can address many problems, including issues with product quality, customer satisfaction, team morale, budget and schedule overruns, funding, portfolio management, and overall project issues.

Finally, highlight some of agile project management's overall benefits. Some of the real and tangible benefits that drive shifts from traditional methods of project management to agile methods include the following:

>> **Happier customers:** Agile projects often have higher customer satisfaction because agile project teams produce working products quickly, can respond to change, and collaborate with customers as partners.

>> **Profit benefits:** Agile approaches allow project teams to deliver functionality to market quicker than with traditional approaches. Agile organizations can realize higher return on investment, often resulting in self-funded projects.

>> **Defect reduction:** Quality is a key part of agile approaches. Proactive quality measures, continuous integration and testing, and continuous improvement all contribute to higher-quality products.

>> **Improved morale:** Agile practices such as sustainable development and self-managing development teams can mean happier employees, improved efficiency, and less company turnover.

You can find more benefits of agile project management in Chapter 19.

Can you make the transition?

You've established many valuable reasons for moving to an agile approach, and your case looks good. But will your organization be able to make the transition? Here are some key questions to consider:

>> **What are the organizational roadblocks?** Does your organization have a value-delivery culture or a risk-management culture? Does it support coaching and mentorship alongside management? Is there support for training? How does the organization define success? Does it have an open culture that will embrace a high visibility of project progress?

>> **How are you doing business today?** How are projects planned at the macro level? Is the organization fixated on fixed scope? How engaged are business representatives? Do you outsource development?

>> **How do your teams work today, and what will need to shift under agile methods?** How ingrained is waterfall? Does the team have a strong command-and-control mentality? Can good ideas come from anywhere? Is there trust in the team? Are people shared across teams? What do you need to ask for to secure a shift? Can you get people, tools, space, and commitment to pilot the change?

>> **What are the regulatory challenges?** Are there processes and procedures that relate to regulatory requirements? Are these requirements imposed upon you from externally or internally adopted regulations and standards? Will you need to create additional documentation to satisfy regulatory requirements? Are you likely to be audited for compliance, and what would be the cost of noncompliance?

As you review your analysis of the roadblocks and challenges, you may uncover the following concerns:

>> **Agile approaches reveal that the organization needs to change.** As you compare agile practices and results with what you have done traditionally, you may reveal that performance has not been all it could have been. You need to tackle this head on. Your organization has been operating within a framework of how projects were expected to be run. Your organization has done its best to produce a result, often in the face of extreme challenges. For all parties involved, you have to acknowledge their efforts and introduce the potential of agile processes to allow them to produce yet greater results.

>> **Project management leaders may misinterpret agile techniques as insufficient.** Often the values and principles of the Agile Manifesto are misinterpreted to mean agile frameworks involve insufficient planning and documentation and attempt to disregard generally accepted project management standards. Experienced project managers may view some of that value slipping away in a transition to agile processes. Take every opportunity to clarify what agile values and principles support and do not support. Show how each principle addresses the same challenges that traditional project management attempts to resolve, and how agile techniques are an extension of project managers' capabilities and career, not as devaluing anything they've worked hard to secure.

>> **Moving from a leadership to a service model can be challenging.** Agile leaders are service oriented. Command and control gives way to facilitation. Servant leadership is a big shift for many project teams and functional managers. Demonstrate how the shift provides more effective outcomes for everyone. You can read more about servant leadership in Chapter 14.

Keep in mind that some resistance will arise; change can't happen without opposition. Be ready for resistance, but don't let it thwart your overall plan.

Timing the transition

Organizationally, you can start your initiative to move to an agile approach at any time. You might consider a few optimal times:

>> **When you need to prove that agile project management is necessary:** Use the end of a large project, when you can see clearly what did not work (for example, during a sunset review). You'll be able to demonstrate clearly the issues with waterfall, and you'll gain a springboard for piloting your first agile project.

>> **When your challenge is doing accurate budgeting:** Run your first agile project in the quarter before the start of the annual budget year (namely, one quarter before the end of the current budget cycle). You'll get metrics from your first project that will allow you to be more informed when planning next year's budget.

>> **When you're starting a new project:** Moving to agile processes when you have a new project lets you start fresh without the baggage of old approaches.

>> **When you're trying to reach a new market or industry:** Agile techniques allow you to deliver quick innovation to help your organization create products for new types of customers.

>> **When you have new leadership:** Management changes are great opportunities for setting new expectations with agile approaches.

Although you can take advantage of any of these opportunities to start using agile processes, they're not required. The best time to become more agile is . . . today!

Choosing the Right Pilot Team Members

Determining the right people to work with, especially in the early stages, is important to agile project success. Here are things to think about when choosing people for the different roles in your organization's first agile project.

The agile champion

At the beginning of an agile transition, the agile champion will be a key person in helping ensure the project team can succeed. This person should be able to effectively and quickly influence each level of the organization that affects the pilot agile teams' chances for success. A good agile champion should be able to do all these tasks:

- » Be passionate about agility and the organizational and market issues agile approaches will address.

- » Make decisions about company processes. If there is a status quo, the agile champion should be able to influence a change.

- » Get the organization excited about what's possible with agile processes.

- » Regularly and directly collaborate with and support the project team as it goes through the steps to establish agile processes.

- » Acquire the project team members necessary for success, both for the first project and in the long term.

- » Be an escalation point to remove unnecessary distractions and non-agile processes.

When choosing an agile champion, look for someone who has authority in the organization — whose voice is respected and who has led change initiatives successfully in the past.

The agile transition team

As important as the agile champion is, one person can't do everything. The agile champion should work together with other organizational leaders whom the agile project team relies on for support in the transition. Together, the agile transition team removes organizational impediments to ensure the success of the pilot team and future agile teams. The agile transition team should

- » Be committed to organizational success through the continuous support of pilot agile teams.

- » Establish a clear vision and roadmap for how the organization will become agile.

- » Be organized like a scrum team, with a product owner (agile champion), development team (leaders who can make organizational changes in support of the pilot scrum teams), and a scrum master (an organizational leader who can focus on helping the agile transition team adopt agile principles and enforce the rules of scrum).

- » Operate as a scrum team, holding all five scrum events and implementing all three scrum artifacts.

Figure 16-1 illustrates how the agile transition team's and pilot scrum team's sprint cadences are aligned. Impediments identified in the sprint retrospective of the pilot team become backlog items for the transition team to resolve as process improvements for the pilot team.

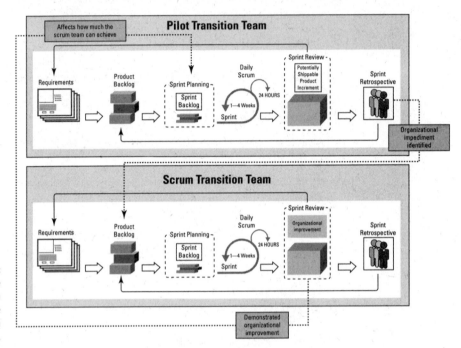

FIGURE 16-1:
Alignment of the agile transition team and the pilot scrum team cadences.

Not only does the agile transition team provide systematic support for the pilot scrum team, but the organizational leadership also becomes more agile by using scrum alongside the pilot team.

The product owner

With an agile champion and an agile transition team in place, the focus turns to pilot scrum teams. The pilot scrum team product owners should come from the business side of the organization, aligning the business with technology. During the first agile project, the product owner may need to acclimate to working on the project daily with the development team. A good product owner should

» Be decisive.

» Be an expert about customer requirements and business needs.

>> Have the business authority and be empowered to prioritize and reprioritize product requirements.

>> Be organized enough to manage ongoing changes to the product backlog.

>> Be committed to working with the rest of the scrum team and to being available to the development team daily throughout a project.

>> Have the ability to obtain project funding and other resources.

When choosing a product owner for your first agile project, find someone who can provide product expertise and commitment to the project.

The development team

On agile projects, the self-managing development team is central to the success of the project. The development team determines how to go about the work of creating the product. Good development team members should be able to do the following:

>> Be versatile.

>> Be willing to work cross-functionally.

>> Plan a sprint and self-manage around that plan.

>> Understand the product requirements and provide effort estimates.

>> Provide technical advice to the product owner so that he or she can understand the complexity of the requirements and make appropriate decisions.

>> Respond to circumstances and adjust processes, standards, and tools to optimize performance.

Intellectually curious developers, eager to learn new things and contribute to project goals in a variety of ways, are most likely to thrive in an agile environment. When choosing a development team for the pilot project, select people who are open to change, enjoy a challenge, like to be in the forefront of new developments, and are willing to do whatever it will take to ensure success, including learning and using new skills outside their existing skill set.

The scrum master

The scrum master on a company's first agile project may need to be more sensitive to potential development team distractions than on later projects. A good scrum master should

- » Have influence (clout).

- » Have enough organizational influence to remove outside distractions that prevent the project team from successfully using agile methods.

- » Know enough about agile project management to be able to help the project team uphold agile processes throughout a project.

- » Have the communication and facilitation skills to guide the development team in reaching consensus.

- » Trust enough to step back and allow the development team to organize and manage itself.

When determining the scrum master for a company's first agile project, you want to select someone who is willing to be a servant-leader. At the same time, the scrum master will need to have a strong enough temperament to help thwart distractions and uphold agile processes in the face of organizational and individual resistance.

The project stakeholders

On an organization's first agile project, good project stakeholders should

- » Be involved.

- » Defer to the product owner for final product decisions.

- » Attend sprint reviews and provide product feedback.

- » Understand agile processes. Sending project stakeholders to the same training as the rest of the project team will help them be more comfortable with new processes.

- » Receive project information in agile formats, such as sprint reviews, product backlogs, and sprint backlogs.

- » Provide details when the product owner and development team have questions.

- » Work collaboratively with the product owner and the rest of the project team.

The project stakeholders for your agile project should be trustworthy, cooperative, and active contributors to a project.

The agile mentor

An agile mentor, sometimes called an agile coach, is key to keeping teams and organizations on track while learning scrum and beginning to establish a more agile environment. A good agile mentor should

- **»** Be experienced.

- **»** Be an expert at agile processes, especially in the agile processes your organization chooses.

- **»** Be familiar with projects of different sizes, large and small.

- **»** Help teams self-manage, ask questions to help them learn for themselves, and provide useful advice and support without taking over a project.

- **»** Guide the project team through its first sprint at the beginning of the project and be available to answer questions as needed throughout the project.

- **»** Work with and relate to the product owner, the development team members, and the scrum master.

- **»** Be a person from outside a department or organization. Internal agile mentors often come from a company's project management group or center of excellence. If the agile mentor comes from inside the organization, he or she should be able to put aside political considerations when making suggestions and providing advice.

A number of organizations offer agile strategy, planning, and mentorship, including our company, Platinum Edge.

Creating an Environment That Enables Agility

When you're laying the foundation for adjusting your approach from traditional methods to agile methods, create an environment where agile projects can be successful and project teams can thrive. An agile environment refers to not only physical environments, such as the one we describe in Chapter 5, but also a good organizational environment. To create a good agile project environment, you should have the following:

- **»** **Good use of agile processes:** This may seem obvious, but using proven agile frameworks and techniques from the beginning. Use the Roadmap to Value in Figure 16-2, using scrum and the other key agile practices to increase your chances of success. Start with the basics; build on them only when the project and your knowledge progress. Progress for the sake of progress doesn't lead to perfection. Remember, practice doesn't make perfect; practice makes permanent. Start out correctly.

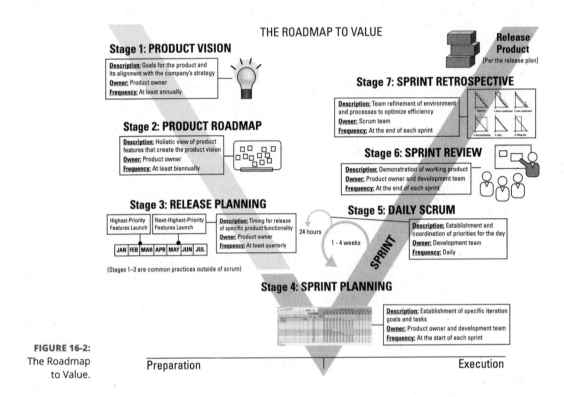

THE ROADMAP TO VALUE

Stage 1: PRODUCT VISION
Description: Goals for the product and its alignment with the company's strategy
Owner: Product owner
Frequency: At least annually

Release Product
[Per the release plan]

Stage 7: SPRINT RETROSPECTIVE
Description: Team refinement of environment and processes to optimize efficiency
Owner: Scrum team
Frequency: At the end of each sprint

Stage 2: PRODUCT ROADMAP
Description: Holistic view of product features that create the product vision
Owner: Product owner
Frequency: At least biannually

Stage 6: SPRINT REVIEW
Description: Demonstration of working product
Owner: Product owner and development team
Frequency: At the end of each sprint

Stage 3: RELEASE PLANNING
Highest-Priority Features Launch | Next-Highest-Priority Features Launch
Description: Timing for release of specific product functionality
Owner: Product owner
Frequency: At least quarterly
JAN FEB MAR APR MAY JUN JUL

(Stages 1–3 are common practices outside of scrum)

24 hours
1 - 4 weeks
SPRINT

Stage 5: DAILY SCRUM
Description: Establishment and coordination of priorities for the day
Owner: Development team
Frequency: Daily

Stage 4: SPRINT PLANNING
Description: Establishment of specific iteration goals and tasks
Owner: Product owner and development team
Frequency: At the start of each sprint

Preparation
Execution

FIGURE 16-2:
The Roadmap to Value.

>> **Unfettered transparency:** Be open about project status and upcoming process changes. People on the project team and throughout the organization should be privy to project details.

>> **Frequent inspection:** Use the regular feedback loop opportunities that scrum provides to see firsthand how the project is going.

>> **Immediate adaptation:** Follow up on inspection by making necessary changes for improvement throughout the project. Take opportunities to improve today; don't wait until the end of a release or the entire project.

>> **A dedicated scrum team:** Ideally, the product owner, development team, and scrum master will be fully allocated to the project.

>> **A collocated scrum team:** For best results, the product owner, development team, and scrum master should sit together, in the same area of the same office.

>> **A well-trained project team:** When the members of the project team work together to learn about agile values and principles and experiment with agile techniques, they have shared understanding and common expectations about where they're headed as an agile organization.

Luckily, many opportunities for training in agile processes are available. You can find formal certification programs as well as non-certification agile courses and workshops. Available agile certifications include the following:

>> From the Scrum Alliance:

- Certified ScrumMaster (CSM)

- Advanced Certified ScrumMaster (A-CSM)

- Certified Scrum Product Owner (CSPO)

- Advanced Certified Scrum Product Owner (A-CSPO)

- Certified Scrum Developer (CSD)

- Advanced Certified Scrum Developer (A-CSD)

- Certified Scrum Professional (CSP) for ScrumMasters (CSP-SM), Product Owners (CSP-PO), and Developers (CSP-D)

- Certified Team Coach (CTC)

- Certified Enterprise Coach (CEC)

- Certified Agile Leadership (CAL)

>> The Project Management Institute Agile Certified Practitioner (PMI-ACP) accreditation

>> From Scrum.org:

- Professional Scrum Master (PSM I, II, III)

- Professional Scrum Product Owner (PSPO I, II)

- Professional Scrum Developer (PSD)

>> From the International Consortium for Agile (ICAgile):

- Various tracks in agile coaching, engineering, training, business agility, delivery management, DevOps, enterprise, agility, and value management

>> Numerous university certificate programs

With a good environment, you have a good chance at success.

Support Agility Initially and Over Time

When you first launch into agile processes, give your agile transition every chance for success by paying attention to key success factors:

- » **Choose a good pilot.** Select a project that's important enough to get everyone's support. At the same time, set expectations: Although the project will produce measurable improvements, the results will be modest while the project team is learning new methods and will improve over time.

- » **Get an agile mentor.** Use a mentor or coach to increase your chances of setting up a good agile environment and maximizing your chances of great performance.

- » **Communicate — a lot.** Keep talking about agile processes at every level of the organization. Use your agile champion to encourage progress through the pilot and toward more extensive agile adaptation.

- » **Prepare to move forward.** Keep thinking ahead. Consider how you'll take the lessons from the pilot to new projects and teams. Also think about how you'll scale from a single project to many projects, including those with multiple teams.

Chapter **17**

Scaling across Agile Teams

Depending on the schedule, scope, and required skills, many small and medium-sized projects can be accomplished with a single scrum team. Larger projects, however, may require more than one scrum team to achieve the product vision and release goals in a reasonable go-to-market time frame. When more than one scrum team is required, the teams need effective inter-team collaboration, communication, and synchronization — they need to be agile at scale. Regardless of project size, if interdependencies exist between multiple teams working together on the same project, or even across a collection of projects, you may need to scale.

TIP

Scale only if you have to. Even though you may have the talent and resources available to deploy multiple teams on your project, multiple teams don't automatically ensure higher quality and faster time to market. Always look for ways to implement the tenth agile principle, "Simplicity — the art of maximizing the amount of work not done — is essential." Less is more.

As an agile framework, scrum helps teams organize their work and expose progress effectively, whether your project comprises one scrum team or one thousand scrum teams. Scaling brings new challenges, however, so you want to implement techniques for coordination and collaboration across teams that not only support agile values and principles, but also address the specific challenges facing your project and organization.

In this chapter, we discuss some of the issues to address when you need multiple teams on an agile project. We also provide overviews of some common agile scaling frameworks and approaches that address the challenges of scaling.

Multi-Team Agile Projects

Organizations determine the need for multiple scrum teams when the product backlog and release plan require a faster speed of development than a single scrum team can achieve.

With agile projects, cross-functional teams work together during every sprint of the project, doing the same types of work each sprint and implementing requirements from the product backlog into completed, working, shippable functionality. When multiple teams work from the same product backlog, however, you have new challenges to address.

Common challenges with more than one scrum team working on the same project include the following:

>> **Project planning:** Agile planning is collaborative, from the beginning. Collaboration for large groups is different than for single scrum teams. Establishing a vision with the broader project team (all scrum teams and stakeholders) and building a product roadmap and product backlog with collaborative input from all parties involved requires a different approach than with single-team projects.

>> **Release planning:** Similar to the challenge of project planning, releases involve more specific planning of scope and release timing. Coordinating who will work on what and when throughout the release cycle is even more critical to ensure that dependencies, scope gaps, and talent allocation match the needs across the project.

>> **Decomposition:** To break down larger requirements in the same backlog, multiple teams may need to be involved in research and refinement discussions and activities. Who initiates these discussions? Who facilitates?

>> **Sprint planning:** Although not the last opportunity to coordinate planning and execution between scrum teams, sprint planning is when scrum teams lock in a certain amount of scope from the product backlog to execute. At this stage, dependencies between scrum teams become reality. If the preceding

activities of developing the product roadmap and release plan have not exposed dependencies, what are some ways scrum teams can expose and address them at sprint planning?

>> **Daily coordination:** Even after effective planning and collaboration from project initiation through sprint planning, scrum teams can and should collaborate each day. Who participates and what can be done while teams are in execution mode?

>> **Sprint review:** With so many teams demonstrating their product increments and seeking feedback, how can stakeholders participate with their limited schedules? How can product owners update the product backlog with all that was learned across multiple scrum teams? How do development teams know what was accomplished by other development teams?

>> **Sprint retrospective:** Multiple scrum teams working together make up a broader project team. How do they identify opportunities for improvement and implement those improvements across the program?

>> **Integration:** All product increments need to work together in an integrated environment. Who does the integration? Who provides the infrastructure to the teams? Who ensures the integrations work?

>> **Architecture decisions:** Who oversees the architecture and technical standards? How can these decisions be decentralized to enable teams to be self-organizing and work as autonomously as possible?

These are some examples; you might be able to identify others based on your experience. Whatever your situation, select solutions to your scaling challenges that address your specific challenge.

TIP

Some scaling frameworks offer solutions to challenges you may not have. Be careful not to bloat your framework fixing things that are not broken.

REMEMBER

Throughout this chapter, we refer to products, projects, programs, and portfolios. In general, a *product* is a set of features that provide some sort of value or usefulness to a customer. A *project* is a planned set of work that requires time, effort, and planning to complete. It has a distinct start and end. A *program* is a collection of projects with an affinity to each other (addressing a certain market segment or rolling into the same product). A *portfolio* is a collection of programs and projects used to meet specific strategic business objectives. The projects or programs of the portfolio may not be directly related to each other but are grouped to facilitate management of the work.

Since the first scrum teams in the mid-1990s, there have been agile projects requiring multiple scrum teams collaborating effectively together. Following are overviews of various scaling frameworks and techniques addressing many of these challenges.

Making Work Digestible through Vertical Slicing

One of the simplest scaling approaches is known as vertical slicing, which provides a straightforward solution for dividing the work across teams so they can incrementally deliver and integrate functionality at every sprint. If your scaling challenge is breaking down the work across teams, vertical slicing is the solution.

REMEMBER

The concept of vertical slicing applies to single team projects, too. Development teams consist of people who collectively possess all skills required to turn a requirement into completed, shippable functionality. The development team swarms on one requirement at a time, which is a vertical slice of the product backlog, potentially touching all aspects of the technology and skills required.

With *vertical slicing,* multiple scrum teams work in synchronized sprints of the same length on a *vertical slice* — a separate portion or module of the overall product — and then those modules are integrated by an integration scrum team after each sprint. The integration scrum team lags the development scrum teams by one sprint and is its own scrum team, with a dedicated product owner, development team members, and scrum master.

Figure 17-1 illustrates how a product backlog is sliced into specific requirements for each scrum team. Then, at the end of each sprint, the individual teams implement working functionality that can be integrated with other working functionality in the broader set of product features. Each individual team's features feed into an integration team's backlog (the scrum team directly above it in the illustration) for architectural and system-level coordination.

The number of integration scrum team levels required depends on the complexity of each project. The figure shows you four levels that a suite of features in Microsoft Office might logically require. (We use Microsoft as an example because it is familiar to most people.)

REMEMBER

Each *integration scrum team* handles all system-level development work for the integration of functionality produced by the teams that feed into it, and provides architectural oversight to unify the individual scrum teams.

With Microsoft Office as an illustration:

>> A single scrum team develops the functionality for the Email feature "compose/transmit messages" (requirement ID 1.1.1.1).

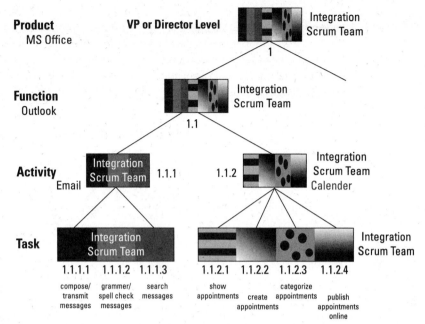

Product
MS Office

VP or Director Level | Integration Scrum Team
1

Function
Outlook

Integration Scrum Team
1.1

Activity
Email

Integration Scrum Team 1.1.1   1.1.2 | Integration Scrum Team Calender

Task

Integration Scrum Team | Integration Scrum Team

1.1.1.1   1.1.1.2   1.1.1.3   1.1.2.1   1.1.2.2   1.1.2.3   1.1.2.4

compose/   grammer/   search   show   categorize
transmit   spell check messages   appointments create appointments publish
messages   messages   appointments   appointments
                                                                             online

FIGURE 17-1: Scrum teams working on vertical slices of product features, using Microsoft Office as an example.

>> A different scrum team develops the functionality for "grammar/spell check messages" (1.1.1.2).

>> A third scrum team develops the functionality for "search messages" (1.1.1.3).

>> The integration scrum team (at the Activity level) does the development work to integrate the functionality from these three scrum teams' functionality into a package (1.1.1) that the Email integration team can integrate into the entire Email module.

>> The Outlook integration team then takes the Email modules, along with the Calendar, Contacts, and other modules, to integrate them into an Outlook package (1.1) that can then be integrated by the MS Office integration team into the entire MS Office suite (1).

In this example, integration teams operate as separate scrum teams, with dedicated team members for each role.

Scrum of scrums

How do these different scrum teams coordinate with each other daily? The *scrum of scrums* model facilitates effective integration, coordination, and collaboration among scrum teams using vertical slicing. Almost all scaling frameworks we show you in this chapter use scrum of scrums to enable daily coordination between scrum teams.

Figure 17-2 illustrates each role of each team coordinating daily with people of the same role in other teams regarding priorities, dependencies, and impediments that affect the broader program team. The scrum of scrums for each role is facilitated by the integration-level person for each role. Thorough integration and release efforts establish a consistent and regular scrum of scrums model.

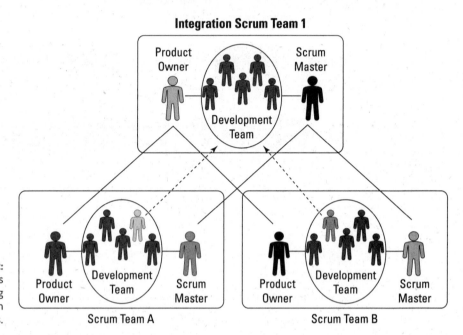

FIGURE 17-2:
Scrum of scrums
for coordinating
between scrum
teams.

Each day, individual scrum teams hold their own daily scrums at approximately the same time, in separate locations. Following these daily scrums, the scrum of scrums meetings described next occur.

Product owner scrum of scrums

Each day, following the individual scrum teams' daily scrums, the product owners from each scrum team meet with the integration team product owner for no longer than 15 minutes. They address the requirements being completed and make any adjustments based on the realities uncovered during the individual scrum team's daily scrum. Each product owner addresses the following:

>> The business requirements that each has accepted or rejected since the last time they met

>> The requirements that should be accepted by the time they meet again

>> Which requirements are impeded and need help from other teams to resolve (such as "John, we won't be able to do requirement 123 until you complete requirement xyz from your current sprint backlog.")

The integration team product owner makes the cross-team prioritization decisions necessary to ensure that the impediments are addressed during the daily scrum of scrums.

Development team scrum of scrums

Each day following the individual scrum teams' daily scrums, one development team member representative from each scrum team attends the integration team's daily scrum (which is the scrum of scrums for developers) and participates with the integration development team members in discussing the following:

>> Their team's accomplishments since the last time they met

>> Their team's planned accomplishments between now and the next meeting

>> Technical concerns with which they need help

>> Technical direction decisions that the team has made and what anyone should be aware of to prevent potential issues

TIP

Consider rotating development team members from the individual scrum teams who attend the scrum of scrums (integration team's daily scrum), either daily or for each sprint, to ensure that everyone stays tuned in to the integration efforts of the portfolio.

Scrum master scrum of scrums

The scrum masters from each scrum team also meet with the integration scrum team scrum master for no longer than 15 minutes to address the impediments that each team is dealing with. Each scrum master addresses the following:

>> The individual team-level impediments resolved since the last time they met and how they were resolved, in case other scrum masters run into the issue

>> New impediments identified since last time they met and any unresolved impediments

>> Which impediments they need help resolving

>> Potential impediments that everyone should be aware of

The integration team scrum master then makes sure that escalated impediments are addressed after the daily scrum of scrums.

With vertical slicing, a single product backlog exists, and team attributes are assigned to those requirements as they are broken down and move to the development scrum team. With this model, you can see the overall program and also quickly filter down to your own team's piece of that overall program.

A common question is "Who is responsible for architecture in a vertically sliced program?" The answer is that it depends on which modules will be affected by the decision.

Your organization should have existing architectural standards, coding standards, and style guides. This way, each team doesn't have to reinvent the wheel.

Consider an architectural decision that needs to be made and that will affect only module A. The development team of module A would make that decision. If it were going to affect multiple teams, the development team at the integration level that all affected teams roll into would make that decision. That integration level might be one level up or four levels up.

Using Figure 17-2 as an example, an architectural decision affecting two of the Email module teams (1.1.1.2 and 1.1.1.3) would be made by the Email integration team (1.1.1). A decision affecting the search messages Email module team (1.1.1.3) and the Calendar integration scrum team (1.1.2) would be made by the Outlook integration scrum team (1.1).

Vertical slicing is a simple way to maintain the autonomy of each scrum team to deliver valuable functionality within a wider program context. It is also effective at helping teams have timely and relevant conversations about constraints and progress.

Aligning through Roles with Scrum at Scale

Agile scaling models vary in complexity and simplicity. The Scrum at Scale approach for two or hundreds of scrum teams working together is a form of basic scrum of scrums model for scrum masters and product owners coordinating communication, impediment removal, priorities, requirement refinement, and planning. Using a scrum of scrums model for the scrum master and product owner roles is how this daily synchronization occurs between teams across programs of varying sizes.

Scaling the scrum master

Following the vertical slicing model of scrum of scrums, Scrum at Scale groups five scrum masters into a scrum master scrum of scrums. It mirrors the daily scrum for individual scrum teams to surface and remove impediments. With Scrum at Scale, narrowing the scope of a scrum of scrums to five scrum masters from each of five scrum teams limits the communication complexities for effective cross-team collaboration on what the scrum teams are working on and how their work might be affecting each other. A scrum master scrum of scrums coordinates release activities as the release team.

Figure 17-3 illustrates the Scrum at Scale scrum of scrums model.

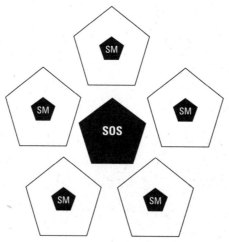

FIGURE 17-3:
Scrum at Scale scrum of scrums model.

With projects of more than five scrum teams, Scrum at Scale implements a scrum of scrums of scrums, where a representative of each scrum master scrum of scrums attends with four other scrum of scrums representatives to surface and remove impediments at the scrum of scrums of scrums level.

Figure 17-4 illustrates the Scrum at Scale scrum of scrums of scrums model.

When a project has more than 25 teams, an executive action team (EAT) supports a third-level scrum of scrums of scrums to remove the organizational impediments the scrum of scrums groups cannot remove themselves.

Figure 17-5 illustrates the Scrum at Scale third-level scrum of scrums of scrums model with an executive action team (EAT).

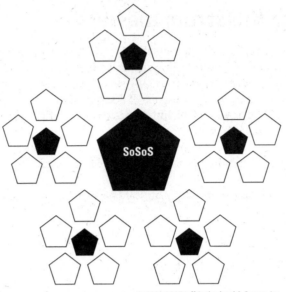

© 1993-2017 Jeff Sutherland & Scrum, Inc.

FIGURE 17-4:
Scrum at Scale
scrum of scrums
of scrums model.

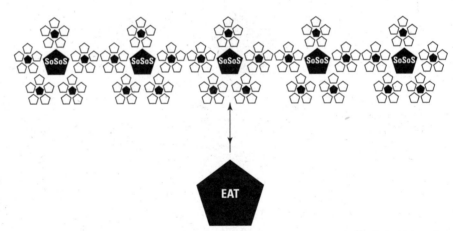

FIGURE 17-5:
Scrum at Scale
third-level scrum
of scrums of
scrums model
with executive
action team (EAT).

© 1993-2017 Jeff Sutherland & Scrum, Inc.

Scaling the product owner

The product owners organize in a similar and aligned way, only instead of labeling them as scrum of scrums, they are meta scrums. A first-level meta scrum brings five product owners together for meta scrum meetings to refine and plan priorities. Each meta scrum has a chief product owner (CPO) who oversees the bigger picture of the vision and product backlog and facilitates the coordination between product owners in the meta scrum.

Figure 17-6 illustrates the Scrum at Scale meta scrum for product owners.

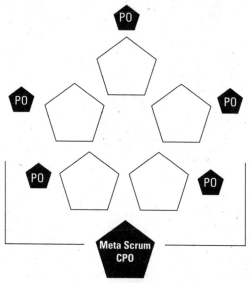

© 1993-2017 Jeff Sutherland & Scrum, Inc.

FIGURE 17-6: Scrum at Scale meta scrum for product owners.

At the second- and third-level meta scrums, the grouping aligns with that of the scrum master scrum of scrums of scrums. An executive meta scrum (EMS) supports the meta scrums by owning and communicating the organization-wide vision, taking in technical priority feedback from the meta scrums and providing overall priority decisions for the program.

Figure 17-7 illustrates the Scrum at Scale third-level meta scrums model with executive meta scrum (EMS).

Figure 17-8 illustrates the aligned grouping of Scrum at Scale's third-level scrum of scrums of scrums and meta scrums model with executive action team (EAT) and executive meta scrum (EMS).

A meta scrum should be a synchronization meeting that includes stakeholders. All stakeholders at the CPO level should be present to ensure alignment across the organization and support of the CPO's product backlog prioritization during every sprint.

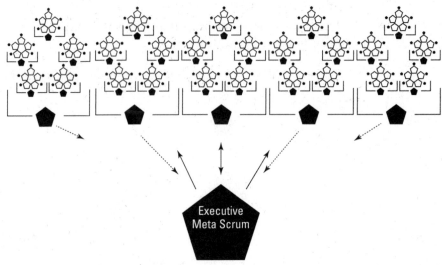

FIGURE 17-7:
Scrum at Scale third-level meta scrum model with executive meta scrum (EMS).

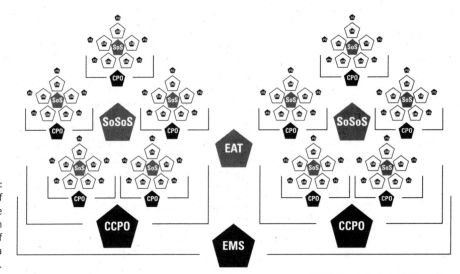

FIGURE 17-8:
Alignment of Scrum at Scale third-level scrum of scrums and meta scrums.

Synchronizing in one hour a day

In an hour or less per day, an entire organization can align priorities for the day and accomplish effective coordination of impediment removal. For instance, at 8:00 a.m., each individual scrum team holds their daily scrums separately. At 8:45 a.m., the scrum masters hold their scrum of scrums and the product owners hold their level-one meta scrum meetings. At 9:00 a.m., scrum masters meet in scrum of scrums of scrums, and the product owners meet in level-two meta scrums. Finally, at 9:15 a.m., the scrum master scrum of scrums of scrums meets with the EAT and the product owner meta scrum representatives meets with the EMS.

Multi-Team Coordination with LeSS

Large-scale scrum (LeSS) is another way to scale scrum across massive projects. *LeSS* is based on principles that support keeping scrum simple when putting multiple scrum teams together to work on the same product backlog. LeSS focuses more on how scrum teams work together than on organizational structures. It also presents a variety of options for addressing each scaling challenge. In this section, we present an overview and then cover a few options that stand out.

LeSS defines two framework sizes: LeSS and LeSS Huge. The difference lies in the size of the total teams involved.

LeSS, the smaller framework

Figure 17-9 illustrates the basic LeSS framework, using three scrum teams as an example. LeSS recommends no more than eight scrum teams follow the basic model.

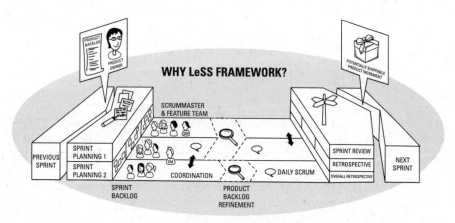

FIGURE 17-9: Basic LeSS framework.

Used with permission, Craig Larman and Bas Vodde.

LeSS outlines how scrum teams work together one sprint at a time, starting with sprint planning, followed by sprint execution and daily scrums, and ending with sprint review and sprint planning. Although much of LeSS remains true to the scrum framework, the following significant differences exist:

REMEMBER

>> In LeSS, scrum masters typically work with one to three teams, and there is only one product owner for up to eight teams.

We strongly recommend dedicating product owners and scrum masters to each scrum team to ensure that development teams have immediate, direct access to business decisions and clarifications and fast impediment resolution, so they can keep moving without interruption.

>> Sprint planning (Part 1) does not require all developers to attend, but at least two members per scrum team, along with the product owner, attend. The representative team members then go back and share their information with their teams.

>> Independent sprint planning (Part 2) and daily scrum meetings occur, and members from different teams can attend each other's meeting to facilitate information sharing.

>> Sprint reviews are usually combined across all teams.

>> Overall sprint retrospectives are held in addition to individual team retrospectives. Scrum masters, product owners, and representatives from development teams inspect and adapt the overall system of the project, such as processes, tools, and communication.

LeSS Huge framework

With LeSS Huge, a few thousand people could work on one project. But the structure remains simple.

The scrum teams are grouped around major areas of customer requirements, called requirement areas. This grouping might be similar to the group of teams who work together under an integration team in vertical slicing.

For each area, you have one area product owner and between four and eight scrum teams (a minimum of four teams in each requirement area prevents too much local optimization and complexity). One overall product owner works with several area product owners, forming a product owner team for the project. Figure 17-10 illustrates LeSS Huge.

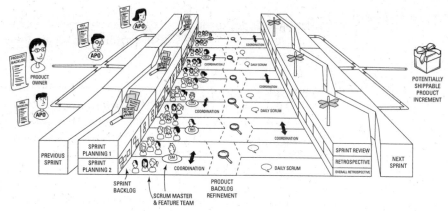

FIGURE 17-10:
The LeSS Huge
framework.

Used with permission, Craig Larman and Bas Vodde.

As in scrum at a single team level, as well as in basic LeSS, you have one product backlog, one definition of done, one potentially shippable product increment, one (area) product owner, and one sprint cadence across teams. LeSS Huge is simply a stacking of multiple smaller LeSS implementations for each requirement area.

To enable these teams to work together effectively across the requirement areas

>> The area PO regularly coordinates with each product owner.

>> Requirement areas are added to the product backlog to identify who is planning to work on which parts of the product.

>> A set of parallel sprint meetings is needed per requirement area. Overall sprint reviews and retrospectives involving all teams are necessary to enable continuous inspection and adaptation beyond single teams. These multi-team events help coordinate the overall work and process across the program.

With the exception of limiting opportunities for developers to work closely with business people (the product owner) on a daily basis, LeSS provides a simple way for scaling scrum across projects. We also find the flexibility of coordination techniques suggested in LeSS to be effective for teams addressing their specific multi-team coordination challenges. In addition to a scrum of scrums (discussed earlier in this chapter) and continuous integration (see Chapter 4), LeSS suggests several options for scrum teams coordinating with other scrum teams, as described in the following sections.

Sprint review bazaar

Multiple teams work toward the same product increment in each sprint, so all teams have something to demonstrate, and all teams need stakeholder feedback for updating their portion of the product backlog. Because all scrum teams are on the same cadence, even a LeSS basic organization would involve a lot of sprint review meetings for stakeholders to attend on the same day.

LeSS recommends a diverge-converge pattern to the sprint review, similar to a science fair or bazaar format. Each scrum team sets up in one part of a room large enough to accommodate all scrum teams. Each scrum team demonstrates what it did during the sprint, collecting feedback from the stakeholders visiting its area. Stakeholders visit their areas of interest. Scrum teams may loop through their demonstrations a few times to accommodate stakeholders visiting multiple teams. This approach also allows scrum team members to see demonstrations of other scrum teams. Note that combined sprint reviews can be held in other ways.

Combining sprint reviews increases transparency and collaboration culture across scrum teams.

Observers at the daily scrum

Although daily scrums are conducted so that the scrum team can coordinate their work for the day, anyone is invited to listen. Transparency is key for agility. The scrum of scrums model described previously in this chapter is a participatory model — developers attending the integration scrum team daily scrum participate in the discussion. However, sometimes other scrum team members just need to be aware of what other teams are doing.

A representative of the development team from one team may attend the daily scrum of another team, observe, and then report back to his or her own team to determine any action to take. This can be a non-disruptive way for other scrum teams to be involved without extra meeting time overhead.

Component communities and mentors

LeSS takes a vertical slicing approach also to dividing up the product backlog across teams, so multiple teams may "touch" the same system or technology components. For instance, multiple teams may work in a common database, user interface, or automated testing suite. Setting up communities of practice (CoP) around these areas gives these people a chance to collaborate informally on the component areas where they spend most of their time.

CoPs are usually organized by someone from one of the scrum teams who has the knowledge and experience to teach people how the component works, monitor the component long-term, and engage the community in regular discussions, work-shops, and reviews of work being done in the component area.

Multi-team meetings

Similar to the combined sprint review model, LeSS scrum teams may benefit from meeting together for other scrum planning events and activities. Product backlog refinement, sprint planning part two, and other design workshops are some examples. LeSS recommends similar formats for each situation, common elements of which include the following:

>> An overall session first, shared among all teams, to identify which teams are likely to take on which product backlog items.

>> Representatives of each team attend overall sessions (all can attend, but attendance is not required).

>> Team-level sessions follow overall sessions to dive into details.

>> Multi-team breakouts follow overall session, as needed, with just those teams involved.

The key to these sessions is that they are face to face, in the same room, allowing for real-time collaboration to break down dependencies. For distributed LeSS groups (one team in one geographic location and other teams in other locations), videoconferencing is key.

Travelers

The more versatile your development team, the fewer bottlenecks your scrum team will experience. Traditional organizations have specialists in technical areas, and there are not enough of them to go around to all the scrum teams when starting an agile transition. To begin bridging skill gaps across teams, technical experts can become travelers, joining scrum teams to coach and mentor in their area of expertise through pairing (see Chapter 4), workshops, and teaching sessions.

As this expertise is shared, the expert mentor continues to lead and grow the skills across the organization (as a CoP organizer). In addition, scrum teams increase their cross-functionality and can develop more efficiently.

Reducing Dependencies with Nexus

Dependencies between teams working on the same product impede the kind of productivity single scrum teams usually experience without those dependencies. *Nexus* is a scaling framework focused on treating multiple teams as a single unit. Reduction of inter-team dependencies is key to scaling success.

Inter-team dependencies usually revolve around how teams structure requirements and the product backlog, the domain knowledge differences between teams, and the software and test artifacts. Mapping requirements, team members' knowledge, and test artifacts to the same scrum teams reduces dependencies.

Nexus is a framework that describes how three to nine scrum teams — a *Nexus* — work together on the same product backlog, and under the guidance of a single product owner, to deliver potentially shippable functionality to every sprint.

Figure 17-11 illustrates the Nexus framework.

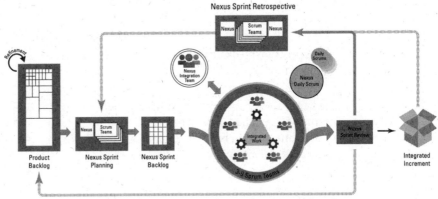

FIGURE 17-11: The Nexus framework.

In addition to scrum roles, artifacts, and events, Nexus introduces one new role, three new artifacts, and five new events to support the larger group of scrum teams operating together.

Nexus helps scrum teams working on the same product identify and resolve dependencies quickly and early, enabling each scrum team to move forward in their work unblocked and unimpeded. Inter-team dependencies are often created when product backlog items are not sufficiently refined, or not broken down into relatively independent items that can be worked on by a single scrum team. Dependencies can also arise from differences in technical skills or domain knowledge between teams. Joint product backlog refinement helps teams identify dependencies and minimize them before they cause conflict.

Nexus role — Nexus integration team

Similar to the vertical slicing model's integration team concept, the Nexus integration team ensures that an integrated product increment is produced at least every sprint for the Nexus. The scrum teams do the work, but the Nexus integration team remains accountable for the integrated product as a whole.

The Nexus integration team's activities may include developing tools and practices that will help with integration or serving as coaches and consultants to help with coordination. To accomplish these activities, Nexus integration team members must have a teaching mindset. Their roles are to help expose issues that need to be solved at the Nexus level, and to help the scrum teams solve the issues.

The Nexus integration team consists of people from the member scrum teams of the Nexus. It is a scrum team that consists of the following:

>> The **product owner** is accountable for ordering and refining the Nexus product backlog so that maximum value is derived from the work created by the Nexus each sprint. The product owner's role does not change from scrum; the scope of the work is simply more complex.

>> **Development team members** are usually also members of scrum teams in the Nexus. The priority for the Nexus integration development team members is the Nexus integration team over the individual scrum teams, with the integrated product increment being the prime goal for each sprint. Over time, the members of the Nexus integration team may change depending on specific integration needs over the life of the project.

REMEMBER

Dedicating scrum team members to one team eliminates the overhead of frequent cognitive demobilization and remobilization due to context switching. Always be aware of the risks of splitting the focus of team members across multiple teams.

>> The **scrum master** has overall responsibility for ensuring the Nexus framework is enacted and understood. This Nexus integration team scrum master may also be a scrum master in one or more of the other scrum teams in the Nexus.

As a last resort, the Nexus integration team members may pull items from the product backlog to implement them as a scrum team, but they undertake this emergency mode behavior only when all other options have been exhausted and the scrum teams are not capable of producing an integrated product increment. As the term *emergency mode* suggests, this situation is highly unusual, highly undesirable, and not sustainable. It is undertaken only when it is the only way to help the scrum teams get back on track.

Nexus artifacts

Three additional artifacts provide transparency at the Nexus level for inspection and adaptation:

>> **Nexus goal:** Although the sprint goal is not a separate artifact in scrum, a Nexus sprint goal is explicitly called out. Having a clear, visible, common purpose for all scrum teams in the Nexus is key to keeping all teams in sync throughout the sprint, working toward the integrated product increment.

>> **Nexus sprint backlog:** Each scrum team has its own sprint backlog of implementation and integration tasks. The Nexus sprint backlog is not an aggregation of these sprint backlogs; it exists to expose and map inter-team dependencies and how work is flowing across all scrum teams in the Nexus. The Nexus sprint backlog is updated daily as part of the Nexus daily scrum.

>> **Integrated increment:** All integrated work completed by all the scrum teams in the Nexus during the sprint is the integrated increment. It meets the definition of done for usable, potentially shippable functionality.

Nexus events

Five additional events enhance inter-team coordination of dependencies at the Nexus level.

Nexus sprint planning

During Nexus sprint planning, the product owner provides priority and business context for the sprint, and sets the sprint goal. The individual scrum teams select work for the sprint while highlighting and minimizing dependencies. Each scrum team then holds its own sprint planning to plan the execution of the work it has pulled from the Nexus sprint backlog. Nexus sprint planning concludes when the last scrum team is finished with its individual sprint planning.

Nexus daily scrum

Nexus does not prescribe who should attend the daily scrum — the right people are members of individual scrums teams who understand how their work may affect, or be affected by, the work of other scrum teams. The questions addressed are similar to a single scrum team's daily scrum but focused on cross-team integration, including the following:

>> Did yesterday's work get successfully integrated?

>> What new dependencies have been discovered?

>> What information needs to be shared across teams?

The Nexus daily scrum is held before each scrum team holds its own daily scrum to provide the scrum teams with input to better help them plan their day's work.

Nexus sprint review

Similar to other scaling frameworks, the Nexus sprint review can replace individual scrum team sprint reviews, because the focus is the integrated increment. You can use a variety of techniques for conducting the meeting to maximize stakeholder feedback, but none are prescribed. Techniques suggested in this chapter can be utilized.

Nexus sprint retrospective

The Nexus sprint retrospective is a formal opportunity to improve the way the Nexus works through inspection and adaption. The Nexus sprint retrospective includes three parts:

>> Representatives from Nexus scrum teams meet to identify cross-team issues and make them transparent across the Nexus.

>> Individual scrum teams hold their own sprint retrospectives.

>> Representatives from the scrum teams meet again to decide what to do to resolve Nexus-wide issues.

Refinement

A Nexus uses refinement to decompose product backlog items so they can be developed as independently as possible by a scrum team. In addition to the general process of progressively elaborating requirements we show you in Chapter 7, the Nexus process for refining them includes the following:

>> Breaking product backlog items down enough to understand which scrum teams might be able to implement them

>> Identifying and visualizing dependencies between product backlog items

Nexus is a lightweight framework, focused on extending scrum's empirical approach to products whose development requires more than one scrum team.

Joint Program Planning with SAFe

Scaled Agile Framework (SAFe) is used to scale scrum and agile principles across multiple layers of an IT and software or systems development organization. SAFe addresses scaling at four levels: portfolio, large solutions, program, and team. Figure 17-12 shows the full SAFe 4.5 big picture.

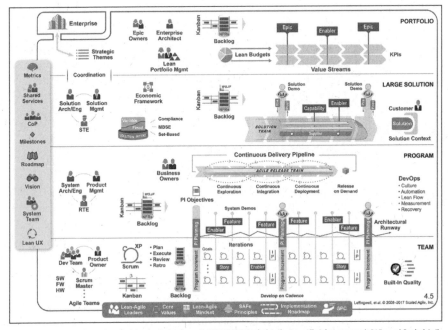

FIGURE 17-12: SAFe 4.5 for lean software and systems engineering.

Reproduced with permission from © 2011-2017 Scaled Agile, Inc. All rights reserved. SAFe and Scaled Agile Framework are registered trademarks of Scaled Agile, Inc.

SAFe has four configurations, utilizing combinations of the four SAFe levels. Full SAFe (refer to Figure 17-12) contains all levels (portfolio, large solution, program, and team). Essential SAFe, shown in Figure 17-13, is a basic starting point for smaller organizations and consists of only the program and team levels. Portfolio SAFe adds the portfolio level to essential SAFe, and is for organizations that have smaller programs within a portfolio. Large solution SAFe adds the large solution level to essential SAFe and is aimed at organizations that are building large solutions that require hundreds of people, but do not require portfolio coordination.

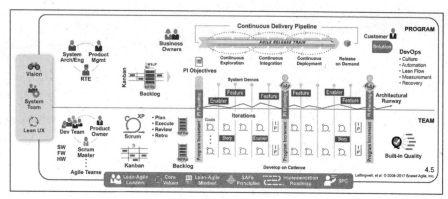

FIGURE 17-13:
Essential SAFe
configuration.

SAFe is underscored by a set of core values, a lean–agile mindset, and the agile values and principles in the Agile Manifesto. Although other scaling frameworks have tactical differences, they also have many similarities, such as the following:

>> Development is done in agile teams.

>> The teams are aligned in sprint length and cadence.

>> A scrum of scrums coordinates at the program level.

We don't go into all details of SAFe here, but we do provide a general overview and highlight a few practices that address some of the scaling challenges discussed previously in this chapter.

Understanding the four SAFe levels

In SAFe, you find up to four prescribed levels of integration and coordination, each aimed at decentralizing decisions to the lower levels. We emphasize *up to four* because not all organizations require all levels, such as the large solution level.

WARNING

Frameworks provide flexibility over rigidity. Although SAFe provides a detailed visualization at all levels of the portfolio organization, avoid implementing structures that are unnecessary for your situation.

The four levels — portfolio, large solution, program, and team — are described next.

Portfolio level

At the *portfolio level,* the vision and roadmap for the entire portfolio are established. Strategic themes are developed to support the vision. Budget, business objectives, and enterprise architecture governance are managed. The portfolio is organized in value streams that align the organization to the value delivered.

SAFe defines a *value stream* as the sequence of steps to deliver value to the customer, from concept to delivery or receipt of payment. It includes the people who do the work, systems, and the flow of materials.

Three portfolio-level roles drive portfolio decisions:

>> **Lean portfolio management (LPM):** This role aligns strategy and execution by communicating strategic themes to the portfolio, establishing value streams, and allocating budgets. LPM is responsible for strategy, investment funding, agile program guidance, and lean governance of the entire portfolio. (Learn more about lean in Chapter 4.) LPM collaborates with many groups across all levels of the organization.

>> **Epic owner:** Epics are introduced in Chapter 8, although SAFe uses a different feature-epic relationship. In SAFe, *epics* are the largest and most long-term initiatives and drive the business value for the organization. They are broken down into features, or capabilities, which are then broken down into user stories that can be executed by single development teams at the team level. Epic owners work with solutions management and product management at the large solution and program levels, and with agile teams at the team level.

>> **Enterprise architect:** The enterprise architect establishes a common technical vision and drives the holistic approach to technology across programs through continuous feedback, collaboration, and adaptive engineering design and engineering practices.

The portfolio backlog in SAFe consists of both business and enabler epics. Enablers are requirements for extending architectural capabilities to support future business functionality. LPM guides the flow of large initiatives using kanban. (Learn more about kanban in Chapter 4.)

Large solution level

The *large solution level* hosts the solution train, which is an organizational construct for coordination of multiple agile release trains (ARTs), defined next in the "Program level" section. The large solution level is for organizations building solutions that require more than 125 people.

Solution trains are coordinated by three roles, similar to the program-level roles, which are all described in the next section, "Program level."

Program level

In line with the portfolio vision and backlog, *programs* establish a vision and road-map to define the outer boundary of their scope of work, focused on selected epics from the portfolio backlog.

At the program level, release and product management occur. This level uses the *agile release train (ART) model*, which is a team of multiple agile teams (50–125 people in total) delivering incremental releases of value. The "train" departs the station on a reliable schedule and features can be loaded onto the train if ready. The ART provides a fixed cadence with which the teams of the program align and synchronize. The rest of the organization, knowing this cadence, can also reliably plan its work around this known release schedule.

If organized at the large solution level, three roles provide coordination for the ARTs in each respective value stream: solution train engineer (STE), solution management, and solution architect/engineer.

Without the large solution level, ARTs are driven by a release train engineer (RTE), product management, and a system architect/engineer. ART roles and solution train roles are similar, so we explain them together:

>> **Release train engineer (or solution train engineer):** ARTs are generally self-organizing, but they need coordination to steer themselves. RTEs facilitate program level processes, impediment escalation, risk management, and continuous improvement. STEs provide a similar service, working with RTEs guiding the work of all ARTs in the solution train. Similar to scrum masters at the team level, RTEs and VSEs are servant-leaders.

>> **Product management (or solution management):** These people continuously define and prioritize requirements for the ART or solution train so that product owners have the information and empowerment they need to make fast decisions and provide instant clarification to the developers on individual scrum teams.

>> **System architect/engineer (or solution architect/engineer):** A cross-discipline team with system view responsibility for overall architectural and engineering design for the respective ART or solution train. Similar to the way architecture decisions are made at the lowest-level integration team in vertical slicing, the architect/engineer provides the standards to enable developers on the individual scrum teams to make in-the-moment technical decisions.

At this level of integration, the ART works at a cadence of five iterations by default to create what is known as program increments (PI).

Team level

ARTs are made up of a certain number of individual agile teams, which make up the team level of SAFe. Agile teams in an ART work in cadence with each other, and their team backlogs each support and align with the program vision and backlog.

SAFe has many aspects, but we find the following to be most valuable in addressing challenges of scaling.

Joint program increment planning

Joint program increment (PI) planning unifies agile teams across an ART. In PI planning, agile teams plan their work for the next PI together, face-to-face, in the same room at the same time.

PI planning includes the following:

>> Setting business context for the PI by a senior executive or business owner.

>> Communicating program vision by product management, and supporting features from the program backlog.

>> Presenting the system architecture vision and any agile-supportive changes to development practices (such as test automation).

>> Outlining the planning process by the RTE.

>> Setting up agile team breakout sessions to determine capacity and backlog items that they will work on in support of the program vision.

>> Reviewing draft plans with all agile teams, with each team presenting key planning outputs, potential risks, and dependencies. Product management and other stakeholders provide input and feedback.

>> Reviewing draft plans by management to identify any issues with scope, talent allocation constraints, and dependencies. Facilitated by the RTE.

>> Breaking out of agile teams to adjust planning based on all feedback.

>> Reviewing the final plan, facilitated by the RTE.

The magic of PI planning is that dependencies are identified and coordinated in the moment during these two-day sessions — two days well spent. If one team identifies a dependency in one of its own requirements during the team breakouts, that team sends a team member to another team to discuss the dependency right there and then. No back-and-forth occurs.

Although no amount of planning can identify every issue upfront, this type of collaboration addresses most issues ahead of time. In addition, it establishes an open line of communication throughout the program increment execution, ensuring teams synchronize and address issues immediately and more effectively than if they had planned as separate teams, sharing documentation without discussion.

Clarity for managers

In Chapters 3 and 14, we discuss ways management changes to enable teams to be more agile and adaptive in nature. For larger organizations, SAFe provides structure for middle management's involvement with agile teams. The portfolio, large solution, and program levels outline roles and functions not fulfilled by individual team members, providing some clarity to how functional, technical, and other leadership types can clear the way and enable the individual agile teams to be as effective and efficient as possible, as well as connect strategy to execution.

Modular Structures with Enterprise Scrum

Of all the scaling models presented in this chapter, Enterprise Scrum (ES) may offer the most modular approach to scaling. The ES framework is highly configurable for the sake of achieving overall business agility.

For larger projects, programs, and portfolios, ES stretches the foundations of single-team scrum practice across many teams and supports self-organization at scale through menus of structuring options. These options allow teams of teams to not only track their work of creating functionality but also specify, test, inspect, and adapt everything that matters to their success, including all their configuration choices, at the end of each iteration.

Some configuration menus include patterns for structuring teams and roles, collaboration style, delivery modes, contract types, and a range of metrics. ES also generalizes some of the core elements of scrum (roles, artifacts, and events). We discuss the ES scrum element generalizations and key configuration menus in this section.

ES scrum elements generalizations

Scaling agility across an organization pulls in people who may not initially be familiar with specific terms used in scrum. ES generalizes some names of scrum roles, artifacts, and events to make them more familiar to members of the broader organization but keeps their functions inline with scrum.

WARNING

The elements of scrum — three roles, three artifacts, five events — are central to the scrum framework. Removing or changing any of them means you're not doing scrum. You don't have to use scrum, but always use the four agile values and 12 agile principles as your litmus test to determine if you're being agile. You can learn more about the agile values and principles in Chapters 1 and 2.

Some examples of ES scrum generalizations include the following:

>> A product owner becomes a *business owner* to highlight that this role applies to the overall business, even on initiatives that may not be product focused, but rather service or initiative-focused.

>> The scrum master role becomes a *coach* to emphasize the enabling nature of the role both within the team and externally with all stakeholders and business units.

>> A product backlog becomes a *value list* to emphasize that each value list item may consist of user stories directly affecting functionality, or anything providing value to the business regarding any items outlined in the canvas. Learn about canvases in the next section, "ES key activities."

TIP

The idea of adding more than just product functionality requirements to a product backlog is introduced in Chapter 7, where we show you examples of product backlog items that include not only requirements (functionality) but also maintenance (development on existing functionality), overhead (required work that does not affect functionality), and improvement (action items from sprint retrospectives to improve structures and processes for the team and organization).

>> A sprint backlog becomes a *scrumboard* to emphasize the value of visualizing the work to be done in a sprint on a wall or a task board. You can learn more about task boards in Chapter 9.

>> A sprint becomes a *cycle*. With software projects, cycles are still one to four weeks, with the same cadence of planning, inspecting, and adapting (review and retrospective) as sprints. Non-software cycles may be longer.

>> Sprint planning and sprint review become *cycle planning* and *cycle review*, respectively, to align with the renaming of *sprint*.

>> Sprint retrospective becomes *improvement* to emphasize the forward-looking direction of inspecting and adapting.

ES key activities

ES has three key activities, which we outline here by how each applies to scaling across multiple teams.

Step 1: Visualize everything that matters

ES offers a growing library of templates for organizing project information, including vision, roadmap, roles, teams involved, resources, value list items, deployment methods, stakeholders, and customers. These templates are called *canvases* and are the foundation for teams visualizing their work. Figure 17-14 illustrates the canvas template for a scaled software development project. (ES canvas templates exist for other types of non-software development, but we focus on the scaled software development canvas here.)

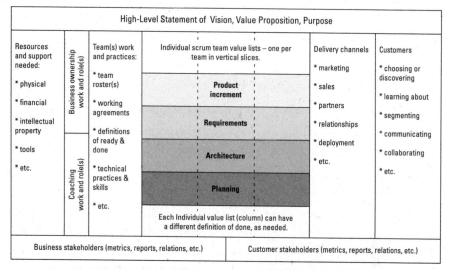

FIGURE 17-14:
ES scaled
software
development
canvas.

Used with permission, © 2017 Enterprise Scrum Inc.

Each section contains the work or issues that need to be addressed for each category. The team pulls the items in each section into the value list and subsets of the list onto the scrumboard for implementation during each cycle.

The ES canvas contains everything that matters for successful delivery. It expands the concept of product backlog into a customized value list of every kind of work required. The contents of the value list start at a high level and are refined to whatever level of detail is needed to complete the work in a cycle. The entire contents of the canvas and value list are reviewed for possible improvements after every cycle.

When scaling with multiple teams, the canvas holds the value list, including all user stories, sliced and detailed as the work progresses (middle section). The value list also includes the full range of surrounding issues and relationships from the canvas, including vision, resources, business ownership, coaching, teams involved, metrics, and interactions with stakeholders, deployment, and customers.

Step 2: Make active configuration choices

At scale, ES also provides options for how the desired outcomes of some roles, artifacts, or events are achieved to address individual circumstances. Drawing on a set of menus that offer a range of options, teams make active choices about their configurations. Some of the most important menus and choices are described in this section.

DELIVERY TARGETS MENU

Understanding the level of scale you need is an important first step to determining what approach you need to take. To begin, ES provides a delivery targets menu, which is a set of guidelines for determining the highest level of coordinated delivery that the set of teams in the scaling effort is targeting:

>> Large project: Two or more teams working together to deliver a project

>> Program: Two or more projects serving the same customer segment

>> Portfolio: Two or more application teams working together on multiple programs in a business unit

>> Enterprise architecture: Two or more business areas requiring the use of common architecture elements

>> Business process: Applying agile techniques to non-software organizational units, such as human resources, finance, marketing, sales, compliance, or finance

>> Business agility: Applying agile principles company wide

In contrast to other scaling models that provide a range of multi-team sizes for specific approaches, ES considers two or more teams to be the basis for considering any options in the menus.

STRUCTURAL PATTERNS MENU

ES focuses on roles rather than titles assigned to individual people. Structural pattern menu options for structuring the business owner and coach roles for each team include the following:

>> Dedicated business owner and dedicated coach for each scrum team (as we outline in Chapter 6)

>> One business owner for all teams and one coach for all teams

>> One business owner for all teams and one coach for each team

>> One business owner for each team and one coach for all teams

REMEMBER

Dedicating each role on a scrum team reduces the risk of lost productivity and defects that often result from task switching, or thrashing.

» Virtual business owner or virtual coach — a business owner or coach steps into the role as needed, while also filling another role as a developer or an external role to the team

» Chief business owner or coach to provide direction to individual team business owners or coaches, respectively

» Virtual teams of business owners or coaches, where either function can be fulfilled by a collaborative, self-managing team of business owners or coaches

WARNING

Having multiple people in the business owner (product owner) or coach (scrum master) roles increases complexity of communication channels, and may introduce confusion for all project team members.

The configuration you choose depends on many factors, including budget, organizational culture, management style, and individual expertise.

COLLABORATION MODES MENU

The collaboration modes menu is used to coordinate business priorities and clarification across teams. Various approaches may be used to support or align with the chosen structural pattern:

» **Centralization:** A business owner makes prioritization decisions and provides clarification to all teams.

» **Delegation:** A chief business owner provides overall prioritization and meets regularly with individual team business owners to empower them to do the same for their teams for their portion of the value list.

» **Collaboration:** Each team's business owner works with the other teams' business owners to make collaborative agreements without the oversight of a chief business owner.

» **Subsumption:** Experts from broader areas of the organization outside developing functionality (such as marketing, finance, and sales) collaborate on everything that the business needs to deliver value to the customer. This scope of collaboration is usually needed to address business process or overall business agility delivery targets outlined previously.

Like other scaling approaches, the scrum of scrums (see the section in this chapter on vertical slicing) is also used in ES to help facilitate the resolution of dependencies across teams, with the encouragement to keep lines of communication always open.

DELIVERY MODES MENU

Each organization will have different requirements and constraints for how often and on what cadence it delivers functionality to the customer. The frequency and type of delivery will also determine the level of coordination needed between teams on a daily basis, during each cycle, and with each release. Delivery modes menu examples include the following:

> **Continuous delivery:** The product increment is continuously integrated and tested but not deployed to production.

> **Continuous deployment:** As each requirement is implemented, it is deployed to production as soon as it is completed.

> **Cycle:** The product increment is deployed to production at the end of each cycle.

> **Release:** The product increment is deployed after multiple cycles.

Organizations may progress or evolve from one of the delivery modes to another as they inspect and adapt over time, without breaking the ES framework. You can learn more about releasing functionality in Chapter 8.

Step 3: Plan, collaborate, review, and improve everything, every cycle

ES is about the continuous inspection and adaptation of all aspects of the canvas as well as all configuration choices made from each of the menus. At the end of each cycle, everything completed and everything yet to be done on the canvas is open for inspection and adaptation.

ES also invites teams to consider metrics toward more balanced agile management, and to provide transparency into the team's or program's progress for inspection and adaptation. You can learn more about agile metrics in Chapter 21.

Each of these scaling models has many things in common. They all aim to address the challenges of coordination, communication, prioritization, execution, and integration that come with complex projects and systems requiring more than a single team. Scaling projects across multiple cross-functional feature teams requires coordination and leadership guidance at the highest level of an organization. Management structures need to change from traditional command and control to distributed decision-making and autonomy to the lowest level possible where the work is being executed.

Making this transition requires organization-wide commitment to long-term changes in mindset and structure, which we discuss in Chapter 18.

Chapter **18**

Being a Change Agent

I f you're contemplating the idea of introducing agile project management to your company or organization, this chapter can help get you started on those changes. Introducing agility means learning and practicing a new mindset, culture, organizational structures, frameworks, and techniques. In this chapter, you learn key principles and steps to implementing agile project management techniques. We also introduce common change models, including the model we use at our company, Platinum Edge. We also cover common pitfalls to avoid in your agile transition.

Becoming Agile Requires Change

Traditional project management is focused on processes, tools, comprehensive documentation, contract negotiation, and following a plan. Although agile project management remains dedicated to addressing each of these, the focus shifts to individuals, interactions, working functionality, customer collaboration, and responding to change.

Waterfall organizations didn't get where they are overnight and won't change overnight. For some organizations, decades of forming habits, establishing and protecting fiefdoms, and reinforcing a traditional mindset are engrained.

The organizational structure will require some type of change, the leadership will need to learn a new way of looking at developing people and empowering them to do their work, and those doing the work will have to learn to work together and manage themselves in ways they may not be used to.

Why Change Doesn't Happen on Its Own

Change is about people more than it is about defining a process. People resist change, and that resistance is based on personal experience, emotion, and fear. We see these reactions firsthand as we help organizations make these changes. Often our first exposure to an organization is when it asks for formal classroom training to learn what it means to be agile and how scrum works. After a two-day class, the level of excitement about implementing this more modern way of thinking and working usually increases, and our students consistently express how much it makes sense.

Scrum is simple. Agile values and principles resonate with almost everyone. But none of it is easy. Scrum for developing products and services is like playing a new game, with new positions, new rules, and a different playing field. Imagine that an American football coach came to his team one day and said, "We're going to learn how to play futbol (American soccer) today. Meet me out on the pitch in 15 minutes with your gear, and we'll get right to work." What would happen? Everyone might know how to play futbol based on what he or she had seen on TV or experienced as a youth, but the team wouldn't be ready to make the change.

A lot of confusion would ensue. Old rules, techniques, training, and thinking would have to be unlearned for the team to learn the new stuff and come together to compete effectively. Immediately, you'd hear questions from the players, such as the following:

>> When can I use my hands?

>> How many timeout calls do we get?

>> Am I on offense or defense during this play?

>> Where do I line up at kick-off?

>> Who holds the ball when we kick a goal?

>> How many tries do we get before the other team gets the ball?

>> Where's my helmet?

>> These shoes make it hard to kick sometimes.

Transitioning to agile techniques won't happen overnight, but it will happen if you and your organization's leadership take a change management approach to your agile transition. For existing waterfall organizations, agile transformation takes at least one to three years from the time management commits to it. It's an ongoing journey, not a destination.

Strategic Approaches to Implementing and Managing Change

Organizational change initiatives typically fail without a strategy and discipline. Here, we define *failure* as not reaching the desired end state goal of what the organization will look like after the change. Failure is often due to being unclear as to the goal or because the change plan doesn't address the highest risk factors and challenges impeding the desired change.

Various approaches exist to managing change. We show you several here, including ours (Platinum Edge), so you know what to expect as you embark on your own change initiative.

Lewin

Kurt Lewin was an innovator in social and organizational psychology in the 1940s and established a cornerstone model for understanding effective organizational change. Most modern change models are based on this philosophy, which is unfreeze — change — refreeze, as illustrated in Figure 18-1.

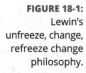
FIGURE 18-1:
Lewin's unfreeze, change, refreeze change philosophy.

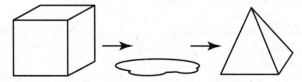

If you want to change the shape of a cube of ice, you first have to change it from its existing frozen state to liquid so that it can be changed or reshaped, then mold the liquid into the new shape you want, then put it through a solidification process to form the new shape. Unfreezing is implied between the first two states in the figure, and the changes made are implied during the unfrozen state.

Unfreeze

The first stage represents the preparation needed before change can take place — challenging existing beliefs, values, and behaviors. Reexamination and seeking motivation for a new equilibrium is what leads to participation and buy-in for meaningful change.

Change

The next stage involves uncertainty and resolving that uncertainty to do things a new way. This transitional stage represents the formation of new beliefs, values, and behaviors. Time and communication are the keys to seeing the changes begin to take effect.

Refreeze

As people embrace new ways, confidence and stability increase, and the change starts to take shape into a solid new process, structure, belief system, or set of behaviors.

This simple pattern provides the foundation for most change management tools and frameworks, including those we discuss in this chapter.

ADKAR's five steps to change

Prosci is one of the leading organizations in change management and benchmarking research. One of Prosci's change management tools, ADKAR, is an acronym for the five outcomes (awareness, desire, knowledge, ability, and reinforcement) individuals and organizations need to achieve for successful change. It is a goal-oriented model for individuals, and a focus model for the discussions and actions organizations need to take together.

Organizational changes still require change for individuals, so the secret to success is affecting change for everyone involved.

ADKAR outlines the individual's successful journey through change. The five steps of the journey also each align with organizational change activities. They should be completed in the order described next.

Awareness

Humans find change difficult. When change initiatives come top-down in an organization, people may verbally agree to them, but their actions tell a different story. Mismatch of actions and words is usually innocent and natural. Without awareness, or an understanding of the factors influencing management's desire to change, or especially without a recognition that something should change, individuals will not be motivated to change. Informing the individuals in an organization, helping them have a shared understanding of the challenges that exist, and then assessing whether awareness is common constitute the first step to successful, lasting change. It is the basis, without which the initiative won't make progress.

Desire

Based on their awareness of a challenge needing to be addressed, individuals will have an opinion on whether or not change is necessary or desired to address it. Making the connection between the awareness of an issue and what could or should be done about it is the next step. After desire exists for the individuals in an organization, there is motivation to move together to change.

Knowledge

Desire is key, but knowledge of how to make the change and where each individual fits into the change make up the next crucial part of the change process. Individuals throughout the organization need to understand what the changes mean for them, and leadership needs to facilitate education and actions in a cooperative way across the organization. Knowledge comes from training and coaching.

Ability

With new knowledge of how to change, implementation requires acquiring skills, redefining roles, and clearly defining new performance expectations. Other commitments may need to be delayed or replaced with new behaviors or responsibilities. Continued coaching and mentoring may be required, and leadership needs to be clear that this reprioritization of commitments is expected and encouraged.

Reinforcement

Changes don't stick after one successful iteration. New behaviors, skills, and processes must be reinforced through continued corrective action and coaching to ensure that old habits don't return.

The ADKAR model surrounds these steps with assessments and action plans to guide leaders and individuals through their change journey. ADKAR should be used iteratively, using scrum, inspecting and adapting until each step is achieved before progressing to the next step.

Kotter's eight steps for leading change

John Kotter's process for leading change identifies eight common but preventable reasons why organizations fail at their change initiatives, and addresses each with actions that should be taken to successfully lead change.

- » **Permitting too much complacency:** The leadership action is to create a sense of urgency. People get used to the status quo, and learn to deal with it. Helping others see the need for change requires the creation of a sense of urgency for change. Leaders must communicate the importance of immediate action.

- » **Lack of a powerful guiding coalition:** The leadership action is to build a guiding coalition. Successful change will require more than just one active supporter, even if that one person is at the highest level of the organization. Executives, directors, managers, and even informal social leaders with influence need to be unified in the need for and vision of a change. This coalition must be formed and drive the change.

- » **Underestimating and undercommunicating the power of vision:** The leadership action is to form a strategic vision and initiatives. Kotter estimates that leadership undercommunicates the vision for change by as much as 1,000 times. Even if people are unhappy with the status quo, they won't always make sacrifices for a change unless they believe in the proposed benefits and that change is possible. As a change coalition, clearly define how the future is different from the past and present, as well as the steps to make that future a reality. We discuss visions and roadmaps for products and services in Chapter 7 — change management also needs to begin with a clear vision of where you're headed.

- » **Lack of rallying around a common opportunity:** The leadership action is to enlist a volunteer army. Change will accelerate and last if people buy in and are internally driven. As a result of leadership's effective communication of vision and need, people should rally around a cause they come to believe in. If they don't rally, reevaluate your messaging, tone, and frequency.

- » **Allowing obstacles to block the vision:** The leadership action is to remove barriers to action. Some obstacles may be only perceived, but others are real. However, both must be overcome. One blocker in the "right" place can be the single reason for failure. Many people tend to avoid confronting obstacles (processes, hierarchies, working across silos), so leadership must act as servant-leaders to identify and remove impediments that are reducing the empowerment of individuals implementing the changes on the front lines.

- » **Lack of short-term wins:** The leadership action is to generate short-term wins. The end transformation goal usually can't be achieved in the short term, so fatigue can set in for everyone involved if successes and progress go unrecognized along the way. Evidence of change should be highlighted and exposed early and regularly. This reinforcement increases morale through difficult times of change, and motivates and encourages continued efforts and progress.

>> **Declaring victory too early:** The leadership action is to sustain acceleration. Celebrating short-term wins sets a false sense of security that change is complete. Each success should build on the previous success. Push on, and push on harder after each success, with increased confidence and credibility. Continue to overcommunicate the vision throughout the transformation.

>> **Neglecting anchoring of changes in organizational culture:** The leadership action is to institute change. Leadership will have the opportunity throughout the change process to connect successes and new behaviors with the culture's evolution and growing strength to keep old habits from returning. These connections should be recognized openly and made visible to everyone as soon as successes and new behaviors are realized.

Platinum Edge's Change Roadmap

Throughout this book, we highlight the fact that agile processes are different from traditional project management. Moving an organization from waterfall to an agile mindset is a significant change. Through our experience guiding companies through this type of change, we've identified the following important steps to take to successfully become an agile organization.

Figure 18-2 illustrates our agile transition roadmap for successful agile transformation.

Step 1: Conduct an implementation strategy with success metrics

An *implementation strategy* is a plan that outlines the following:

>> Your current strengths to build on as you transition

>> The challenges you'll face based on your current structure

>> Action items for how your organization will transition to agile project management

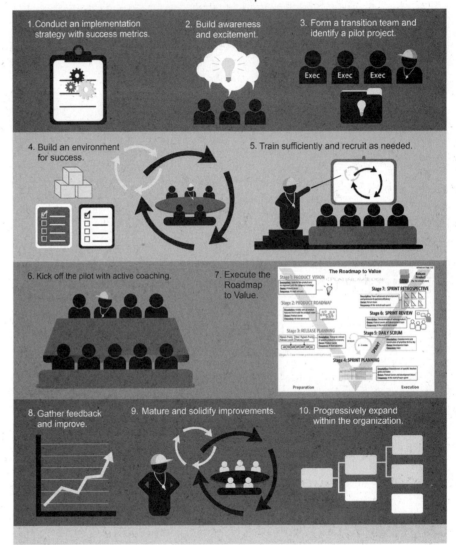

SCRUM TRANSITION
Roadmap

1. Conduct an implementation strategy with success metrics.

2. Build awareness and excitement.

3. Form a transition team and identify a pilot project.

4. Build an environment for success.

5. Train sufficiently and recruit as needed.

6. Kick off the pilot with active coaching.

7. Execute the Roadmap to Value.

8. Gather feedback and improve.

9. Mature and solidify improvements.

10. Progressively expand within the organization.

FIGURE 18-2:
Platinum Edge agile transition roadmap.

TIP

Implementation strategies are most effectively performed by external agile experts in the form of an assessment or a current state audit.

Whether you engage with a third party or conduct the assessment yourself, make sure the following questions are addressed:

>> **Current processes:** How does your organization run projects today? What does it do well? What are its problems?

>> **Future processes:** How can your company benefit from agile approaches? What agile methods or frameworks will you use? What key changes will your organization need to make? What will your transformed company look like from a team and process perspective?

>> **Step-by-step plan:** How will you move from existing processes to agile processes? What will change immediately? In six months? In a year or longer? This plan should be a roadmap of successive steps getting the company to a sustainable state of agile maturity.

>> **Benefits:** What advantages will the agile transition provide for the people and groups in your organization and the organization as a whole? Agile techniques are a win for most people; identify how they will benefit.

>> **Potential challenges:** What will be the most difficult changes? What departments or people will have the most trouble with agile approaches? Whose fiefdom is being disrupted? What are your potential roadblocks? How will you overcome these challenges?

>> **Success factors:** What organizational factors will help you while switching to agile processes? How will the company commit to a new approach? Which people or departments will be agile champions?

A good implementation strategy will guide your company through its move to agile practices. A strategy can provide supporters with a clear plan to rally around and support, and it can set realistic expectations for your organization's agile transition.

For your first agile project, identify a quantifiable way to recognize project success. Using metrics will give you a way to instantly demonstrate success to project stakeholders and your organization. Metrics provide specific goals and talking points for sprint retrospectives and help set clear expectations for the project team.

TIP

Metrics related to people and performance work best when related to teams rather than to individuals. Scrum teams manage themselves as a team, succeed as a team, fail as a team — and should be evaluated as a team.

Keeping track of project success measurements can do more than help you improve throughout the project. Metrics can provide clear proof of success when you move past your first project and start to scale agile practices throughout your organization.

Chapter 21 describes metrics for success in detail.

Step 2: Build awareness and excitement

After you have a roadmap showing you the "how" of your agile transition, you need to communicate the coming changes to people in your organization. Agile approaches have many benefits; be sure to let all individuals in your company know about those benefits and get them excited about the coming changes. Here are some ways to build awareness:

>> **Educate people.** People in your organization may not know much — or anything — about agile project management. Educate people about agile principles and approaches and the change that will accompany the new approaches. You can create an agile wiki, hold lunchtime learning sessions, and even have hot-seat discussions (face-to-face discussions with leadership where people can talk safely about concerns and get their questions answered about changes and agile topics) to address concerns with the transition.

>> **Use a variety of communication tools.** Take advantage of communication channels such as newsletters, blogs, intranets, email, and face-to-face workshops to get the word out about the change coming to your organization.

>> **Highlight the benefits.** Make sure people in your company know how an agile approach will help the organization create high-value products, lead to customer satisfaction, and increase employee morale. Chapter 19 has a great list of the benefits of agile project management for this step.

>> **Share the implementation plan.** Make your transition plan available to everyone. Talk about it, both formally and informally. Offer to walk people through it and answer questions. We often print the transition roadmap on posters and distribute it throughout the organization.

>> **Involve the initial scrum team.** As early as you can, let the people who may work on your company's first agile project know about the upcoming changes. Involve the initial scrum team members in planning the transition to help them become enthusiastic agile practitioners.

>> **Be open.** Drive the conversation about new processes. Try to stay ahead of the company rumor mill by speaking openly, answering questions, and quelling myths about agile project management. Structured communications like the hot-seat sessions we mention earlier are a great example of open communication.

Building awareness will generate support for the upcoming changes and alleviate some of the fear that naturally comes with change. Communication will be an important tool to help you successfully implement agile processes.

Step 3: Form a transformation team and identify a pilot project

Identify a team in your company that can be responsible for the agile transformation at the organization level. This agile transition team, which is described in Chapter 16, is made up of executives and other leaders who will systematically improve processes, reporting requirements, and performance measurements across the organization.

The transformation team will create changes within sprints, just like the development team creates product features within sprints. The transformation team will focus on the highest-priority changes supporting agility in each sprint and will demonstrate its implementation, when possible, during a sprint review with all stakeholders, including the pilot scrum team members.

Starting your agile transition with just one pilot project is a great idea. Having one initial project allows you to figure out how to work with agile methods with little disruption to your organization's overall business. Concentrating on one project to start also lets you work out some of the kinks that inevitably follow change. Figure 18-3 shows the types of projects that benefit most from the agile approach.

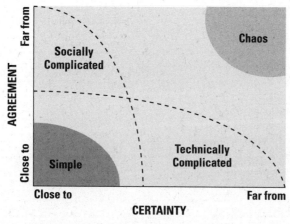

FIGURE 18-3: Projects that can benefit from agile techniques.

When selecting your first agile project, look for an endeavor with these qualities:

>> **Appropriately important:** Make sure the project you choose is important enough to merit interest within your company. However, avoid the most important project coming up; you want room to make and learn from mistakes. See the note on the blame game in the later section "Avoiding Pitfalls."

>> **Sufficiently visible:** Your pilot project should be visible to your organization's key influencers, but don't make it the most high-profile item on the agenda. You will need the freedom to adjust to new processes; critical projects may not allow for that freedom on the first try of a new approach.

>> **Clear and containable:** Look for a product with clear requirements and a business group that can commit to defining and prioritizing those requirements. Try to choose a project that has a distinct end point, rather than one that can expand indefinitely.

>> **Not too large:** Select a project that you can complete with no more than two scrum teams working simultaneously to prevent too many moving parts at once.

>> **Tangibly measurable:** Choose a project that you know can show measurable value within sprints.

TECHNICAL STUFF

People need time to adjust to organizational changes of any type, not just agile transitions. Studies have found that with large changes, companies and teams will see dips in performance before they see improvements. *Satir's Curve,* shown in Figure 18-4, illustrates the process of teams' excitement, chaos, and finally adjustment to new processes.

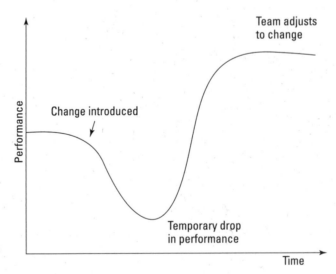

FIGURE 18-4:
Satir's Curve.

After you've successfully run one agile project, you'll have a foundation for future successes.

Step 4: Build an environment for success

One of the agile principles states, "Build projects around motivated individuals. Give them the environment and support they need, and trust them to get the job done."

We outline what it means to create an environment to enable success in Chapter 5. Study the 4 agile values and the 12 agile principles carefully (see Chapter 2) and seriously to determine whether you're creating an environment for success or rationalizing that the status quo is good enough.

Start fixing and improving your environment as early as possible.

Step 5: Train sufficiently and recruit as needed

Training is a critical step when shifting to an agile mindset. The combination of face-to-face training with experienced agile experts and the ability to work through exercises using agile processes is the best way to help the project team to absorb and develop the knowledge needed to successfully begin an agile project.

Training works best when the members of the project team can train and learn together. As agile trainers and mentors, we've had the opportunity to overhear conversations between project team members that start, "Remember when Mark showed us how to . . .? That worked when we did it in class. Let's try it and see what happens." If the product owner, development team, scrum master, and project stakeholders can attend the same class, they can apply lessons to their work as a team.

Recruiting talent to fill gaps in the roles you need avoids the obvious problems you'll have at the start of the transition. Without a dedicated product owner and his or her clear direction to the team, how likely is your project to succeed? How will that affect the team's ability to self-organize? Who will facilitate the many interactions if you're missing a scrum master? What will the first sprint look like if you're missing a key skill on the development team required to minimally achieve the first sprint goal?

Work with your human resources department as early as possible to start the recruiting process. Work with your agile expert advisers to tap into their network of experienced agile practitioners.

Step 6: Kick off the pilot with active coaching

When you have a clear agile implementation strategy, an excited and trained project team, a pilot project with a product backlog, and clear measures for success, congratulations! You're ready to run your first sprint.

Don't forget, though — agile approaches are new to the pilot team. Teams need coaching to become high performing. Engage with agile experts for agile coaching to start the project right.

TIP

Practice doesn't make perfect. Practice makes permanent.

As the scrum team plans its first sprint, it should not bite off too many requirements. Keep in mind that you're just starting to learn about a new process and a new product. New scrum teams often take on a smaller amount of work than they think they can complete in their first sprints. A typical progression follows.

REMEMBER

After you establish overall goals through the product's vision statement, product roadmap, and initial release goal, your product backlog needs only enough user-story level requirements (see Chapter 8) for one sprint for the scrum team to start development.

>> **In sprint 1,** scrum teams take on 25 percent of the work they think they can complete during sprint planning.

>> **In sprint 2,** scrum teams take on 50 percent of the work they think they can complete during sprint planning.

>> **In sprint 3,** scrum teams take on 75 percent of the work they think they can complete during sprint planning.

>> **In sprint 4 and beyond,** scrum teams take on 100 percent of the work they think they can complete during sprint planning.

By sprint 4, the scrum team will be more comfortable with new processes, will know more about the product, and will be able to estimate tasks with more accuracy.

WARNING

You can't plan away uncertainty. Don't fall victim to analysis paralysis; set a direction and go!

Throughout the first sprint, be sure to consciously stick with agile practices. Think about the following during your first sprint:

>> Have your daily scrum meeting, even if you feel like you didn't make any progress. Remember to state roadblocks, too!

>> The development team may need to remember to manage itself and not look to the product owner, the scrum master, or anywhere besides the sprint backlog for task assignments.

>> The scrum master may have to remember to protect the development team from outside work and distractions, especially while other members of the organization get used to having a dedicated agile project team around.

>> The product owner may have to become accustomed to working directly with the development team, being available for questions, and reviewing and accepting completed requirements immediately.

In the first sprint, expect the road to be a little bumpy. That's okay; agile processes are about learning and adapting.

In Chapter 8, you can see how the scrum team can plan the sprint. Chapter 9 provides the day-to-day details on running the sprint.

Step 7: Execute the Roadmap to Value

When you've chosen your pilot project, don't fall into the trap of using a plan from an old methodology or set of habits. Instead, use agile processes from the project's start.

We outline the Roadmap to Value throughout this book, introducing it in Chapter 7 and leading you through each of the seven stages in Chapters 7 through 10.

Step 8: Gather feedback and improve

You'll naturally make mistakes at first. No problem. At the end of your first sprint, you gather feedback and improve with two important events: the sprint review and the sprint retrospective.

In your first sprint review, it will be important for the product owner to set expectations about the format of the meeting, along with the sprint goal and completed product functionality. The sprint review is about product demonstration — fancy presentations and handouts are unnecessary overhead. Project stakeholders may initially be taken aback by a bare-bones approach. However, those stakeholders will soon be impressed as they find a working product replacing the fluff of slides and lists. Transparency and visibility — show, rather than tell.

The first sprint retrospective may require setting some expectations as well. It will help to conduct the meeting with a preset format, such as the one in Chapter 10, both to spark conversation and avoid a free-for-all complaining session.

In your first sprint retrospective, pay extra attention to the following:

>> Keep in mind how well you met the sprint goal, not how many user stories you completed.

>> Go over how well you completed requirements to meet the definition of done: defined, tested, integrated, and documented.

>> Discuss how you met your project success metrics.

>> Talk about how well you stuck with agile principles. We start the journey with principles.

>> Celebrate successes, even small gains, as well as examine problems and solutions.

>> Remember that the scrum team should manage the meeting as a team, gain consensus on how to improve, and leave the meeting with a plan of action.

You can find more details about both sprint reviews and sprint retrospectives in Chapter 10.

Step 9: Mature and solidify improvements

Inspecting and adapting enables scrum teams to grow as a team and to mature with each sprint.

Agile practitioners sometimes compare the process of maturing with the martial arts learning technique of *Shu Ha Ri*, a Japanese term that can be translated to "maintain, detach, transcend." The term describes three stages in which people learn new skills:

>> **In the *Shu* stage,** students follow a new skill as they were taught, without deviation, to commit that skill to memory and make it automatic.

New scrum teams can benefit from making a habit of closely following agile processes, until those processes become familiar. During the Shu stage, scrum teams may work closely with an agile coach or mentor to follow processes correctly.

>> **In the *Ha* stage,** students start to improvise as they understand more about how their new skill works. Sometimes the improvisations will work, and sometimes they won't. The students will learn more about the skill from these successes and failures.

As scrum teams understand more about how agile approaches work, they may try variations on processes for their own project. During the Ha stage, scrum teams will find that the sprint retrospective is a valuable tool for talking about how their improvisations worked or did not work. In this stage, scrum team members may still learn from an agile mentor, but they may also learn from one another, from other agile professionals, and from starting to teach agile skills to others.

>> **In the *Ri* stage,** the skill comes naturally to the former student, who will know what works and what doesn't. The former student can now innovate with confidence.

With practice, scrum teams will get to the point where agile processes are easy and comfortable, like riding a bicycle or driving a car. In the Ri stage, scrum teams can customize processes, knowing what works in the spirit of the Agile Manifesto and 12 Agile Principles.

At first, maturing as a scrum team can take a concentrated effort and commitment to using agile processes and upholding agile values. Eventually, however, the scrum team will be humming along, improving from sprint to sprint, and inspiring others throughout the organization.

With time, as scrum teams and project stakeholders mature, entire companies can mature into successful agile organizations.

Step 10: Progressively expand within the organization

Completing a successful project is an important step in moving an organization to agile project management. With metrics that prove the success of your project and the value of agile methodologies, you can garner commitment from your company to support new agile projects.

To progressively scale agile project management across an organization, start with the following:

>> **Seed new teams.** An agile project team that has reached maturity — the people who worked on the first agile project — should now have the expertise and enthusiasm to become agile ambassadors in the organization. These people can join new agile project teams and help those teams learn and grow.

>> **Redefine metrics.** Identify measurements for success, across the organization, with each new scrum team and with each new project.

>> **Scale methodically.** It can be exciting to produce great results, but company-wide improvements require significant process changes. Don't move faster than the organization can handle. Check out Chapter 17 for different ways of scaling agile projects across multiple teams.

>> **Identify new challenges.** Your first agile project may have uncovered roadblocks that you didn't consider in your original implementation plan. Update your strategy and maturity roadmap as needed.

>> **Continue learning.** As you roll out new processes, make sure that new team members have the proper training, mentorship, and resources to effectively run agile projects.

The preceding steps work for successful agile project management transitions. Use these steps and return to them as you scale, and you can make agile practices thrive in your organization.

Avoiding Pitfalls

Project teams can make a number of common but serious mistakes when implementing agile practices. Table 18-1 provides an overview of some typical problems and ways to turn them around.

As you may notice, many of these pitfalls are related to a lack of organizational support, the need for training, and falling back on old project management practices. If your company supports positive changes, if the project team is trained, and if the scrum team makes an active commitment to upholding agile values, you'll have a successful agile transition.

TABLE 18-1   **Common Agile Transition Problems and Solutions**

Problem	Description	Potential Solution
Faux agile or double work agile or both	Sometimes organizations will say that they are "doing agile." They may go through some of the practices used on agile projects, but they haven't embraced agile principles and continue creating waterfall deliverables and products. This is sometimes called *faux agile* and is a sure path to avoiding the benefits of agile techniques. Trying to complete agile processes in addition to waterfall processes, documents, and meetings is another faux agile approach. *Double work agile* results in quick project team burnout. If you're doing twice the work, you aren't adhering to agile principles.	Insist on following one process — an agile process. Garner support from management to avoid non-agile principles and practices.
Lack of training	Investment in a hands-on training class will provide a quicker, better learning environment than even the best book, video, blog, or white paper. Lack of training often indicates an overall lack of organizational commitment to agile practices. Keep in mind that training can help scrum teams avoid many of the mistakes on this list.	Build training into your implementation strategy. Giving teams the right foundation of skills is critical to success and necessary at the start of your agile transition.
Ineffective product owner	The product owner role is non-traditional. Agile project teams need a product owner who is an expert on business needs and priorities and can work well with the rest of the scrum team on a daily basis. An absent or indecisive product owner will quickly sink an agile project.	Start the project with a person who has the time, expertise, and temperament to be a good product owner. Ensure the product owner has proper training. The scrum master can help coach the product owner and may try to clear roadblocks preventing the product owner from being effective. If removing impediments doesn't work, the scrum team should insist on replacing the ineffective product owner with a product owner — or at least an agent — who can make product decisions and help the scrum team be successful.

(continued)

TABLE 18-1 *(continued)*

Problem	Description	Potential Solution
Lack of automated testing	Without automated testing, it may be impossible to fully complete and test work within a sprint. Manual testing requires time that fast-moving scrum teams don't have.	You can find many low-cost, open-source testing tools on the market today. Look into the right tools and make a commitment as a development team to using those tools.
Lack of transition support	Making the transition successfully is difficult and far from guaranteed. It pays to do it right the first time with people who know what they are doing.	When you decide to move to agile project management, enlist the help of an agile mentor — either internally from your organization or externally from a consulting firm — who can support your transition. Process is easy, but people are hard. It pays to invest in professional transition support with an experienced partner who understands behavioral science and organizational change.
Inappropriate physical environment	When scrum teams are not collocated, they lose the advantage of face-to-face communication. Being in the same building isn't enough; scrum teams need to sit together in the same area.	If your scrum team is in the same building but not sitting in the same area, move the team together. Consider creating a room or annex for the scrum team to continually collaborate. Try to keep the scrum team area away from distracters, such as the guy who can talk forever or the manager who needs just one small favor. Before starting a project with a dislocated scrum team, do what you can to enlist local talent. If you must work with a dislocated scrum team, take a look at Chapter 14 to see how to manage dislocated teams.
Poor team selection	Scrum team members who don't support agile processes, don't work well with others, or don't have capacity for self-management will sabotage a new agile project from within.	When creating a scrum team, consider how well potential team members will enact the agile principles. The keys are versatility and a willingness to learn.

Problem	Description	Potential Solution
Discipline slips	Remember that agile projects still need requirements, design, development, testing, and releases. Doing that work in sprints requires discipline.	You need more, not less, discipline to deliver working functionality in a short iteration. Progress needs to be consistent and constant. The daily scrum helps ensure that progress is occurring throughout the sprint. Use the sprint retrospective as an opportunity to reset approaches to discipline.
Lack of support for learning	Scrum teams succeed as teams and fail as teams; calling out one person's mistakes (known as the *blame game*) destroys the learning environment and destroys innovation.	The scrum team can make a commitment at the project start to leaving room for learning and to accepting success and failures as a group.
Diluting until dead	Watering down agile processes with old waterfall habits erodes the benefits of agile processes until those benefits no longer exist.	When making process changes, stop and consider whether those changes support the Agile Manifesto and the 12 Agile Principles. Resist changes that don't work with the manifesto and principles. Remember to maximize work not done.

Signs Your Changes Are Slipping

The following list of questions helps you see warning signs and provide ideas on what to do if problematic circumstances arise:

>> **Are you doing "scrum, but . . ."?**

"ScrumBut occurs when organizations partially adopt scrum. Some agile purists say that ScrumBut is unacceptable; other agile practitioners allow room for gradual growth into a new method. Having said that, beware of old practices that thwart agile principles, such as finishing sprints with incomplete functionality.

Scrum is three roles, three artifacts, and five events. If you find your team tweaking those basic framework components, ask why. Is scrum exposing something you're not willing to inspect and adapt?

REMEMBER

» Are you still documenting and reporting in the old way?

If you're still burning hours on hefty documentation and reporting, it's a sign that the organization has not accepted agile approaches for conveying project status. Help managers understand how to use existing agile reporting artifacts and quit doing double work!

» A team completing 50 story points in a sprint is better than another team doing 10, right?

No. Keep in mind that story points are relative and consistent within one scrum team, not across multiple scrum teams. Velocity isn't a team comparison metric. It is simply a post-sprint fact that scrum teams use to help them in their own planning. You can see more about story points and velocity in Chapter 8.

» When will the stakeholders sign off on all the specifications?

If you're waiting for sign-offs on comprehensive requirements to start developing, you're not following agile practices. You can start development as soon as you have enough requirements for one sprint.

» Are we using offshore to reduce costs?

Ideally, scrum teams are collocated. The ability for instant face-to-face communication saves more time and money and prevents more costly mistakes than the initial hourly savings you may see with some offshore teams.

If you do work with offshore teams, invest in good collaboration tools such as individual video cameras and persistent, virtual team rooms.

» Are development team members asking for more time in a sprint to finish tasks?

The development team may not be working cross-functionally or swarming on priority requirements. Development team members can help one another finish tasks, even if those tasks are outside of a person's core expertise.

This question can also indicate outside pressures to underestimate tasks and fit more work into a sprint than the development team can handle.

» Are development team members asking what they should do next?

After a sprint is planned and development work is under way, if the developers are waiting for direction from the scrum master or product owner, they aren't self-organizing. The development team should be telling the scrum master and the product owner what it's doing next, not the other way round.

» Are team members waiting until the end of the sprint to do testing?

Agile development teams should test every day in a sprint. All development team members are testers.

» Are the stakeholders showing up for sprint reviews?

If the only people at sprint reviews are the scrum team members, it's time to remind stakeholders of the value of frequent feedback loops. Let stakeholders know that they're missing their chance to review working product functionality regularly, correct course early, and see firsthand how the project is progressing.

» Is the scrum team complaining about being bossed around by the scrum master?

Command-and-control techniques are the antithesis of self-management and are in direct conflict with agile principles. Scrum teams are teams of peers — the only boss is the team. Have a discussion with the agile mentor and act quickly to reset the scrum master's expectations of his or her role.

» Is the scrum team putting in a lot of overtime?

If the end of each sprint becomes a rush to complete tasks, you aren't practicing sustainable development. Look for root causes, such as pressure to underestimate. The scrum master may need to coach the development team and shield its members from product owner pressure if this is the case. Reduce the story points for each sprint until the development team can get a handle on the work.

» What retrospective?

If scrum team members start avoiding or cancelling sprint retrospectives, you're on the slide back to waterfall. Remember the importance of inspecting and adapting and be sure to look at why people are missing the retrospective in the first place. If you're not progressing, complacency usually results in sliding backwards. Even if the scrum team has great velocity, development speed can always be better, so keep the retrospective, and keep improving.

6

The Part of Tens

Communicate the benefits of agile project management.

Address key factors for agile project success.

Measure progress in appropriately inspecting and adapting to become more agile as an organization.

Become an agile professional by learnin g, with support from valuable resources.

Chapter **19**

Ten Key Benefits of Agile Project Management

I n this chapter, we provide ten important benefits that agile project management provides to organizations, project teams, and products.

REMEMBER

To take advantage of agile project management benefits, you need to trust in agile practices, learn more about different agile approaches, and use what's best for your project team.

Better Product Quality

Projects exist to build great products and purpose-driven outcomes. Agile methods have excellent safeguards to make sure that quality is as high as possible. Agile project teams help ensure quality by doing the following:

» Take a proactive approach to quality to prevent product problems.

» Embrace technological excellence, good design, and sustainable development.

- >> Define and elaborate requirements just in time so that knowledge of product features is as relevant as possible.

- >> Build acceptance criteria into user stories so that the development team better understands them and the product owner can accurately validate them.

- >> Incorporate continuous integration and daily testing into the development process, allowing the development team to address issues while they're fresh.

- >> Take advantage of automated testing tools to develop during the day, test overnight, and fix defects in the morning.

- >> Conduct sprint retrospectives, allowing the scrum team to continuously improve processes and work.

- >> Complete work using the definition of done: developed, tested, integrated, and documented.

You can find more information about project quality in Chapter 15.

Higher Customer Satisfaction

Agile project teams are committed to producing products that satisfy customers. Agile approaches for happier project sponsors include the following:

- >> Collaborate with customers as partners and keep customers involved and engaged throughout projects.

- >> Have a product owner who is an expert on product requirements and customer needs. (Check out Chapters 6 and 9 to find out more information about the product owner role.)

- >> Keep the product backlog updated and prioritized to respond quickly to change. (You can find out about the product backlog in Chapter 8 and its role in responding to change in Chapter 12.)

- >> Demonstrate working functionality to customers in every sprint review. (Chapter 10 shows you how to conduct a sprint review.)

- >> Deliver products to market quicker and more often with every release.

- >> Possess the potential for self-funding projects. (Chapter 13 tells you about self-funding projects.)

Reduced Risk

Agile project management techniques virtually eliminate the chance of absolute project failure — spending large amounts of time and money with no return on investment. Agile project teams run projects with lower risk by doing the following:

» Develop in sprints, ensuring a short time between initial project investment and either failing fast or knowing that a product or an approach will work.

» Always have a working, integrated product, starting with the first sprint, so that some value is added as shippable functionality every sprint, ensuring an agile project won't fail completely.

» Develop requirements according to the definition of done in each sprint so that project sponsors have completed, usable functionality, regardless of what may happen with the project in the future.

» Provide constant feedback on products and processes through the following:

- Daily scrum meetings and constant development team communication

- Regular daily clarification about requirements and review and acceptance of features by the product owner

- Sprint reviews, with stakeholder and customer input about completed product functionality

- Sprint retrospectives, where the development team discusses process improvement

- Releases, where the end user can see and react to new features on a regular basis

» Generate revenue early with self-funding projects, allowing organizations to pay for a project with little up-front expense.

You can find more information about managing risk in Chapter 15.

Increased Collaboration and Ownership

When development teams take responsibility for projects and products, they can produce great results. Agile development teams collaborate and take ownership of product quality and project performance by doing the following:

» Make sure that the development team, the product owner, and the scrum master work closely together on a daily basis.

>> Conduct goal-driven sprint planning meetings, allowing the development team to commit to the sprint goal and organize its work to achieve it.

>> Hold daily scrum meetings led by the development team, where development team members organize around work completed, future work, and roadblocks.

>> Conduct sprint reviews, where the development team can demonstrate and discuss the product directly with stakeholders.

>> Conduct sprint retrospectives, allowing development team members to review past work and recommend better practices with every sprint.

>> Work in a collocated environment, allowing for instant communication and collaboration among development team members.

>> Make decisions by consensus, using techniques such as estimation poker and the fist of five.

You can find out how development teams estimate effort for requirements, decompose requirements, and gain team consensus in Chapter 7. To discover more about sprint planning and daily scrum meetings, see Chapter 9. For more information about sprint retrospectives, check out Chapter 10.

More Relevant Metrics

The metrics that agile project teams use to estimate time and cost, measure project performance, and make project decisions are often more relevant and more accurate than metrics on traditional projects. Agile metrics should encourage sustainable team progress and efficiency in a way that works best for the team to deliver value to the customer early and often. On agile projects, you provide metrics by doing the following:

>> Determine project timelines and budgets based on each development team's actual performance and capabilities.

>> Make sure that the development team that will be doing the work, and no one else, provides effort estimates for project requirements.

>> Use relative estimates, rather than hours or days, to accurately tailor estimated effort to an individual development team's knowledge and capabilities.

>> Refine estimated effort, time, and cost on a regular basis, as the development team learns more about the project.

>> Update the sprint burndown chart every day to provide accurate metrics about how the development team is performing within each sprint.

>> Compare the cost of future development with the value of that future development, which helps project teams determine when to end a project and redeploy capital to a new project.

WARNING

You might notice that velocity is missing from this list. *Velocity* (a measure of development speed, as detailed in Chapter 13) is a tool you can use to determine timelines and costs, but it works only when tailored to an individual team. The velocity of Team A has no bearing on the velocity of Team B. Also, velocity is great for measurement and trending, but it doesn't work as a control mechanism. Trying to make a development team meet a certain velocity number only disrupts team performance and thwarts self-management.

If you're interested in finding out more about relative estimating, be sure to check out Chapter 7. You can find out about tools for determining timelines and budgets, along with information about capital redeployment, in Chapter 13. Chapter 21 shows you ten key metrics for agile project management.

Improved Performance Visibility

On agile projects, every member of the project team has the opportunity to know how the project is going at any given time. Agile projects can provide a high level of performance visibility by doing the following:

>> Place a high value on open, honest communication among the scrum team, stakeholders, customers, and anyone else in an organization who wants to know about a project.

>> Provide daily measurements of sprint performance with sprint backlog updates. Sprint backlogs can be available for anyone in an organization to review.

>> Provide daily insight into the development team's immediate progress and roadblocks through the daily scrum meeting. Although only the development team may speak at the daily scrum meeting, any member of the project team may attend.

>> Physically display progress by using task boards and posting sprint burndown charts in the development team's work area every day.

>> Demonstrate accomplishments in sprint reviews. Anyone within an organization may attend a sprint review.

Improved project visibility can lead to greater project control and predictability, as described in the following sections.

Increased Project Control

Agile project teams have numerous opportunities to control project performance and make corrections as needed because of the following:

>> Adjusting priorities throughout the project allows the organization to have fixed-time and fixed-price projects while accommodating change.

>> Embracing change allows the project team to react to outside factors such as market demand.

>> Daily scrum meetings allow the scrum team to quickly address issues as they arise.

>> Daily updates to sprint backlogs mean sprint burndown charts accurately reflect sprint performance, giving the scrum team the opportunity to make changes the moment it sees problems.

>> Face-to-face conversations remove roadblocks to communication and issue resolution.

>> Sprint reviews let project stakeholders see working products and provide input about the products before release.

>> Sprint retrospectives enable the scrum team to make informed course adjustments at the end of every sprint to enhance product quality, increase development team performance, and refine project processes.

The many opportunities to inspect and adapt throughout agile projects allow all members of the project team — the product owner, development team, scrum master, and stakeholders — to exercise control and ultimately create better products.

Improved Project Predictability

Agile project management techniques help the project team accurately predict how things will go as the project progresses. Here are some practices, artifacts, and tools for improved predictability:

>> Keeping sprint lengths and development team allocation the same throughout the project allows the project team to know the exact cost for each sprint.

>> Using individual development team speed allows the project team to predict timelines and budgets for releases, the remaining product backlog, or any group of requirements.

>> Using the information from daily scrum meetings, sprint burndown charts, and task boards allows the project team to predict performance for individual sprints.

You can find more information about sprint lengths in Chapter 8.

Customized Team Structures

Self-management puts decisions that would normally be made by a manager or the organization into scrum team members' hands. Because of the limited size of development teams — which consist of three to nine people — agile projects can have multiple scrum teams on one project if necessary. Self-management and size-limiting mean that agile projects can provide unique opportunities to customize team structures and work environments. Here are a few examples:

>> Development teams may organize themselves into groups with specific skills or that work on specific parts of the product system and features.

>> Development teams may organize their team structure around people with specific work styles and personalities. Organization around work styles provides these benefits:

- Allows team members to work the way they want to work

- Encourages team members to expand their skills to fit into teams they like

- Helps increase team performance because people who do good work like to work together and naturally gravitate toward one another

>> Scrum teams can make decisions tailored to provide balance between team members' professional and personal lives.

>> Ultimately, scrum teams can make their own rules about whom they work with and how they work.

REMEMBER

The idea of team customization allows agile workplaces to have more diversity. Organizations with traditional management styles tend to have monolithic teams where everyone follows the same rules. Agile work environments are much like the old salad bowl analogy. Just like salads can have ingredients with wildly different tastes that fit in to make a delicious dish, agile projects can have people on teams with very diverse strengths that fit in to make great products.

Higher Team Morale

Working with happy people who enjoy their jobs can be satisfying and rewarding. Agile project management improves the morale of scrum teams in these ways:

>> Being part of a self-managing team allows people to be creative, innovative, and acknowledged for their contributions.

>> Focusing on sustainable work practices ensures that people don't burn out from stress or overwork.

>> Encouraging a servant-leader approach assists scrum teams in self-management and actively avoids command-and-control methods.

>> Having a dedicated scrum master, who serves the scrum team, removes impediments, and shields the development team from external interferences.

>> Providing an environment of support and trust increases people's overall motivation and morale.

>> Having face-to-face conversations helps reduce the frustration of miscommunication.

>> Working cross-functionally allows development team members to learn new skills and to grow by teaching others.

You can find out more about team dynamics in Chapter 14.

Chapter **20**

Ten Key Factors for Project Success

H ere are ten key factors that determine whether an agile transition will succeed. You don't need all issues resolved before you begin. You just need to be aware of them and have a plan to address them as early in your journey as possible.

TIP

We have found that the first three are the strongest indicators for success. Get those right and the likelihood of your success increases dramatically.

Dedicated Team Members

In Chapter 6, we talk about the importance of dedicating team members — product owner, development team members, as well as scrum master — to a single project at a time. This is especially critical at the beginning, when the scrum team and the rest of the organization are still learning what it means to value agility and embody agile principles.

If team members are jumping between project contexts hourly, daily, weekly, or even monthly, the focus on getting agile techniques right is minimized at the expense of just trying to keep up with multiple task lists. Also, the time lost due to the continual cognitive demobilization and remobilization involved with task switching is very costly to each project involved.

TIP

If you think you don't have enough people to dedicate to your scrum teams, you definitely don't have enough people to thrash them across multiple projects simultaneously. The American Psychological Association reports that task switching wastes as much as 40 percent of time.

Collocation

The Agile Manifesto lists individuals and interactions as the first value. The way you get this value right is by collocating team members to be able to have clear, effective, and direct communication throughout a project.

In Chapter 5, we talk about collocation as the first crucial element of an agile environment. Bell Laboratories showed a fifty-fold improvement in productivity simply by getting individuals and interactions right through collocation. With this success factor addressed adequately, customer collaboration, working functionality, and responding effectively to change become much more of a reality.

Automated Testing

Development teams cannot develop at the rate technology and market conditions change if they have to manually test their work every time they integrate new pieces of functionality throughout the sprint. The longer teams rely on manual testing, the larger the holes in test coverage become — manual testing simply takes too long and in reality becomes spot-checking. Without automation, scrum teams will struggle to completely deliver value in every sprint.

In Chapter 4, we discuss extreme programming practices aimed at building in quality upfront; automated testing is one of the primary practices. Chapter 15 also discusses building in quality through automation and continuous integration.

Enforced Definition of Done

Ending sprints with non-shippable functionality is an anti-pattern to becoming more agile. Your definition of done should clarify the following:

>> The environment in which the functionality should be integrated

>> The types of testing

>> The types of required documentation

The scrum team should also enforce its definition of done. If scrum teams tell their stakeholders that they are done after a sprint, but an aspect of the definition of done is not met, the work to finish meeting the definition of done must be added to the next sprint, taking capacity away from working on new valuable product backlog items. This scenario is a Ponzi scheme.

Development teams get to done by swarming on user stories — working on one user story together at a time until it is complete before starting the next. Developers hold each other accountable by ensuring that all rules for their definition of done are satisfied before starting a new user story. Product owners review completed work against the scrum team's definition of done (as well as the user story's acceptance criteria — see Chapter 8) as soon as developers complete it, and the scrum master ensures that developers resolve issues rejected by the product owner before moving on to new user stories.

Swarming to follow a clear definition of done makes sprints successful. See Chapters 2, 8, 10, and 15 for more on the definition of done.

Clear Product Vision and Roadmap

Although the product owner owns the product vision and product roadmap, many people have the responsibility to ensure the clarity of these agile artifacts. Product owners need access to stakeholders and customers at the beginning during project planning as well as throughout the project to ensure that the vision and roadmap continually reflect what the customer and market need. Purpose-driven development delivers business and customer value and mitigates risk effectively.

Without a clear purpose, people wander and lack ownership. When all team members understand the purpose, they come together. Remember the agile principle, "The best architectures, requirements, and designs emerge from self-organizing teams."

We discuss the mechanics of developing the vision and product roadmap in Chapter 7.

Product Owner Empowerment

The product owner's role is to optimize the value produced by the development team. This product owner responsibility requires someone to be knowledgeable about the product and customer, available to the development team throughout each day, and empowered to make priority decisions and give clarification in the moment so that development teams don't wait or make inappropriate decisions for the product's direction.

Although all roles on the scrum team are vital and equally important, an unempowered and ineffective product owner usually causes scrum teams to ultimately fail at delivering the value customers need from the team. See Chapter 6 for more on the product owner role.

Developer Versatility

You probably won't start your first agile project with a development team that has the ideal level of skills required for every requirement on your product backlog. However, the goal should be to achieve skill coverage as soon as possible. Your team will also be challenged to meet its sprint goal if you have single points of failure on any one skill, including testing.

From day one, you need developers on your team with the intellectual curiosity and interest to learn new things, to experiment, to mentor and to receive mentoring, and to work together as a team to get things to done as quickly as possible. This versatility is discussed more in Chapter 6.

Scrum Master Clout

As you depart from command and control leadership to empower the people doing the work to make decisions, servant leadership provides the solution. With formal authority, a scrum master would be viewed as a manager — someone to report to. Scrum masters should not be given formal authority but should be empowered by leadership to work with members of the scrum team, stakeholders, and other third parties to clear the way so that the development team can function unhindered.

If scrum masters have organizational clout, which is informal and is a socially earned ability to influence, they can best serve their teams to optimize their working environment. In Chapter 6, we talk more about different types of clout. Provide training and mentorship to ensure that your scrum masters develop the soft skills of servant leadership and put off the tendencies of commanding and directing.

Management Support for Learning

When executive leaders decide to become agile, their mindset has to change. Too often we see leadership directives without any follow-through for supporting the learning process to implement the changes. It is unrealistic to expect all the benefits of following agile principles after the first sprint. In Chapter 18, we talk about choosing an appropriate agile pilot project, one with leeway to stumble a bit at first as everyone learns a new way of working together.

The bottom line: If support for learning is merely lip service, scrum teams will pick up on it early, will lose motivation to try new things, and will go back to waiting for top-down directives on how to do their job.

Transition Support

Chapter 18 compares an agile transition to a sports team transitioning to play a different sport. Good coaching at leadership and team levels increases your chances to succeed. Coaching provides support in the following forms:

>> In-the-moment course correction when discipline starts to slip or mistakes are made

>> Reenforcing training

>> One-on-one mentoring for specific role-based challenges

>> Executive leadership style and mindset adjustments

See our Platinum Edge agile transition roadmap in Chapter 18 for specific steps to take alongside your trusted agile expert coaches.

Chapter **21**

Ten Metrics for Agile Organizations

O n an agile project, metrics can be powerful tools for planning, inspecting, adapting, and understanding progress over time. Rates of success or fail-ure can let a scrum team know whether it needs to make positive changes or keep up its good work. Time and cost numbers can highlight the benefits of agile projects and provide support for an organization's financial activities. Metrics that quantify people's satisfaction can help a scrum team identify areas for improvement with customers and with the team itself.

This chapter describes ten key metrics to help guide agile project teams.

Return on Investment

Return on investment (ROI) is income generated by the product less project costs: money in versus money out. ROI is fundamentally different in agile projects than it is in traditional projects. Agile projects have the potential to generate income with the first release and can increase revenue with each new release.

To fully appreciate the difference between ROI on traditional and agile projects, compare the examples in Tables 21-1 and 21-2. The projects for both examples have the same project costs and take the same amount of time to complete. Both products have the potential to generate $100,000 in income every month when all the requirements are finished.

First, look at the ROI on a traditional project in Table 21-1.

TABLE 21-1 ## ROI on a Traditional Project

Month	Monthly Income	Monthly Costs	Monthly ROI	Total Income	Total Costs	Total ROI
January	$0	$80,000	–$80,000	$0	$80,000	–$80,000
February	$0	$80,000	–$80,000	$0	$160,000	–$160,000
March	$0	$80,000	–$80,000	$0	$240,000	–$240,000
April	$0	$80,000	–$80,000	$0	$320,000	–$320,000
May	$0	$80,000	–$80,000	$0	$400,000	–$400,000
June (project launch)	$0	$80,000	–$80,000	$0	$480,000	–$480,000
July	$100,000	$0	$100,000	$100,000	$480,000	–$380,000
August	$100,000	$0	$100,000	$200,000	$480,000	–$280,000
September	$100,000	$0	$100,000	$300,000	$480,000	–$180,000
October	$100,000	$0	$100,000	$400,000	$480,000	–$80,000
November (breakeven)	$100,000	$0	$100,000	$500,000	$480,000	$20,000
December	$100,000	$0	$100,000	$600,000	$480,000	$120,000

Here are some key points of the traditional project in Table 21-1:

>> The project first generated income in July, after the project launch the end of June.

>> The project finally had a positive total ROI in November, 11 months after the project started.

>> By the end of one year, the project generated $600,000 in revenue.

>> At the year's end, the project's total ROI was $120,000.

Now look at the ROI for an agile project in Table 21-2.

TABLE 21-2 **ROI on an Agile Project**

Month	Monthly Income	Monthly Costs	Monthly ROI	Total Income	Total Costs	Total ROI
January	$0	$80,000	–$80,000	$0	$80,000	–$80,000
February	$15,000	$80,000	–$65,000	$15,000	$160,000	–$145,000
March	$25,000	$80,000	–$55,000	$40,000	$240,000	–$200,000
April	$40,000	$80,000	–$40,000	$80,000	$320,000	–$240,000
May	$70,000	$80,000	–$10,000	$150,000	$400,000	–$250,000
June (project end)	$80,000	$80,000	$0	$230,000	$480,000	–$250,000
July	$100,000	$0	$100,000	$330,000	$480,000	–$150,000
August	$100,000	$0	$100,000	$430,000	$480,000	–$50,000
September (breakeven)	$100,000	$0	$100,000	$530,000	$480,000	$50,000
October	$100,000	$0	$100,000	$630,000	$480,000	$150,000
November	$100,000	$0	$100,000	$730,000	$480,000	$250,000
December	$100,000	$0	$100,000	$830,000	$480,000	$350,000

Pay special attention to these points of the agile project in Table 21-2:

>> The project first generated income in February, shortly after the project start.

>> The project had a positive total ROI in September — two months earlier than the traditional project.

>> By the end of one year, the project generated $830,000 in revenue, nearly 40 percent more than the traditional project.

>> At the year's end, the total ROI was $350,000, almost threefold the ROI on the traditional project.

REMEMBER

Like time to market, ROI metrics are a great way for an organization to appreciate the ongoing value of an agile project. ROI metrics help justify projects from the start because companies can fund projects based on ROI potential. Organizations can track ROI for individual projects as well as for the organization as a whole.

New requests in ROI budgets

An agile project's capability to quickly generate high ROI provides organizations with a unique way to fund additional product development. New product functionality may translate to higher product income.

For example, suppose that in the example project from Table 21-2, the project team were to identify a new feature that would take one month to complete and would boost the product income from $100,000 a month to $120,000 a month. Here's what the effect would be on ROI:

>> The project would still have its first positive ROI in September, with an ROI of $110,000 instead of $50,000.

>> By the end of the year, the project would have generated a total income of $950,000 — 14 percent more than if it generated $100,000 a month.

>> By the end of the year, the total ROI would be $470,000 — 34 percent higher than the original project.

If a project is already generating income, it can make sense for an organization to roll that income back into new development and see higher revenue.

Capital redeployment

On an agile project, when the cost of future development is higher than the value of that future development, it's time for the project to end.

The product owner prioritizes requirements, in part, by their capability to generate revenue or value. If only low-revenue or low-value requirements remain in the backlog, a project may end before the project team has used its entire budget. The organization may then use the remaining budget from the old project to start a new, more valuable project. The practice of moving a budget from one project to another is called *capital redeployment*.

To determine a project's end, you need the following metrics:

>> The value (V) of the remaining requirements in the product backlog

>> The actual cost (AC) for the work to complete the requirements in the product backlog

>> The opportunity cost (OC), or the value of having the scrum team work on a new project

When V < AC + OC, the project can stop. The cost you would sink into the project would be more than the value you would receive from the project.

Capital redeployment allows an organization to spend efficiently on valuable product development and maximize the organization's overall ROI. You can find the details on capital redeployment in Chapter 13.

Satisfaction Surveys

On agile projects, a scrum team's highest priority is to satisfy the customer early and often. At the same time, the scrum team strives to motivate individual team members and promote sustainable development practices.

A scrum team can benefit from digging deeper into customer and team member experiences. One way to get measurable information about how well a scrum team is embodying agile principles is through satisfaction surveys:

>> **Customer satisfaction surveys:** Measure the customer's experience with the project, the process, and the scrum team.

  The scrum team may want to use customer surveys multiple times during a project. The scrum team can use customer survey results to examine processes, continue positive practices, and adjust behavior as necessary.

>> **Team satisfaction surveys:** Measure the scrum team members' experience with the organization, the work environment, processes, other project team members, and their work. Everyone on the scrum team can take team surveys.

  As with the customer survey, the scrum team may choose to give team surveys throughout a project. Scrum team members can use team survey results to regularly fine-tune and adjust personal and team behaviors. The scrum team can also use results to address organizational issues. Customer survey results over time can provide a quantitative look at how the scrum team is maturing as a team.

TIP

Survey results will be more honest and freely given if the organization fosters a culture of openness, transparency, and support for learning.

You can put together informal paper surveys, or use one of the many online survey tools. Some companies even have survey software available through their human resources department.

Defects in Production

Defects are a part of any project. However, testing and fixing them can be time-consuming and costly, especially when they reach production. Agile approaches help development teams proactively minimize defects.

As development teams iterate through the development of a requirement, they test and find defects. The sprint cycle facilitates fixing those defects immediately before they reach production. Ideally, defects in production don't occur due to automated testing and continuous integration, as discussed in Chapters 7 and 15.

Tracking defect metrics can let the development team know how well it's preventing issues and when to refine its processes. To track defects, it helps to look at the following numbers:

>> **Build defects:** If the development team uses automated testing and continuous integration, it can track the number of defects at the build level in each sprint.

By understanding the number of build defects, the development team can know whether to adjust development processes and environmental factors to be able to catch defects even sooner in their development process.

>> **User acceptance testing (UAT) defects:** The development team can track the number of defects the product owner finds when reviewing completed functionality in each sprint.

By tracking UAT defects, the development team and the product owner can identify the need to refine processes for understanding requirements. The development team can also determine whether adjustments to automated testing tools are necessary.

>> **Release defects:** The development team can track the number of defects that make it past the release to the marketplace.

TIP

Development teams can also track the number of days between user story acceptance and defect discovery. The fewer days passed since a developer worked on the functionality, the lower the cost to fix the defect.

By tracking release defects, the development team and the product owner can know whether changes to the UAT process, automated testing, or the development process are necessary. Large numbers of defects at the release level may indicate bigger problems in the scrum team.

The number of defects and whether defects are increasing, decreasing, or staying the same are good metrics to spark discussions on project processes and development techniques at sprint retrospectives.

You can find out more about proactive quality management and testing in Chapter 15.

Sprint Goal Success Rates

One way to measure agile project performance is the rate of achieving the sprint goal.

REMEMBER

The sprint may not need all the requirements and tasks in the sprint backlog to achieve the goal. However, a successful sprint should have a working product increment that fulfills the sprint goals and meets the scrum team's definition of done: developed, tested, integrated, and documented.

Throughout the project, the scrum team can track how frequently it succeeds in reaching the sprint goals and use success rates to see whether the team is maturing or needs to correct its course. Sprint success rates are a useful launching point for inspection and adaptation.

You can find out more about setting sprint goals in Chapter 8.

Time to Market

Time to market is the amount of time an agile project takes to provide value by releasing working functionality to users. Organizations may perceive value in a couple of ways:

>> When a product directly generates income, its value is the money it can make.

>> When a product is for an organization's internal use, its value will be the employees' ability to use the product and will contain subjective factors based on what the product can do.

When measuring time to market, consider the following:

>> Measure the time from the project start until you first show value.

>> Some scrum teams deploy new product features for use at the end of each sprint. For scrum teams that release with every sprint, the time to market is simply the sprint length, measured in days.

>> Other scrum teams plan releases after multiple sprints and deploy product features in groups. For scrum teams that use longer release times, the time to market is the number of days between each release.

Time to market helps organizations recognize and quantify the ongoing value of agile projects. Time to market is especially important for companies with revenue-generating products because it aids in budgeting throughout the year. It's important also if you have a self-funding project — a project being paid for by the income from the product.

You can find out more about product-income generation and self-funding projects in Chapter 13.

Lead and Cycle Times

Lead time is the average amount of time between receiving a request for a requirement and delivering it finished. *Cycle time* is the average time between when development on a requirement begins and when it is delivered.

Agile teams work in a lean environment, one that seeks to eliminate waste. Constraints exist in every flow of work or stream of creating value. Agile teams continually seek ways to identify and remove constraints to maximize the flow of work through their system.

Lead and cycle time provide not only a measurement of where bottlenecks may exist but also expectations for stakeholders regarding how long a request they submit may take to be completed, on average.

If the lead time for a particular scrum team is 45 days but the cycle time is only 5 days, this discrepancy may alert the team to evaluate its planning and product backlog refinement process to see how it might tighten the 40-day difference. Likewise, if the lead time is 45 days and the cycle time is 40 days, the team may want to evaluate its development workflow for bottlenecks. In any case, scrum teams should always be looking at removing constraints to decrease both lead and cycle time appropriately.

Cost of Change

Agile leaders and teams embrace change for the customer's competitive advantage. But acceptance of change should not mean acceptance of unnecessary costs associated with changes. As agile teams inspect and adapt the product and their processes, their goal should be to continuously minimize the effect of change.

Increasing product flexibility is a common way of reducing the cost of change. With software development, using a service oriented architecture (SOA) strategy allows agile teams to make each component of an application independent of others, so that the entire system doesn't require changes when one component must be changed. Development, testing, and documentation require significantly less effort.

In manufacturing, standardization and modularization of parts has allowed car manufacturers such as Toyota and more recently WikiSpeed to build cars more quickly and with less wasteful rework due to incompatibility. (See Chapter 4 for more on the Toyota Production System.)

Value stream mapping is a common technique for identifying constraints in a system or a workflow. By visualizing (on a whiteboard, for instance) each step in a process, agile teams can identify where introducing changes forces the most stress or cost on its processes. When a constraint is identified, the scrum master and other organizational change agents can work to remove that constraint to decrease the cost of future changes in the system.

Team Member Turnover

Agile projects tend to have higher morale. One way of quantifying morale is by measuring turnover. Although turnover isn't always directly tied to satisfaction, it can help to look at the following metrics:

>> **Scrum team turnover:** Low scrum team turnover can be one sign of a healthy team environment. High scrum team turnover can indicate problems with the project, the organization, the work, individual scrum team members, burnout, ineffective product owners forcing development team commitments, personality incompatibility, a scrum master who fails to remove impediments, or overall team dynamics.

>> **Company turnover:** High company turnover, even if it doesn't include the scrum team, can affect morale and effectiveness. High company turnover can be a sign of problems in the organization. As a company adopts agile practices, it may see turnover decrease.

When the scrum team knows turnover metrics and understands the reasons behind those metrics, it may be able to take actions to maintain morale and improve the work environment. If turnover is high, start asking why.

Skill Versatility

Mature scrum teams are typically more cross functional than less mature scrum teams. By eliminating single points of failure in a scrum team, you increase its ability to move faster and produce higher-quality products. Tracking skill versatility allows scrum teams and functional managers to gauge the growth of cross-functionality.

When starting out, capture the existing skills and levels contained at each of the following organizational structures:

» Per person skills and levels

» Per team skills and levels

» Per organization skills and levels

Over time, as each person increases his or her quantity and level of skills, the constraints and delays due to skill gaps disappear. Agile teams are about skills, not titles. You want team members who can contribute to the sprint goal each and every day without the risk of single points of failure.

Manager-to-Creator Ratio

Larger organizations likely have developed a heavy middle layer of managers. Many organizations haven't figured out how to function well without multiple managers handling personnel, training, and technical direction on development issues. However, you need to strike the right balance of managers and individuals who produce product.

Imagine two professional rival futbol (American soccer) teams of 11 players each who both train intensively and prepare for a match against each other. Team B beats Team A 1-0.

Both teams go back to train for the next match. Team A's management calls on an analyst to provide a solution. After careful analysis of both teams, he sees that

Team B has one player as goalkeeper, and ten spread across the field as defenders, midfielders, and forwards, while Team A plays ten goalkeepers at once and one forward to maneuver the ball down the field to the goal without any team members getting in the way.

Team A's management calls in a consultant to restructure the team. She finds what seems obvious: Team A is playing way too many goalkeepers. The consultant recommends that the team play half as many goalkeepers (five), and play five defenders who can relay instructions to the forward from the goalkeepers who have a view of the entire field. She also suggests doubling the assistant coaching staff to increase training and motivation of the forward to score goals.

At the next match, Team B again beats Team A, but this time 2-0.

The forward gets cut, the assistant coaches and defenders get recognized for their motivation strategy, but management calls for another analysis. As a result of the analysis, they build a more modern practice facility and invest in the latest shoe technology for the next season.

REMEMBER

Every dollar spent on someone who manages organizational processes is a dollar not spent on a product creator.

Track your manager-to-creator ratio to identify bloat and ways to minimize the investment you're making in people who don't create product.

Chapter **22**

Ten Valuable Resources for Agile Professionals

M any organizations, websites, blogs, and companies exist to provide information about and support for agile project management. To help you get started, we compiled a list of ten resources that we think are valuable to support your journey to agile project management.

Agile Project Management For Dummies Online Cheat Sheet

www.dummies.com

You can use our online cheat sheet as a companion to this book as you start implementing the agile values and principles from the Agile Manifesto, as well as models outlined throughout the book. You'll find how-to guides, tools, templates, and other helpful resources for your agile toolkit. To get to the cheat sheet, go to www.dummies.com, and then type *Agile Project Management For Dummies* in the Search box.

Scrum For Dummies

In 2014, we published *Scrum For Dummies* (Wiley) as a field guide not only to scrum but also to scrum in industries and business functions outside information technology (IT) and software development. Scrum can be applied in any situation where you want early empirical feedback on what you're building or pursuing on a project.

Learn about scrum in industries such as game software development and tangible goods production (construction, manufacturing, hardware development) and in services such as healthcare, education, and publishing.

Explore scrum's applications in business functions, including operations, portfolio management, human resources, finance, sales, marketing, and customer service.

And in everyday life, see how scrum can help you organize your pursuits of dating, family life, retirement planning, and education.

The Scrum Alliance

www.scrumalliance.org

The Scrum Alliance is a nonprofit professional membership organization that promotes the understanding and usage of scrum. The alliance achieves this goal by promoting scrum training and certification classes, hosting international and regional scrum gatherings, and supporting local scrum user communities. The Scrum Alliance site is rich in blog entries, white papers, case studies, and other tools for learning and working with scrum. Chapter 16 lists many of the Scrum Alliance certifications.

The Agile Alliance

www.agilealliance.org

The Agile Alliance is the original global agile community, with a mission to help advance the 12 Agile Principles and common agile practices, regardless of approach. The Agile Alliance site has an extensive resources section that includes articles, videos, presentations, and an index of independent agile community groups across the world.

The Project Management Institute Agile Community

www.projectmanagement.com/practices/agile

The Project Management Institute (PMI) is the largest nonprofit project management membership association in the world. It has more than 400,000 members and a presence in more than 200 countries. PMI supports an agile community of practice and an agile certification, the PMI Agile Certified Practitioner (PMI-ACP).

The PMI website provides information and requirements for certification along with access to papers, books, and seminars about agile project management. PMI members can also access PMI's agile community website, with an extensive knowledge center including blog posts, forums, webinars, and information about local agile networking events.

International Consortium for Agile (ICAgile)

icagile.com

ICAgile is a community-driven organization helping people become agile through education, awareness, and certification. Its learning roadmap provides career path development support in business agility, enterprise and team agile coaching, value management, delivery management, agile engineering, agile testing, and DevOps.

InfoQ

www.infoq.com/agile

InfoQ is an independent online community with a prominent agile section offering news, articles, video interviews, video presentations, and minibooks, all written by domain experts in agile techniques. The resources at InfoQ tend to be high quality, and the content is both unique and relevant to the issues facing agile project teams.

Lean Enterprise Institute

www.lean.org

Lean Enterprise Institute publishes books, blogs, knowledge bases, news, and events for the broader community of lean thinkers and practitioners. As you pursue agile project management, remember to incorporate lean thinking in all that you do. Lean.org is a good launching pad for you to explore the lean topics relevant to your situation.

Extreme Programming

ronjeffries.com/xprog/what-is-extreme-programming/

Ron Jeffries was one of the originators of the extreme programming (XP) development approach, along with Kent Beck and Ward Cunningham. Ron provides resources and services in support of XP's advancement on his ronjeffries.com site. The "What Is Extreme Programming?" section of the site summarizes the core concepts of XP. Other articles and extreme programming resources are also available in wiki format at http://wiki.c2.com/?ExtremeProgrammingCorePractices.

Platinum Edge

www.platinumedge.com

Since 2001, our team at Platinum Edge has been helping companies maximize organizational return on investment (ROI). Visit our blog to get the latest insights on practices, tools, and innovative solutions emerging from our work with Global 1000 companies and the dynamic agile community.

We also provide the following services, which are outlined in more detail in Chapter 18:

>> **Agile audits:** Auditing your current organizational structure and processes to create an agile implementation strategy that delivers bottom-line results.

>> **Recruiting:** With access to the best agile and scrum talent — because we've trained them — we help you find the right people to bootstrap your scrum projects, including scrum masters, scrum product owners, and scrum developers.

>> **Training:** Public and private customized corporate agile and scrum training and certification, regardless of your level of knowledge. In addition to custom and non-certified training options, we offer the following certifications:

- Certified ScrumMaster classes (CSM)

- Certified Scrum Product Owner classes (CSPO)

- Certified Scrum Developer classes (CSD)

- SAFe Scaled Agile training and implementations

- PMI Agile Certified Practitioner (PMI-ACP) test preparation classes

>> **Transformation:** Nothing is a larger factor of future success than proper coaching. We follow up on agile training with embedded agile coaching and mentoring to ensure that the right practices occur in the real world.

Index

A

ability, in ADKAR, 347

acceptance criteria, user stories, 140, 278–279

accountability, in team dynamics, 248

adaptation
  in agile approach, 16, 59
  in agile project environment, 308
  in empirical approach, 14, 66
  in Enterprise Scrum, 342
  in just-in-time planning, 120–121
  in quality management, 280–281
  in scrum framework, 73–74
  in self-managing development teams, 112
  sprint retrospective, 191

ADKAR change management tool, 346–347

affinity estimating, 150–152

after-party, 165

Agile Alliance, 18, 396

agile audits, 398

agile champion, 300, 302–303

agile coach. *See* agile mentor; scrum master

agile litmus test, 41–42

Agile Manifesto
  agile litmus test, 41–42
  changes resulting from, 40–41
  customer collaboration, 20, 24–25
  defined, 18
  general discussion, 17–20
  individuals and interactions, 19, 20–22
  overview, 13
  responding to change, 20, 25–26
  working functionality, 19, 22–24

agile mentor, 75, 102, 125, 307, 310

Agile Principles
  agile litmus test, 41–42
  changes resulting from, 40–41
  of customer satisfaction, 27–30
  defined, 18
  overview, 13, 26–27
  Platinum Principles, 37–40

  of project management, 33–36
  of quality, 30–31
  of teamwork, 31–33

agile project management. *See also specific agile approaches and features*
  approaches, overview, 65–69
  approaches, similarities between, 80
  benefits of, 57–61, 300, 369–376
  certifications, 77, 309
  commitment to, 297–299
  defined, 7
  double work agile, 267, 361
  as empirical approach, 13–14, 66
  environment enabling, creation of, 307–309
  failure in, 57
  faux agile, 361
  flexibility and stability of, 49–51
  versus historical approaches, 43–48
  history of, 11–13
  integrated approach in organizations, 40
  key factors for success, 377–381
  nonproductive tasks as reduced in, 51–53
  overview, 1–3
  project control with, 56
  quality and delivery with, 53–54
  resources for, 395–399
  superiority of, 14, 16
  support for, 310
  team performance in, 54–56
  transition to, 300–302, 343–344, 360–363, 381
  versus waterfall methodology, 15, 45–46

agile release train (ART) model, 335–336

agile transition team, 303–304, 353

anchor story, 149

architecture, 313, 318

artifacts
  accessibility of, 162
  in agile communication, 264–265
  cost management, 244
  defined, 134
  Nexus, 330

artifacts *(continued)*

  overview, 263

  risk management, 292–293

  scope management, 213–214

  scrum, 75

  time management, 236–237

assembly-line management, 188

audits, Platinum Edge, 398

automated testing, 176, 281–283, 362, 378

average velocity, 230

awareness, 346–347, 352

B

barely sufficient documentation, 23

Beck, Kent, 76

big bang development, 44

blame game, 363

Blanchard, Kenneth, 253

bloat, scope, 10–11, 207, 238

budget, 228, 239–240

bugs, 271

build defects, tracking, 388

burndown chart, 87, 157, 167–169, 267–268

business owner, in Enterprise Scrum, 338

business value and risk, assessing, 133

C

canvases, Enterprise Scrum, 339

capital redeployment, 243–244, 386–387

certifications, 77, 309, 399

change. *See also* Platinum Edge change roadmap;
    scope management

  adaptation to as benefit of agile, 59

  becoming agile as requiring, 343–344

  challenges related to, 344–345

  cost of, 391

  lack of, as failure, 206

  pitfalls, avoiding, 360–363

  responding to, in Agile Manifesto values, 20, 25–26

  stability and flexibility of agile approach, 48–50

  strategic approaches to, 345–349

  warning signs related to, 363–365

cheat sheet, 2, 395

chief product owner (CPO), 320–321

CI (continuous integration), 31, 79, 176, 277

Cirillo, Francesco, 105

clout, of scrum master, 100, 178, 380–381

coaching, 338, 356–357, 381. *See also* agile mentor;
    scrum master

Cockburn, Alistair, 83, 263–264

coding, in XP, 78, 79

collaboration

  communication channels, 265

  customer, in Agile Manifesto values, 20, 24–25

  in elaboration process, 175

  as key benefit of agile, 371–372

  in procurement management, 214, 219–221

  in self-organizing development teams, 110–111

collaboration modes menu, ES, 341

collaboration websites, 89–90, 261

collective code ownership, 79, 277

collocation

  agile trouble signs, 364

  creating agile project environment, 308

  as key factor for success, 378

  role in teamwork, 33, 55

  setting up, 82–83

  success of, 260

command and control approach, 247

commitment, 103, 297–299

communication

  agile methods, 263–266

  collocation, role in, 82–83

  in dislocated teams, 260–261

  in extreme programming, 78

  high-tech, 88–90

  low-tech, 86–88

  overview, 245

  in Platinum Edge change roadmap, 352

  proactive quality practices, 279

  in self-managing teams, 250

  in self-organizing development teams, 110

  status and progress reporting, 266–268

  in success of agile, 310

  in teamwork, 32–33

  traditional versus agile, 262–263

communication fidelity, 82–83

communication plan, 23

communities of practice (CoP), in LeSS, 326

E

F

G

H

Ha stage, *Shu Ha Ri* technique, 359
high-level time frames, determining, 135
high-tech communication, 88–90
Huge framework, LeSS, 324–325

I

icons, explained, 2
immediate adaptation, 14, 66
implementation strategy, 349–351
InfoQ, 397
information radiators, 87
innovation, 51, 254
inspection
  creating agile project environment, 308
  in empirical approach, 14, 66
  in Enterprise Scrum, 342
  in just-in-time planning, 120–121
  overview, 16
  in quality management, 280–281
  in scrum framework, 73–74
  in self-managing development teams, 112
  sprint retrospective, 191
instant messaging, 89
integrated agile approach, 40
integrated increment, Nexus, 330
integrated scrums, 260
integration teams, 314–315, 316–318, 328–329
integration testing, 283
interactions, in Agile Manifesto, 19, 20–22
International Consortium for Agile (ICAgile), 309, 397
INVEST approach, 147
isolated scrums, 259
IT operations, DevOps model, 198
iteration, in waterfall methodology, 67–68
iterations, 14, 28, 46, 155. *See also* sprints
iterative development, 53, 55, 59, 65

J

Jeffries, Ron, 398
joint program increment (PI) planning, 336–337
just-in-time (JIT) elaboration, 60, 69–70
just-in-time (JIT) planning. *See* planning

K

kanban board, 72, 87–88, 89
kanban practices, 71–72
knowledge, in ADKAR, 347
Kotter, John, 348–349

L

large solution SAFe®, 332, 334, 335
large-scale scrum (LeSS), 323–327
Larsen, Diana, 190–191
lead time, 72, 390
leadership, 111. *See also* servant leadership
leading change, 348–349
Lean Enterprise Institute, 398
lean portfolio management (LPM), 334
lean product development, 66, 69–72, 80, 188
lean-kanban, 71–72
learning, 70, 363, 381
legal department, 128
Less complicated burndown pattern, 169
Lewin, Kurt, 345–346
load testing, 283
long-range costs, 242–244
low-balling vendors, 219
low-tech communication, 86–88
Lying burndown pattern, 169

M

maintenance work, 197–199
management, 60–61, 85, 337, 381
manager-to-creator ratio, 392–393
manufacturing, 8, 69–70
Mark II Aiken Relay Calculator, 271
marketing department, 128, 201
marketplace, preparing for release, 200–201
marshmallow challenge, 44
mass production methods, 69–70
maturing improvements, 358–359
meetings. *See also* daily scrum
  agile approaches to, 52
  in agile communication, 264–265
  in dislocated teams, 260–261
  multi-team, in LeSS, 327

About the Authors

Mark C. Layton, known globally as *Mr. Agile,* is an organizational strategist and Scrum Alliance certification instructor with over 20 years in the project/program management field. He is the Los Angeles chair for the Agile Leadership Network, the author of the international *Scrum For Dummies* and *Agile Project Management For Dummies* book series (both published by Wiley), the creator of the *Agile Foundations Complete Video Course* with Pearson Education, and the founder of Platinum Edge, LLC — an organizational improvement company that supports businesses making the waterfall-to-agile transition.

Prior to founding Platinum Edge in 2001, Mark developed his expertise as a consulting firm executive, a program management coach, and an in-the-trenches project leader. He also spent 11 years as a Cryptographic Specialist for the US Air Force, where he earned both Commendation and Achievement medals for his accomplishments.

Mark holds MBAs from the University of California, Los Angeles, and the National University of Singapore; a B.Sc. (*summa cum laude*) in Behavioral Science from Pitzer College/University of La Verne; and an A.S. in Electronic Systems from the Air Force's Air College. He is also a Distinguished Graduate of the Air Force's Leadership School, a Certified Scrum Trainer (CST), a certified Project Management Professional (PMP), a recipient of Stanford University's advanced project management certification (SCPM), and a certified Scaled Agile Framework Program Consultant (SAFe SPC).

In addition to his books and videos, Mark is a frequent speaker at major conferences on Lean, Scrum, XP, and other agile solutions.

Additional information can be found at platinumedge.com.

Steven J Ostermiller is a coach, mentor, and trainer empowering leaders, teams, and individuals to become more agile. Steve is co-founder and organizer of Utah Agile (sponsored by Agile Alliance, Scrum Alliance, and Agile Leadership Network), a professional community committed to increasing agility for Utah businesses, technology, and individuals. He developed and taught a business college's agile project management curriculum and serves on its project management advisory board. Steve was also technical editor on projects such as *Scrum For Dummies* and Pearson Education's *Agile Foundations Complete Video Course.* He also occasionally speaks and writes about his experience with agile techniques for households.

Steve facilitates Platinum Edge, LLC's agile transformation engagements through audit, recruiting, training, and embedded coaching. He has worked with executive leadership and individual teams in finance, healthcare, media, entertainment, defense and energy, local and state government, logistics, ecommerce, manufacturing, ERP implementations, PMO development, startups, and nonprofits. He is a Certified Scrum Professional (CSP) and a Project Management Professional (PMP), and holds a B.S. in Business Management/Organizational Behavior from the Marriott School of Management at Brigham Young University.

Steve spends as much time as possible with his adorable wife and their five charming children in Utah living their dreams, one home-cooked meal at a time.

Dedications

To the friends, family, and special loved ones who tirelessly love and support as I pursue these wild ideas. Your time is now. — Mark

To Gwen, my complete and final answer. And to our five littles, who give me every reason to continuously inspect and adapt. — Steve

Authors' Acknowledgments

We'd like to again thank the numerous people who contributed to the first edition of this book and helped make it a reality.

We are also very grateful to those who helped make this second edition a more valuable field guide: David Morrow for his insight and technical editing; Caroline Patchen for ensuring that these concepts are more easily understood through clear visualization; Jeff Sutherland, Ken Schwaber, Kurt Bittner, Patricia Kong, Dean Leffingwell, Alex Yakyma, Inbar Oren, Craig Larman, Bas Vodde, Mike Beedle, and Michael Herman for providing scaling options to the public and for their valuable feedback with the new scaling chapter; and to Amy Fandrei, Susan Pink, and the broader John Wiley & Sons team. You are all fantastic professionals; thank you for the opportunity to make this book even better.

And a shout-out to the signers of the Agile Manifesto. Thanks for coming together, finding common ground, and kickstarting the discussion that inspires us to keep becoming more agile.

Publisher's Acknowledgments

Acquisitions Editor: Amy Fandrei
Project Editor: Susan Pink
Copy Editor: Susan Pink
Technical Editor: David Morrow
Sr. Editorial Assistant: Cherie Case

Production Editor: Antony Sami
Cover Image: © wsfurlan/iStockphoto